D1765544

Handbook of Bipolar Disorder

Medical Psychiatry

1. Handbook of Depression and Anxiety: A Biological Approach, *edited by Johan A. den Boer and J. M. Ad Sitsen*
2. Anticonvulsants in Mood Disorders, *edited by Russell T. Joffe and Joseph R. Calabrese*
3. Serotonin in Antipsychotic Treatment: Mechanisms and Clinical Practice, *edited by John M. Kane, H.-J. Möller, and Frans Awouters*
4. Handbook of Functional Gastrointestinal Disorders, *edited by Kevin W. Olden*
5. Clinical Management of Anxiety, *edited by Johan A. den Boer*
6. Obsessive-Compulsive Disorders: Diagnosis • Etiology • Treatment, *edited by Eric Hollander and Dan J. Stein*
7. Bipolar Disorder: Biological Models and Their Clinical Application, *edited by L. Trevor Young and Russell T. Joffe*
8. Dual Diagnosis and Treatment: Substance Abuse and Comorbid Medical and Psychiatric Disorders, *edited by Henry R. Kranzler and Bruce J. Rounsaville*
9. Geriatric Psychopharmacology, *edited by J. Craig Nelson*
10. Panic Disorder and Its Treatment, *edited by Jerrold F. Rosenbaum and Mark H. Pollack*
11. Comorbidity in Affective Disorders, *edited by Mauricio Tohen*
12. Practical Management of the Side Effects of Psychotropic Drugs, *edited by Richard Balon*
13. Psychiatric Treatment of the Medically Ill, *edited by Robert G. Robinson and William R. Yates*
14. Medical Management of the Violent Patient: Clinical Assessment and Therapy, *edited by Kenneth Tardiff*
15. Bipolar Disorders: Basic Mechanisms and Therapeutic Implications, *edited by Jair C. Soares and Samuel Gershon*
16. Schizophrenia: A New Guide for Clinicians, *edited by John G. Csernansky*

17. Polypharmacy in Psychiatry, *edited by S. Nassir Ghaemi*
18. Pharmacotherapy for Child and Adolescent Psychiatric Disorders: Second Edition, Revised and Expanded, *David R. Rosenberg, Pablo A. Davanzo, and Samuel Gershon*
19. Brain Imaging In Affective Disorders, *edited by Jair C. Soares*
20. Handbook of Medical Psychiatry, *edited by Jair C. Soares and Samuel Gershon*
21. Handbook of Depression and Anxiety: A Biological Approach, Second Edition, *edited by Siegfried Kasper, Johan A. den Boer, and J. M. Ad Sitsen*
22. Aggression: Psychiatric Assessment and Treatment, *edited by Emil Coccaro*
23. Depression in Later Life: A Multidisciplinary Psychiatric Approach, *edited by James Ellison and Sumer Verma*
24. Autism Spectrum Disorders, *edited by Eric Hollander*
25. Handbook of Chronic Depression: Diagnosis and Therapeutic Management, *edited by Jonathan E. Alpert and Maurizio Fava*
26. Clinical Handbook of Eating Disorders: An Integrated Approach, *edited by Timothy D. Brewerton*
27. Dual Diagnosis and Psychiatric Treatment: Substance Abuse and Comorbid Disorders: Second Edition, *edited by Henry R. Kranzler and Joyce A. Tinsley*
28. Atypical Antipsychotics: From Bench to Bedside, *edited by John G. Csernansky and John Lauriello*
29. Social Anxiety Disorder, *edited by Borwin Bandelow and Dan J. Stein*
30. Handbook of Sexual Dysfunction, *edited by Richard Balon and R. Taylor Segraves*
31. Borderline Personality Disorder, *edited by Mary C. Zanarini*
32. Handbook of Bipolar Disorder: Diagnosis and Therapeutic Approaches, *edited by Siegfried Kasper and Robert M. A. Hirschfeld*

Handbook of Bipolar Disorder

Diagnosis and Therapeutic Approaches

edited by

Siegfried Kasper

Department of General Psychiatry
Medical University of Vienna
Austria

Robert M. A. Hirschfeld

Department of Psychiatry and Behavioral Sciences
University of Texas Medical Branch
Galveston, Texas, U.S.A.

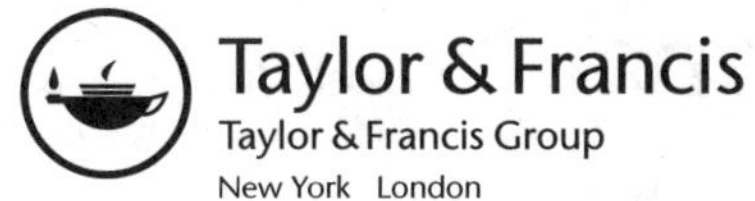
Taylor & Francis
Taylor & Francis Group
New York London

Published in 2005 by
Taylor & Francis Group
6000 Broken Sound Parkway NW, Suite 300
Boca Raton, FL 33487-2742

Printed in the United States of America on acid-free paper
10 9 8 7 6 5 4 3 2 1

International Standard Book Number-10: 0-8247-2935-8 (Hardcover)
International Standard Book Number-13: 978-0-8247-2935-6 (Hardcover)

Library of Congress Cataloging-in-Publication Data

Catalog record is available from the Library of Congress

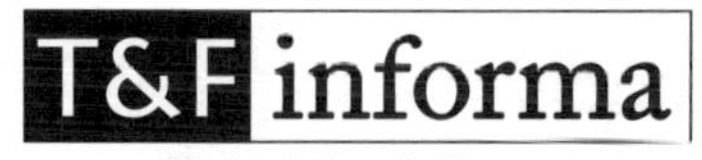

Taylor & Francis Group
is the Academic Division of T&F Informa plc.

Visit the Taylor & Francis Web site at
http://www.taylorandfrancis.com

Foreword

Over the last 10 to 15 years, so much knowledge about bipolar disorder has exploded on all fronts that even academic specialists, let alone clinicians, struggle to keep up. This handbook makes that struggle substantially easier, especially for clinicians.

These 27 chapters are authored by an international "who's who" in bipolar disorder research, and the depth of coverage fits the intended audience—primarily clinicians—quite well.

Some edited books on bipolar disorder organize treatment chapters around specific clinical situations, i.e., the treatment of mania, depression, etc. while others choose to organize chapters by the different treatments used, i.e., lithium, anticonvulsants, etc. This handbook employs both organizational schema.

As with any multi-authored book, it is best to read the chapters as they were written, that is, independent of one another. In this way, the reader can appreciate the differences in emphasis that should be expected when over 20 experts in bipolar treatment are assigned to approach overlapping topics. For example, one can compare how lithium's role in bipolar depression is handled in lithium pioneer Paul Grof's chapter, with how it is treated in Bob Hirschfeld's and Vornik's chapter on bipolar depression. Such inevitable differences in perspective are also evident in the first section dealing with diagnosis, epidemiology, and course. Consider, for example, the approach to diagnosis taken by Charles Bowden compared with the approach of Hagop Akiskal in the chapter on spectrum, or of Zoltan Rihmer and Jules Angst in the chapter on epidemiology.

A certain unity of perspective is achievable in a book with one or two authors (somehow *Manic Depressive Illness* by Goodwin and Jamison, 1990, comes to mind). While this has its virtues, there is also real value in being exposed to diverse points of view, as long as one makes the effort to read all the overlapping chapters—an effort that is, by the way, well worth it.

Frederick K. Goodwin, MD
Research Professor of Psychiatry
George Washington University Medical Center
Washington D.C., U.S.A.

Preface

Bipolar disorder is one of the most frequent psychiatric diseases and together with other bipolar spectrum disorders, affects three to five percent of the population. If untreated or improperly treated, patients with bipolar disorder face a lower life expectancy and an altogether lower quality of life. Recent data on diagnosis and epidemiology reveal that, apart from Bipolar I and Bipolar II, further diseases of the bipolar spectrum that are of broad clinical relevance can be diagnosed. Recent data indicate that if patients remain untreated, as is all too often the case, they have a higher morbidity and mortality even if psychiatric causes such as suicidality are excluded.

The underlying biology of bipolar disorder recently revealed new insights into neuropeptides and signal transduction. The importance of intracellular mechanisms has further been substantiated by molecular biology techniques. Brain imaging is a link to everyday clinical practice since it demonstrates where changes are located in patients. Using the technique of newer brain imaging methodology, it is possible to uncover small and functionally important changes, which together with molecular genetics—now termed molecular neuroimaging—shape a promising new field of research.

There is a huge amount of literature available on new treatments for bipolar disorder in various clinical states. These situations include mania, bipolar depression, mixed state, rapid cycling, and also the long-term perspective with the goal of mood stabilization. The treatment of patients with schizoaffective disorder and the treatment of bipolar disorder in children, as well as those in late life, add another important perspective to specific treatment procedures.

In the past, only lithium and antiepileptics of the first generation and mood stabilizers were available, while now there are a number of new antiepileptic medications as well as atypical antipsychotics on the market. Despite sometimes being in a quite deteriorated state, a large number of manic patients still receive typical neuroleptics, mostly in a depot fashion. However, this practice has been questioned recently with the newer compounds available. Antidepressants are used in bipolar disorder together with atypical antipsychotics and mood stabilizers, and there is a question of when to use and of how long to use this group of medications. New treatment options include the group of atypical antipsychotics and mood stabilizers, probably together as a combination therapy.

Besides pharmacotherapeutic approaches, psychotherapeutic interventions such as social role therapy or social rhythm therapy have also been studied for bipolar disorder in a controlled design.

This book provides an accessible and expert summary of state-of-the-art knowledge in various currently relevant issues regarding diagnosis and treatment of bipolar disorder, with a special emphasis on novel treatment applications. The existing theories are reviewed and clinically relevant applications given. The book is structured in four main parts; diagnosis and epidemiology, biology, treatment in typical clinical situations, and treatment approaches by the different methodology used. This enables the reader to focus either on diagnostic procedures, underlying biology, or most importantly the treatment perspectives.

The chapters have been written by authorities in various aspects of psychiatric research and aim to reach an audience comprising physicians and basic scientists in various psychiatric specialties as well as doctors in neurology and hope to be of importance for public health considerations. The book should be of particular interest also for policy makers who seek a comprehensive and current source of basic spectra and treatment implications of this disorder. Such a volume should, from our point of view, prove to be attractive for individuals as well as libraries around the world.

Siegfried Kasper
Robert M. A. Hirschfeld

Contents

Contributors

Hagop S. Akiskal Department of Psychiatry, and International Mood Center, University, of California at San Diego and VA Hospital, San Diego, California, U.S.A.

Jules Angst Zurich University Psychiatric Hospital, Zurich, Switzerland

Celso Arango Servicio de Psiquiatria, Hospital General "Gregorio Maranon," Madrid, Spain

Maria-Teresa Bascaran Departamento de Psiquiatria, Facultad de Medicina, Universidad de Oviedo, Oviedo, Spain

Helmut Beckmann Department of Psychiatry and Psychotherapy, University of Würzburg, Würzburg, Germany

Zubin Bhagwagar University Department of Psychiatry, Warneford Hospital, Oxford, U.K.

Julio Bobes Departamento de Psiquiatria, Facultad de Medicina, Universidad de Oviedo, Oviedo, Spain

Robert J. Boland Department of Psychiatry and Human Behavior, Brown University and Miriam Hospital/LifeSpan, Providence, Rhode Island, U.S.A.

Manuel Bousoño Departamento de Psiquiatria, Facultad de Medicina, Universidad de Oviedo, Oviedo, Spain

Charles L. Bowden Department of Psychiatry, The University of Texas Health Science Center at San Antonio, San Antonio, Texas, U.S.A.

Paolo Brambilla Department of Pathology and Experimental and Clinical Medicine, Section of Psychiatry, University of Udine School of Medicine, Udine, Italy

Peter Brieger Klinik und Poliklinik für Psychiatrie, Martin-Luther-Universität Halle-Wittenberg, Germany

John Cookson The Royal London Hospital, St. Clement's, London, U.K.

Dimitris G. Dikeos Department of Psychiatry, Athens University Medical School, Athens, Greece

Andreas Erfurth Department of General Psychiatry, Medical University of Vienna, Vienna, Austria

Peter Fahnestock Department of Psychiatry, Washington University School of Medicine, St. Louis, Missouri, U.S.A.

Nuri B. Farber Department of Psychiatry, Washington University School of Medicine, St. Louis, Missouri, U.S.A.

Gerardo Florez Centro Asistencial "As Burgas," Ourense, Spain

Maria-Paz Garcia-Portilla Departamento de Psiquiatria, Facultad de Medicina, Universidad de Oviedo, Oviedo, Spain

Guy M. Goodwin University Department of Psychiatry, Warneford Hospital, Oxford, U.K.

Jack Gorman Mount Sinai School of Medicine, New York, New York, U.S.A.

Paul Grof Bipolar Research Unit, University of Ottawa, Royal Ottawa Hospital, Ottawa, Ontario, Canada

Heinz Grunze Department of Psychiatry, Ludwig-Maximilians University, Munich, Germany

Dan Haupt Department of Psychiatry, Washington University School of Medicine, St. Louis, Missouri, U.S.A.

Robert M. A. Hirschfeld Department of Psychiatry and Behavioral Sciences, University of Texas Medical Branch, Galveston, Texas, U.S.A.

Siegfried Kasper Department of General Psychiatry, Medical University of Vienna, Wien, Austria

Martin B. Keller Department of Psychiatry and Human Behavior, Brown University, Butler Hospital and Brown Affiliated Hospitals, Providence, Rhode Island, U.S.A.

M. Kosel Department of Psychiatry, University of Bonn, Bonn, Germany

Adrian J. Lloyd School of Neurology, Neurobiology and Psychiatry, University of Newcastle upon Tyne, Royal Victoria Infirmary, Newcastle upon Tyne, U.K.

Husseini K. Manji Laboratory of Molecular Pathophysiology, National Institute of Mental Health, Bethesda, Maryland, U.S.A.

Andreas Marneros Klinik und Poliklinik für Psychiatrie, Martin-Luther-Universität, Halle-Wittenberg, Germany

H. J. Möller Department of Psychiatry, Ludwig-Maximilians University, Munich, Germany

John W. Newcomer Department of Psychiatry, Washington University School of Medicine, St. Louis, Missouri, U.S.A.

Nga Anh Nguyen Department of Psychiatry and Behavioral Sciences, University of Texas Medical Branch, Galveston, Texas, U.S.A.

George N. Papadimitriou Department of Psychiatry, Athens University Medical School, Athens, Greece

Lori Pellegrino Mount Sinai School of Medicine, New York, New York, U.S.A.

Giulio Perugi Department of Psychiatry, University of Pisa, Pisa, Italy

Bruno Pfuhlmann Department of Psychiatry and Psychotherapy, University of Würzburg, Würzburg, Germany

Jorge A. Quiroz Laboratory of Molecular Pathophysiology, National Institute of Mental Health, Bethesda, Maryland, U.S.A.

Mark Rapoport Department of Psychiatry, Sunnybrook & Women's College Health Sciences Centre, University of Toronto, Toronto, Canada

Zoltán Rihmer National Institute for Psychiatry and Neurology, Budapest, Hungary

Pilar-Alejandra Saiz Departamento de Psiquiatria, Facultad de Medicina, Universidad de Oviedo, Oviedo, Spain

Jose Sanchez-Moreno Bipolar Disorders Program, Hospital Clinic, University of Barcelona, Barcelona, Spain

Ayal Schaffer Department of Psychiatry, Sunnybrook & Women's College Health Sciences Centre, University of Toronto, Toronto, Canada

Thomas E. Schlaepfer Department of Psychiatry, University Hospital, Bern, Switzerland, University of Bonn, Bonn, Germany, and Johns Hopkins University, Baltimore, Maryland, U.S.A.

Kenneth I. Shulman Department of Psychiatry, Sunnybrook & Women's College Health Sciences Centre, University of Toronto, Toronto, Canada

Jaskaran Singh Laboratory of Molecular Pathophysiology, National Institute of Mental Health, Bethesda, Maryland, U.S.A.

Jair C. Soares Division of Mood and Anxiety Disorders, Department of Psychiatry, University of Texas Health Science Center at San Antonio, San Antonio, Texas, U.S.A.

Constantin R. Soldatos Department of Psychiatry, Athens University Medical School, Athens, Greece

Michael E. Thase Department of Psychiatry, University of Pittsburgh School of Medicine, Western Psychiatric Institute and Clinic, Pittsburgh, Pennsylvania, U.S.A.

Eduard Vieta Bipolar Disorders Program, Hospital Clinic, University of Barcelona, Barcelona, Spain

L. A. Vornik Department of Psychiatry and Behavioral Sciences, University of Texas Medical Branch, Galveston, Texas, U.S.A.

Karen Dineen Wagner Division of Child and Adolescent Psychiatry, Department of Psychiatry and Behavioral Sciences, University of Texas Medical Branch, Galveston, Texas, U.S.A.

Allan H. Young School of Neurology, Neurobiology and Psychiatry, University of Newcastle upon Tyne, Royal Victoria Infirmary, Newcastle upon Tyne, U.K.

Carlos A. Zarate Jr. Laboratory of Molecular Pathophysiology, National Institute of Mental Health, Bethesda, Maryland, U.S.A.

1

Concept of Bipolar Disorder: A Historical Perspective

George N. Papadimitriou, Dimitris G. Dikeos, and Constantin R. Soldatos
Department of Psychiatry, Athens University Medical School, Athens, Greece

INTRODUCTION

Bipolar disorder is a chronic psychiatric disease often causing disability and significant functional impairment with considerable consequences on the quality of life not only of the patients themselves, but also of their family members and others in their environment (1). The disorder represents a major public-health problem; it frequently requires hospitalization and is associated with significant mortality due to suicide, the rate of which (15–20%) is higher than that in the general population and other psychiatric or medical patient populations (2–4).

The concept of affective disorder is very old. Literary and clinical descriptions of depression (often referred to as "melancholia") and mania date back to the antiquity. The word mania is the very first word of Homer's most celebrated epic, *The Iliad*, where it is used to describe the uncontrollable rage of Achilles against Agammemnon (5). Descriptions of both mania and depression also appear elsewhere in the epic, for example in the description of Bellerophontes' depression and of Ajax's mood fluctuation between a condition that resembles psychotic mania and great sadness ending to suicide.

FROM HIPPOCRATES TO THE PREDECESSORS OF KRAEPELIN

Medical thinking of ancient Greeks constitutes one of the earliest attempts to move from the demonic or divine etiology of the various disorders into an attempt of biological explanations. Hippocrates of Cos (460–377 B.C.), the most prominent figure of Hellenic medicine, considered that individual characteristics such as temperament and disease were related to the balance among the four main humors (blood, yellow bile, black bile, phlegm) of the human body. "Melancholia," the term of which first appears in Hippocratic scripts, was associated with the over-secretion of black bile ("melaina chole") from the liver. Hippocrates considered the brain as the site of origin of all emotions and thus rejected the earlier theories professing that mental phenomena are a result of divine intervention. The term mania is mentioned as a mental illness in the *Corpus Hippocraticum*. In addition, Hippocrates had observed that mood fluctuations sometimes had a seasonal component (6).

On the basis of Hippocratic tradition, Galen (129 or 130–199 A.D.) considered abnormalities in the secretion of black bile as the cause of melancholy. He used the term "hypochondria" to describe a combination of physical illness with psychological symptomatology. For Aretaeus of Cappadocia (practicing in Rome during the second century A.D.), the rising of black bile in the stomach or the diaphragm was responsible for the manifestation of melancholy, which he considered to have both physical and mental symptoms, such as sadness, psychomotor retardation, and suicidal ideation. He had made the observation that euphoria (which he considered as a sort of "catharsis" leading to amelioration of the clinical picture) may follow melancholy, thus describing, for the first time, the two phases and the periodic course of bipolar illness (7–10).

Melancholy seems to have been constantly recognized during the period between the Classical Times and Renaissance, although during the Dark Ages it was frequently associated to magic influence or sin. The contribution of somatic functions in its etiology emerged again during Renaissance. First, the ancient humoral theories regarding mental disease were combined with theology by Paracelsos (1391–1431), who also describes mania as a periodic illness. He believed that the etiology of mental illness might be endogenous or exogenous or based on "obsession" (11). Descartes' theories on human emotions ("passions") and mental disorders stressed the division between body and soul ("Cartesian dualism") and attempted to explain psychiatric disease as the result of untoward childhood experiences or transmission of feelings from the mother to the unborn child. These theories were among the first ones after Medieval times to offer a non-mystical approach to human soul and disease (12).

Biological theories of depression prevailed throughout the 16th and most of the 17th centuries; the main theories for the causation of depression were attempting to provide biological explanations similar to the Hippocratic ones. This is particularly demonstrated in the famous works by Vesalius (1514–1564) and Burton (1577–1640) who in 1621 published the *Anatomy of Melancholy* (13). Towards the end of the 17th century, a conceptual change occurred in psychiatry with the prominence being hitherto given to the description of symptomatology and not in the attempts of biological explanations, similarly to the prevailing attitude among the other medical fields. Different writers gave various definitions to the word "melancholy" at that time. It has been considered as an affective disease with depressive and euphoric moods [by Gullen (1710–1790)] or it was used [by Pinel (1745–1826) and Heinroth (1773–1843)] as a term for a state that resembles residual schizophrenia, with "mania" describing agitated schizophrenic symptomatolgy (14). In Pinel's (1818) *Nosographie* (15), mania was considered to be a part of the broader family of "insanities" and it was subcategorized into delusional and nondelusional. At the same time, Heinroth considered that "mania" could be divided into simplex (pure rage), ecstatica (insane), ecnoa (rage accompanied by folly), and catholica (common rage) (16). During the 19th century, questions were raised among scientists regarding the clusters of mental functions and their disorders. The main hypothesis was that there are three clusters of mental functions (intellectual, emotional, and volitional), each of which might manifest a disorder independently of the others. Melancholia was considered to be a disorder of the intellectual function, although there were also writers [such as Esquirol (1772–1830)] who believed that this was not true and that the condition was related to temperament (17,18).

Until the middle of the 19th century, the clinical course was not taken into account when describing a psychiatric condition, but diagnosis was based on the manifest symptoms at the time of the examination. This, however, was changed after many patients started to be hospitalized for long periods of time in the psychiatric asylums established in the second half of the 18th century, allowing for longitudinal observations of the disorders. Thus, Pinel proposed that the course of the disease is important in its description and Falret (1794–1870) and Baillarger (1809–1890) observed the circularity of mania and depression interspersed with symptom-free periods; this observation leads them to coin the terms "folie circulaire" (19) and "folie à double forme" (20–22).

The 19th century also saw the development of an integrated nosologic approach. This approach is best represented in psychiatry by the works of Kahlbaum (1828–1899), who proposed that patients with the same diagnosis should share similar symptoms, common etiology of their disease, the same therapeutic response to particular interventions, as well as a common prognosis, biochemical aberrations, and pathology. Kraepelin was particularly influenced by this "holistic" description of disease. Kahlbaum also proposed the terms "dysthymia" (chronic form of melancholia) and "cyclothymia" while noted that the "cyclic psychoses" are separate entities from "typical insanity," which was characterized by severe and progressive course (23,24).

THE ERA OF KRAEPELIN AND THE FIRST HALF OF THE 20TH CENTURY

At the end of the 19th century, keeping in line with the then widely supported "degeneration theory," Kraepelin (1856–1926), suggested that mental illness should be considered either as "endogenous" (which was believed to be due to a "degeneration of the human seed") or "exogenous." In 1896 (25), he further divided the "endogenous psychoses" into "manic-depressive illness" and "dementia praecox" (what today is called "schizophrenia"), whereas in 1899 he proposed the use of the term "manic-depressive insanity" to describe all forms of recurrent psychoses. "Manic-depressive insanity" was considered to have a good prognosis (not evolving into dementia), even if the existence of mild residual symptoms after recovery from the episodes was acknowledged. Kraepelin (26) also mentioned that the inter-episode periods were likely to become progressively shorter after the first three episodes of manic-depressive insanity.

Kraepelin's separation of "manic-depressive insanity" from "dementia praecox" was based on symptomatology, course, and family history and is being considered as the basis of modern psychiatric nosology (27–29). Another contribution of Kraepelin to modern nosologic terminology was the substitution of the term "melancholy" with that of "depression" to describe the mood disorder that is part of the manic-depressive illness. Kraepelin's "melancholia" was not part of manic-depressive illness but could take three forms: simplex, activa, and atonita. The first two were characterized by sadness, the first without, and the second with anxiety and psychomotor activation, whereas the third has, as its prominent feature, an extreme psychomotor retardation ("stupor") and a prognosis, which resembled that of dementia praecox (16,30).

Freud and Meyer were among the other influential psychiatrists of the first-half of the 20th century who contributed to our conceptual understanding of mood disorders. Freud (1856–1939) (31) considered melancholy to be due to low self-esteem stemming from a disturbed childhood and as the result of the withdrawal of libido invested in the object and retroflexion of the hostility directed at the lost object onto the self. Adolf Meyer (1866–1950) introduced Kraepelin's classification in the United States pointing out at the same time that many types of depression should not be considered as a part of manic-depressive insanity (32).

MODERN CLASSIFICATIONS AND DIAGNOSTIC CRITERIA

Until about the 1960s, Kraepelin's view that all affective illness belonged to the category of manic-depressive insanity dominated diagnostic classification. In 1957, however, Leonhard (33) proposed a new distinction, that of unipolar vs. bipolar illness. This distinction was based on the existence or not of manic episodes during the course of the disease, thus introducing the element of "polarity" in the classification of affective disorders. Patients who had only depressive episodes were to be considered as unipolar, whereas any patient who had ever had a manic episode as bipolar. A patient is still considered bipolar even if only manic episodes have occurred, being actually considered as a bipolar disorder during which a depressive episode has not yet occurred. Leonhard's suggestion has taken firm footing in the modern classification of affective disorders, particularly after being supported by the works of Angst (34), Perris (35,36), and Winokur et al. (37).

The diagnosis of bipolar disorder seems to correspond to an underlying nosologic entity much better than that of unipolar disorder. This was consistently shown by several lines of research on its genetics, neurobiology, and response to biological treatments. For unipolar disorder, it is suggested that the category must be considered as potentially including various conditions resulting in depression, among which bipolar disorder is a strong candidate. For this reason, it has been suggested that at least three episodes of depression need to have taken place before a patient is considered as unipolar (35,38,39); other studies, however, have shown that perhaps more episodes are needed, as the possibility of a manic episode after three depressive ones is still in the range of 13–16%, dropping to 4% after a fourth depressive episode (36). On the basis of epidemiological and family studies, it has also been proposed that recurrent depression with well-defined episodes, clearly separated by periods of unquestionable normothymia, should be considered as a form of bipolar disorder (40). On the other hand, according to current knowledge, there is no distinction between the features of a major depressive episode based on whether it is part of bipolar disorder or part of unipolar major depressive disorder (41), although there have been some findings that point towards certain differences regarding vegetative symptoms such as sleep and appetite (42,43).

A systematic effort to enhance reliability among psychiatrists for the diagnosis of mental disorders and to develop a consistent classification was launched with the introduction, in 1965, of the eighth revision of the WHO International Classification of Diseases (ICD-8) (44) that was followed, in 1978 (45), by the ninth revision (ICD 9). Both these systems, however, offered only relatively vague diagnostic guidelines and did not help much regarding diagnostic reliability of psychiatric illnesses. It must be noted that in ICD-9, the distinction between unipolar and bipolar affective disorders is implied but not clearly stated, whereas the term bipolar appears only in the glossary (45).

Similar efforts to incorporate findings from research and clinical experience into a coherent diagnostic system led, in the United States, to the development of the classifications by the American Psychiatric Association (46). In the third edition of the

Diagnostic and Statistical Manual of the American Psychiatric Association (DSM-III) (47), major affective disorders were subdivided into bipolar disorder and major depression. According to the DSM-III definition, whether or not a manic episode has ever occurred is the distinguishing feature; patients who had one or more manic episodes and did not yet had any depressive ones are considered to be bipolar. The revised edition of DSM-III (DSM-III-R) (48), the fourth edition of the manual in its original and its text-revised version (DSM-IV, APA, 1994; DSM-IV-TR, APA, 2000) (49,50), and the 10th edition of the International Classification of Diseases (ICD-10) (51) followed the same guidelines as DSM-III for the classification of affective (mood) disorders. The term "mood disorders" was preferred to that of "affective disorders" in DSM-IV and ICD-10 in order to imply that there is a clear differentiation between mood states and anxiety disorders, which could be considered as not being clearly differentiated from "affective" states. Another interesting feature of these two classification systems is that while they retain the notion of unipolar–bipolar distinction, the term unipolar has been dropped in favor of the term "major depression" (52,53).

The use of modern classification systems and manuals has come along with the development of standardized criteria aiming at enhancing reliability of psychiatric diagnosis. To this end, various standardized questionnaires and rating scales have been introduced, usually reflecting the diagnostic guidelines of DSM and ICD or other criteria, such as those introduced by Feighner et al. (54) or Spitzer et al. (55). Various of these questionnaires are accompanied by computer programs for the establishment of diagnosis; most widely known among these is the Present State Examination and its computerized system CATEGO (56).

In the quest of identification of the purest possible nosologic entities, in order to study separately epidemiological, familial, biologic, and other clinical characteristics, further subdivisions of bipolar disorder have been proposed. Bipolar disorder is thus subdivided, on the basis of history of hospitalization for mania and/or significant loss of functioning in major life roles during a manic episode, into bipolar I (patients who needed hospitalization and/or had loss of functioning in major roles) and bipolar II (57). The periods of manic symptoms of bipolar II patients, which have not required hospitalization nor have lead to a significant impairment in major roles, are considered as "hypomanic" episodes; a patient is considered as bipolar II when, hypomanic and depressive episodes have occurred. On the same lines, it has been proposed to consider as "bipolar III" the patient who has had episodes of depression only, but a family history of mania (58), or has developed hypomania following the use of antidepressants, other somatic therapies, or the abrupt discontinuation of a mood stabilizer. It has also been proposed that patients with a history of major depressive but not manic or hypomanic episodes who are outside their periods of depression extroverted, cheerful, optimistic, confident, and energetic ("trait hypomania" or "hyperthymic temperament") should be classified as part of the bipolar spectrum, perhaps as bipolar type IV (28). It is, however, questionable to which extent these subgroups of bipolar disorder patients correspond to true nosologic entities, given the fact that even bipolar II disorder seems to be heterogeneous with some patients resembling bipolar I, some unipolar, and some "breeding true" (59) and that the NIMH Collaborative Program on the Psychobiology of Depression (60) provided no evidence that the course of bipolar II disorder differed from that of bipolar I, confirming other similar findings (61).

Other subdivisions that have been proposed for bipolar disorder are based on the presence or absence of psychotic features (congruent and incongruent), whether the episode frequency shows a rapid cycling pattern, the age of onset, the overall severity of the disease, and presence or absence of deterioration, the symptom pattern, and the co-morbidity with other disorders. Specifically for rapid cycling bipolar disorder, the DSM-IV now lists clear criteria for its definition while it is supported that patients prone to rapid cycling usually exhibit higher depressive morbidity than other bipolar patients and are at high risk for serious suicidal attempts (62). It is not, however, clear whether the patient with rapid cycling can be considered as belonging to a separate group, as the pattern is a transient phenomenon in the majority of cases (62). The same uncertainty exists for another distinction, that of the "mixed states," which is based on the co-existence of manic and depressive symptomatology during the same episode and can be viewed as temperament intruding into an episode of opposite polarity (63).

Finally, it has been suggested that a dimensional approach could be used (64–66), instead of attempting to divide mood disorders into a number of distinct and mutually exclusive categories. It follows the assumption that, due to the high multiformity of psychiatric disorders, subordinating an individual to strict diagnostic criteria derived from standardized instruments, and ascribing a patient to a taxonomic group may result in an impoverishment of information (52). On the basis of this approach, it is proposed that each patient could be described by a number of different descriptive dimensions (or "factors") of symptomatology. Dimensional characteristics are often used in studies focusing on neuropsychology, statistical analysis, or an empirical approach to classification (66). The dimensional approach provides useful information for research into developing new diagnostic concepts and categories, but it is too complex to be applicable in clinical practice; an additional disadvantage of it being that since the time of Hippocrates, nosologists are used to function within a typological or categorical model, which conceptualizes illnesses as discrete entities (66,67).

CONCLUSIONS

Although since ancient times, there have been descriptions of bipolar mood disorder, the differentiation of this nosological entity from other mental illnesses was made in the 20th century, following Leonhard's differentiation of bipolar illness from unipolar major depression. In spite of its establishment, however, as a separate diagnosis in the modern classification systems, the diagnosis of bipolar disorder is symptom-based, lacking firm validating criteria such as specific biological markers that, if they existed, could prove that the clinical diagnosis really corresponds to a specific disease entity (52,68,69). On the other hand, even if biological indices cannot concretely validate it, this diagnosis serves important functions, as it delineates phenomenologically more homogeneous groups, improves diagnostic reliability among clinicians, infers meaningful clinical distinctions, helps in the prediction of the clinical course, and also predicts the response to treatment. In addition, the establishment of diagnostic guidelines and standard operational diagnostic criteria with the subsequent development of standardized questionnaires and scales further contributes to the improvement of reliability of diagnoses that assists considerably in clinical practice as well as in research.

REFERENCES

1. Angst J, Sellaro R. Historical perspectives and natural history of bipolar disorder. Biol Psychiatry 2000; 48:445–457.
2. Chen YW, Dilsaver SC. Lifetime rates of suicide attempts among subjects with bipolar and unipolar disorders relative to subjects with other axis I disorders. Biol Psychiatry 1996; 39:896–899.
3. Judd LL, Akiskal HS, Schettler PJ, Endicott J, Maser J, Solomon DA, Leon AC, Rice JA, Keller MB. The long-term natural history of the weekly symptomatic status of bipolar I disorder. Arch Gen Psychiatry 2002; 59:530–537.
4. Kupfer DJ, Frank E, Grochocinski VL, Cluss PA, Houck PR, Stapf DA. Demographic and clinical characteristics of individuals in a bipolar disorder case registry. J Clin Psychiatry 2002; 63:120–125.
5. Lattimore R. (Transl.). The Iliad of Homer. Chicago: University of Chicago Press, 1961.
6. Hippocrates. Samtliche Werke. München: H. Luneburg, 1897.
7. Lewis AJ. Melancholia: a historical review. J Ment Sci 1934; 80:1–42.
8. Kotsopoulos S. Aretaeus the Cappadocian on mental illness. Compr Psychiatry 1986; 27:171–179.
9. Georgotas A. Evolution of the concepts of depression and mania. In: Georgotas A, Cancro R, eds. Depression and Mania. New York: Elsevier, 1988:3–12.
10. Angst J, Marneros A. Bipolarity from ancient to modern times: conception, birth and rebirth. J Affect Dis 2001; 67:3–19.
11. Pauleicof B. Das Menschenbild im Waldel der Zeit. Ideen-genschichte der Psychiatrie und Klinishen Psychologie. Hurtgenwald: Pressler, 1983.
12. Albuquerque J, Deshauer D, Grof P. Descartes' passions of the soul—seeds of psychiatry? J Affect Dis 2003; 76:285–291.
13. Burton R. The anatomy of melancholy. In: Dell F, Jordan-Smith P, eds. New York: Tudor Publishing Co, 1621/1938.
14. Schmidt-Degenhard M. Melancholie und Depression. Stuttgart: Kohlhammer, 1983.
15. Pinel Ph. Nosographie philosophique ou la methode de l'analyse appliquée à lamédecine. 6th ed. Paris: Brosson, 1818.
16. Berrios GE. Depressive and manic states during the nineteenth century. In: Georgotas A, Cancro R, eds. Depression and Mania. New York: Elsevier, 1988:13–25.
17. Esquirol E. Des Maladies Mentales. Paris: Raillire, 1838.
18. Tellenbach H. Melancholie. Berlin: Springer, 1961.
19. Falret JP. De la folie circulaire ou forme de maladie mentale caracterisée par l'alternative regulierè de la manie et de la melancholie. Bull Acad Med (Paris), 1854; 19:382–415.
20. Baillarger J. De la folie à double-forme. Ann Med Psychol (Paris) 1854; 6:367–391.
21. Ritti A. Folie avec conscience. In: Dechambre A, ed. Dictionnairc Encyclopedique des Sciences Médicaaales. Paris: P. Asselin, G. Masson, 1879:520–559.
22. Pichot P. The birth of the bipolar disorder. Eur Psychiatry 1995; 10:1–10.
23. Kahlbaum KL. Die Gruppirung der Psychischen Krankheiten und Die Eintheilung der Seelenst; Oerungen: Entwurf einer Historish-Kritischen Darstellung der Bisherigen Eintheilungen und Versuch zur Anbahnung einer Empirisch-Wissenschaftlichen Grundlage der Psychiatrie als Klinischer Disciplin. Danzig: Kafemann, 1863.
24. Baethge C, Salvatore MD, Baldessarini RJ. "On Cyclic Insanity" by Karl Ludwig Kahlbaum, MD: a translation and commentary. Harv Rev Psychiatry 2003; 11:78–90.
25. Kraepelin E. Psychiatrie. 5th ed. Leipzig: Barth, 1896.
26. Kraepelin E. Psychiatrie. Ein Lehrbuch fur Studierende und Arzte. Vol. III. 8th ed. Leipzig: JA Barth, 1913.
27. Kraepelin E. Manic-Depressive Insanity and Paranoia. Edinburg, Scotland: E&S Livingstone, 1921.
28. Akiskal HS, Pinto O. The evolving bipolar spectrum. Prototypes I, II, III, and IV. Psychiatr Clin North Am 1999; 22:517–534.

29. Berrios GE, Hauser R. The early development of Kraepelin's ideas on classification: a conceptual history. Psychol Med 1988; 18:813–821.
30. Lanczik M, Beckmann H. Historical aspects of affective disorders. In: Feighner JP, Boyer WF, eds. The Diagnosis of Depression. Chichester: John Wiley & Sons Ltd, 1991:1–16.
31. Freud S. Mourning and Melancholia. In: Strachey J, ed. Standard Edition of the Complete Psychological Works of Sigmund Freud. Vol. 14. London: Hogarth Press, 1957.
32. Meyer A. The problems of mental reaction types, mental causes and diseases. Psychol Bull 1908; 5:245.
33. Leonhard K. Aufteilung der Endogenen Psychosen und Ihre Differenzierte Aetiologie. Berlin: Akademie-Verlag, 1957.
34. Angst J. Zur Aetiologie und Nosologie Endogener Depressiver Psychosen. Eine Genetische, Sociologische und Klinische Studie. Berlin: Springer, 1966.
35. Perris C. A study of bipolar (manic-depressive) and unipolar recurrent depressive psychoses. Acta Psychiatr Scand 1966; 42 (suppl 194):172–188.
36. Perris C. The distinction between bipolar and unipolar affective disorders. In: Paykel ES, ed. Handbook of Affective Disorders. Edinburgh: Churchill Livingstone, 1982:43–58.
37. Winokur G, Clayton P, Reich T. Manic Depressive Illness. St Louis: Mo C.V. Mosby, 1969.
38. Bertelsen A, Harvard B, Hauge M. A Danish twin study of manic-depressive disorders. Br J Psychiatry 1977; 130:330–351.
39. Smeraldi E, Negri F, Melica AM. A genetic study of affective disorders. Acta Psychiatr Scand 1978; 56:382–398.
40. Angst J. Historical aspects of the dichotomy between manic-depressive disorders and schizophrenia. Schizophrenia Res 2002; 57:5–13.
41. Kasper S. Issues in the treatment of bipolar disorder. Eur Neuropsychopharmacol 2003; 13:37–42.
42. Papadimitriou GN, Dikeos DG, Daskalopoulou E, Soldatos CR. Co-occurrence of disturbed sleep and appetite loss differentiates between unipolar and bipolar depressive episodes. Prog Neuropsychopharmacol & Biol Psychiatry 2002; 26:1041–1045.
43. Papadimitriou GN, Dikeos DG, Soldatos CR. Sleep disturbance in unipolar and bipolar depression: Relationship to psychiatric family history. Neuropsychobiology 2003; 48:131–136.
44. World Health Organization. Mental Disorders: Manual of the International Statistical Classification of Diseases, Injuries and Causes of Death. Geneva: World Health Organization, 1967.
45. World Health Organization. Mental Disorders: Glossary and Guide to Their Classification in Accordance with the Ninth Revision of the International Classification of Diseases. Geneva: World Health Organization, 1978.
46. Klerman GL. History and development of modern concepts of affective illness. In: Post RM, Ballenger JC, eds. Neurobiology of Mood Disorders. Baltimore/London: Williams & Wilkins, 1984:1–19.
47. American Psychiatric Association. Diagnostic and Statistical Manual of Mental Disorders (DSM-III). 3rd ed. Washington, DC: American Psychiatric Association, 1980.
48. American Psychiatric Association. Diagnostic and Statistical Manual of Mental Disorders. 3rd ed. (revised). Washington, DC: American Psychiatric Association, 1987.
49. American Psychiatric Association. Diagnostic and Statistical Manual of Mental Disorders. 4th ed. Washington, DC: American Psychiatric Association, 1994.
50. American Psychiatric Association. Diagnostic and Statistical Manual of Mental Disorders. 4th ed. (text rev.). Washington, DC: American Psychiatric Association, 2000.
51. World Health Organization. International Statistical Classification of Diseases and Related Health Problems (10th rev.). Geneva: World Health Organization, 1992.

52. Stefanis CN, Dikeos DG, Papadimitriou GN. Clinical strategies in genetic research. In: Mendlewicz J, Papadimitriou GN, eds. Genetics of Mental Disorders. Part I: Theoretical Aspects. Vol. I. London: Bailliere Tindal, 1995;1–18.
53. Stefanis CN, Stefanis NC. Diagnosis of depressive disorders: a review. In: Maj M, Sartorius N, eds. Depressive Disorders. Chichester: John Wiley & Sons Ltd, 1999:1–51.
54. Feighner JP, Robins E, Guze SB, Woodruff RA, Winokur G. Diagnostic criteria for use in psychiatric research. Arch Gen Psychiatry 1972; 26:56–73.
55. Spitzer RL, Endicott J, Robins E. Research diagnostic criteria: Rationale and reliability. Arch Gen Psychiatry 1978; 35:773–782.
56. Wing JK, Cooper JE, Sartorius N. The Measurement and Classification of Psychiatric Symptoms. London, New York, Melbourne: Oxford University Press, 1974.
57. Fieve RR, Dunner DL, Kumbaraci T, Stallone F. Lithium carbonate prophylaxis of depression in three subtypes in primary affective disorder. Pharmakopsychiatr Neuropsychopharmakol 1976; 9:100–107.
58. Depue RA, Monroe SN. The unipolar–bipolar distinction in the depressive disorders. Psychol Bull 1978; 85:1001–1029.
59. Coryell W, Winokur G, Shea T, Maser JD, Endicott J, Akiskal HS. The long-term stability of depressive subtypes. Am J Psychiatry 1994; 151:199–204.
60. Coryell W, Keller M, Endicot J, Andreasen N, Clayton P, Hirschfeld R. Bipolar II illness: course and outcome over a five-year period. Psychol Med 1989, 19:129–141.
61. Angst J. The course of major depression, atypical bipolar disorder, and bipolar disorder. In: Hippius H, Klerman GL, Matussek N, eds. New Results in Depression Research. Berlin: Springer, 1986:26–35.
62. Coryell W, Solomon D, Turvey C, Keller M, Leon AC, Endicott J, Schettler P, Judd L, Mueller T. The long-term course of rapid-cycling bipolar disorder. Arch Gen Psychiatry 2003; 60:914–920.
63. Marneros A. Origin and development of concepts of bipolar mixed states. J Affect Dis 2001; 67:229–240.
64. Eysenck HJ. The classification of depressive illnesses. Br J Psychiatry 1970; 117:241–250.
65. Kendell RE. The classification of depressions: a review of contemporary confusion. Br J Psychiatry 1976; 129:15–28.
66. Andreasen NC. Concepts, diagnosis and classification. In: Paykel ES, ed. Handbook of Affective Disorders. Edinburgh: Churchill Livingstone, 1982:25–44.
67. Goldberg D. Plato vs. Aristotle: categorical and dimensional models for common mental disorders. Compr Psychiatry 2000; 2(suppl 1):8–13.
68. Holzer CP III, Nguyen HT, Hirschfeld RMA. Reliability of diagnosis in mood disorders. Psychiatr Clin North Am 1996; 19:73–84.
69. Kendler KS, Gardner CO Jr. Boundaries of major depression: an evaluation of DSM-IV criteria. Am J Psychiatry 1998; 155:172–177.

2
Diagnosis of Bipolar Disorder

Charles L. Bowden
Department of Psychiatry, The University of Texas Health Science Center at San Antonio, San Antonio, Texas, U.S.A.

INTRODUCTION

Recent studies both in the United States and in Europe have resulted in an increased interest in making earlier and more accurate diagnoses of bipolar disorders. The findings from these studies can also be utilized to change clinical practices and thereby improve patient outcomes. The three fundamental findings from these studies are (i) bipolar disorder is often misdiagnosed as major depression; (ii) both bipolar I and, particularly, bipolar II disorder are characterized by much more time spent with depressive than manic symptomatology, and (iii) the prevalence of bipolar disorders is at least in the 3–4% range, approximating that of major depression (1–5). We shall examine ways to improve on accuracy and timeliness of making a diagnosis of bipolar disorder.

FUNDAMENTAL AND RELATIVELY SPECIFIC SYMPTOMS AND ILLNESS COURSE FEATURES OF BIPOLAR DISORDERS

Impulsivity appears to be a factor present in nearly all studies of bipolar patients (5–8). Decreased inhibition was present in 71% of bipolar II patients (9). In addition, impulsivity appears to persist as a trait characteristic in depression, euthymia, as well as hypomania (10).

Manic episodes are less likely to be euphoric or pure in type than to have various mixed features (11). These features are not only those of DSM-IV defined depressive episodes, as is now the DSM-IV requirement for a mixed manic episode. Symptoms of anxiety often coassociate with depression in mixed states (7,12). Irritability is common in all forms of bipolar disorder, is a distinct factor from hyperactivity or grandiosity, and is inadequately captured in most rating scales (7,12–14). These components of bipolar disorders are substantially consistent with what Kraepelin (15) defined, a century ago, as psychobiological roots of personality or temperament: hyperthymia, irritability, cyclothymia, or mood instability, and dysthymia.

Onset of depression before the age of 30 years is suggestive of bipolar disorder (16). Geller found that 10 years following prepubertal diagnosis of unipolar major depression, even with initial careful attention to exclusion of persons with bipolar disorders, 48.6% of subjects had been diagnosed as having bipolar I or II disorder, compared with 7.1% of healthy controls also followed for 10 years ($p = 0.0001$) (17). Importantly, history of mania in a parent or grandparent was significantly predictive of development of bipolar I disorder in these youths. Depressive symptoms that persist for more than half of a period of ≥ 1 year are more likely to be present in bipolar disorder, particularly bipolar II disorder, than major depression (18–20).

Similarly, comorbidity of bipolar disorders with certain other disorders is so common that presence of illness features of anxiety disorders, substance dependence, or migraine should cause the clinician to assess for evidence of bipolar disorder (21,22). Even in psychoses, unless the negative symptoms characteristic of schizophrenia are present (23), consideration of bipolar disorder is inherently important (13,23–25). Mood disturbances that occur during the post-partum period are most often indicative of bipolar conditions, although, in this instance, information comes largely from small case series (26,27).

Rather than ignoring these characteristic relationships in the process of diagnosis of psychiatric disorders, when there is evidence of such symptoms and illness course features, a careful cross-sectional and longitudinal assessment for bipolar disorder should be conducted. The DSM-IV approach of separating manic episodes occurring in association with medication use from the group of bipolar disorders, as well as some other features, such as borrowing the criteria for depression from unipolar major depression, which authorities agree warrants correction, tends to discourage such diagnostic considerations. However, the DSM-IV introductory commentary makes clear that the clinician is to use the explicit criteria as "guidelines to be informed by clinical judgment" and to factor in other evidence-based information in the diagnosis recorded (page xxiii). The psychiatrist of other mental health clinician needs to keep in mind that DSM-IV criteria were based on evidence last systematically reviewed in 1992 (28). Thus, as of this writing, the criteria do not factor in any of the information developed over more than one dozen years from randomized, prospectively conducted, large-scale studies in many countries, and in many instances, confirmed by more than one study. It is reasonable to incorporate reliable, confirmed information of over a decade into diagnostic processes rather than literally to the DSM-IV listed criteria, and—as indicated—the DSM manual allows for this.

FEATURES OF DEPRESSION INDICATIVE OF BIPOLAR DISORDER

Certain characteristics of depression are relatively specific for bipolar disorders, albeit not sufficiently reliable to base diagnosis on them alone. Nonetheless, their presence warrants heightened concern about a possible bipolar condition in a person with depression. These are listed in Table 1.

Table 1 Symptom Differences in Bipolar Vs. Unipolar Depression

Total sleep time	BP > UP
Hypersomnia	BP > UP
Psychomotor retardation	BP > UP
Post-partum episodes	BP > UP
Weight loss	UP > BP

Slowed psychomotor activity is common in bipolar but not unipolar depression (29,30). Hypersomnia is common in bipolar depression but not unipolar depression (31,32). As indicated earlier, bipolar disorder is more likely to appear first as a depressive episode, and the first depressive episode is likely to occur before age of 30 years (33). In particular, depression that begins pre-pubertally is likely to ultimately prove to be bipolar in type. The high frequency of initial diagnosis of a depressive disorder, rather than bipolar depression, leads both to treatment with antidepressants without use of mood stabilizers and to lack of attention in treatment to stress factors for bipolar disorder (34). The delay in accurate diagnosis and in associated appropriate treatment, in turn, leads to poorer social functioning, more hospitalizations, and more suicide attempts (35). Depressions that are refractory to standard treatments, including ones that worsen with antidepressant treatments, should raise concerns about bipolar disorders, as mood destabilization from antidepressants is essentially limited to bipolar disorders and can be misinterpreted as non-response (1).

The 13-item Mood Disorder Questionnaire (MDQ), which requires < 5 minutes for self-administration, can aid in early identification of fundamentally bipolar conditions. It is useful in primary-care settings, as it does not require professional administration (36). The MDQ can also be accessed by any individual at dbsa@.org

MANIC SYMPTOMS WITH HIGH SPECIFICITY AND SENSITIVITY

Certain characteristics of mania are more sensitive and more specific for manic/hypomanic episodes than others. Reduced need for sleep is not characteristic of any other psychiatric disorder and is highly prevalent in manic and hypomanic states. Increased sexuality is less prevalent but highly specific. DSM-IV does not list impulsivity per se as a symptom of mania/hypomania (16). It does list complex behaviors that are likely to have an impulsive component, most specifically "excessive involvement in high-risk activities." In our view, criteria should when possible be defined in terms of the fundamental behavioral disturbance, not principally as characteristic examples carried out in daily life. Were all of the DSM so defined in terms of behavioral examples, we would have a criterion for "believes he is a more important person than is supported by the evidence" than the concise and meaningful word "grandiosity."

EFFECTIVE ASSESSMENT STRATEGIES FOR BIPOLAR DISORDER

In the forthcoming sections, we review the DSM-IV criteria for bipolar disorder, those criteria that more recent evidence indicates should be modified, even though the fundamental inclusion in syndromal criteria is valid, and strategies for eliciting information on the behavior, or course of illness, that can improve accuracy of diagnosis.

We encourage a relatively structured approach to diagnostic assessment for possible bipolar disorder. Bipolar disorder is the only condition we know of where a substantial number of important symptoms of the illness are viewed, accurately, as desirable characteristics, rather than problems. The listing of symptoms of hypomania in Table 2 underscores this unusual feature of the disease (9). This point is made in DSM-IV for bipolar II disorder, as it is the only axis I disorder that does not require functional impairment for diagnosis. Persons with increased activity,

Table 2 Most Common Manifestations of Hypomania

Increased activity	97%
Increased energy	96%
Increased plans, ideas	91%
Increased self-confidence	86%
Decreased sleep	84%
Increased talkativeness	72%
Decreased inhibition	71%
Increased optimism	68%

speeded thinking, grandiosity, and the ability to function seemingly well on 4 hours of sleep are not necessarily denying symptomatology when they do not complain of these features. A structured approach that asks about the behavior independent of its subjective dysfunctional aspects will often yield information that will otherwise not be immediately obtained. A structured approach is particularly important for milder forms of bipolar disorder. Persons who are so ill that they are hospitalized for a manic state essentially telegraphs evidence of the condition sufficient to make the diagnosis. Persons with earlier and milder symptomatology will not do so. This is an especially important consideration for those symptoms for which the patients may be more subjectively aware of their presence than is evident to the professional. These include irritability, evening mood escalation, and the sense that one's thoughts are racing (37). Examples of the type and form of questions that have been found useful in structured rating instruments to establish diagnosis and symptom severity in studies of bipolar disorder are listed in Table 3.

MANIA OR HYPOMANIA

The criteria for mania are listed in Table 4. These are generally satisfactory, with most not requiring either editorial clarification or change in any restructuring of criteria. However, some are problematic as written. The requirement that fewer symptoms be evident for a form of mania (variously described as euphoric, euthymic, pure, or classical mania) that is substantially less frequent than irritability, with or without specific mixed features, seems inconsistent to most authorities with a reasoned set of criteria (38). Some of the criteria are principally observable: increased talkativeness, pressured speech, and distractibility. Therefore, sufficient time with a patient, securing information from family members or from observers, e.g., teachers, co-workers, nurses, can aid in assessing these areas.

Other criteria require some exploration. It is often best to state that you recognize that the patient may not find actions risky, or grandiose, but that friends and family have viewed them thusly. Sleep is similarly complex. To a simple question of "How is your sleep?" patients may respond that their sleep is fine in actuality, when they are sleeping 4 hr or perhaps 7 hr, but only with a sleep cycle that starts at 3 a.m. Therefore, it is important to ask about actual time asleep and when the sleep occurred. In addition, endeavor to have the patients respond to questions about sleep with reference back to a time when they were not in their current mood state and when their functions were not impaired. As indicated earlier, irritability can be observable during an interview, but patients often are more sensitive to

Table 3 Questions Used in Structured Rating Scales to Assess for Prototypical Symptoms Mania/Hypomania

Irritability
How irritated, angry, or resentful have you felt—whether you showed it or not?
How strongly did you feel this way?
How much of the time did you feel this way?
How did you show your anger, annoyance, and irritability?
Increased energy
Have you had more energy than usual to do things?
More than just a return to normal or usual level?
Did it seem like too much energy?
Elevated evening energy
Have your mood, interest, and energy been about the same throughout the day?
Have you had any tendency to be more active or take on projects in the evening or at night?
(Have these kept you up past your usual hour of going to bed or beyond midnight)?
Has it ever been difficult to stop what you are doing?
Impulsivity
Have you been patient or impatient when you have had to stand in line, say at a check out counter? Have you cut in line?
Have you bought things that you did not need? Have you talked when you should have kept quiet or have you taken on a project without thinking it through?
Have you made any decisions without thinking the situation through? Have you made any snap judgments?
Have you been able to control your responses when placed in a situation where a decision or choice is needed?
Affective lability
How steady has your mood been?
Do your emotions shift fairly suddenly at times?
How much of the time are you this way? When this happens can you put a halt to it? Does it interfere in your daily life?

recognition of felt irritability that they did not express. The probe questions on irritability in Table 3 can help in such an inquiry.

The criteria for mania or hypomania are also problematic in that they are cross-sectional, except for the durational requirement. The criteria do not require that all of a period be spent in expression of a symptom. Although the requirement for duration is somewhat unclear in DSM-IV, most authorities recognize that many of the behaviors characteristic of mania come and go with rapidity and may not be present for most of the hours of a day, yet cause great distress and functional disturbance.

Table 4 Manic Episode

Elevated, expansive, or irritable mood for $\geq$1 week with more than three symptoms (more than four symptoms if irritability is the only symptom)
- Inflated self-esteem or grandiosity
- Decreased need for sleep
- More talkative than usual or pressured speech
- Flight of ideas/racing thoughts
- Distractibility
- Increased goal-directed activity or psychomotor agitation
- Excessive involvement in high-risk activities

Some symptoms of mania/hypomania are simply not included in the stated criteria (Table 3). In the author's view, it is important to inquire about all of these, as well as less prevalent, but diagnostically useful actions, e.g., hypersexuality, evening mood escalation, and substance abuse. In particular, it is odd that affective lability (or if one prefers, mood instability) was not incorporated into the DSM, as descriptions of bipolar disorders have consistently described this as a core element, and contributed to introduction of the phrase mood stabilizer. Geller and associates have published very useful results of studies that indicate which symptoms are most specific to bipolar disorders, which, though limited to youth, likely have some general relevance. For example, they indicate that hypersexuality and impulsivity are specific to and sensitive as indicators of bipolar disorders.

A final problem principally applies to bipolar II disorder and by extension cyclothymia. The durational criterion for bipolar II disorder was set at 4 days at a time that studies now published had not been conducted. These studies make a solid case that hypomania tends to have much shorter modal periods, with 1 or 2 days supported by evidence, and even shorter expressions recognized as common in youth with bipolar disorder (38). Authorities making decisions on the threshold for a syndrome have inherent difficulties in gray areas such as this, but it is apparent that the decisions of the early 1990s warrant shortening of time requirements. This similarly applies to the current time and episode sequence for rapid cycling, with several studies indicating that shorter periods of symptoms, and a less rigid requirement than for 8 weeks of euthymia between episodes in the same mood direction would almost certainly provide more illness course descriptor utility (39).

DEPRESSION

The criteria for depression (Table 5) are quite consistent with most recent studies of depression in bipolar disorder. Although recent studies indicate that depression in bipolar disorder may have two or three fundamental components, e.g., depressed mood and anxiety, depressive cognitions, and motor retardation, these data have been collected in the context of drug treatment, principally with lamotrigine, and require further study regarding their specificity (25). The one behavioral component that is most strongly identifiable with bipolar depression is motor retardation, even including evidence of association with disturbed amine metabolism in bipolar disorder (25,29). Irritability is a symptom that is common in bipolar depression

Table 5 Major Depressive Episode

More than five symptoms during a 2-week period and more than one of which is either depressed mood or loss of interest/pleasure

- Depressed mood (e.g., feels sad or empty, appears tearful)
- Markedly diminished interest/pleasure in activities
- Significant weight loss or decrease or increase in appetite
- Insomnia or hypersomnia
- Psychomotor agitation or retardation
- Fatigue or loss of energy
- Feelings of worthlessness or excessive or inappropriate guilt
- Diminished ability to think or concentrate, or indecisiveness
- Suicidal ideation

but not included in the listed criteria, perhaps because it is also relatively common in mania. However, the purpose of operational criteria is to track the evidence regarding the expression of a disorder. On that basis, irritability should be inquired about and expected often in bipolar depression.

Recent studies suggest that the form of depression seen in bipolar II disorder is somewhat at variance with that seen in bipolar I disorder. The evidence is strongest for the proportion of time depressed and the duration of depressive episodes, both of which are greater in bipolar II disorder, and definitely longer than the average duration for unipolar depression (5,40,41). There is some evidence that anxiety is more common in bipolar II disorder and is fundamentally linked to depressed mood (7). It is, therefore, unreasonable that anxiety in some form is not included as a criterion for bipolar depression. The evidence for this is further supported by epidemiological studies that report high comorbidity between bipolar and anxiety disorders and by recent evidence that a history of anxiety is associated with poor long-term outcome of bipolar depression (42).

Some bipolar patients with depressed features do not subjectively experience these as sadness, or pessimism, but as loss of energy, worry, and anxiety. If this appears to be the case, it may be preferable to organize the inquiry around the symptom domains to which the patient does subscribe.

MIXED STATES

DSM-IV lists one form of mixed states, namely, a full depressive episode for at least 1 week in the context of a full manic episode. In fact, and with substantial recent evidence for the point, many patients have other admixtures of manic and other symptoms, sometimes at a syndromal level, but not invariably so (43–47). It is generally advisable to start an inquiry with a focus on the symptoms that are known, or appear to be dominant, and then add inquiry in the other areas of symptoms of bipolar disorder.

INVOLVING THE PATIENT AND FAMILY IN DIAGNOSIS

Much of the difficulty in diagnosis of bipolar disorder is consequent to the changing illness expression of the disorder, inherent in the characteristic mood instability of the illness. Therefore, rather than expect to make a conclusive diagnosis cross-sectionally, it is often advisable to explain the fluctuating course to the patient and an involved family member, indicating what types of behavior would indicate bipolar disorder, and seek active collaboration in exploring the possibilities over time.

REFERENCES

1. Ghaemi SN, Boiman EE, Goodwin FK. Diagnosing bipolar disorder and the effect of antidepressants: a naturalistic study. J Clin Psychiatry 2004; 61(10):804–808.
2. Hantouche EG, Akiskal HS, Lancrenon S, Allilaire JF, Sechter D, Azorin JM, et al. Systematic clinical methodology for validating bipolar-II disorder: data in med-stream from a French national multi-site study (EPIDEP). J Affect Disord 1998; 50(2–3):163–173.

3. Lewinsohn PM, Klein DN, Seeley JR. Bipolar disorders in a community sample of older adolescents: prevalence, phenomenology, comorbidity, and course. J Am Acad Child Adolesc Psychiatry 1995; 34(4):454–463.
4. Lish JD, Dime-Meenan S, Whybrow PC, Price RA, Hirschfeld RMA. The National Depressive and Manic-depressive Association (DMDA) survey of bipolar members. J Affect Disord 1994; 31:281–294.
5. Akiskal HS, Maser JD, Zeller PJ, Endicott J, Coryell W, Keller M. Switching from 'unipolar' to bipolar II. An 11-year prospective study of clinical and temperamental predictors in 559 patients. Arch Gen Psychiatry 1995; 52(2):114–123.
6. Johnstone EC, Crow TJ, Frith CD, Owens DG. The Northwick Park "functional" psychosis study: diagnosis and treatment response. Lancet 1988; 2(8603):119–125.
7. Swann AC, Janicak PL, Calabrese JR, Bowden CL, Dilsaver SC, Morris DD, et al. Structure of mania: depressive, irritable, and psychotic clusters with distinct course of illness in randomized clinical trial participants. J Affect Disord 2001; 67:123–132.
8. Hollander E, Tracy KA, Swann AC, Coccaro EF, McElroy SL, Wozniak P, et al. Divalproex in the treatment of impulsive aggressive: efficacy in cluster B personality disorders. Neuropsychopharmacology 2003; 28(6):1186–1197.
9. Wicki W, Angst J. The Zurich Study. X. Hypomania in a 28 to 30 year old cohort. Eur Arch Psychiatry Clin Neurosci 1991; 240(6):339–348.
10. Janowsky DS, Morter S, Hong L, Howe L. Myers Briggs Type Indicator and Tridimensional Personality Questionnaire differences between bipolar patients and unipolar depressed patients. Bipolar Disord 1999; 1(2):98–108.
11. Swann AC, Bowden CL, Morris D, Calabrese JR, Petty F, Small J, et al. Depression during mania: treatment response to lithium or divalproex. Arch Gen Psychiatry 1997; 54:37–42.
12. Cassidy F, Forest K, Murry E, Carroll BJ. A factor analysis of the signs and symptoms of mania. Arch Gen Psychiatry 1998; 55(1):27–32.
13. Geller B, Luby J. Child and adolescent bipolar disorder: review of the past 10 years. J Am Acad Child Adolesc Psychiatry 1997; 36(9):1168–1176.
14. Altman EG, Hedeker DR, Janicak PG, Peterson JL, Davis JM. The Clinician-Administered Rating Scale for Mania (CARS-M): development, reliability, and validity. Soc Biol Psychiatry 1994; 36:124–134.
15. Kraepelin E. Manic-Depressive Insanity and Paranoia. Edinburg: E & S Livingstone, 1921.
16. Akiskal HS. Depressive onset in pre-pubertal, pubertal, and possibly teenage and early adult years (age 21 and earlier) has been shown to presage eventual bipolarity. J Am Acad Adolesc Psychiatry 1995; 34:754–763.
17. Geller B, Zimerman B, Williams M, Bolhofner K, Craney JL. Bipolar disorder at prospective follow-up of adults who had prepubertal major depressive disorder. Am J Psychiatry 2001; 158(1):125–127.
18. Keller MB, Lavori PW, Coryell W, Andreasen NC, Endicott J, Clayton PJ, et al. Differential outcome of pure manic, mixed/cycling, and pure depressive episodes in patients with bipolar illness. J Am Med Assoc 1986; 255:3138–3142.
19. Joffe RT, Young LT, MacQueen GM. A two-illness mode of bipolar disorder: a commentary. Bipolar Disord 1999; 1(1):25–30.
20. Judd LL, Akiskal HS, Schttler PJ, Coryell W, Endicott J, Maser JD, et al. A prospective investigation of the natural history of the long-term weekly symptomatic status of bipolar II disorder. Arch Gen Psychiatry 2003; 60(3):261–269.
21. Merikangas KR, Stevens DE. Comorbidity of migraine and psychiatric disorders. Neurol Clin 1997; 15(1):115–123.
22. Kessler RC, McGonagle KA, Zhao S, Nelson CB, Hughes M, Eshleman S, et al. Lifetime and 12-month prevalence of DSM-III-R psychiatric disorders in the United States. Arch Gen Psychiatry 1994; 51:8–19.
23. Marder SR, Davis JM, Chouinard G. The effects of risperidone on the five dimensions of schizophrenia derived by factor analysis: combined results of the North American trials. J Clin Psychiatry 1998; 58(12):538–546.

24. Winokur G, Wesner R. From unipolar depression to bipolar illness: 29 who changed. Acta Psychiatr Scand 1987; 76(1):59–63.
25. Mitchell PB, Wilhelm K, Parker G, Austin MP, Rutgers P, Malhi GS. The clinical features of bipolar depression: a comparison with matched major depressive disorder patients. J Clin Psychiatry 2002; 63(1):77–78.
26. Kadrmas A, Winokur G, Crowe R. Postpartum mania. Br J Psychiatry 1979; 135: 551–554.
27. Reich T, Winokur G. Postpartum psychoses in patients with manic-depressive disease. J Nerv Ment Dis 1970; 151:60–68.
28. American Psychiatric Association. Diagnostic and Statistical Manual of Mental Disorders. 4th ed., Washington D.C.: American Psychiatric Association, 2000 (text revision).
29. Swann AC, Katz MM, Bowden CL, Berman NG, Stokes PE. Psychomotor performance and monoamine function in bipolar and unipolar affective disorders. Biol Psychiatry 1999; 45:979–988.
30. Brockington IF, Altman E, Hillier V, Meltzer HY, Nand S. The clinical picture of bipolar affective disorder in its depressed phase: a report from London and Chicago. Br J Psychiatry 1982; 141:558–562.
31. Hartman E. Longitudinal studies of sleep and dream patterns in manic-depressive patients. Arch Gen Psychiatry 1968; 19(3):312–329.
32. Kupfer DJ, Himmelhoch JM, Swartzburg M, Anderson C, Byck R, Detre TP. Hypersomnia in manic-depressive disease (a preliminary report). Dis Nerv Syst 1972; 33:720–724.
33. Roy-Byrne P, et al. The longitudinal course of recurrent affective illness: life chart data from research patients at the NIMH. Acta Psychiatr Scand 1985; 71:34.
34. Ghaemi SN, Goodwin FK. Long-term naturalistic treatment of depressive symptoms in bipolar illness with divalproex vs lithium in the setting of minimal antidepressant use. J Affect Disord 2001; 65(3):281–287.
35. Goldberg JF, Ernst CL. Features associated with the delayed initiation of mood stabilizers at illness onset in bipolar disorder. J Clin Psychiatry 2002; 63(11):985–991.
36. Hirschfeld RMA, Williams JBW, Spitzer RL, Calabrese JR, Flynn L, Keck PE Jr, et al. Development and validation of a screening instrument for bipolar spectrum disorder: the Mood Disorder Questionnaire [report]. Am J Psychiatry 2000; 157(11):1873–1875.
37. Secunda SK, Swann A, Katz MM, Koslow SH, Croughan J, Chang S. Diagnosis and treatment of mixed mania. Am J Psychiatry 1987; 144(1):96–98.
38. Angst J, Gamma A. A new bipolar spectrum concept: a brief review. Bipolar Disord 2002; 4S:11–14.
39. Maj M, Magliano L, Pirozzi R, et al. Validity of rapid-cycling as a course specifier for bipolar disorder. Am J Psychiatry 1994; 7(151):1015–1019.
40. Judd LL, Akiskal HS, Schettler PJ, Endicott J, Maser J, Solomon DA, et al. The long-term natural history of the weekly symptomatic status of bipolar I disorder. Arch Gen Psychiatry 2002; 59(6):530–537.
41. Judd LL, Schettler PJ, Akiskal HS, Maser J, Coryell W, Solomon D, et al. Long-term symptomatic status of bipolar I vs. bipolar II disorders. Int J Neuropsychopharmacol 2003; 6(2):127–137.
42. Kessler RC, Nelson CB, McGonagle KA, Liu J, Swartz M, Blazer DG. Comorbidity of DSM-III-R major depressive disorder in the general population: results from the US National Comorbidity Survey. Br J Psychiatry 1996; 30(suppl):17–30.
43. Swann AC, Secunda SK, Katz MM, Croughan J, Bowden CL, Koslow SH, et al. Specificity of mixed affective states: clinical comparison of dysphoric mania an agitated depression. J Affect Disord 1993; 28(2):81–89.
44. Swann AC. Mixed of dysphoric manic states: psychopathology and treatment. J Clin Psychiatry 1995; 56(suppl 3):6–10.
45. Bowden CL, Calabrese JR, Wallin BA, Swann AC, McElroy SL, Risch SC, et al. Illness characteristics of patients in clinical drug studies of mania. Psychopharmacol Bull 1995; 31(1):103–109.

46. Cassidy F, Murry E, Forest K, Carroll BJ. Signs and symptoms of mania in pure and mixed episodes. J Affect Disord 1998; 50(2–3):187–201.
47. Benazzi F. Depressive mixed states: testing different definitions. Psychiatry Clin Neurosci 2001; 55:646–652.

3
Epidemiology of Bipolar Disorder

Zoltán Rihmer
National Institute for Psychiatry and Neurology, Budapest, Hungary

Jules Angst
Zurich University Psychiatric Hospital, Zurich, Switzerland

INTRODUCTION

Historical Background

Owing to the great development in the classification and treatment of mood disorders, in the second-half of the 20th century, clinical studies of this period clearly show that bipolar disorders are much more common than previously believed. The two main sources of this change are the steady and substantial decrease of misdiagnosis of classical manic-depressive (bipolar I) disorder as schizophrenia, as well as the fact that the most recent classification systems such as DSM-IV (1), DSM-IV-TR (2), and ICD-10 (3) have made the diagnosis of manic-depressive (bipolar I) disorders more inclusive. The subdivision of bipolar mood disorders further into bipolar I (depression with a history of mania) and bipolar II (depression with a history of hypomania, but not with mania) was proposed almost 30 years ago (4,5). Since then, several studies have demonstrated that bipolar II disorder represents a quite common, clinically and biologically distinct form of major mood disorders that should be separated from both bipolar I and unipolar major depressive disorder (6–11), and that bipolar II disorders show the same—or even worse—psychiatric and social consequences as do bipolar I and unipolar patients (4,12–16).

The recently increased interest in psychiatric epidemiology owes much to the development of methodology. With the introduction of operational diagnostic criteria from DSM-III (17) to DSM-IV-TR (2) or to ICD-10 (3), it has become possible to perform large scale, cross-sectional longitudinal, and cross-national community surveys either in different medical settings or in the general population. Specific new instruments for assessing different psychiatric disorders and to generate DSM/ICD diagnoses were developed such as Diagnostic Interview Schedule (DIS) (18), Composite International Diagnostic Interview Schedule (CIDI) (19), the Mini International Neuropsychiatric Interview (MINI) (20), the Schedule for Clinical Assessment in Neuropsychiatry (SCAN) (21), and the Structured Psychopathological Interview and Rating of the Social Consequences for Epidemiology (SPIKE) (22).

Recent Developments Beyond DSM-IV

The recent epidemiological studies, applying the earlier-mentioned instruments, have found higher prevalence rates for specific mood (and other) disorders than earlier studies, on the basis of unstructured clinical interviews. However, these new diagnostic systems (including DSM-IV-TR and ICD-10) are not free from shortcomings. Inaccurate recall and memory loss of interviewed person can bias the lifetime- and period-prevalence rates, and most of them cannot detect the "subthreshold" syndromes.

Patients may show major depression and some hypomanic symptoms that do not reach the severity and/or duration thresholds for official hypomania (bipolar II disorder) in the DSM-IV system. However, external validators strongly suggest that these patients (major depressives with hypomania lasting <4 days and major depressives with some hypomanic symptoms not reaching the DSM-IV severity threshold of hypomania) could be correctly classified as bipolar II cases (12,13,16).

On the other hand, it has also been demonstrated that not only the elevated/irritable mood (a stem criteria for hypomania in DSM-IV and in DSM-IV-TR), but also the over-activity are equally valid and clinically useful leading symptoms of hypomania (23,24). In other words, in contrast to the fact that the DSM-IV(-TR) criteria for hypomania have been never validated, recent findings mentioned earlier strongly suggest that beside elevated/irritable mood, over-activity and a minimum duration of hypomanic episode of 1 or 2 days rather than 4 days are also reliable and valid stem criteria for hypomania (12,13,16,23,24). Moreover, while according to DSM-IV/DSM-IV-TR (1,2) and ICD-10 (3), "antidepressant-associated" hypomania does not belong to the category of bipolar II disorder, several lines of evidences strongly suggest that these patients (also called as bipolar III) are much closer to bipolar II disorder than to unipolar major depression (25,26). There is no statistical evidence for the existence of drug-induced hypomania in unipolar depression: all these cases can be considered as bipolar disorders (bipolar II and minor bipolar disorders) (25,27).

As DSM-IV/DSM-IV-TR cyclothymic disorders do not cover all bipolar patients with subthreshold level of psychopathology, an additional bipolar spectrum disorder diagnosis (minor bipolar disorders) has been recently introduced (12,13). Minor bipolar disorder is defined as the presence of mild depression (dysthymia, minor depression, or recurrent brief depression) plus hypomanic symptoms, including recurrent brief hypomania (soft criteria) or hypomanic syndromes with consequences (hard criteria). Cyclothymic disorder in this context is considered to be a chronic form of minor bipolar disorders. Minor bipolar disorders constitute a milder form of bipolar mood disorders, intermediate between bipolar II disorders, and controls in most external validators (12,13). Minor bipolar disorders seem to be the attenuated forms and frequently the precursors of major bipolar (mostly bipolar II) disorders, as it has been found that a significant part of patients with cyclothymia develop major bipolar (first of all bipolar II) disorder during a 2- to 3-year follow-up (26).

The correct identification of broadly defined bipolar II disorder and minor bipolar disorders is not as sterile exercises with the diagnostic border between the unipolar and bipolar realms of mood disorders and has important implications but not only for the epidemiological research. In the absence of mood stabilizers, antidepressants alone may worsen (destabilize) the course of bipolar disorders inducing (hypo)mania, rapid cycling, and "treatment resistant" depressive mixed states (10,28–30).

PREVALENCE AND INCIDENCE OF BIPOLAR DISORDERS IN THE COMMUNITY

Lifetime Prevalence of Bipolar Disorders in the Adult Population

Before the last decade, in most epidemiological studies, bipolar disorder was equated with classical (bipolar I) disorder, and it was found that the lifetime prevalence of bipolar disorder was around ≤1% (14). The study of the Cross-National Collaborative Group on the epidemiology of major depression and bipolar I disorder found relatively consistent lifetime rates for bipolar I disorder across the seven countries studied. As in the case of major depression, the lowest figures for DSM-III bipolar I disorder were found in the far eastern countries (0.3% in Taiwan and 0.4% in Korea), whereas the highest rates emerged in New Zealand (1.5%) and in the United States (0.9%). In the remaining three sites (Canada, Puerto Rico, and Germany), the figures were 0.6%, 0.6%, and 0.5%, respectively (31). However, if the diagnosis of bipolar II disorder was considered, much higher lifetime prevalence rates up to 6% were reported (14). Using the recently developed Mood Disorder Questionnaire, a validated, highly sensitive, and specific screening instrument for bipolar I and bipolar II disorders in the community, it has also been found that at least 3.7% of American adults may suffer from DSM-IV bipolar I and bipolar II disorders (32).

Table 1 shows the main findings of the four largest, nationally representative community surveys that analyzed separately the lifetime prevalences of DSM-III/III-R bipolar I, bipolar II, and unipolar major depressive disorder (33–37). Except the ECA study (33), the lifetime prevalence of DSM-III/III-R unipolar major depressive disorder is very similar in the remaining three studies (15.1%, 15.4%, and 15.8%, respectively): bipolar I disorder shows greater (between 0.8% and 3.0%) variation, and bipolar II disorder shows the greatest (between 0.2% and 2.0%) variation. The proportion of all bipolar (I + II) patients among all major mood disorders ranges between 10% and 25%, respectively.

Figures presented in Table 1 also show that the lifetime prevalence of the conservatively defined (i.e., DSM-III/III-R) bipolar II disorder was much lower than that of the bipolar I disorder in all the four studies. However, the re-analysis of the ECA database, taking into account the subthreshold cases of hypomania (broadly defined bipolar II disorder), has shown that the lifetime prevalence rate of bipolar II disorder (mainly in the expense of unipolar depression) raised from 0.5% to 5.6%, yielding a total 6.4% lifetime prevalence for the combined group of bipolar I and bipolar II disorders (Table 2) (16).

In addition, the data of the Zurich Cohort Study also have demonstrated that, if the Zurich hard and soft criteria for hypomania were applied and minor bipolar disorders were also considered, the lifetime prevalence rates of the bipolar II disorder and the total bipolar spectrum disorders raised up to 11% and 24%, respectively, resulting in a 1:1 ratio of total bipolar spectrum disorders to unipolar depressions (12,38–40) (Table 3).

Using the data generated from the ECA and NCS clinical significance questions (seeking professional help or taking medication for the illness and substantial interface of the symptoms with the everyday life), the 1-year prevalence rates of mental and substance use disorders were substantially reduced in both studies (41). However, applying these criteria for bipolar I and bipolar II disorders, the 1-year prevalence in NCS remained the same (1.3% and 0.2%, respectively) but decreased markedly in the ECA study (from 0.9% to 0.5% and from 0.4% to 0.2%, respectively) (41). Methodological differences in clinical significance questions and in diagnostic

Table 1 Lifetime Prevalence of Bipolar I, Bipolar II, and Major Depressive Disorders in Selected Epidemiological Surveys

Source, country	*N*	Diagnosis	Lifetime prevalence (%)			Percentage of all BPs among all mood disorders
			Bipolar I	Bipolar II	Unipolar major depressives	
Ref. 33, ECA study, USA	18,572	DIS DSM-III	0.8	0.5	4.4	23
Ref. 34, NCS, USA	8,098	CIDI DSM-III-R	1.6	0.2	15.8	10
Ref. 35, Hungary	2,953	DIS DSM-III-R	3.0	2.0	15.1	25
Refs. 36,37, The Netherlands	7,076	CIDI DSM-III-R	1.3	0.6	15.4	11

Table 2 Lifetime Prevalence Rates (%) of Threshold and Subthreshold Cases of Bipolar I and Bipolar II Disorders in the ECA Study, $N = 18,572$

Diagnosis	Threshold cases	Subthreshold cases	Total
Bipolar I	0.8	—	0.8
Bipolar II	0.5	5.1	5.6
Total	1.3	5.1	6.4

Source: From Ref. 16.

procedure between the ECA study and NCS can explain this difference. Although the main source of the revised prevalence estimation is the more appropriate service planning, this restrictive view can be seriously questioned by the fact that patients with subthreshold level of mood disorder can have similar degree of disability and social consequences as do DSM-III/IV threshold cases (12,13,16). Clinical significance in the foregoing sense (41) and severity of the given disorder, as well as the subjective perception of the symptoms, seem to be three, only partially overlapping dimensions that require further attention.

Relationship Between Lifetime, 1-Year, and 1-Month Prevalence Rates

The relationship between the lifetime, 1-year, and 1-month (current) prevalence rates is quite complex. Because of memory loss over time, lifetime prevalence rates are less reliable. However, it might be true primarily for ambulatory-treated or not-treated depressions, rather than for manic states, which result in hospitalization or medical treatment (by definition). In the case of a chronic, non-fluctuating illness, the lifetime, 1-year, and 1-month prevalence rates are very close to one another. However, as bipolar disorders are highly recurrent conditions (5,42), it means also that the recovery rate is also high. Therefore, relatively large differences between the lifetime, 1-year, and 1-month prevalence rates of bipolar disorder are expected.

The lifetime, 1-year, and 1-month prevalence rates of bipolar disorders (types I and II combined) in two epidemiological surveys with the same diagnostic procedure are shown in Table 4 (33,35). Given the 5% lifetime, the 0.9% 1-year, and the 0.5% 1-month prevalence rates of bipolar disorders in the Hungarian study (35), it means that out of 1000 persons studied, 50 had lifetime, nine had past-year, and five had past-month prevalence of any episode of bipolar disorder. Out of these 50 patients

Table 3 Lifetime Prevalence Rates (%) of Bipolar Disorder Subtypes as a Function of Definition in the Zurich Cohort Study, $N = 591$

Diagnosis	DSM-IV criteria	Zurich hard criteria	Zurich soft criteria
Bipolar I	0.5	0.5	0.5
Bipolar II	1.1	5.3	11.0
Minor bipolar disorder	—	3.2	9.4
Hypomania + cylcothymia	1.5	3.3	3.3
Total prevalence	3.1	12.3	24.2

Source: From Refs. 39, 40.

Table 4 Lifetime, 1-Year, and 1-Month Prevalence Rates (%) of Bipolar (I + II) Disorders in Two Epidemiological Studies with Similar Diagnostic Procedure

				Prevalence (%)		
Source, country	*N*	Diagnosis	Age range	Lifetime	1-year	1-month
Ref. 33, ECA study, USA	18,572	DIS DSM-III	≥18 years	1.2	1.0	0.8
Ref. 35, Hungary	2,953	DIS DSM-III-R	18–64 years	5.0	0.9	0.5

with lifetime history of bipolar disorders, every fifth (nine patients) experienced an acute episode of their illness in the past year, and nearly half of them (four out of nine) recovered from their mania/hypomania or major depression in the first 11 months of the preceding year. Considering the fact that the average duration of the affective episodes in bipolar disorders are between 3 and 4 months (42) (and in treated cases even less) and that bipolar I and II patients are symptomatically ill above the DSM-IV threshold level in 16–22% of their lifetime (43,44), the great differences between the 1-month, 1-year, and lifetime prevalence's in the Hungarian study (35) might reflect a real clinical situation. Because the two compared studies (33,35) used the same diagnostic procedure, the greatest difference in the prevalence rates (i.e., lifetime prevalence's are 5.0% in the Hungarian study and 1.2% in the ECA study) could be explained—at least in part—by the different age-range of the subjects interviewed. While the Hungarian study included only persons aged between 18 and 64 years (35), about 15% of the participants in the ECA study (33) were older than 65 years, which makes a greater likelihood for a biasing effect of memory loss, resulting in lower lifetime prevalence rates in the latter survey.

Prevalence of Bipolar Disorders in Primary Care

The point prevalence of major depressive disorder in primary care is around 10–15% (45–47), which three to six times exceeds its point prevalence in the general population (33,35,37,48). Although the literature on the prevalence of depressive and anxiety disorders in primary care is voluminous, there are only few surveys looking for the prevalence of bipolar disorders in primary-care practice. The three studies shown in Table 5 indicate that the point prevalence of bipolar (I and II) disorders in primary care is between 1% and 1.9% (45–47), which also means a two to four times

Table 5 Point Prevalence Rates (%) of Bipolar (I + II) Disorders in Primary Care

Source, country	*N*	Diagnosis	Point prevalence (%)
Ref. 45, USA	1,000	PRIME-MD DSM-III	1.0
Ref. 46, Hungary	301	DIS DSM-III	1.3
Ref. 47, Belgium	2,316	PRIME-MD DSM-IV	1.9

over-representation, compared with the figures of point prevalence of bipolar disorders in the general population (33,35,37).

Prevalence of Bipolar Disorders in Young and Old Age

Before the last decade, bipolar disorders in childhood and adolescence have been less intensively studied. Although the prepubertal onset of bipolar disorders is rare, an American community-based school survey in adolescents aged between 14 and 18 years reported a lifetime prevalence rate of bipolar I and II disorders for the first two waves of 1.4% (49): the third wave at the age of 23 years added another 0.7%. Very important was the finding that subthreshold bipolar disorder was present in a further 4.5% (50). The threshold and subthreshold groups showed comparable psychosocial impairment and suicide attempt rates (50). A German study, including more than 3,000 14 to 24-year-old girls and boys (the period in which bipolar disorders start most frequently), has reported a lifetime rate of DSM-IV bipolar disorder of 1.8% (bipolar I: 1.4%, bipolar II: 0.4%) (51).

Similarly, relatively little is known about the prevalence, incidence, and phenomenology of bipolar disorders in old age, but recent evidences suggest that there is a significant decline in the prevalence of mania (bipolar I disorder) among old people (42,52).

The special characteristics of bipolar disorders in children and adolescents and in old age, including the topic of epidemiology, are presented in more detail in Chapters 6 and 7 in this volume.

Incidence of Bipolar Disorders

Incidence data are very difficult to obtain, particularly in the case of bipolar affective disorders. There are relatively few data on the annual incidence of bipolar disorder, and the majority of the studies presents incidence rates based on different information-gathering methods. Annual first hospitalization rates for (conservatively defined, e.g., type I) bipolar disorder have been reported between 0.03% and 0.06% (53–55), and the same figure based on bipolar patients seeking any kind of treatment has been found to be between 0.011% and 0.021% (54,56). Because only a fraction of bipolar patients are under treatment (16,32,42) and subthreshold cases are also quite common (12,16,39), the real annual incidence figures might be much higher, particularly in young age cohorts.

DEMOGRAPHIC FACTORS

Gender

In contrast to unipolar depression (in which the female to male ratio is 2–2.5:1), the gender ratio in bipolar disorders (all forms combined) is around 1:1 (31,33–37,42). However, among bipolar II patients (10,36,42,44) and in special subpopulations such as mixed/dysphoric mania (42,57), depressive mixed states/agitated depression (10,58), winter depression (42), bipolar depression with atypical features (59), and rapid cycling bipolar disorder (29,60), females are more or less over-represented.

Across the mania-depression continuum as a spectrum, there is a clear correlation between female gender and increasing rate of the depression component either cross-sectionally (e.g., dysphoric mania) or longitudinally (e.g., bipolar II, unipolar depression).

Recent population-based epidemiological surveys showed that the lifetime and one-year prevalences of bipolar disorders (types I and II combined) were much higher among people with same-sex sexual behavior, particularly in the case of males (61).

Age

The age of onset of bipolar disorder is substantially (about 8–10 years) lower than in unipolar major depression, being most commonly around 18 to 20 years of age (31,33,35,42). In contrast to this, first-onset mania is quite rare among elderly people (42,52). The age of onset of bipolar I and bipolar II patients is similar with a slight tendency for higher age of onset in bipolar II patients (11,12,42,44). Like unipolar major depressives, bipolar patients with positive family history of mood (mostly bipolar) disorders are significantly younger at the beginning of the illness and need less stressors to precipitate it than those lacking such history (42,62,63). More than half of bipolar patients have depression as the first episode of their illness (42,64), and unfortunately, first of all, these bipolar patients are misdiagnosed as unipolars (28,32).

Recent findings indicate that there are three (rather than two) age-at-onset subgroups of bipolar patients: the greatest peak is around 17, the smaller one at 25, and the smallest one at 40 years of age. Affected siblings were more likely to belong to the same age-at-onset subgroup (62), reflecting probably the different intensity (and/or nature) of underlying genetic vulnerability.

Recently, an interesting historical trend in the age of onset of bipolar disorders has been reported: the median age-at-onset of bipolar disorder was lower by 4.5 years in patients born after 1940, compared with patients born before that date (64).

Ethnicity

The prevalence of bipolar I disorder does not show a significant variation by ethnicity if social class, education, and residency are controlled (34,42,65). However, compared with African-Americans, Caucasian subjects are three-times over-represented in dysphoric (mixed) mania, whereas the same ratio among patients with pure mania is about 1:1 (66).

The significant effect of sociocultural factors over ethnicity is supported by recent findings, according to which Mexican immigrants, living in California, had lifetime rate of manic episode (bipolar I disorder) similar to those of Mexican citizens living in Mexico City (1.4% and 1.3%, respectively), while the same rate for native-born Mexican Americans was much higher (2.7%) (67).

SOCIAL VARIABLES

Marital Status

The relationship between marital status and mood disorders is very complex. Being single or divorced/separated, for example, can be either a risk factor for mood disorder or the consequence of the negative life events generated by depressive and/or manic states. Major mood disorder patients are over-represented among divorced, and the rate of family breakdown (separation, divorce, chaotic family life) is elevated substantially in major depressive and markedly in bipolar I and bipolar II patients (14,16,35,42,68). Bipolar patients generate more negative life events and more interpersonal conflicts than patients with other diagnoses. In NCS, the odds ratio for subsequent divorce in the first marriage was 1.5 for dysthymic disorder, 1.7 for major depression, and 3.2 for bipolar I disorder (68). Major depressions, but first of all mania and hypomania, are powerful predictors either for being never married (16,35) or for future divorce (14,35,68), which can cause serious distress for the patients and for their spouses and may generate negative life events for their children.

Socio-Economic Factors

Because persons with lower socio-economic status have lower educational level, lower income, poorer living conditions, higher rate of unemployment (and ultimately homelessness) and vice versa, the relationship between the socio-economic factors and mood disorders is also complex and multidimensional. However, as in the case of marital status and mood disorders, cause and effect may be reversed here too. Mood disorders (and particularly bipolar illness) can easily lead to unemployment, low income, divorce, substance abuse, etc. (11,14,68), resulting in regression on the social hierarchy scale. However, mood disorders seem to have negative impact in psychosocial sense: several evidences suggest that, in contrast to schizophrenia, unipolar depression, and bipolar I disorder, patients with bipolar II disorder (and their first-degree relatives) belong to higher social classes, tend to have higher educational level (35,42,69) and are over-represented among socially active, prominently creative persons (42,69,70).

Residence

As urban communities are more stressful than rural ones, it is not surprising that most studies performed in Western societies found that either unipolar major depression or bipolar disorder was more frequent in urban residents than in their rural counterparts, even after controlling for age, socio-economic, and marital status and ethnicity (42,65). However, it should be noted that differences in the prevalence rates of mood disorders might have to do with the interplay of several factors rather than simply one variable.

The urban–rural distinction provides little information about the real living and social conditions in general, but it can be a good marker for the density of population reflecting indirectly the amount and the nature of psychosocial stressors.

PSYCHOSOCIAL STRESSORS AND SOCIAL SUPPORT

Social stressors and low-level social support have been well recognized as risk factors for unipolar and bipolar disorders (42,63,71). However, different kinds of stressors (childhood vs. adulthood life events, acute vs. chronic stressors, positive vs. negative life events) can play different roles in the predisposition for, and precipitation of, different affective episodes. In patients with unipolar major depression and bipolar disorders, the association of acute stressors and the onset of the illness episode become progressively weaker with the increasing number of previous episodes (42,63). On the other hand, it has also been demonstrated that not only negative, but also positive life events can precipitate either depressive or (hypo)manic episodes in vulnerable individuals during the vulnerable time-periods (42,63).

It is also important to note that negative life events can be considered not only as predisposing or precipitating factors, as they are frequently the consequences of the own behavior of unipolar depressives and particularly of bipolar patients. On the other hand, however, it has also been reported that adequate social support may decrease the risk of relapse for patients with bipolar disorder (71).

SEASONAL AND GEOGRAPHIC FACTORS

In spite of the fact that about two-thirds of patients with recurrent major mood disorders show irregular seasonal patterns individually, in a statistical sense it is spring and fall that are the peak times for major depression. On the other hand, the peak for mania is in late spring and summer, and the incidence of mania is less frequent in winter (42,72,73). However, depressive episodes of unipolar and bipolar disorders may show different seasonal patterns (42), and if bipolar I and bipolar II patients are analyzed separately, a significantly different seasonal occurrence of depression between these two subgroups is also reported (73).

The seasonal profiles of committed and attempted suicide, and the prescription of antidepressants and ECT are quite similar to the seasonal onset of major depression and of mixed depressive episodes (42,72,74,75), but as long-term pharmacotherapy of mood disorders (or its cessation) may dampen the seasonal pattern of episodes (76), this fact should be taken into account in planning studies and in the interpretation of the results.

There is a positive correlation between the prevalence of winter depression (which is mostly bipolar II) (42) and latitude in North America and Europe, and the geographic distribution of summer depression (which is also commonly bipolar) across the latitudes shows the opposite tendency (42,77). Regarding the West–East dimension, the lower prevalence of bipolar I disorder in Far Eastern countries (31) may be related primarily to methodological problems and to cultural (including dietary) differences. A recent study showing that greater rates of seafood consumption (intake of ω-3 essential fatty acids) were significantly associated with lower lifetime prevalence rates of bipolar I, bipolar II, and bipolar spectrum disorders (but not with the prevalence of schizophrenia) in 12 different countries. Interestingly, all the three Far Eastern populations that were included in that study (Hong-Kong, Korea, Taiwan) have very high seafood consumption (78), which suggests that the prevalence of bipolar disorders in these countries may really be lower.

COMORBIDITY AND COMPLICATIONS

Patients with major mood disorders are at increased risk of having one or more additional (comorbid) psychiatric or medical disorders. Compared with unipolar depressives, bipolar patients show more frequently comorbid anxiety disorders (30,78), substance-use disorders (79), suicidal behavior (15,42), as well as migraine headache (80) and type 2 diabetes mellitus (81). If bipolar I and bipolar II subgroups are analyzed separately, bipolar II patients have the highest rate of anxiety disorder comorbidity (11,30,80,82), suicidal behavior (15,16,80), and migraine headache (80), whereas bipolar I patients show most frequently comorbid substance-use disorders (11,83).

The topic of comorbidity in bipolar disorders is discussed in detail in the chapter by Wittchen in this volume.

PUBLIC SIGNIFICANCE OF BIPOLAR DISORDERS

The prevalence of bipolar disorders, particularly when bipolar II and minor bipolar disorders are also considered, is much higher than previously believed and may be as common as that of unipolar major depressive disorder. In spite of the great clinical and public significance of bipolar disorders (suicide, loss of productivity, secondary substance use, criminal behavior increased somatic morbidity, etc.) (15,79,84,85), they are still under-referred, under-diagnosed and under-treated (12,14,16,28,32, 36,84). A recent large-scale community survey in the United States showed that among persons with positive screens for bipolar I and II disorders, only 20% had received the diagnosis of bipolar disorder previously, 31% had received the diagnosis of unipolar depression, and nearly half of the sample (49%) reported having received no diagnosis of either bipolar or unipolar depression (32). Particularly bipolar II subjects and patients with minor bipolar disorders are under-referred (16,36) and/ or misdiagnosed, mostly as unipolar depressives (27,28,84,85), resulting in no treatment or inadequate treatment and consequently worsening the short- and long-term prognosis. The importance of correct diagnosis is underlined by the recent findings of Hirschfeld et al. (86), who have investigated the prevalence of bipolar disorder in patients being treated for depression with antidepressants in a family medicine clinic. Twenty-one percentage of the patients taking antidepressants for depression screened positive for bipolar disorder on the Mood Disorder Questionnaire. Almost two-thirds of those patients screened positive had never received a diagnosis of bipolar disorder. These results suggest that screening for bipolar disorder in such patients improves the recognition and appropriate treatment of mood and particularly bipolar disorders.

REFERENCES

1. American Psychiatric Association. Diagnostic and Statistical Manual of Mental Disorders. 4th ed. (DSM-IV). Washington, DC: American Psychiatric Association, 1994.
2. American Psychiatric Association. Diagnostic and Statistical Manual of Mental Disorders. 4th ed. Text revision. (DSM-IV-TR). Washington, DC: American Psychiatric Association, 2000.
3. World Health Organization. The ICD-10 Classification of Mental and Behavioural Disorders. Geneva: World Health Organization, 1992.
4. Dunner DL, Gershon ES, Goodwin FK. Heritable factors in the severity of affective illness. Biol Psychiatry 1976; 11:31–42.
5. Angst J. The course of affective disorders. II. Typology of bipolar manic-depressive illness. Arch Psychiatr Nervenkr 1978; 226:65–73.
6. Akiskal HS, Mallya G. Criteria for the "soft" bipolar spectrum: treatment implications. Psychopharmacol Bull 1987; 23:68–73.
7. Angst J, Frey R, Lohmeyer B, Zerbin-Rüdin E. Bipolar manic-depressive psychoses: results of a genetic investigation. Hum Genet 1980; 55:237–254.
8. Rihmer Z, Bagdy Gy, Arató M. Serum dopamine-beta-hydroxylase activity in manic-depressive patients. Biol Psychiatry 1984:423–427.
9. Coryell W. Bipolar II disorder: a progress report. J Affect Disord 1996; 41:159–162.
10. Benazzi F, Akiskal HS. Clinical and factor-analytic validation of depressive mixed states: a report from the Ravenna–San Diego collaboration. Curr Opin Psychiatry 2003; 16(suppl 2):s71–s78.

11. Judd LL, Akiskal HS, Schettler PJ, Coryell W, Maser J, Rice JA, Solomon DA, Keller MB. The comparative clinical phenotype and long term longitudinal episode course of bipolar I and II: a clinical spectrum or distinct disorders? J Affect Disord 2003; 73:19–32.
12. Angst J, Gamma A, Benazzi F, Ajdacic V, Eich D, Rössler W. Diagnostic issues in bipolar disorder. Eur Neuropsychopharmacol 2003; 13:s43–s50.
13. Angst J, Gamma A, Benazzi F, Ajdacic V, Eich D, Rössler W. Toward a re-definition of subthreshold bipolarity: epidemiology and proposed criteria for bipolar-II, minor bipolar disorders and hypomania. J Affect Disord 2003; 73:133–146.
14. Angst J. The emerging epidemiology of hypomania and bipolar II disorder. J Affect Disord 1998; 50:143–151.
15. Rihmer Z, Kiss K. Bipolar disorders and suicide risk. Clin Appr Bipol Disord 2002; 1:15–21.
16. Judd LL, Akiskal HS. The prevalence and disability of bipolar spectrum disorders in the US population: re-analysis of the ECA database taking into account the subthreshold cases. J Affect Disord 2003; 73:123–131.
17. American Psychiatric Association. Diagnostic and Statistical Manual of Mental Disorders. 3rd ed. (DSM-III). Washington, DC: American Psychiatric Association, 1980.
18. Robins LN, Heltzer J, Croughan J. National Institute of Mental Health Diagnostic Interview Schedule: its history, characteristics and validity. Arch Gen Psychiatry 1981; 38: 381–389.
19. World Health Organization. Composite International Diagnostic Interview (CIDI), Version 1.0. Geneva: World Health Organization, 1990.
20. Lecrubier Y, Sheehan DV, Weiler E, Amorim P, Bonora I, Sheehan HK, Janavs J, Dunbar GC. The MINI International Neuropsychiatric Interview (M.I.N.I.), a short diagnostic structured interview: reliability and validity according to the CIDI. Eur Psychiatry 1997; 12:224–231.
21. World Health Organization. SCAN: Schedule for Clinical Assessment in Neuropsychiatry. Geneva: WHO, 1992.
22. Angst J, Dobler-Mikola A, Binder J. The Zurich Cohort Study. A prospective epidemiological study of depressive, neurotic and psychosomatic syndromes. Part 1. Problem, methodology. Eur Arch Psychiatry Neurol Sci 1984; 234:13–20.
23. Akiskal HS, Bourgeois ML, Angst J, Post R, Möller H-J, Hischfeld R. Re-evaluating the prevalence and diagnostic composition within the broad clinical spectrum of bipolar disorders. J Affect Disord 2000; 59:s5–s30.
24. Benazzi F, Akiskal HS. Refining the evaluation of bipolar II: beyond the strict SCID-CV guidelines for hypomania. J Affect Disord 2003; 73:33–38.
25. Akiskal HS, Hantouche E-G, Allilare J-F, Sechter D, Bourgeois ML, Azorin J-M, Chatenet-Duchéne L, Lancrenon S. Validating antidepressant-associated hypomania (bipolar III): a systematic comparison with spontaneous hypomania (bipolar II). J Affect Disord 2003; 73:65–74.
26. Akiskal HS, Djenderedjian AH, Rosenthal RH, Khani MK. Cyclothymic disorder: validating criteria for inclusion in the bipolar affective group. Am J Psychiat 1977; 134: 1227–1233.
27. Chun BJDH, Dunner DL. A review of antidepressant-induced hypomania in major depression: suggestions for DSM-V. Bipol Disord 2004; 6:32–42.
28. Benazzi F. How could antidepressants worsen unipolar depression? Psychother Psychosom 2003; 72:107–108.
29. Koukopoulos A, Sani G, Koukopoulos AE, Minnai GP, Pani L, Albert MJ, Reginaldi D. Duration and stability of the rapid-cycling course: a long-term personal follow-up of 109 patients. J Affect Disord 2003; 73:75–85.
30. Henry C, Sorbara F, Lacoste J, Gindre C, Leboyer M. Antidepressant-induced mania in bipolar patients: identification of risk factors. J Clin Psychiatry 2001; 62:249–255.
31. Weissman MM, Bland RC, Canino GJ, Faravelli C, Greenwald S, Hwu H-G, Joyce PR, Karam EG, Lee C-K, Lellouch J, Lépine J-P, Newman SC, Rubio-Stipec M, Wells E,

Wickramaratane PJ, Wittchen H-U, Yeh E-K. Cross-national epidemiology of major depression and bipolar disorder. JAMA 1996; 276:293–299.
32. Hirschfeld RMA, Calabrese JR, Weissman MM, Reed M, Davies MA, Frye MA, Keck PE, Lewis L, McElroy SL, McNulty JP, Wagner KD. Screening for bipolar disorder in the community. J Clin Psychiatry 2003; 64:53–59.
33. Weissman MM, Leaf PJ, Tsichler GL, Blazer DG, Karno M, Bruce ML, Florio LP. Affective disorders in five United States communities. Psychol Med 1988; 18:141–153.
34. Kessler RC, McGonaglc KA, Zhao S, Nelson CB, Hughes M, Eshleman S, Wittchen H-U, Kendler KS. Lifetime and 12-month prevalence of DSM-III-R psychiatric disorders in the United States. Arch Gen Psychiatry 1994; 51:8–19.
35. Szádóczky E, Papp Zs, Vitrai J, Rihmer Z, Füredi J. The prevalence of major depressive and bipolar disorders in Hungary. Results from a national epidemiologic survey. J Affect Disord 1998; 50:153–162.
36. Ten Have M, Vollebergh W, Bijl R, Nolen WA. Bipolar disorder in the general population in the Netherlands (prevalence, consequences and care utilization): results from The Netherlands Mental Health Survey and Incidence Study (NEMESIS). J Affect Disord 2002; 68:203–213.
37. Bijl RV, Ravelli A, van Zersen G. Prevalence of psychiatric disorder in the general population: results of the Netherlands Mental Health Survey and Incidence Study (NEMESIS). Soc Psychiatry Psychiatr Epidemiol 1998; 33:587–595.
38. Angst J, Gamma A. A new bipolar spectrum concept. a brief review. Bipol Disord 2002; 4(suppl 1):11–14.
39. Angst J, Gamma A. Prevalence of bipolar disorders: traditional and novel approaches. Clin Appr Bipol Disord 2002; 1:10–14.
40. Angst J. The evolving epidemiology of bipolar disorder. World Psychiatry 2002; 1: 146–148.
41. Narrow WE, Rae DS, Robins LN, Regier DA. Revised prevalence estimates of mental disorders in the United States. Arch Gen Psychiatry 2002; 59:115–123.
42. Goodwin FK, Jamison KR. Manic-Depressive Illness. New York: Oxford University Press, 1990.
43. Judd LL, Akiskal HS, Schettler PJ, Endicott J, Maser J, Solomon DA, Leon AC, Rice JA, Keller MB. The long-term natural history of the weekly symptomatic status of bipolar I disorder. Arch Gen Psychiatry 2002; 59:530–537.
44. Judd LL, Akiskal HS, Schettler PJ, Coryell W, Endicott J, Maser JD, Solomon DA, Leon AC, Keller MB. A prospective investigation of the natural history of the long-term weekly symptomatic status of bipolar II disorder. Arch Gen Psychiatry 2003; 60:261–269.
45. Spitzer RL, Williams JBW, Kroenke K, Linzer M, deGruy FV, Hahn SR, Brody D, Johnson JG. Utility of a new procedure for diagnosing mental disorders in primary care. The PRIME-MD 1000 Study. JAMA 1994:1749–1756.
46. Szádóczky E, Rihmer Z, Papp Zs, Füredi J. The prevalence of affective and anxiety disorders in primary care practice in Hungary. J Affect Disord 1997; 43:239–244.
47. Ansseau M, Dierick M, Buntinkx F, Cnockaert P, De Smedt J, Van Den Haute M, Mijnsbrugge DV. High prevalence of mental disorders in primary care. J Affect Disord 2004; 78:49–55.
48. Blazer DG, Kessler RC, McGonagle KA, Swartz MS. The prevalence and distribution of major depression in a national community sample: The National Comorbidity Survey. Am J Psychiatry 1994; 151:979–986.
49. Lewinshon PM, Seeley J, Klein DN. Bipolar disorder in adolescents. Epidemiology and suicidal behavior. In: Geller B, Del Bello M, eds. Bipolar Disorder in Childhood and Early Adolescence. New York: Guilford Press, 2003:7–24.
50. Lewinsohn PM, Seeley JR, Buckley ME, Klein DN. Bipolar disorder in adolescence and young adulthood. Child Adolesc Psychiatr Clin N Am 2002; 11:461–475.
51. Wittchen H-U, Nelson CB, Lachner G. Prevalence of mental disorders and psychosocial impairments in adolescents and young adults. Psychol Med 1998; 28:109–126.

52. Shulman KL, Herrmann N. The nature and management of mania in old age. Psychiatr Clin North Am 1999; 22:649–665.
53. Leff JP, Fischer M, Bertelsen AC. A cross-national epidemiological study of mania. Br J Psychiatry 1976; 129:428–442.
54. Nielsen JA, Biorn-Henriksen T. Prevalence and disease expectancy for depressive psychoses in a geographically delimited Danish rural population. In: Schou M, Strömgren E, eds. Origin, Prevention and Treatment of Affective Disorders. London: Academic Press, 1979:199–206.
55. Weeke A. Admission pattern and diagnostic stability among unipolar and bipolar manic-depressive patients. Acta Psychiatr Scand 1984; 70:603–613.
56. Helgason T. Epidemiological investigations concerning affective disorders. In: Schou M, Strömgren E, eds. Origin, Prevention and Treatment of Affective Disorders. London: Academic Press, 1979:241–255.
57. McElroy SL, Keck PE, Pope HG, Hudson JI, Faedda GL, Swann AC. Clinical and research implications of the diagnosis of dysphoric or mixed mania or hypomania. Am J Psychiatry 1992; 149:1633–1644.
58. Maj M, Pirozzi R, Magliano L, Bartoli L. Agitated depression in bipolar I disorder: prevalence, phenomenology, and outcome. Am J Psychiatry 2003; 160:2134–2140.
59. Angst J, Gamma A, Sellaro R, Zhang H, Merikangas K. Toward validation of atypical depression in the community: results of the Zurich Cohort Study. J Affect Disord 2002; 72:125–138.
60. Coryell W, Endicott J, Keller M. Rapidly cycling affective disorder. Demographics, diagnosis, family history, and course. Arch Gen Psychiatry 1992; 49:126–131.
61. Standfort TGM, de Graaf R, Bijl R, Schnabel P. Same-sex sexual behavior and psychiatric disorders. Arch Gen Psychiatry 2001; 58:85–91.
62. Bellivier F, Golmard J-L, Rietschel M, Schultze TG, Malafosse A, Preisig M, McKeon P, Mynett-Johnson L, Henry C, Leboyer M. Age at onset in bipolar I affective disorder: further evidence for three subgroups. Am J Psychiatry 2003; 160:999–1001.
63. Johnson L, Anderson-Lundman G, Aberg-Wistedt A, Mathé A. Age of onset in affective disorder: its correlation with heredity and psychosocial factors. J Affect Disord 2000; 59:139–148.
64. Chengappa KNR, Kupfer DJ, Frank E, Houck PR, Grochinski VJ, Cluss PA, Stapf DA. Relationship of birth cohort and early age at onset of illness in a bipolar disorder case registry. Am J Psychiatry 2003; 160:1636–1642.
65. Blazer DG, George LK, Landerman R, Pennybacker M, Melville ML, Woodbury M, Manton KG, Jordan K, Locke B. Psychiatric disorders. A rural/urban comparison. Arch Gen Psychiatry 1985; 42:651–656.
66. Cassidy F, Carroll BJ. The clinical epidemiology of pure and mixed manic episodes. Bipol Disord 2001; 3:35–40.
67. Vega WA, Kolody B, Aguliar-Gaxiola S, Alderete E, Catalano R, Caravco-Anduaga J. Lifetime prevalence of DSM-III-R psychiatric disorders among urban and rural Mexican Americans in California. Arch Gen Psychiatry 1988; 55:771–778.
68. Kessler RC, Walters EE, Forthofer MS. The social consequences of psychiatric disorders. III. Probability of marital instability. Am J Psychiatry 1998; 155:1092–1096.
69. Verdoux H, Bourgeois M. Social class in unipolar and bipolar probands and relatives. J Affect Disord 1995; 33:181–187.
70. Akiskal HS, Akiskal K. Reassessing the prevalence of bipolar disorders: clinical significance and artistic creativity. Psychiatr Psychobiol 1988; 3:s29–s36.
71. Johnson L, Lundström O, Aberg-Wistedt M, Mathé A. Social support in bipolar disorder: its relevance to remission and relapse. Bipol Disord 2003; 5:129–137.
72. Cassidy F, Carroll BJ. Seasonal variation of mixed and pure episodes of bipolar disorder. J Affect Disord 2002; 68.
73. Rihmer Z. Season of birth and season of hospital admission in bipolar depressed female patients. Psychiatr Res 1980; 3:247–251.

74. Preti A. Seasonal variation and meteotropism in suicide: clinical relevance of findings and implications for research. Acta Neuropsychiatrica 2002; 14:17–28.
75. Rihmer Z, Rutz W, Pihlgren H, Pestality P. Decreasing tendency of seasonality in suicide may indicate lowering rate of depressive suicides in the population. Psychiatr Res 1998; 81:233–240.
76. Barbini B, Di Molfetta D, Gasperini M, Manfredonia MG, Smeraldi E. Seasonal concordance of recurrence in mood disorder patients. Eur Psychiatry 1995; 10:171–175.
77. Mersch PPA, Middendrop HM, Bouhuys AL, Beersma DGM, van den Hoofdakker RH. Seasonal affective disorder and latitude: a review of the literature. J Affect Disord 1999; 53:35–48.
78. Noaghiul S, Hibbeln JR. Cross-national comparisons of seafood consumption and rates of bipolar disorders. Am J Psychiatry 2003; 160:2222–2227.
79. Brown ES, Suppes T, Adinoff B, Thomas NR. Drug abuse and bipolar disorder: comorbidity or misdiagnosis? J Affect Disord 2001; 65:105–115.
80. Oedegard KJ, Fasmer OB. Is migraine in unipolar depressed patients a bipolar spectrum trait? J Affect Disord. In press.
81. Regenold WT, Thapar RK, Marano C, Gavirneni S, Kondapavuluru PV. Increased prevalence of type 2 diabetes mellitus among psychiatric inpatients with bipolar I affective and schizoaffective disorders independent of psychotropic drug use. J Affect Disord 2002; 70:19–26.
82. Rihmer Z, Szádóczky E, Füredi J, Kiss K, Papp Zs. Anxiety disorders comorbidity in bipolar I, bipolar II and unipolar major depression: results from a population-based study in Hungary. J Affect Disord 2001; 67:175–179.
83. Frye MA, Altshuler LL, McElroy SL, Suppes T, Keck PE, Denicoff K, Nolen WA, Kupka R, Leverich GS, Pollio C, Grunze H, Walden J, Post RM. Gender differences in prevalence, risk and clinical correlates of alcoholism comorbidity in bipolar disorder. Am J Psychiatry 2003; 160:883–889.
84. Dunner DL. Clinical consequences of under-recognized bipolar spectrum disorder. Bipol Disord 2003; 5:456–463.
85. Goldberg JE, Ernst CL. The economic and social burden of bipolar disorder: a review. In: Maj M, Akiskal HS, Lopez-Ibor JJ, Sartorius N, eds. Bipolar Disorder. Chichester: John Wiley and Sons, 2002:441–467.
86. Hirschfeld RMA, Cass AR, Holt DCL, Carlson CA. Screening for bipolar disorder in patients treated for depression in a family medicine clinic. J Am Board Fam Pract. In press.

4

Re-examining the Bipolar–Schizophrenia Dichotomy

Helmut Beckmann and Bruno Pfuhlmann
Department of Psychiatry and Psychotherapy, University of Würzburg, Würzburg, Germany

KRAEPELIN'S DICHOTOMY AND THE PROBLEM OF "ATYPICAL" PSYCHOSES

Kraepelin's dichotomy of endogenous psychoses (1) into manic-depressive insanity and dementia praecox introduced, without doubt, a certain order into the chaos that had previously reigned in the classification of mental illnesses. Psychoses with a favorable prognosis were assigned to the group of manic-depressive disorders while those with an unfavorable prognosis were termed dementia praecox. This dichotomy was, however, confronted with the problem of "atypical psychoses" that concerned the classification of psychoses, which could be assigned neither to dementia praecox nor to manic-depressive insanity due to their "atypical" symptomatology. Furthermore, it was often impossible to determine the long-term prognosis of a psychosis from its momentary clinical picture, and it was found that psychoses resembling each other in the initial stages could either remit or result in more or less states of mental deficiency. Eugen Bleuler (2), therefore, replaced Kraepelin's concept of dementia praecox by his concept of a group of "schizophrenias," because "many diseases that could not be distinguished in their psychopathological appearance from psychoses leading to "imbecility" have a good prognosis, as does manic-depressive insanity. A term needed to be devised that would link together the disease forms with like symptomatology, even though some of them end in recovery, others in mental deficiency, and yet others in imbecility" (p. 47).

This broadening of the concept of schizophrenia proved to be less than fully adequate either for clinical or for research purposes and considerably reduced the heuristic value of the diagnosis. As a consequence, the concept of schizophrenia as a nosological entity was abandoned as it is reflected in Kurt Schneider's "anosological" diagnostic classification (3): "Among the numerous varieties of experience that arise in schizophrenia, there are some that we call symptoms of the first rank, not because we think of them as fundamental disorders but because they have special importance for this diagnosis (...). Nothing is thereby said about the theory of schizophrenia (...). Wherever such varieties of experience are determined to exist and no underlying physical diseases are to be found, we speak in all modesty of schizophrenia" (p. 135). Schneider's view is, to a large extent, also that of the currently used operationalized classification systems DSM-IV (4) and ICD-10 (5). These, without doubt, are able to produce high inter-rater reliability, though not uncommonly at the expense of clinical validity.

CONCEPT OF CYCLOID PSYCHOSES AS A SOLUTION OF THE PROBLEM OF "ATYPICAL" PSYCHOSES

In contrast to the earlier-mentioned development of a broadening of the schizophrenia concept, which inevitably resulted in a decrease of clinical validity and lack of prognostic significance, Karl Leonhard (6) elaborated building on the earlier work of Carl Wernicke (7) and Karl Kleist (8), a differentiated nosology of endogenous psychoses that was also prognostically meaningful. Leonhard sub-divided Kraepelin's two major forms of psychoses into further nosologically independent disease entities on the basis of extended longitudinal empirical studies of a great number of patients. Within Leonhard's nosology, the problem of "atypical" psychoses was accommodated by the idea that there might be an independent group of endogenous psychoses in addition to schizophrenias and manic-depressive illness, i.e., the cycloid psychoses. These "atypical" psychoses fell into the manic-depressive insanity group of Kraepelin due to their favorable prognosis, but belong to the schizophrenic psychoses according to Bleuler's and Schneider's viewpoints, as the patients show "schizophreniform" symptoms in the cross-sectional clinical picture. Ever since Bleuler's time, the diagnosis of schizophrenia has been associated with an uncertain prognosis. This contributed to the ascendance of the term "schizoaffective psychoses," which, however, proved to be a rather vague diagnostic category of little clinical utility that was never elaborated to a stringent clinical entity but instead comprised different conceptions in the course of time. In actual classification systems like DSM-IV and ICD-10, "schizoaffective psychoses" represent a kind of "mixed psychoses" that are located between the two great entities of the former Kraepelinian dichotomy, but which have no nosological or prognostic significance.

In contrast, cycloid psychoses according to Leonhard are by no means only mixed forms in the kind of schizoaffective psychoses but form a clinically and nosologically distinct group of psychoses that can be delineated from affective, as well as from schizophrenic, psychoses. Within the affective and schizophrenic psychoses, Leonhard also introduced further nosological differentiations resulting in five nosologically distinct major groups of endogenous psychoses. Thus, this classification goes far beyond Kraepelin's dichotomy despite maintaining his prognostical differentiation. Table 1 gives an overview of Leonhard's nosological conception in relation to Kraepelin's dichotomy and the classifications of Bleuler and ICD-10/DSM-IV, which abstain from a prognostical differentiation.

SYMPTOMATOLOGY OF CYCLOID PSYCHOSES

Cycloid psychoses had already been distinguished from manic-depressive insanity and schizophrenic psychoses by Kleist (9) and his co-worker Fünfgeld (10), but Leonhard (6) was the first to provide precise symptomatological criteria for their accurate diagnosis. He distinguished three clinical sub-forms: anxiety–happiness psychosis,

Table 1 Nosology of Endogenous Psychoses: Leonhard's Differentiated Classification in Relation to Kraepelin's Dichotomy and the Classifications of Bleuler and DSM-IV/ICD-10

	Favorable prognosis		Unfavorable prognosis
Kraepelin	Manic-depressive insanity		Dementia praecox
Bleuler	Manic-depressive insanity	Group of schizophrenias	
DSM/ICD	Affective disorders	Schizoaffective disorders	Schizophrenia
Leonhard	Monopolar affective psychoses Manic-depressive illness Cycloid psychoses		Unsystematic schizophrenias Systematic schizophrenias

excited–inhibited confusion psychosis, and hyperkinetic–akinetic motility psychosis. The clinical syndromes are polymorphous but nevertheless typical in that they allow establishing the diagnosis of a specific sub-form for most cases just relying on the cross-sectional presentation of the syndrome. If the differential diagnosis between the sub-forms is complicated in the acute condition, careful observation for a sufficiently long time usually facilitates a precise diagnosis of one of the sub-syndromes. Table 2 gives an overview of the characteristic clinical manifestations of each sub-form.

Leonhard repeatedly stressed that the illness of a given patient belongs to the group of cycloid psychoses only insofar as it can be diagnosed as one of the sub-types. Therefore, the assembly of diagnostical criteria for singular "cycloid psychosis" as proposed by Perris and Brockington (11) may be a hazardous over-simplification. Moreover, the diagnosis should, by no means, be established only because the course is favorable. Cycloid psychoses, as originally described by Leonhard, are found in various diagnostic categories of the current operationalized classification systems, depending on their particular manifestations and, despite some overlap, are not identical to any of the defined categories. In particular, they are not identical with the "acute transient polymorphous psychotic disorders" of ICD-10 or with the "schizophreniform psychoses" or "brief psychotic disorder" of DSM-IV. These diagnoses are all characterized by rather arbitrary criteria of duration, lack of precise differentiation of symptom clusters, and an absence of a clear prognostic judgment (12–14). For these reasons, it still seems advantageous to use Leonhard's original descriptions of the sub-forms of cycloid psychoses as a diagnostic guideline.

All three sub-types of cycloid psychosis are characterized by bipolarity and a phasically remitting course even if a given episode may sometimes last for a long period of time. Primary deficit or genuine residual syndromes never occur in cycloid psychoses. Leonhard conceded that a certain degree of impairment of internal energy or mental tension might develop after multiple episodes and hospitalizations, but considered this to be a reactive phenomenon due to the severe mental stress and psychosocial problems associated with a multiply remitting psychic illness. In this regard, one must not misinterpret issues related to coping strategies of the patients as indicating formation of a residuum.

Leonhard's differentiated classification is applicable with high reliability if the investigators are trained sufficiently (15,16). In order to examine the nosological

Table 2 Symptomatology of Cycloid Psychoses

Anxiety–happiness psychosis
Anxiety pole
- Severe anxiety with distrust and ideas of reference
- Anxious paranoid ideas: threat, persecution, destruction, anxious misinterpretation of environment
- Affect-congruent illusory or hallucinatory phenomena (mostly phonemes)
- Anxiously colored somatic sensations

Happiness pole
- Ecstatic mood with ideas of calling, happiness, or salvation, reflecting an altruistic component of the ecstasy
- Affect-generated illusory or hallucinatory phenomena: e.g., divine inspirations (phonemes, divine visions)
- Pathetic gesture, ecstatic facial expression

Both poles
- Ideas of self sacrifice combining anxiety and ecstasy

Excited inhibited confusional psychosis
Excited pole
- Incoherence of thought with compulsive speech at high degrees of excitation, at lower degrees incoherence of thematic choice or digressive theme choice
- Fleeting misrecognitions of persons (no misrecognitions of an absurd character)
- Ideas of reference, fleeting hallucinations

Inhibited pole
- Inhibition of thought, perplexedness
- Ideas of meaning, ideas of reference
- Hallucinations, mainly acustic, occasionally visual or somatopsychic

Hyperkinetic–akinetic motility psychosis
Hyperkinetic pole
- Increase in expressive and reactive motions, which only in high degrees of hyperkinesis lose their natural value and become exaggerated but not particularly distorted
- Severe distractibility by environmental conditions with continued senseless motor activity (hypermetamorphosis according to Wernicke)

Akinetic pole
- Disappearing of reactive motions, stiffness of expressive motions
- In severe cases reduction or standstill of voluntary movements
- Mostly lack of spontaneous speech

Facultative
- Incoherent speech resulting from blurting out of unrelated utterances, expelling of unarticulated sounds of an expressive character (screaming, howling, etc.)
- Ideas of reference, hallucinations, mood alterations from anxious to ecstatic, often with rapid changes

validity of the concept of cycloid psychoses, a whole series of studies was undertaken that aimed at an external validation of the concept by clinical, genetic-epidemiological, and biological data.

RESEARCH FINDINGS REGARDING CYCLOID PSYCHOSES

Long-Term Course and Prognosis

Additionally to Leonhard's own catamnestic studies (17), Beckmann et al. (18) demonstrated a high prognostic validity of the diagnostic category of cycloid psychoses by means of a prospective follow-up study. They were able to observe 26 out of 31 patients with a cycloid psychosis over a period of four years and found no residual states. All but two patients, who were actually in an acute phase of their cycloid psychosis, showed a complete remission. Studies of Perris (19) and Maj (20) could also confirm that prognosis and outcome are favorable.

Jabs et al. (21) reported a significantly higher satisfaction with the global quality of life (measured by the German version of the Lancaster quality of life profile) in patients with cycloid psychoses than in patients with schizophrenic psychoses. In both groups, the mean duration of illness was about 13 years. Concerning outcome and social functioning, patients suffering from cycloid psychosis also reached significantly higher scores in the Strauss–Carpenter-Outcome Scale and Global-Assessment-of-Functioning Scale than schizophrenic patients.

Etiology and Clinical Genetics

With regard to the etiology of cycloid psychoses, Leonhard (6) postulated a prominent role of somatic factors in these psychoses, whereas a hereditary predisposition seemed to play only a subordinate role. In his family studies, Leonhard found a frequency of 4–5% of endogenous psychoses among the patient's first-degree relatives. Leonhard's original observations were further substantiated by a recent family study that has been performed to a high methodological standard by means of a personal examination of all traceable first-degree relatives by an experienced psychiatrist blind to the diagnosis of the index cases (22). Morbidity risks of first-degree relatives of 45 patients with cycloid psychoses, 32 patients with manic-depressive illness, and 27 healthy controls were calculated using the life-table method. Out of a total of 431 first-degree relatives, 353 could be traced and examined personally (82%). Information about not traceable relatives was obtained by the "Family-History" method. Whereas 24.4% of the index probands with cycloid psychoses had at least one first-degree relative with an endogenous psychosis; this was the case in 62.5% of the manic-depressive index probands and in 14.8% in the control persons. The age-corrected morbidity risk for first-degree relatives to suffer from an endogenous psychosis was 10.8% in cycloid psychoses vs. 35.2% in manic-depressive illness ($p < 0.0001$) and 5.7% in the control group (Fig. 1). The difference between cycloid psychoses and controls was not significant. In relatives of cycloid psychotic probands, the morbidity risk for homonymous psychoses was 4.4% and the risk for affective disorders was 5.8%. The results of this family study correspond well with the figures of Maj (20) who reported familial morbidity risks of 4.2% for affective disorders and 4.8% for "mixed psychosis" in relatives of patients with cycloid psychoses.

These findings contradict the thesis of a continuous spectrum of bipolar disorders, as given a genetic continuum ranging from slighter bipolar affective forms to more serious cycloid forms, the higher familial loadings were to be expected in cycloid psychoses due to their more serious symptomatology. On the contrary, cycloid psychoses showed a considerably lower familial morbidity than manic-depressive illness indicating that these forms of psychoses have to be differentiated etiologically and nosologically.

A particularly suitable method to address the question of the relative importance of genetic versus environmental factors in the etiology of cycloid psychoses is a twin study, in which pairs of twins with at least one affected member are systematically recruited. The classical twin study method is based on a comparison of monozygotic and dizygotic twin pairs assuming that both kinds of twins are subject

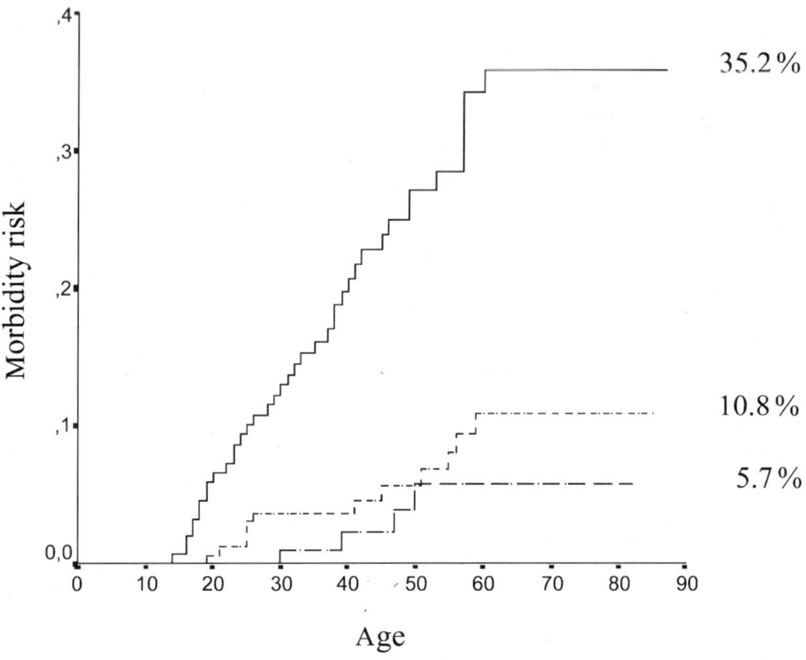

Figure 1 Morbidity risk of endogenous psychoses in relatives. ———, manic-depressive illness (153 relatives); - - - - - -, cycloid psychosis (172 relatives); and — — —, controls (106 relatives).

to the same environmental influences but differ in their genetic similarity. If genetically identical monozygotic twins are concordant for a particular trait more often than dizygotic twins, heritability is implied according to Galton's rule. Conversely, all phenotypic differences between monozygotic twins are assumed to be due to environmental factors. Here, it is important that twin studies take possible complications of pregnancy and delivery into account. Owing to such factors, the prenatal "environments" of twins may be markedly different as is shown by the well-known twin-transfusion syndrome. Franzek and Beckmann (23,24) conducted a systematic twin study meeting all these methodological requirements. They found 12 monozygotic and 11 dizygotic twin pairs in which at least one twin suffered from a sub-form of a cycloid psychosis. Regarding the proband-associated concordance rates, 36% of affected monozygotic twins and 31% of affected dizygotic twins had an ill co-twin; these figures did not differ significantly. The corresponding low heritability index of 0.14 (maximum value 1) and low monozygotic/dizygotic ratio of 1.16 (minimum value 1) indicate that genetic influences do not play an important etiological role in cycloid psychoses. In contrast, concordance rates in monozygotic and dizygotic twins with unsystematic schizophrenias were significantly different suggesting a primary genetic predisposition in the etiology of these psychoses. Interestingly, monozygotic twins with systematic schizophrenias were not at all detected, a finding that was already reported by Leonhard (6) and is difficult to interpret (25), but nevertheless shows that cycloid psychoses have to be distinguished from systematic schizophrenias, as well as from unsystematic schizophrenias, regarding etiological aspects.

The apparently minor role of a genetic predisposition gives rise to the question which kind of environmental factors might be important for the causation of cycloid psychoses. Twin studies may give evidence for such factors in the form of environmental differences between affected and unaffected monozygotic twins. In this situation, genetically identical individuals are subject to environmental differences. Franzek and Beckmann's systematic twin study (23) also addressed this question. In the nine discordant monozygotic pairs with a cycloid psychosis, the affected index twins showed significantly more frequent and more severe birth complications than their healthy co-twins, and in concordant pairs, the more seriously ill twin showed more such complications. These twin findings emphasize the relevance of environmental influences in the causation of cycloid psychoses and suggest prenatally or perinatally operating biological noxes to be of remarkable etiological importance in cycloid psychoses.

These clinical genetic findings are supplemented by the results of other studies that also suggest an important role of somatic factors in the pathogenesis of cycloid psychoses. Franzek et al. (26), in a comparison study of psychiatric patients with unspecific abnormalities on cerebral computed tomography (CCT) and a matched control group with normal CCT, found a significantly higher number of patients with cycloid psychoses among the patients with abnormal CCT scans. The CCT abnormalities consisted mainly in ventricular asymmetry and/or enlargement and were judged by an independent neuroradiologist to be the likely result of pre- or perinatal insults. Although the described structural abnormalities cannot be interpreted as specific for cycloid psychoses, the question arises as to what the nature of these insults might be. An observation directly relevant to this question is the seasonality of birth, i.e., excess births in winter and spring months, which were observed particularly among patients with schizophrenic spectrum psychoses without affected relatives (27,28). Franzek and Beckmann (29) studied the phenomenon of birth seasonality in a large group of patients with psychoses of the schizophrenic spectrum applying the differentiated classification of Leonhard. They found that the excess was limited to patients with cycloid psychoses and systematic schizophrenias—both forms of psychoses that do not show a high familial loading. The highly familial unsystematic schizophrenias even showed a deficit of births in winter and spring months. The favored explanation for birth seasonality is that insults arising preferentially in the colder seasons may affect a vulnerable phase of fetal brain development in such a way that the individual is proposed to develop a psychosis in adulthood. Therefore, Franzek and Beckmann (29) assumed that individuals with primary genetic impairment might be less likely to survive if they sustain a further, exogenous insult to the central nervous system.

A possible cause of exogenous insults in the prenatal cerebral development is maternal viral infections, as they may damage the fetus directly or indirectly through a number of mechanisms (26). Stöber et al. (30) were the first to examine the relationship between maternal infectious diseases and the later occurrence of cycloid psychoses. They reported that mothers of patients with a cycloid psychosis suffered in the first trimester of gestation significantly more often from febrile infectious diseases—usually of the respiratory tract—than mothers of controls as well as mothers of patients with manic-depressive illness and mothers of patients with unsystematic schizophrenias, both illnesses with high familial loading. Among mothers of patients with systematic schizophrenias, which, like cycloid psychoses, show no essential heredity in their etiology, infections occurred more often in the second trimester of pregnancy. Therefore, it is hypothesized that the timing, localization, and extent of cerebral damage seems to determine the degree to which the individual becomes vulnerable to the respective forms of environmentally caused psychosis. These hypotheses are in agreement with the "neurodevelopmental concept" of schizophrenic psychoses that is underpinned by the finding of circumscribed cytoarchitectonic abnormalities indicating disturbances of cerebral development (31,32).

Neurophysiological investigations, such as the measurement of P300, have also revealed significant differences between patients with cycloid psychosis and patients with either manic-depressive illness or schizophrenic psychoses (33). Regarding the topography of P300, both cycloid psychoses and controls showed a dislocation of the mean P300 peak away from the midline towards the left hemisphere, whereas in schizophrenic patients, P300 peaks were located within the right hemisphere. Additionally, significantly higher amplitude of P300 was found in patients with cycloid psychoses compared with age- and sex-matched controls. In contrast, schizophrenic patients showed significantly lower amplitude than controls, whereas manic-depressive individuals did not differ significantly from controls in this respect. The elevated amplitudes in cycloid psychoses may probably reflect a state of increased arousal of the central nervous system.

Other functional correlates of cycloid psychoses, i.e., global and regional cerebral perfusion at rest, were up to now studied by research groups around Warkentin et al. (34) and Bartsch (unpublished data). Warkentin et al. measured the mean hemispheric blood flow and its regional distribution in acute phases of cycloid psychoses, as well as after one week of treatment, and finally at discharge by ^{133}Xe-inhalation cerebrography. Their results suggested a global "hyperactivity" during the acute phases of cycloid psychoses favoring occipital on cost of frontal perfusion, particularly on the right side of the brain. On average, initial hyperperfusion of both hemispheres at admission was found to decrease within 1 week by more than 10% and in seven out of eight patients under neuroleptic treatment. Thereafter, cerebral perfusion did not differ significantly from control subjects.

However, a recently ongoing study using ^{99m}Tc-HMPAO-SPECT (Bartsch et al., unpublished data) did not yet yield any evidence for acute elevations of the global perfusion estimator in neither cycloid psychoses ($n = 8$) nor hebephrenias ($n = 7$). Differential diagnoses of non-systematic schizophrenias according to Leonhard, as well as the medication history, may be crucial in these regards. In contrast to chronic schizophrenias, some cases of cycloid psychoses may present an "acute hyperfrontality" that is redistributed to occipito–temporo–parietal areas upon their treatment and remission. In comparison with hebephrenias at admission, as well as at their discharge, acute cycloid psychoses presented a significantly pronounced perfusion of the left dorsolateral prefrontal cortex and within the anterior cingulum. Interestingly, the latter survived a small volume correction centered on the Talairach space co-ordinates given by Liddle et al. (35) for maximum positive correlations with "schizophrenic disorganization." Moreover, cycloid psychoses exhibited a significantly steeper decrease of perfusion than hebephrenias according to Leonhard in the dorsolateral prefrontal cortex bilaterally, along the corpus callosum and in the right anterior cingulum from admission to discharge. Again, the latter survived a small volume correction centered on the Talairach space co-ordinates given by the group around Liddle (35) for increasing "schizophrenic disorganization."

CONCLUSION: CYCLOID PSYCHOSES AS A CHALLENGE FOR THE BIPOLAR–SCHIZOPHRENIA DICHOTOMY

The Kraepelinian dichotomy of endogenous psychoses into affective and schizophrenic types has failed to bring about a decisive breakthrough either in clinical practice or in the scientific study of these illnesses. Psychoses that do not fit neatly into either category are designated as "atypical psychoses," "schizophreniform" psychoses, "schizoaffective disorders," "brief psychotic disorders," or "acute transient polymorphic psychotic disorders" and are assigned to either an "affective spectrum," a "bipolar spectrum," or a "schizophrenic spectrum" of psychoses, depending on which of the "classical" basic orientations is preferred, that of Kraepelin or its modification along the lines of Bleuler. However, none of the concepts mentioned earlier enables a delimitation of symptomatologically sharply characterized clinical syndromes with a prognostical significance and an external validation by means of epidemiological, clinical-genetic, and biological findings. Therefore, these concepts of "atypical psychoses" seem not to represent valid diagnostic entities, and their assignment to one of the categories of Kraepelinian dichotomy seems not well founded.

In contrast, Leonhard's differentiated nosological classification offers a promising alternative for the resolution of this problem of "atypical" psychoses. Leonhard's concept of the cycloid psychoses as an independent nosological entity distinct from both manic-depressive illness and schizophrenic psychoses may help to overcome the restrictions and problems of the Kraepelinian dichotomy that obviously cannot adequately reflect clinical reality. The referred research findings regarding cycloid psychoses support the assumption that these psychoses may form an independent nosological entity and, therefore, constitute a challenge for a Kraepelinian dichotomy of endogenous psychoses. The nosological diversification of endogenous psychoses beyond a mere dichotomy provides seminal perspectives for a better scientific understanding of the etiology, genetics, prognosis, and differential treatment of the endogenous psychoses.

REFERENCES

1. Kraepelin E, Lange J. Psychiatrie. Klinische Psychiatrie. Vol. 3. 8th ed. Leipzig: Barth, 1923.
2. Bleuler E. Dementia praecox oder die Gruppe der Schizophrenien. In: Aschaffenburg G, ed. Handbuch der Psychiatrie. Leipzig: Deuticke, 1911.
3. Schneider K. Klinische Psychopathologie. 8th ed. Stuttgart: Thieme, 1967.
4. American Psychiatric Association. Diagnostic and Statistical Manual of Mental Disorders. 4th ed. Washington, DC: American Psychiatric Press, 1994.
5. World Health Organization. Tenth revision of the International Classification of Diseases. Chapter V (F): mental and behavioural disorders (including disorders of psychological development). Clinical Descriptions and Diagnostical Guidelines. Geneva: WHO, 1991.
6. Leonhard K. In: Beckman H, ed. Classification of Endogenous Psychoses and Their Differentiated Etiology. Second, revised and enlarged edition. Wien, New York: Springer, 1999.
7. Wernicke C. Grundriß der Psychiatrie in klinischen Vorlesungen. ThiemeLeipzip1900.
8. Kleist K. Cycloid, paranoid, and epileptoid psychoses and the problem of degenerative psychoses. In: Hirsch SR, Shepherd M, eds. Themes and Variations in European Psychiatry. An Anthology. Bristol: Wright, 1974:297–331.
9. Kleist K. Über zykloide Degenerationspsychosen, besonders Verwirrtheiten und Motilitätspsychosen. Zentralbl ges Neurol Psychiatr 1926; 44:265–267.
10. Fünfgeld E. Die Motilitätspsychosen und Verwirrtheiten. Berlin: Karger, 1936.
11. Perris C, Brockington IF. Cycloid psychoses and their relation to the major psychoses. In: Perris C, Struwe G, Jansson B, eds. Biological Psychiatry. Amsterdam: Elsevier, 1981:447–450.

12. Peralta V, Cuesta MJ. Diagnostic significance of Schneider's first-rank symptoms in schizophrenia. Comparative study between schizophrenic and non-schizophrenic psychotic disorders. Br J Psychiatry 1999; 174:243–248.
13. Harrow M, Grossman LS, Herbener ES, Davies EW. Ten-year outcome: patients with schizoaffective disorders, schizophrenia, affective disorders and mood-incongruent psychotic symptoms. Br J Psychiatry 2000; 177:421–426.
14. Marneros A, Pillmann F, Haring A, Balzuweit S. Die akuten vorübergehenden psychotischen Störungen. Fortschr Neurol Psychiatr 2000; 68 (suppl 1):S22–S25.
15. Franzek E, Beckmann H. Reliability and validity of the Leonhard classification tested in a five-year follow-up study of 50 chronic schizophrenics. In: Ferrero FP, Haynal AE, Sartorius N, eds. Schizophrenia and Affective psychoses. Nosology in Contemporary Psychiatry. New York: John Libbey CIC, 1992:67–72.
16. Pfuhlmann B, Franzek E, Stöber G, Cetkovich-Bakmas M, Beckmann H. On interrater-reliability for Leonhard's classification of endogenous psychoses. Psychopathology 1997; 30:100–105.
17. Trostorff Sv, Leonhard K. Catamnesis of endogenous psychoses according to the differential diagnostic method of Karl Leonhard. Psychopathology 1990; 23:259–262.
18. Beckmann H, Fritze J, Lanczik M. Prognostic validity of the cycloid psychose. A prospective follow-up study. Psychopathology 1990; 23:205–211.
19. Perris C. A study of cycloid psychoses. Acta Psychiatr Scand 1974; (suppl 253):1–77.
20. Maj M. Cycloid psychotic disorder: validation of the concept by means of a follow-up and a family study. Psychopathology 1990; 23:196–204.
21. Jabs BE, Krause U, Althaus G, Stöber G, Pfuhlmann B. Vergleichsuntersuchung zur Lebensqualität bei Probanden mit zykloiden und schizophrenen Psychosen Nervenarzt. Nervenarzt 2004; 75:460–466.
22. Pfuhlmann B. Familienbefunde bei Zykloiden Psychosen und Manisch-Depressiver Erkrankung. Darmstadt: Steinkopff, 2003.
23. Franzek E, Beckmann H. The different genetic background of schizophrenic spectrum psychoses. A twin study. Am J Psychiatry 1998; 155:76–83.
24. Franzek E, Beckmann H. Psychoses of the schizophrenic spectrum in twins. A Discussion on the Nature-Nurture Debate in the Etiology of Endogenous Psychoses. Wien, New York: Springer, 1999.
25. Pfuhlmann B, Franzek E, Beckmann H. Absence of a subgroup of chronic schizophrenias in monozygotic twins—consequences for etiological considerations. Eur Arch Psychiatry Clin Neurosci 1999; 249:50–54.
26. Franzek E, Becker T, Hofmann E, Flöhl W, Stöber G, Beckmann H. Is computerized tomography ventricular abnormality related to cycloid psychosis? Biol Psychiatry 1996; 40:1255–1266.
27. D'Amato D, Dalery J, Rochet T, Terra JL, Marie-Cardine M. Saisons de naissance et psychiatrie. Etude rétrospective d'une population hospitière. Encéphale 1991; 17:67–71.
28. O'Callaghan E, Gibson T, Colohan HA, Walshe D, Buckley B, Larkin C, Waddington JL. Season of birth in schizophrenia. Evidence for confinement of an excess of winter births to patients without a family history of mental disorder. Br J Psychiatry 1991; 158:764–769.
29. Franzek E, Beckmann H. Season-of-birth effect reveals the existence of etiologically different groups of schizophrenia. Biol Psychiatry 1992; 32:375–378.
30. Stöber G, Kocher I, Franzek E, Beckmann H. First-trimester maternal gestational infection and cycloid psychosis. Acta Psychiatr Scand 1997; 95:319–324.
31. Jakob H, Beckmann H. Prenatal developmental disturbances in the limbic allocortex in schizophrenia. J Neural Transm 1986; 65:303–326.
32. Beckmann H, Jakob H. Prenatal disturbances of nerve cell migration in the entorhinal region: a common vulnerability factor of functional psychoses? J Neural Transm (Gen Sect) 1991; 84:155–164.

33. Strik WK, Fallgatter AJ, Stöber G, Franzek E, Beckmann H. Specific P300 features in patients with cycloid psychosis. Acta Psychiatr Scand 1996; 94:471–476.
34. Warkentin S, Nilson A, Karlson S, Risberg J, Franzen G, Gustafson L. Cycloid psychoses: regional cerebral blood flow correlates of a psychotic episode. Acta Psychiatr Scand 1992; 85:23–29.
35. Liddle PF, Friston KJ, Frith CD, Hirsch SR, Jones T, Frackowiak RSJ. Patterns of cerebral blood flow in schizophrenia. Br J Psychiatry 1992; 160:179–186.

5

The Bipolar Spectrum: History, Description, Boundaries, and Validity

Hagop S. Akiskal
Department of Psychiatry, and International Mood Center, University of California at San Diego and VA Hospital, San Diego, California, U.S.A.

INTRODUCTION

This chapter reviews evidence in favor of a broad "bipolar spectrum" (1–3) beyond ICD-10 (4) and DSM-IV (5) formulations for bipolar disorders. This expanded spectrum includes mania, but also considers new bipolar subtypes linked together by various degrees of hypomania, excitatory phenomena, and underlying temperamental dysregulation along cyclothymic and hyperthymic lines (6,7). Since much of the research in the enlargement of the boundaries of bipolar disorder has come through the work of the present author and his collaborators, the bibliography of this article reflects key references from this work. The more extensive literature on the subject can be found in recent reviews by the author (2,8–10), as well as in a recent monograph published as a special issue of the *Journal of Affective Disorders* (11).

THE CONCEPT OF THE BIPOLAR SPECTRUM

To the best of our knowledge, the rubric "bipolar spectrum" first appeared in the psychiatric literature in our paper on cyclothymic disorder in 1977 (12). This was a study of the clinical, familial, treatment–response, and course of 46 cyclothymic outpatients, subsequently expanded to a total sample of 50 (13). These individuals who presented to a community mental health center in Memphis with history of tempestuous interpersonal relationships and associated social disturbances were found to have mood swings that failed to meet the symptomatologic and duration criteria for depression and mania as described by Feighner et al. (14): in effect, they alternated cyclically from subdepressive to hypomanic periods lasting no more than a few days at a time. Compared with a personality disorder comparison group, these probands had a significant excess of bipolar disorder in their first-degree relatives, thereby providing external validating support to our formulation of a sub-bipolar thesis. Our prospective follow-up of these outpatients revealed the occurrence of (in increasing frequency) of manic, hypomanic, and depressive episodes, as well as

Table 1 Prospective Course of Cyclothymic Temperament

Manic episodes	(3/46)	6%
Hypomanic episodes	(6/46)	12%
Depressive episodes	(11/46)	24%
Cycling on TCAs	(11/25)	44%

Source: From Refs. 12 and 13.

cycling on antidepressants (Table 1). Overall, our data provided "evidence for a cyclothymic-bipolar spectrum" (12, p. 107). Although "cyclothymic disorder" did officially make it into DSM-III (16), the conservative stance of the nosologic formulations of mood disorder in that edition of the manual did not formally refer to a spectrum concept.

ICD-10 and DSM-IV

There is much current disagreement about the boundaries of affective disorder subtypes. This is not a new phenomenon, as the debate about affective subtypes is at least 100 years old (15). But those who hoped that classification, with the use of operational criteria as embodied in the official nomenclature of the American Psychiatric Association [of which DSM-IV-TR (5) is the latest version], would clarify matters have much to be disappointed about. This manual basically adheres to the unipolar–bipolar distinction, with strong bias in favor of these non-bipolar conditions. Thus, major depressive disorder (MDD) dominates mood disorders of which residual and chronic depressive, dysthymic, and double depressive course variants are recognized.

The DSM-IV focus on bipolar disorder is largely limited to manic-depressive illness (bipolar I). True, DSM-IV has formally endorsed the category of "bipolar II," and both "bipolar not otherwise specified (NOS)" and cyclothymia complete the bipolar roster. This gradient of bipolar conditions can be viewed as being closer to a veritable "bipolar spectrum" compared with their DSM-III counterparts (16), but again such terminologic conceptualization is avoided by DSM-IV (5). In the latter more up-to-date manual, in principle, the entire breadth of bipolarity should be diagnosable. Yet such bipolar subclassification is difficult to translate into practice, because the definitions of mania and hypomania are phrased in nearly identical language (except for psychosis for the former and relative lack of impairment for the latter), bipolar NOS is basically left undefined, and cyclothymia is likely to be misclassified as an erratic personality disorder (7,12,13,17). In brief, the entire range of bipolarity in the less-than-manic domain is at risk for being relegated to MDD and/or Axis II, Cluster B. Two decades earlier, the main diagnostic errors were in favoring schizophrenia over mania (1), but this appears to be less of a problem today; instead, bipolar disorder is now diagnosed as "unipolar" MDD (7,18,19) by clinicians. Nonetheless, it is noteworthy that DSM-IV does not refer to a "unipolar" disorder—it refers only to MDD, perhaps out of tacit acknowledgment that MDD may change over time to bipolar disorder? Thus, some wisdom appears buried in its terminologic avoidance of the "unipolar" rubric.

The World Health Organization Classification of Diseases in its 10th revision of the Mental and Behavioral Disorders (ICD-10) is more limited in the breadth of bipolar subtypes (3). Thus, bipolar II is only parenthetically mentioned as more or less equivalent to atypical bipolar disorder. Furthermore, mild post-depressive elated symptomatology is permitted as being part of depressive disorder! This extreme restriction of the territory of bipolar disorders in a basically European classification is all the more surprising, given that broad concepts of manic depression have their origins in Germany (see Ref. 2 for a review).

HISTORICAL ROOTS

A brief review of the historical background of the development of the concepts of affective illness and personality disorders may point to the sources of our current confusion, and could thereby suggest how a new order might emerge from insights that classical observers in psychiatry have provided us.

Although Aretaeus (20) had observed the intimate relationship between melancholic and manic conditions in the first century AD, the modern conceptualization of these disorders as specific nosologic entities was formulated 18 centuries later in France by Falret (21) and Baillarger (22). This 150th anniversary was commemorated in the French National Academy of Medicine (23,24). These two French alienists described a cyclic alternation of manic and melancholic episodes, followed by a free interval. "Falret's discovery" (25) referred to a triphasic course, whereas Baillarger described a biphasic course before a free interval. Subsequently, their disciple, Magnan (reviewed in Refs. 23 and 24), observed that the two course patterns could occur in the same patient, linked by a "mixed state" (manic features during melancholia or melancholic features during mania). These pioneering contributions paved the way to the Kraepelinian (26) synthesis of most mood conditions into a unitary rubric.

Kraepelin (26) subsumed much of what today we call mood disorders (including recurrent depressions) under the rubric of "manic depression." He observed that many depressed patients, when followed longitudinally, developed hypomania or mania, while other depressives had a family history for manic-depressive psychosis. He further noted that just as depressive symptoms could occur during mania, hypomanic intrusions into depressive episodes did occur in a considerable number of patients; these were Kraepelin's categories for mixed states, more broadly defined than in the present official diagnostic schema of ICD-10 (4) and DSM-IV (5). More importantly, Kraepelin believed that constitutionally determined personal dispositions—which today we call "temperament"—represent the fundamental states from which different affective states arose. Kraepelin's conceptualization involved affective dysregulation, which he believed generated a multitude of clinical pictures, including acute confusional psychoses, acute and chronic manic states, retarded depressions, depressions which switched to brief elations, agitated melancholias, anxious-depressive mania, depression with flight of ideas, and other affective states with mood lability in continuum with normality.

Kraepelin's approach was further developed by Kretschmer (27), who expressed the view that "endogenous psychoses are nothing but exaggerated forms of temperament." He believed that there was a central cyclothymic disposition that, in some individuals, manifested in irritable or depressive traits, and in others, in hypomanic traits. His formulation has a very modern ring to it. As modern molecular genetics (28) is concerned with oligogenic traits, the high prevalence of affective traits with near-normal distribution in the community (29,30) is of great theoretical, genetic, and preventive significance. In such a formulation (2,24), bipolar disorder will be at the extreme end of the positive distribution, imperceptibly separated from more normative affective temperaments (Fig. 1).

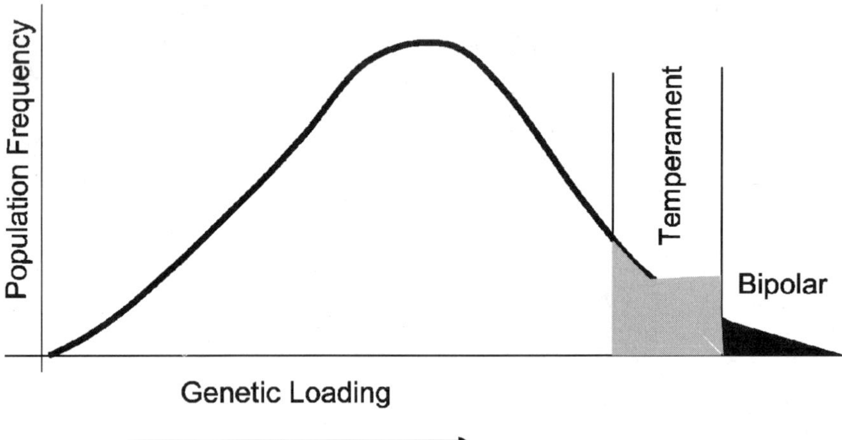

Figure 1 An evolutionary and population genetics perspective on the bipolar spectrum.

Another German psychiatrist, Kurt Schneider (31), who had a profound influence on the field through his writings on what he termed "psychopathic personality" (abnormal personality in today's parlance), believed that such dispositions as the depressive, labile, and hyperthymic had little to do with the "cyclothymic" disorders (his term for manic depression). Schneider's position is similar to the one taken by DSM-IV (5), namely that abnormal personalities are orthogonal to what we today term "bipolar disorder."

Although Schneider's descriptions of individual personality types are phenomenologically superb [we have used them in our operational definitions of the affective temperaments (6)], his legacy—to the extent it is reflected in DSM-IV—is conceptually confusing (32,33). The DSM-IV schema also derives from psychodynamic thinking. In this schema, patients presenting with unmistakable affective signs and symptoms, instead of being considered cyclothymic, would receive such labels as "psychopathic," "histrionic," or "borderline." Likewise, patients with double depression could receive personality characterization as "passive," "avoidant," or "obsessoid," rather than being considered "depressive" in temperament. The main problem with the DSM-IV (5) conceptualization is that today patients still are at risk of being considered character flawed, rather than having constitutionally based affective disorders. The net effect of the current conceptualization of Axis II on psychiatric practice is to discourage diagnosis of affective illness in those with significant interpersonal dysfunction, thereby limiting major mood disorders to relatively straightforward periodic or cyclic cases.

TEMPERAMENT IN BIPOLARITY

Three decades of clinical research, based on longitudinal observations of patients in the setting of mood clinics (2,7,8,34), indicates that a subclassification based on temperament can help demystify the vast terrain of what some people consider personality-disordered depression, but which the present author prefers to consider "soft bipolar disorders" (6). Temperament is natural to the language of mood disorders as it refers to emotionality, reactivity or lack thereof, impulse control, shifts in energy level, and circadian changes (32). Much of what in the psychosocial literature is considered high or low "expressed emotion" and the related construct of hypercritical attitudes, reflects a clash between the temperament of the patient and that of significant others (35). In brief, temperament as a construct appears proximal to the chain of the charged emotional atmosphere and the resultant personal adversity, which define the psychosocial context of affective disorders. We submit that temperament has a fundamental role in helping us, not only in the classification of affective subtypes, but also in understanding their evolution and complications.

How does temperament shed light on the spectrum of bipolarity beyond classic mania (3)? In essence, our thesis is that a great many depressions are bipolar by virtue of temperament (6–8). Indeed, progression from temperament to full-blown episodes has been shown in prospective follow-up of the offspring and kin of manic-depressive probands (36).

DESCRIPTION OF THE BIPOLAR SPECTRUM

As shown in Table 2, there exist types I, II, III, and IV, and as one would expect in a spectrum, types ½ , I ½ , II ½ , III ½ (7). The spectrum includes manic-depressive (bipolar I), bipolar II, bipolar III, and hyperthymic depressive (type IV) prototypes. These are proposed as "categorical" phenotypes, suitable for genetic investigations. However, as expected in a spectrum conceptual framework, intermediary phenotypes are encountered in clinical practice: For instance, ½ or schizobipolar, I ½ or depressions with protracted hypomania (between bipolar I and II), and II ½ or cyclothymic depressions (between bipolar II and bipolar III). The main characteristics of each of these conditions within the spectrum follow.

Bipolar I: This is classically defined by the presence of mania that is often of psychotic proportions. There are those (mostly male) characterized with a predominant manic course, many of whom have a hyperthymic temperament (37,38). Such research has also shown that those who suffer dysphoric manic episodes are

Table 2 A Proposed Clinical Spectrum of Bipolar Disorders

Bipolar ½	Schizobipolar disorder
Bipolar I	Manic-depressive illness
Bipolar I½	Depression with protracted hypomania
Bipolar II	Depression with spontaneous discrete hypomanic episodes
Bipolar II½	Depression superimposed on cyclothymic temperament
Bipolar III	Repeated depression plus hypomania occurring solely in association with antidepressant or other somatic treatment
Bipolar III½	Depression, mood swings, and hypomania occurring in the context of substance and/or alcohol (ab)use
Bipolar IV	Depression superimposed on a hyperthymic temperament
Bipolar V	Recurrent depressions ($\geq$5 episodes)

Source: Expanded from Ref. 7.

characterized by the intrusion of a depressive temperament (more prevalent in women) into a manic episode.

We classify as *bipolar I ½* patients whose illness is characterized by frequent depressive episodes, and few protracted hypomanic episodes lasting weeks but without developing psychotic symptoms and marked social disruption (7). Hypothetically, these patients are genotypically most closely related to bipolar I patients.

Bipolar II: This type was delineated in the pioneering study by Dunner et al. (39) at NIMH. The hallmark here is recurrent anergic depression with hypomania, which often occurs at the tail end of a depression, though less commonly the reverse sequence can also occur. These, particularly the latter, are "sunny" bipolar IIs (40) with infrequent episodes, who often benefit from adaptive hypomanic periods (7) characterized by increased (from baseline) of cheerfulness, gregariousness and people seeking, sexual drive and behavior, talkativeness, confidence and optimism, disinhibition and carefree attitudes, eutonia and vitality, and overinvolvement in new projects; sleep need, on the other hand, is reduced. These manifestations of hypomania are more clearly separable from mania than the non-descript list of hypomanic signs and symptoms in DSM-IV. Hypomania in these patients occurs in discrete episodes that represent changes from the patient's baseline. Such patients are more likely to conform to the narrow (DSM-IV) concept of bipolar II with hypomania 4 days.

However, research conducted in Memphis dating to the late 1970s (12,13,41), and more recent epidemiological research in Zurich (42), have demonstrated that the modal duration of hypomania is 2 days (rather than the 4-day arbitrary threshold of DSM-IV). This lower duration threshold has been validated in outpatient private practice in collaboration with Benazzi and Akiskal (43). A trans-Atlantic consensus statement (9) from centers specializing in bipolarity concluded that for a first episode depression, it would be the best to use the more conservative hypomania cutoff 4 days, but that in most others with recurrent depression, the 2 hypomania duration cutoff was more appropriate. For Angst and Gamma (44), even shorter duration of hypomania is sufficient. It is noteworthy that the Research Diagnostic Criteria defined a floor duration of hypomania of 2 days and a more strict duration of 7 days, which in a recently published NIMH collaborative study on the course of bipolar II were shown to be indistinguishable in most parameters related to bipolarity (45), supporting the inclusion of brief hypomanias within the bipolar spectrum.

Bipolar II ½ represents the more unstable ("darker") side of a putative bipolar II phenotype with high recurrence of both depression and irritable hypomania superimposed upon an interepisodic cyclothymic temperament (40). Here, the mood dysregulation is more severe than in ordinary bipolar II, such that affective states and temperament are not easily discriminable; labile–hostile moods intermixed with depression generate unstable mixed states; hence, the roller-coaster course for both patient and significant others, which in the DSM-IV schema (5) can be mistaken for or labeled as "borderline personality." A prospective study conducted by us within the framework of the NIMH collaborative study (46) has demonstrated that cyclothymic mood lability is the best predictor of which clinically depressed patients will switch into bipolar II. Also, in Italian collaboration with Savino et al. (47) and Perugi et al. (48), we have shown that both panic and social phobic states commonly occur in the context of cyclothymic depressions. Such patients also tend to be suicidal (49). Finally, in support for the foregoing clinical observations, a team of researchers from the Johns Hopkins University (50) has shown that panic attacks with bipolar II disorder might represent a specific genetic subtype of bipolar disorder.

Bipolar III: In these patients, hypomania typically becomes evident during pharmacotherapy with antidepressants [also other somatic treatments such as phototherapy, sleep deprivation, and ECT (9)]. Such hypomania is usually brief and exhibits a low rate of recurrence. Studies conducted in collaboration with Memphis colleagues during the early 1980s (51), and more recently with French collaboration in the EPIDEP study (52), indicate that these individuals are temperamentally depressive or dysthymic, often conforming to the double depressive pattern, yet give evidence for bipolar family history. This is not to say that all double depressions are bipolar, but familial bipolarity represents a clinical marker for predicting which patients with dysthymic or depressive temperament will experience brief reversible switches into hypomania.

In *bipolar III ½*, periods of excitement and depression are so closely linked with substance and alcohol abuse that it is not easy to decide whether these periods would have occurred in the absence of such abuse (7). The occurrence of frequent affective shifts over many years in these patients is the key to differential diagnosis, especially if family history is positive for bipolar affective disorder. Research in this interface of bipolarity and stimulant and alcohol abuse is sorely needed. It is of great relevance for genetics and public health. Their tentative inclusion in the soft bipolar spectrum opens therapeutic opportunities (e.g., with anticonvulsants) for a very large universe of patients with "comorbid" bipolar and stimulant-alcohol features (53).

Bipolar IV: This category includes depressive states superimposed on a hyperthymic temperament. Familial bipolarity supports their inclusion in the bipolar spectrum (54). The prototypical presentation is that of a late onset (>50 years) anergic depressive episode necessitating multiple brief courses of antidepressants (none of which work beyond a few months), and subsequent development of an excited ("agitated") depressive mixed state with psychomotor restlessness, racing thoughts, and/or intense sexual excitement (6). History will often reveal that many of these individuals were extremely successful executives (usually male) with lifelong drive, ambition, high energy, confidence, and extroverted interpersonal skills. Unlike bipolar II, these hypomanic features do not occur as isolated brief episodes, but constitute the stable temperamental baseline of these hyperthymic depressions. I submit that it is this intrusion of an "unwelcome" depression into a hyperthymic temperament that gives rise to the mixed state. Clinically, this is an extremely dangerous condition, because hyperthymic individuals are intolerant of even low levels of depression, and poorly tolerate the affective dysfunction associated with a depressive mixed state. Many mysteries about suicide, and suicides that one reads about in the newspaper (such and such "extremely successful and happy person, who had everything, put the pistol in his mouth") may well belong to this category. These patients might be considered "narcissistic" in the DSM-IV Axis-II schema, but are better characterized as hyperthymic with the following *lifelong* features that are not episode bound, i.e., they are traits (32): upbeat and exuberant, articulate and jocular, overoptimistic and carefree, overconfident and boastful, high energy level, full of plans and improvident activities, versatile with broad interests, overinvolved and meddlesome, uninhibited and risk-taking, and an habitual short sleeper.

Thus far, I have documented a spectrum of affective manifestations with muted manic manifestations that merge into temperament. I have provided the justification for their inclusion within a broad bipolar spectrum beyond classic bipolar I. In our current nomenclature, because of lack of explicit characterization, many of these patients are likely to be considered "unipolar," "borderline," "substance-induced," or "psychopathic" (7,12,55). Instead, I have argued that their depressions are, in clinical reality, pseudounipolar (1,8). Although in referring to the muted, less-than-manic bipolar manifestations, we have employed the terminology of "soft bipolar" (6), types II–IV have actually received considerable "hard" research support (reviewed in Refs. 2,11).

DO RECURRENT "UNIPOLAR" DEPRESSIONS BELONG TO THE BIPOLAR SPECTRUM (TYPE V)?

High rates of recurrence are characteristic of patients who, during prospective observation, would switch to bipolar disorder. This is true for both bipolar I (56) and II (46) disorders. Family history is an external validator of bipolarity in these patients—even in the absence of discrete episodes of hypomania. These patients can be considered to be "phenotypically unipolar" and "genotypically bipolar" (1). That some apparently "unipolar" patients, having failed to respond to tricyclic antidepressants, but subsequently respond to lithium (57) can be interpreted to further support the foregoing formulation. It is indeed plausible that lithium augmentation in antidepressant-resistant unipolar depression refers to the same pseudounipolar subtype (6,58,59). Such patients are not only recurrent (5 episodes), but often display hypomanic features during depressive episodes (60). It would, therefore, be reasonable to expand the bipolar spectrum to include a type V.

OTHER PUTATIVE BIPOLAR SPECTRUM CONDITIONS

There probably also exist conditions within and beyond the spectrum outlined here, which are part of the broader bipolar terrain. Both the late Klerman (61) and, more recently, Noble Endicott (62) have written about these far outreaches of bipolarity. In the main, their categories are similar to the types I–V defined in by us (7), but without the operationalization provided by us. Ghaemi et al. (63) limit the "bipolar spectrum disorder" to all bipolars with subtle levels of bipolarity beyond bipolar I and II (i.e., pharmacologic hypomania, hyperthymic temperament, high depressive recurrence, antidepressant resistance). These are nearly identical to the terrain of bipolar types III and IV in the Akiskal–Pinto schema (7).

In our clinical experience (7), other putative bipolar conditions include atypical and seasonal depressions without discernible hypomanic states, but which exhibit periodicity. Some bulimic states (64) might represent a variant from this seasonal pattern; other patients may present with episodic obsessive–compulsive symptoms, periodic states of irritability or acute suicidal crises in the absence of a fully defined affective syndrome. Many paraphilias and so-called "sexual addictions" with periodic exacerbations are also at some level bipolar; perhaps related to these are other impulse-controlled disorders such as gambling (see Ref. 65). Finally, there are patients with episodic neurasthenic or sleep complaints, and those with non -menstrually related recurrent brief depressions (7). This is not an exhaustive list, but conditions that should be further studied as putative bipolar variants. Their relationship to bipolar disorder is not presently established.

It is beyond the scope of this paper to discuss the complex interplay of attention-deficit hyperactivity disorder (ADHD) and juvenile bipolarity. According to some authorities, one pathway to juvenile bipolar disorder is childhood hyperactivity. This is not to say that childhood hyperactivity is an obligatory precursor of bipolar disorder—nor that all cases of ADHD are bipolar—but to suggest that up to a third of juvenile onsets of bipolar disorder give history of some form of "hyper-activity" prior to the more overt bipolar manifestations. The interested reader may refer to the work of Biederman et al. (66) at Harvard. Here again, the proposed link of ADHD and bipolar spectrum disorders is tentative and in need of further investigation. Suffice it to say that these issues in the interface of bipolarity and ADHD are not mere constructs developed in the research literature as a byproduct of overlapping definitions of the disorders in their operational format. Clinical observation (67) supports the notion of bipolar-ADHD as a putative spectrum childhood subtype of bipolar disorder.

CRITIQUE OF THE BIPOLAR SPECTRUM

The concept of the "bipolar spectrum" is a hot topic in both clinical psychiatry and in research into the genetic origins of bipolar disorder. It can, however, be criticized on the grounds that it is largely a concept driven by clinical-therapeutic considerations. For instance, we have elsewhere presented the thesis that broad concepts of bipolarity help in identifying patients on the border of bipolar disorder who might be destabilized by antidepressants and could potentially benefit from therapeutic interventions developed for classical bipolar disorder (7).

As far as genetic investigations, some authorities believe that it would be easier to identify the molecular basis of the illness by focusing on the "hard core" euphoric manic phenotype (68), while others (28) contend that the most prevalent expressions of bipolar disorder belong to a "soft spectrum," the inclusion of which in genetic investigations would facilitate in the discovery of the oligogenic basis for bipolarity (9).

A recent commentary by Baldessarini (69) has critiqued the broadening of the concept of bipolar disorder on methodological grounds, fearing that the dilution of the classical concept would introduce too much heterogeneity to be manageable in research. It is nonetheless noteworthy that essentially all authors cited by Baldessarini throughout history (Table 3) who have described the phenomenology of this

Table 3 Historical Evolution of the Bipolar Concept[a]

150 AD	Aretaeus	Melancholia→mania
1854	Falret and Baillarger	Circular and double insanity
1867	Griesinger	Unitary mental disorder
1882	Kahlbaum	Cyclothymia
1899	Kraepelin	Manic-depressive psychosis
1960s	Leonhard, Angst, Winokur and Clayton	Unipolar–bipolar distinction
1976	Dunner et al	Bipolar II
1976	Mendels	Pseudounipolar depression
1978	Pope and Lipinski	"Schizophrenic" symptoms in MDP
1983	Akiskal	Bipolar Spectrum
1990	Goodwin and Jamison	Manic-depressive illness

[a]Abstracted from Ref. 69, deleting all but those with focus on nosologic and phenomenologic aspects.

Table 5 Primary Affective Diagnoses in 102 Patients in a Community Health Center

Diagnoses	Percentage	Total (%)
Bipolar I	18	50
Bipolar II	18	
Bipolar III	9	
Cyclothymia	5	
Unipolar	44	50
Dysthymia	8	

Source: Summarized from Ref. 6.

questionnaire that is most relevant to the classic end of the spectrum, has reported a community prevalence of 3.7%. The various studies summarized in Table 4 suggest a modal figure of 5%.

The definition of bipolar II in the foregoing studies deviates from that in DSM-IV (16), which is based on a hypomania threshold of 4 or more days. As discussed earlier, there is now substantial evidence (reviewed in Ref. 9) that depressions with hypomania of 2 or more days belong to the bipolar spectrum: The validation of the 2-day threshold is based on age at onset, rate of depressive recurrence, rates of atypical depressive features and, most importantly, bipolar family history. The varying rates of bipolarity in the population are largely due to the varying definitions of bipolar II and related subthreshold bipolar conditions.

How about clinical populations? In response to inquiries by the American Psychiatric Association's whether DSM-III (—) covered all affectively ill patients in clinical practice, we were the first to report (6) UP:BP ratio of 1:1 from a mental health center (6); it is noteworthy too that BP-II at least as prevalent as BP-I. These data are shown in Table 5. There is now converging data from many studies both in the U.S. and Europe, which indicate that 30–70% of patients presenting with major depressive episodes meet criteria for bipolar II (reviewed in Ref. 9). The systematic French National Study EPIDEP has the virtue of reporting national data from four different regions of France, in which 40% of major depressives were diagnosed as bipolar II (82). If we were to add, upon further examination of the data (83), the remaining types (II 1/2-IV) in the EPIDEP study, the rate of bipolarity would be 65% (Table 6). In the Ravenna–San Diego Collaborative Study, the full spectrum of bipolar II and beyond, including depressive mixed states, yielded a rate of 70% (60).

As far as studies on subclinical bipolar temperaments, the best data derives from an Italian national interview study of "clinically well" students (84), which

Table 6 Bipolar Spectrum Subtypes in the French EPIDEP Study ($n = 493$)[a]

	N	Percentage
Bipolar I	41	8.4
Bipolar II	61	12.4
Bipolar II-½	164	33.5
Bipolar III	28	5.7
Bipolar IV	22	4.5
Total	319	64.5

[a]Validation by bipolar family history (83).

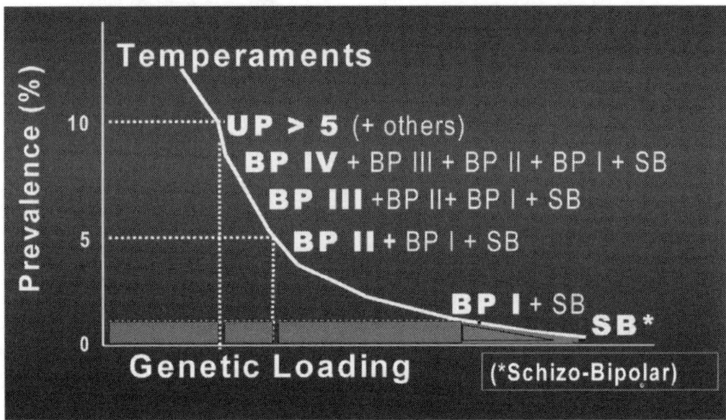

Figure 2 Community prevalence of bipolar phenotypes as a function of genetic loading.

have revealed a relatively high prevalence of those with extreme scores (based on *z*-scores higher than the 2 standard deviation) on such trait measures as cyclothymia (6.3%), depressiveness (3.6%), and irritable temperament (2.2%). Cyclothymia is the most validated temperament whose relevance to bipolar disorder is validated by prospective follow-up and family history (12). If we add the cyclothymia rate of 6.3% in the student population (84) to the modal figures of 5%, we obtain an estimated population rate of 10–11% for the bipolar trait [nearly identical to the broad figure reported by Angst et al. (70)]. The foregoing considerations suggest that bipolar disorder extends from the relatively rare severe psychotic disorder to a highly prevalent cyclothymic disposition which is subclinical (Fig. 2).

FAMILIAL-GENETIC CONSIDERATIONS

In family studies of bipolar disorder, the most common phenotype in first-degree family members is depression (85). Adoption studies have demonstrated that the biological kin of patients with bipolar disorder raised by parents without affective illness, exhibit milder and "neurotic" forms of depression (86). Most importantly, monozygotic cotwins of manic-depressant patients are not only concordant for the strict phenotype of the illness, but they also exhibit an excess of schizophrenoform psychoses, as well as "moody persons" (87). Such data suggest that the genotype of the illness extends from extremely psychotic mania that requires hospitalization to temperamental dysregulation that remains largely ambulatory and untreated.

Molecular genetic studies have also shown some overlap between schizophrenia and bipolar disorder (88), further supported by convergent functional genomics (89). Another study has shown overlap between bipolar II and panic disorder (50). These provocative data suggest that the dysregulation in bipolar disorder extends beyond mood disturbance in the narrow sense, to include activation into psychosis, and even broader affective dysregulation which subsumes anxiety (90). Putative molecular bases for such broad dysregulation have been reported (91,92). Excellent theoretical discussion on putative oligogenic contributions to bipolarity can be seen in reviews by Gershon (88) and Kelsoe (28).

Referring back to Figure 2, we can better place epidemiologic and genetic considerations into graphic representation, for a model of bipolar spectrum which at the one extreme subsumes relatively rare forms of schizobipolar and bipolar I disorders, and at the other extreme, subsumes the large terrain of soft bipolarity, bipolar II with 4- and 2-day hypomanias, as well as recurrent depressions, plus the cyclothymic trait. The concept of a clinical spectrum of bipolar phenotypes—as plotted in Figure 2 as a function of oligogenic loading—does not rule out the possibility of variants within the spectrum resulting from distinct specific genes.

In examining the juvenile offspring and first-degree kin of bipolar adults in a mood clinic (36), we encounter more affected cases with MDDs, dysthymia and mixed states than full-blown mania. Prospective follow-up of such juvenile patients without clear-cut bipolarity often reveals transformation into bipolar II and bipolar I disorders in many, but not all offspring. Such data are best understood in a spectrum model. They have tremendous importance in preventive psychiatry. This conclusion is further buttressed by the fact that many such offspring display cyclothymic moodiness before progressing to clinical bipolarity. New data in support for such a concept are being developed in pediatric bipolarity (93).

CLINICAL CONSIDERATIONS

Table 6 summarizes the clinical validating principles (94) that can be used to establish the bipolar nature of an affective condition (95). Of these, the most important are family history, temperament, and switching. The presence of a bipolar temperament (e.g., cyclothymia) is an indication of an early-onset disorder, which is most often familial (96). The evidence for the remaining principles is documented elsewhere (2,9). Although still controversial, and while DSM-IV (5) continues to deny it, there is actually extensive international evidence (reviewed in Refs. 9,52), that switches into hypomania and mania occurring on antidepressants strongly indicate a bipolar diathesis. In clinical practice, pending further clarification through follow-up, we recommend that such patients be provisionally classified as bipolar III.

On the basis of the foregoing validating principles and an emerging literature (summarized in Ref. 97), the following "depressive" clinical presentations should be considered as putative soft bipolar conditions: Depression + intraepisode "hypomania" (depressive mixed state); agitated depression (severe depressive mixed state); postpartum depression, especially those with psychotic features; atypical depression and/or episodic neurasthenic complaints; refractory depression (failed antidepressant from three different classes); depression with bipolar family history (pseudounipolar depression); and depression with erratic personality disorder(s). The conditions described are often misconstrued as recurrent major depressive in nature. The author submits that they have affinity to bipolar disorder, yet surprisingly they are not listed in the bipolar NOS category in DSM-IV. There is also recent evidence that anxious inhibition may partly replace the depressive phase in certain patients with hyperthymic and cyclothymic tendencies, resulting in social phobic, panic, and obsessive–compulsive variants of bipolarity (48,98); these patients are often considered to have anxious depressions with mood instability. This is an area of great public health significance, because these pseudounipolar patients with soft bipolar features may develop mixed states with suicidal impulses, unless prevented by mood stabilizers (67). We submit that the recent FDA warning about suicidality on SSRIs pertains to these activated yet labile depressive (99) patients. This is not an indictment of SSRIs, which have led to a worldwide decline in suicidality (100), but to highlight the importance of avoiding antidepressant monotherapy in soft bipolar patients.

Such patients typically require mood stabilizer or atypical antipsychotic augmentation (59,101). This is an area that would benefit from more rigorous studies to demonstrate the efficacy of mood stabilizer augmentation in such patients.

CONCLUDING REMARKS

The concept of a bipolar spectrum is a heuristic concept that is rooted in the descriptive clinical tradition, and is validated by a new wave of epidemiologic studies demonstrating the high prevalence of subthreshold cases, familial aggregation studies, high-risk offspring studies, analysis of monozygotic "discordance," and molecular linkage studies. Family history for bipolar disorder, cyclothymic temperament, and switching on antidepressants represent the most useful validating principles in clinical practice when examining depressed patients without antecedent frank hypomania. Early age at onset, postpartum onset, mixity, high rate of recurrence, cyclicity, and seasonality can also serve as clinical validators (Table 7). Specific comorbid patterns of depression with alcohol and stimulant abuse, as well as that of social phobic, panic and OCD should also raise clinical suspicion of a bipolar diathesis. The thrust of arguments made in this chapter suggests that the clinical management of affective disorders will not improve significantly until there is recognition that many, if not most, depressions presenting clinically are, at some level, bipolar (102). As counterintuitive as this suggestion might be, there is increasing evidence in its support summarized in this chapter. This might even be true for primary care settings, where one out of three depressives might be pseudounipolar (103).

This exercise in limiting unipolarity and expanding bipolarity is in the service of treatment, especially the necessity of avoiding antidepressants or antidepressant monotherapy in such patients. The art of clinically managing these patients goes much beyond anticonvulsant concoctions. It requires the art of caring for temperamentally restless—albeit charming—individuals with troubled lives. This topic cannot be covered in the space provided here, but for those who believe that a good prognosis illness has turned into a poor prognosis illness (104). We would suggest that a major reason why this has happened is because the field of psychiatry—in the current "managed care" climate—has abandoned the mood clinics that used to provide access to sophisticated clinical care for the affectively ill and their families (105).

Table 7 Course, Clinical, and Familial Characteristics Suggestive of Bipolar Spectrum Disorders

Early age of onset
High recurrence (at least five episodes)
Rapid onset and offset of episodes
Postpartum depression
Marked seasonality
Atypical features (hypersomnia and overeating)
Hostile and labile mood
Mixity (isolated hypomanic symptoms during depression)
Cycling on antidepressants
Refractoriness (at least three antidepressants from different classes)
Bipolar family history
Family history of mood disorder in three generations

Table 8 Validating the Bipolar Spectrum

Clinical--phenomenological
Prospective follow-up
Familial
Oligogenic model
Ethological model
Therapeutic considerations
Public health significance

Source: Summarized from Ref. 102.

It would be instructive to sign off where we started: on the necessity of incorporating temperament into our conceptual frame of affective disorders. This is not just a terminological preference in a nosological sense. I submit that much of what goes into Axis II is pejorative to patients and generates a distance—if not blatant countertransference—between patient and doctor. Temperament, which defines the long-term, unstable underpinnings of the affective spectrum presented here, also encompasses much of what is positive and desirable about the person suffering from this spectrum of disorders. Temperament helps in the affective bond between patient and doctor, and thereby makes caring possible.

The positive traits of bipolar patients are even more characteristic of their first-degree relatives (106–110). The presence of achievement, success, and creativity in the "well" relatives of bipolar patients indicates that the "dilute" genotypes of the illness may have evolved to subserve adaptive functions such as exploration and risk taking. Such an evolutionary perspective (102,110) represents the ultimate theoretical underpinnings of the concept of bipolar spectrum. The temperaments themselves, particularly the cyclothymic and hyperthymic, may further subserve such functions as interpersonal charm and sexual selection, and territoriality. Table 8 summarizes the validating multidimensional approach to bipolarity (102), in which the author heralds a new paradigm (111).

REFERENCES

1. Akiskal HS. The bipolar spectrum: new concepts in classification and diagnosis. In: Grinspoon L, ed. Psychiatry Update: The American Psychiatric Association Annual Review. Vol. 2. Washington, DC: American Psychiatric Press, 1983:271–292.
2. Akiskal HS. Classification, diagnosis and boundaries of bipolar disorders. In: Maj M, Akiskal HS, Lopez-Ibor JJ, Sartorius N, eds. Bipolar Disorder. London: John Wiley & Sons, 2002:1–52.
3. Akiskal HS, ed. Bipolarity: Beyond Classic Mania. WB Saunders, Psychiatric Clinics of North America, September 1999.
4. World Health Organization. The ICD-10 Classification of Mental and Behavioural Disorders. Geneva: World Health Organization, 1992.
5. American Psychiatric Association. Diagnostic and Statistical Manual of Mental Disorders, Ed. 4 Text Revision (DSM-IV-TR). Washington DC: APA Press, 2000.
6. Akiskal HS, Mallya G. Criteria for the "soft" bipolar spectrum: treatment implications. Psychopharmacol Bull 1987; 23:68–73.
7. Akiskal HS, Pinto O. The evolving bipolar spectrum: prototypes I, II, III, IV. Psychiatr Clin N Am 1999; 22:517–534.

8. Akiskal HS. The prevalent clinical spectrum of bipolar disorders: Beyond DSM-IV. J Clin Psychopharmacol 1996; 16(suppl 1):4s–14s.
9. Akiskal HS, Bourgeois ML, Angst J, Post R, Moller HJ, Hirschfeld RMA. Re-evaluating the prevalence of and diagnostic composition within the broad clinical spectrum of bipolar disorders. J Affect Disord 2000; 59(suppl 1):5s–30s.
10. Akiskal HS. The bipolar spectrum in psychiatric and general medical practice. Primary Psychiatry 2004; 11:35–40.
11. Akiskal HS, ed. Validating the Bipolar Spectrum. J Affect Disord 2003;73:1–205.
12. Akiskal HS, Djenderedjian AH, Rosenthal RH, Khani MK. Cyclothymic disorder: validating criteria for inclusion in the bipolar affective group. Am J Psychiatry 1977; 134:1227–1233.
13. Akiskal HS, Khani MK, Scott-Strauss A. Cyclothymic temperamental disorders. Psychiatr Clin N Am 1979; 2:527–554.
14. Feighner JP, Robins E, Guze SB, Woodruff RA Jr, Winokur G, Munoz R. Diagnostic criteria for use in psychiatric research. Arch Gen Psychiatry 1972; 26:57–63.
15. Kendell RE. The classification of depressions: a review of contemporary confusion. Br J Psychiatry 1976; 129:15–28.
16. American Psychiatric Association. Diagnostic and Statistical Manual of Mental Disorders. 3rd ed. Washington, DC: American Psychiatric Association Press, 1980.
17. Levitt AJ, Joffe RT, Ennis J, MacDonald C, Kutcher SP. The prevalence of cyclothymia in borderline personality disorder. J Clin Psychiatry 1990; 51:335–339.
18. Lish JD, Dime-Meenan S, Whybrow PC, Price RA, Hirschfeld RM. The National Depressive and Manic-Depressive Association (DMDA) survey of bipolar members. J Affect Disord 1994; 31:281–294.
19. Ghaemi SN, Boiman EE, Goodwin FK. Diagnosing bipolar disorder and the effect of antidepressants: a naturalistic study. J Clin Psychiatry 2000; 61(10):804–808.
20. Aretaeus of Cappadoccia. The Extant Works of Aretaeus the Cappadocian. London: Sydenham Society, 1856.
21. Falret JP. Mémoire sur la folie circulaire. Bull Acad Natl Méd 1854; 19:382–415.
22. Baillarger J. Notes sur un genre de folie dont les accès sont caractérisés par deux périodes régulières, l'une de dépression, l'autre d'excitation. Bull Acad Natl Méd 1854; 19:340.
23. Pichot P. [Circular insanity 150 years on]. Bull Acad Natl Med 2004; 188:275–284.
24. Akiskal HS. [From circular insanity (in double form) to the bipolar spectrum: the chronic tendency for depressive recurrence]. Bull Acad Natl Med 2004; 188:285–296.
25. Sedler MJ. Falret's discovery: the origin of the concept of bipolar affective illness (Trans. by Sedler MJ and Dessain EC). Am J Psychiatry 1983; 140:1127–1133.
26. Kraepelin E. Manic-Depressive Insanity and Paranoia. Edinburgh: E&S Livingstone, 1921.
27. Kretschmer E: Physique and Character. London: Kegan, Paul, Trench, Trubner and Co. Ltd., 1936.
28. Kelsoe JR. Arguments for the genetic basis of the bipolar spectrum. Affect Disord 2003; 73:183–197.
29. Erfurth A, Gerlach AL, Michael N, Boenigk I, Hellweg I, Signoretta S, Akiskal K, Akiskal HS. Distribution and gender effects of the subscales of a German version of the temperament autoquestionnaire brief TEMPS-M in a university student population. J Affect Disord 2005; 85:53–69.
30. Karam EG, Mneimenh Z, Solamoun M, Akiskal K, Akiskal HS. Psychometric properties of the Lebanese-Arabic TEMPS-A: a national epidemiologic study. J Affect Disord. In press.
31. Schneider K. Psychopathic Personalities. Springfield, IL: Charles C. Thomas, 1958.
32. Akiskal HS. Delineating irritable and hyperthymic variants of the cyclothymic temperament. J Personal Disord 1992; 6:326–342.

33. Akiskal HS. Temperament and Mood Disorders. Harvard Mental Health Letter 2000; 16, Article #175.
34. Akiskal HS, Akiskal K. Cyclothymic, hyperthymic and depressive temperaments as subaffective variants of mood disorders. In: Tasman A, Riba MB, eds. Annual Review. Vol. 11. Washington, DC: American Psychiatric Press, 1992:43–62.
35. Akiskal HS. The temperamental foundations of mood disorders. In: Mundt CH, ed. Interpersonal Factors in the Origin and Course of Affective Disorders. London: Gaskell, 1996:3–30.
36. Akiskal HS, Downs J, Jordan P, Watson S, Daugherty D, Pruitt DB. Affective disorders in the referred children and younger siblings of manic-depressives: mode of onset and prospective course. Arch Gen Psychiatry 1985; 42:996–1003.
37. Perugi G, Akiskal HS, Micheli C, Musetti L, Paiano A, Quilici C, Rossi L, Cassano GB. Clinical subtypes of bipolar mixed states: validating a broader European definition in 143 cases. J Affect Disord 1997; 43:169–180.
38. Akiskal HS, Hantouche E, Bourgeois M, Azorin JM, Sechter D, Allilaire JF, Lancrenon S, Fraud JP, Chatenet-Duchene L. Gender, temperament and the clinical picture in dysphoric mixed mania: findings from a French national study (EPIMAN). J Affect Disord 1998; 50:175–186.
39. Dunner DL, Gershon ES, Goodwin FK. Heritable factors in the severity of affective illness. Biol Psychiatry 1976; 11:31–42.
40. Akiskal HS, Hantouche EG, Lancrenon S. Bipolar II with and without cyclothymic temperament: "dark" and "sunny" expressions of soft bipolarity. J Affect Disord 2003; 73:49–57.
41. Akiskal HS, Rosenthal RH, Rosenthal TL, Kashgarian M, Khani MK, Puzantian VR. Differentiation of primary affective illness from situational, symptomatic, and secondary depressions. Arch Gen Psychiatry 1979; 36:635–643.
42. Wicki W, Angst J. The Zurich Study. X. Hypomania in a 28- to 30-year-old cohort. Eur Arch Psychiatry Clin Neurosci 1991; 240:339–348.
43. Benazzi F, Akiskal HS. Refining the evaluation of bipolar II: beyond the strict SCID-CV guidelines for hypomania. J Affect Disord 2003; 73:33–38.
44. Angst J, Gamma A. A new bipolar spectrum concept: a brief review. Bipolar Disord 2002; 4(suppl 1):11–14.
45. Judd LL, Akiskal HS, Schettler PJ, Coryell W, Endicott J, Maser JD, Solomon DA, Leon AC, Keller MB. A prospective investigation of the natural history of the long-term weekly symptomatic status of bipolar II disorder. Arch Gen Psychiatry 2003; 60: 261–269.
46. Akiskal HS, Maser JD, Zeller P, Endicott J, Coryell W, Keller M, Warshaw M, Clayton P, Goodwin FK. Switching from "unipolar" to bipolar II: an 11-year prospective study of clinical and temperamental predictors in 559 patients. Arch Gen Psychiatry 1995; 52: 114–123.
47. Savino M, Perugi G, Simonini E, Soriani A, Cassano GB, Akiskal HS. Affective comorbidity in panic disorder: is there a bipolar connection? J Affect Disord 1993; 28: 155–163
48. Perugi G, Akiskal HS, Ramacciotti S, Nassini S, Toni C, Milanfranchi A, Musetti L. Depressive comorbiduty of panic, social phobic and obsessive–compulsive disorders: is there a bipolar II connection? Psychiatr Res 1999; 33:53–61.
49. Young LT, Cooke RG, Robb JAC, Levitt AJ, Joffe RT. Anxious and non-anxious bipolar disorder. J Affect Disord 1993; 29:49–52.
50. MacKinnon DF, Xu J, McMahon FJ, Simpson SG, Stine OC, McInnis MG, DePaulo JR. Bipolar disorder and panic disorder in families: an analysis of chromosome 18 data. Am J Psychiatry 1998; 155:829–831.
51. Rosenthal TL, Akiskal HS, Scott-Strauss A, Rosenthal RH, David M. Familial and developmental factors in characterological depressions. J Affect Disord 1981; 3:183–192.

52. Akiskal HS. Validating antidepressant-associated hypomania (bipolar III): a systematic comparison with spontaneous hypomania (bipolar II). J Affect Disord 2003; 73:65–74.
53. Camacho A, Akiskal HS, Proposal for a bipolar-stimulant spectrum: temperament, diagnostic validation and therapeutic outcomes with mood stabilizers. J Affect Disord 2005; 85:217–230.
54. Cassano GB, Akiskal HS, Savino M, Musetti L, Perugi G. Proposed subtypes of bipolar II and related disorders: with hypomanic episodes (or cyclothymia) and with hyperthymic temperament. J Affect Disord 1992; 26:127–140.
55. Deltito J, Martin L, Riefkohl J, Austria B, Kissilenko A, Corless C, Morse P. Do patients with borderline personality disorder belong to the bipolar spectrum? J Affect Disord 2001; 67:221–228.
56. Akiskal HS, Walker PW, Puzantian VR, King D, Rosenthal TL, Dranon M. Bipolar outcome in the course of depressive illness: phenomenologic, familial, and pharmacologic predictors. J Affect Disord 1983; 5:115–128.
57. Kupfer DJ, Pickar D, Himmelhoch JM, Detre TP. Are there two types of unipolar depression? Arch Gen Psychiatry 1975; 32:866–871.
58. Akiskal HS. A proposed clinical approach to chronic and "resistant" depressions: evaluation and treatment. J Clin Psychiatry 1985; 46(Sec. 2):32–36.
59. Hantouche EG, Akiskal HS, Lancrenon S, Chatenêt-Duchêne L. Mood stabilizer augmentation in apparently "unipolar" MDD: predictors of response in the naturalistic French national EPIDEP study. J Affect Disord 2005; 84:243–249.
60. Akiskal HS, Benazzi F. Family history validation of the bipolar nature of depressive mixed states. J Affect Disord 2003; 73:113–122.
61. Klerman GL. The spectrum of mania. Compr Psychiatry 1981; 22:11–20.
62. Endicott NA. Psychophysiological correlates of 'bipolarity'. J Affect Disord 1989; 17: 47–56.
63. Ghaemi SN, Ko JY, Goodwin FK. "Cade's disease" beyond: misdiagnosis antidepressant use a proposed definition for bipolar spectrum disorder. Can J Psychiatry 2002; 47: 125–134.
64. McElroy SL, Kotwal R, Keck PE Jr, Akiskal HS. Comorbidity of bipolar and eating disorders: distinct or related disorders with shared dysregulations? J Affect Disord. In press.
65. McElroy SL, Pope HG Jr, Keck PE Jr, Hudson JI, Phillips KA, Strakowski SM. Are impulse–control disorders related to bipolar disorder? Compr Psychiatry 1996; 37: 229–240.
66. Biederman J, Mick E, Faraone SV, Spencer T, Wilens TE, Wozniak J. Pediatric mania: a developmental subtype of bipolar disorder? Biol Psychiatry 2000; 48:458–466.
67. Dilsaver SC, Henderson-Fuller S, Akiskal HS. Occult mood disorders in 104 consecutively presenting children referred for the treatment of attention-deficit/hyperactivity disorder in a community mental health clinic. J Clin Psychiatry 2003; 64:1170–1176.
68. Duffy A, Grof P. Psychiatric diagnoses in the context of genetic studies of bipolar disorder. Bipolar Disord 2001; 3:270–275.
69. Baldessarini R. A plea for integrity of the bipolar disorder concept. Bipolar Disord 2000; 2:3–7.
70. Angst J, Gamma A, Benazzi F, Ajdacic V, Eich D, Rossler W. Toward a re-definition of subthreshold bipolarity: epidemiology proposed criteria for bipolar-II minor bipolar disorders hypomania. J Affect Disord 2003; 73:133–146.
71. Paris J. Borderline or bipolar? Distinguishing borderline personality disorder from bipolar spectrum disorders. Harv Rev Psychiatry 2004; 12:140–145.
72. Akiskal HS. Demystifying borderline personality: critique of the concept and unorthodox reflections on its natural kinship with the bipolar spectrum. Acta Psychiatr Scand 2004; 110:401–407.

73. Akiskal HS, Yerevanian BI, Davis GC, King D, Lemmi H. The nosologic status of borderline personality: clinical and polysomnographic study. Am J Psychiatry 1985; 142:192–198.
74. Regier DA, Boyd JH, Burke JD Jr, Rae DS, Myers JK, Kramer M, Robins LN, George LK, Karno M, Locke BZ. One-month prevalence of mental disorders in the United States. Based on five epidemiologic catchment area sites. Arch Gen Psychiatry 1988; 45:977–986.
75. Kessler RC, McGonagle KA, Zhao S, Nelson CB, Hughes M, Eshleman S, Wittchen HU, Kendler KS. Lifetime and 12-month prevalence of DSM-III-R psychiatric disorders in the United States. Results from the National Comorbidity Survey. Arch Gen Psychiatry 1994; 51:8–19.
76. Weissman MM, Bland RC, Canino GJ, Faravelli C, Greenwald S, Hwu HG, Joyce PR, Karam EG, Lee CK, Lellouch J, Lepine JP, Newman SC, Rubio-Stipec M, Wells JE, Wickramaratne PJ, Wittchen H, Yeh EK. Cross-national epidemiology of major depression and bipolar disorder. J Am Med Assoc 1996; 276:293–299.
77. Lewinsohn PM, Klein DN, Seeley JR. Bipolar disorders in a community sample of older adolescents: prevalence, phenomenology, comorbidity, and course. J Am Acad Child Adolesc Psychiatry 1995; 34:454–563.
78. Szadoczky E, Papp Z, Vitrai J, Rihmer Z, Furedi J. The prevalence of major depressive and bipolar disorders in Hungary. Results from a national epidemiologic survey. J Affect Disord 1998; 50:153–162.
79. Angst J. The emerging epidemiology of hypomania and bipolar II disorder. J Affect Disord 1998; 50:143–151.
80. Judd LL, Akiskal HS. The prevalence and disability of bipolar spectrum disorders in the U.S. population: reanalysis of the ECA database taking into account subthreshold cases. J Affect Disord 2002; 73:123–131.
81. Hirschfeld RM, Calabrese JR, Weissman MM, Reed M, Davies MA, Frye MA, Keck PE Jr, Lewis L, McElroy SL, McNulty JP, Wagner KD. Screening for bipolar disorder in the community. J Clin Psychiatry 2003; 64:53–59.
82. Hantouche EG, Akiskal HS, Lancrenon S, Allilaire JF, Sechter D, Azorin JM, Bourgeois M, Fraud JP, Châtenet-Duchêne L. Systematic clinical methodology for validating bipolar-II disorder: Data in mid-stream from a French national multisite study (EPIDEP). J Affect Disord 1998; 50:163–173.
83. Akiskal HS, Hantouche EG, Allilaire JF, Akiskal KK. Validation of the new bipolar spectrum: overview of the phenomenology and the relative prevalence of clinical subtypes in the French National EPIDEP Study. J Affect Disord In press.
84. Placidi GF, Signoretta S, Liguori A, Gervasi R, Maremmani I, Akiskal HS. The semi-structured affective temperament interview (TEMPS-I): reliability and psychometric properties in 1010 14–26 year students. J Affect Disord 1998; 47:1–10.
85. Gershon ES, Hamovit J, Guroff JJ, Dibble E, Leckman JF, Sceery W, Targum SD, Nurnberger JI Jr, Goldin LF, Bunney WE Jr. A family study of schizoaffective, bipolar I, bipolar II, unipolar and control probands. Arch Gen Psychiatry 1982; 39:1157–1167.
86. Mendlewicz J, Rainier JD. Adoption study supporting genetic transmission in manic-depressive illness. Nature 1977; 268:327–329.
87. Bertelsen A, Haovald B, Hauge M. A Danish twin study of manic-depressive disorders. Br J Psychiatry 1977; 130:330–351.
88. Gershon ES. Bipolar illness and schizophrenia as oligogenic disease: implications for the future. Biol Psychiatry 2000; 47:240–244.
89. Niculescu AB, Segal DS, Kuczenski R, Barrett T, Hauger RL, Kelsoe JR. Identifying a series of candidate genes for mania and psychosis: a convergent functional genomics approach. Physiol Genomics 2000; 4:83–91.
90. Akiskal HS, Azorin JM, Hantouche EG. Proposed multidimensional structure of mania: beyond the euphoric–dysphoric dichotomy. J Affect Disord 2003; 73:7–18.

91. Kelsoe JR, Spence MA, Loetscher E, Foguet M, Sadovnick AD, Remick RA, Flodman P, Khristich J, Mroczkowski-Parker Z, Brown JL, Masser D, Ungerleider S, Rapaport MH, Wishart WL, Luebbert H. A genome survey indicates a possible susceptibility locus for bipolar disorder on chromosome 22. Proc Natl Acad Sci USA 2001; 98:585–590.
92. Barrett TB, Hauger RL, Kennedy JL, Sadovnick AD, Remick RA, Keck PE, McElroy SL, Alexander M, Shaw SH, Kelsoe JR. Evidence that a single nucleotide polymorphism in the promoter of the G protein receptor kinase 3 gene is associated with bipolar disorder. Mol Psychiatry 2003; 8:546–557.
93. Geller B, Zimerman B, Williams M, Bolhofner K, Craney JL. Bipolar disorder at prospective follow-up of adults who had prepubertal major depressive disorder. Am J Psychiatry 2001; 158:125–127.
94. Robins E, Guze SB. Establishment of diagnostic validity in psychiatric illness: its application to schizophrenia. Am J Psychiatry 1970; 126:983–986.
95. Akiskal HS. Validating 'hard' and 'soft' phenotypes within the bipolar spectrum: continuity of discontinuity?. J Affect Disord 2003; 73:1–5.
96. Musetti L, Perugi G, Soriani A, Rossi VM, Cassano GB, Akiskal HS. Depression before and after age 65: a re-examination. Br J Psychiatry 1989; 155:330–336.
97. Akiskal HS. The dark side of bipolarity: detecting bipolar depression in its pleomorphic expressions. J Affect Disord. In press.
98. Himmelhoch JM. Social anxiety, hypomania and the bipolar spectrum: data, theory and clinical issues. J Affect Disord 1998; 50:203–213.
99. Akiskal HS, Benazzi F, Perugi G, Rihmer Z. The nosologic status of agitated "unipolar" depression: re-conceptualization as a depressive mixed state and implications for the antidepressant suicide controversy. J Affect Disord 2005; 85:245–258.
100. Rihmer Z. Decreasing national suicide rates-fact or fiction? World J Biol Psychiatry 2004; 5:55–56.
101. Ghaemi S. Long-term naturalistic treatment of depressive symptoms in bipolar illness with divalproex vs. lithium in the setting of minimal antidepressant use. J Affect Disord 2001; 65:281–287.
102. Akiskal HS. The Jean Delay Prize Paper: from dysthymia to the bipolar spectrum: bridging practice and research. Published address at the opening ceremony of the XII World Congress of Psychiatry in Yokahama, Japan, World Psychiatric Association, 2002.
103. Manning JS, Haykal RF, Connor PD, Akiskal HS. On the nature of depressive and anxious states in a family practice setting: the high prevalence of bipolar II and related disorders in a cohort followed longitudinally. Compr Psychiatry 1997; 38:102–108.
104. Goldberg J, Harrow M, eds. Bipolar Disorder: Outcome. Washington, DC: American Psychiatric Press, 1999.
105. Akiskal HS. "bipolar disorder: outcome." New Eng J Med 1999; 341:1861–1862
106. Akiskal HS, Akiskal K. Re-assessing the prevalence of bipolar disorders: clinical significance and artistic creativity. Psychiatr Psychobiol 1988; 3:29s–36s.
107. Richards R, Kinney DK, Lunde I, Benet M, Merzel AP. Creativity in manic-depressives, cyclothymes, their normal relatives, and control subjects. J Abnorm Psychol 1988; 97:281–288.
108. Coryell W, Endicott J, Keller M, Andreasen N, Grove W, Hirschfeld RM, Scheftner W. Bipolar affective disorder and high achievement: a familial association. Am J Psychiatry 1989; 146:983–988.
109. Verdoux H, Bourgeois M. Social class in unipolar and bipolar probands and relatives. J Affect Disord 1995; 33:181–187.
110. Akiskal HS. Dysthymia, cyclothymia and related chronic subthreshold mood disorders. In: Gelder M, Lopez-Ibor J, Andreasen N, eds. New Oxford Textbook of Psychiatry. London: Oxford University Press, 2000:736–749.
111. Akiskal HS. The bipolar spectrum—the shaping of a new paradigm. Curr Psychiatry Rev 2002; 4:1–3.

6

Bipolar Disorder in Children and Adolescents: Diagnosis, Epidemiology, and Clinical Course

Nga Anh Nguyen
Department of Psychiatry and Behavioral Sciences, University of Texas Medical Branch, Galveston, Texas, U.S.A.

Karen Dineen Wagner
Division of Child and Adolescent Psychiatry, Department of Psychiatry and Behavioral Sciences, University of Texas Medical Branch, Galveston, Texas, U.S.A.

INTRODUCTION

Pediatric bipolar disorder is a severe, chronic, and disabling illness that adversely impacts the child's psychosocial development including family, social, and academic functioning. Prevalence of bipolar disorder is about 1% in adolescents. Diagnosis of bipolar disorder in children and younger adolescents is a challenge, as symptoms may differ from those typically observed in late adolescence and adulthood. One main area of debate centers around the core mood symptom of pediatric mania. The presence of classic cardinal symptoms of euphoria and/or grandiosity characterized by distinctive developmental expressions is emphasized by one view, while another view stresses the distinctly assaultive and persistent irritability of pediatric mania. The non-episodic, continuous, rapid cycling pattern and the high rate of mixed mania pose additional diagnostic challenge, as clinicians may not be able to rely on the typical presence of mood swings to make the diagnosis. Frequent occurrence of comorbid disorders exhibiting symptom overlap with pediatric mania, such as attention deficit hyperactivity disorder (ADHD) may further complicate the diagnosis. Appreciation of current evidence combined with exercise of good clinical judgment may help clinicians optimally diagnose a substantial number of psychiatrically referred youths who present with a complex and severe symptomatology suggestive of bipolar disorder.

There is accumulating evidence that bipolar disorder has an early age of onset, yet there is ongoing confusion and controversy about the diagnosis of bipolar disorder in children, as its clinical presentation is different from that found in adult bipolar disorder. Leading experts disagree on its atypical phenomenology, and it is often difficult to differentiate developmental expressions of pediatric mania from normal development variants. Its symptom overlap with ADHD makes the differential diagnosis and the diagnosis of comorbidity challenging. This chapter addresses the epidemiology, diagnosis, comorbidity, differential diagnosis, and course of illness in pediatric bipolar disorder.

EPIDEMIOLOGY

There is a growing body of clinical information that challenges the previous view that pediatric bipolar disorder is very rare. However, there is a paucity of epidemiological studies on pediatric bipolar disorder. While lifetime prevalence of adult bipolar disorder is about 2%, lifetime prevalence of bipolar disorder in adolescents in a community sample is 1%; additionally, 5% of adolescents meet criteria for subsyndromal bipolar disorder (1,2). The prevalence of bipolar disorder in prepubertal children is unknown. However, Geller and Luby (3) suggested that the prevalence of bipolar disorder in children and adolescents is at least similar to that of adults, if not higher. This estimation was based on a variety of data, including case reports, inpatient studies, rates of mania switching in youths, and uninvestigated rate of bipolar disorder in offspring of undiagnosed bipolar parents. Furthermore, there was documentation of a "secular trend," by which onset of bipolar disorder becomes earlier with later years of birth (4), thus increasing the prevalence of pediatric bipolar disorder.

Bipolar disorder is common in psychiatrically referred youths. In a review of case reports of 157 children with severe psychopathology, it was found that 12% had been diagnosed with bipolar disorder, and another additional 12% who had a previous diagnosis of psychosis/schizophrenia met the diagnosis of bipolar disorder on careful rediagnosis (5). Other studies documented fairly substantial rates of prepubertal bipolar disorder in referred clinical samples, ranging from 6.3% (6) to 16% (7).

Demographic data on socioeconomic status and gender are scarce, but there are some findings on age of onset of bipolar disorder. As many as 59% of adults with bipolar disorder dated the onset of their first episode to younger than 18 years of age (8). Some adults with bipolar disorder dated their first manic episode back to as early as the age of 5 to 9 years (9).

DIAGNOSIS

The Diagnostic and Statistical Manual-IV (DSM-IV) (10) criteria for diagnosing bipolar disorder are the same for adults and children. Presence of discrete episodes of mania and depression that are interspersed by normal periods of euthymia is required. Manic mood of at least 1 week duration must be predominantly elated and/or irritable, and accompanied by at least three of the following associated symptoms: grandiosity, decreased need for sleep, pressured speech, flight of ideas, distractibility, increased goal-directed activities, and excessive engagement in pleasurable activities without regard of painful consequences.

Children and adolescents often do not meet full DSM-IV criteria for bipolar disorder, yet their severe and pervasive mood instability cause them to be seriously impaired in their daily functioning. They may not have clearly demarcated episodes of depression and mania, which can be mixed. The manic mood state may consist of extreme irritability rather than elation, with continuous and fast cycling as rapidly as daily.

To address the controversy about the diagnosis of pediatric bipolar disorder, a National Institute of Mental Health round table discussion on child and adolescent bipolar disorder (11) was convened to arrive at an agreement on a definition of child and adolescent bipolar disorder. The agreement was to include bipolar disorder I (manic episode meets full duration of 1 week) and bipolar disorder II (hypomania with shorter duration of $\geq$4 days), and the "working diagnosis" of bipolar disorder, NOS.

Recently, Leibenluft et al. (12) proposed four clinical phenotypes of pediatric bipolar disorder: one narrow, one broad, and two intermediate. In the narrow phenotype, the child meets full DSM-IV criteria for mania or hypomania, including the hallmark symptoms of elated mood and/or grandiosity, clear demarcation of episodes as well as episode duration. The two intermediate phenotypes are characterized by presence of clear mood episodes, with either shorter episode duration of 1–3 days (mania or hypomania NOS) or presence of irritable mood only ("irritable mania or hypomania"). The broad phenotype is characterized by non-episodic, chronic, and severe irritability, with symptoms of hyperarousal (insomnia, agitation, distractibility, racing thought, pressured speech, and intrusiveness), and mood and behavioral dysregulation (prolonged temper tantrum, verbal rage, and physical aggression). Further investigation is needed to test the reliability and validity of these proposed phenotypes, particularly to assess whether or not they differ in course of illness and treatment response. Determination of the ultimate course of children with subsyndromal clinical presentation in the broad phenotype is also of interest. It is not yet known whether the children will develop classic features of mania, continue with subsyndromal symptoms, or experience symptom remission.

The clinical presentation of bipolar disorder in prepubertal children and adolescents was investigated by Geller et al. (6). In a sample of 93 outpatient children with bipolar disorder I or II, ages 7–16 years, mean age of onset of bipolar disorder was 7 years, and episode duration was 3.5 years. Clinical symptoms consisted of mixed mania (55%), rapid cycling (87%), grandiose delusions (50%), and suicidality (25%). There was a high rate of elated mood (89%) as well as irritable mood (97%) and co-occurring irritable and elated mood (87%). These investigators stressed that classic cardinal symptoms of euphoria and/or grandiosity must be present to make the diagnosis of pediatric bipolar disorder.

Elated or expansive mood and grandiosity in pediatric mania may be difficult to detect, as there may be developmental differences in symptom expression in children. Geller et al. (13) provide guidelines for distinguishing normal from manic euphoria and grandiosity. In general, the behaviors associated with manic symptomatology are inappropriate to the situation and impair functioning. For example, parents and teachers often complain about the annoying and inappropriate behavior of their manic children, whose silly and clownish behavior is out of context and cannot be controlled, even with the threat of school suspension or grounding. Although children without mania can be silly at times, it is unlikely that their silliness persists to the point of becoming impervious to the consequence of a school suspension or grounding. Grandiosity in a manic child may present as bragging behavior. For example, an eight-year-old boy with mania, who bragged about being able to bicycle from Texas to Canada (while being fully aware of the thousands miles that separate the two locations) confidently took to the road on his bicycle, and had to be stopped by his mother. Although a normal eight-year-old boy may fantasize and brag about his bicycling feats, he is unlikely to act out this fantasy in real life to the point of putting himself in a high-risk situation. At times, grandiosity may also present itself as an oppositional defiant behavior, taking on what some described as "grandiose defiance" (14). A manic child, who refuses to comply with the teachers' instructions out of belief that they are "stupid" and beneath him, may be labeled as having "an attitude problem" (14). Thus, when faced with the chief complaint of "an attitude problem" in a child, clinicians may consider ruling out the possibility of manic grandiosity, and not automatically presume that it is a symptom of oppositional defiant disorder (ODD), or dismiss it as part of a rebellious phase of a normal child.

While Geller and colleagues emphasized that presence of the classic cardinal symptoms of elated mood and/or grandiosity is required for the diagnosis of pediatric mania, Biederman and colleagues stressed that severe irritability, and not euphoria, is its core mood characteristic. In a sample of 43 children with mania, 77% ($n = 33$) had irritability, only 5% ($n = 2$) had elated mood, and 9% ($n = 4$) had co-occurring irritable and elated mood, while the remaining 9% ($n = 4$) were reported to meet criteria for mania due to excessive energy or having too many thoughts (7).

While irritability is present in a variety of childhood disorders (ODD, conduct disorder (CD), and depression), the irritability of manic children exhibits clearly distinctive features. Parents and teachers report that these children "go off" with minor or no provocations, screaming, yelling obscenities, destroying and throwing things, punching holes in the walls, assaulting, and attacking teachers, peers, and family members. These "affective storms" (15) are difficult to calm down, may occur daily, and are prolonged, sometimes lasting hours. Between explosions, these children remain persistently irritable, causing others to live in the fear of the next unpredictable rage outburst.

Recent family study data provides some support for the view of distinctive severe irritability as the core mood symptom in pediatric bipolar disorder. In a sample of 60 children of bipolar parents, Chang et al. (16) found that classic symptoms of mania, such as elated mood, grandiosity, and decreased need for sleep, were not associated with either bilineal risk (one parent is bipolar, the other may have bipolar disorder or depression) or unilineal risk (one parent with bipolar disorder). Instead, mood and behavior dysregulation characterized by severity of irritable and depressed mood, rejection sensitivity, and lack of mood reactivity (negative mood unresponsive to external consolation) was associated with bilineal risk.

Mixed mania (symptoms of depression and mania are mixed, co-occurring simultaneously) occurs frequently in pediatric bipolar disorder, ranging from 55% (6) to 84% (14). Although mixed mania is considered atypical by adult standards, a meta-analysis of 17 adult studies documented that about 1 in 3 adults with bipolar disorder experienced mixed states (17). Adult mixed mania was found to be often associated with childhood onset bipolar disorder, severity and frequency of episodes, high comorbidity, and familial bipolar disorder (17). Thus, this form of adult bipolar disorder has been likened to pediatric bipolar disorder.

Some manic children are described by their parents as cycling in and out of irritable, sad, and/or silly mood throughout the day. This atypical cycling pattern of pediatric bipolar disorder has been investigated by Geller et al. (18). In its most rapid form, the ultradian rapid cycling type, cycling is essentially continuous, with a mean of four cycles per day, and episode frequency of at least 365 episodes per year. Thus, these children may be best described as showing abnormal moods almost every day, most of the day, for a majority of the time (14). This atypical presentation may be most confusing to the clinicians who rely on the classic requirement of a full week of euphoria or irritable mood for the diagnosis of mania.

A strong family history of bipolar disorder may be another potential clue to the diagnosis of pediatric bipolar disorder, as familial bipolar disorder was documented as a strong risk factor for pediatric bipolar disorder. Offspring of two bipolar parents were found to be at higher risk of developing bipolar disorder than those with one bipolar parent (74% vs. 27%, respectively) (19). In a study of 37 families with 60 offspring (mean age of 11 years) of at least one parent with bipolar disorder, Chang et al. (16) found that 51% of the offspring had a psychiatric disorder, most commonly ADHD (27%), followed by bipolar disorder (15%) and major depression (15%). It is important to recognize that, although children of bipolar parents are at risk for developing bipolar disorder, they may present more commonly with ADHD. Significantly, the earlier the onset of parental bipolar disorder, the greater risk for bipolar disorder in the offspring.

Clinicians should be aware that children with prepubertal major depression may subsequently develop bipolar disorder. In a follow-up study into young adulthood of a sample of 72 children with prepubertal major depression who had participated in a nortriptyline study, Geller et al. (20) found that, as compared to 28 normal controls, 33% of these children with prepubertal depression had developed bipolar I disorder compared to 0% of the normal controls. Bipolar spectrum disorder (bipolar I, II, and NOS) was significantly higher in the prepubertal major depression group than in the normal controls, 48% versus 7%, respectively.

There is the emergence of investigations in neuropathology and temperament precursors of pediatric bipolar disorder aimed at unraveling its diagnostic complexities. Neuroimaging findings showed significant increased rate of deep white matter hyperintensities in a group of bipolar adolescents as compared to a schizophrenic adolescent group and a healthy adolescent comparison group (21). This magnetic resonance imaging (MRI) finding is consistent with that reported in adults with bipolar disorder. With regard to temperament precursors to pediatric bipolar disorder, behavior disinhibition and emotional dysregulation have been proposed as early temperamental features (22). Behavior disinhibition is characterized by high approach, absence of restraint, disinhibited speech and action in novelty situations. Emotional dysregulation is conceptualized as intense, inconsolable, and uncontrollable negative emotional reaction to minor provocations.

DIFFERENTIAL DIAGNOSIS AND COMORBIDITY

Pediatric bipolar disorder is difficult to differentiate from several conditions with which it often shows high rates of comorbidity, including ADHD, CD, substance use disorder (SUD), and anxiety disorders. Additionally, symptom overlap of pediatric bipolar disorder with most of these conditions, especially ADHD, complicates the differential diagnosis and the diagnosis of comorbidity.

Differential Diagnosis and Comorbidity with ADHD

Geller et al. (6) investigated clinical characteristics that differentiate pediatric bipolar disorder from ADHD. Their outpatient sample consisted of 93 children with bipolar disorder (mean age, 10.9 years), 81 with ADHD (mean age, 9.7 years), and 94 community controls (mean age, 11 years). All of these children were given thorough assessment including interview with the child and mother, and review of diagnostic instruments, medical records, school documents, and agency reports. They found five mania-specific symptoms that clearly differentiated children with bipolar disorder from those with ADHD: elevated mood (89% vs. 14%), grandiosity (86% vs. 5%), flight of ideas/racing of thoughts (71% vs. 10%), decreased need for sleep (40% vs. 6%), and hypersexuality (43% vs. 6%). The symptoms that did not distinguish bipolar disorder from ADHD were distractibility and being hyperenergetic. Indeed, overlapping symptoms of distractibility and hyperactivity, as well as impulsivity, make the differential diagnosis between pediatric mania and ADHD a diagnostic challenge.

There are, however, subtle clinical clues that may help to differentiate hyperactivity and impulsivity in a manic child versus in a child with ADHD. A hyperactive child with ADHD is in constant motion, sometimes moving around aimlessly from the time he/she gets up until bedtime. By contrast, overactivity in a bipolar child often acutely emerges as a clear change from previous activity level, and is often expressed selectively during the goal-directed activities of the manic episode (7). For example, a manic child may be up most of the night to cook, clean the house, write poems, and do drawings. Or a child who is usually uninterested about homework is suddenly up all night and makes her friend stay up with her to study and to give one another pop quizzes, when there is no homework or any immediate need to study for a test.

Impulsivity in a child with ADHD may involve kicking a cat because it is on the way of his walking path, breaking a pencil out of frustration at not being able to solve math problems, or grabbing a peer's candy bar when hungry. It tends to be random, whereas impulsivity in pediatric mania usually involves pleasure-seeking behavior with potential for painful consequences. For example, a common scenario is that of a manic youth in a hypersexual arousal state who makes repeated sexual propositions to a classmate with complete disregard of a potential for being suspended and/or given a charge of sexual misconduct.

Rating scales have been reported to be useful screening tools to differentiate pediatric mania from ADHD. While the Conner's Rating Scales did not differentiate ADHD from mania, youths with mania scored significantly higher than those with ADHD on the Young Mania Rating Scale (23). They also scored higher than youths with ADHD on the Child Behavior Check List (CBCL) subscales of Delinquent Behavior, Aggressive Behavior, Anxious/Depressed, and Thought Problems (24).

Comorbidity of pediatric bipolar disorder with ADHD is very high in children, ranging from 87.1% (25) to an almost universal rate of 98% (7). It is lower in adolescent-onset ADHD. In a sample of 36 adolescents hospitalized with mania, 69% were found to have comorbid ADHD. In these adolescents with comorbid bipolar disorder and ADHD, onset of ADHD predated that of bipolar disorder by an average of 5.4 years (26). Thus, it has been suggested that ADHD may be the initial presentation of early onset pediatric bipolar disorder.

High comorbidity between two disorders characterized by symptom overlap generated a great deal of controversy, which was addressed by Milberger et al. (27). After using the subtraction method to correct for symptom overlap, they found that 80% of children with comorbid pediatric bipolar disorder and ADHD continued to meet bipolar disorder criteria, and all of them (100%) continued to meet ADHD criteria.

Family genetic studies also provide support for high comorbidity of pediatric bipolar disorder with ADHD, showing that these two disorders cosegregate in relatives of probands with comorbid bipolar disorder and ADHD (28).

There is also evidence that pediatric bipolar disorder comorbid with ADHD presents an exceptionally severe clinical picture characterized by high rate of psychiatric hospitalization, psychosis, comorbid depression, academic difficulties, and suicide (7). This severe morbidity may even lead to increased risk for mortality. Indeed, it was found that, compared to suicide attempters, adolescents who completed suicide had a significantly higher rate of mania comorbid with ADHD (29). Given the malignant course of illness of pediatric bipolar disorder comorbid with ADHD, failure to diagnose comorbid mania in a child with ADHD may result in treatment resistance and chronicity of course of illness (30).

There is also a bidirectional but asymmetrical overlap between pediatric bipolar disorder and ADHD. As opposed to the above-mentioned approximate rate of >90% of comorbid ADHD in primary pediatric bipolar disorder, the comorbid rate of bipolar disorder in youths with primary ADHD is only 23% (31). However, it was shown that in children with a primary diagnosis of ADHD, manic symptoms did not persist over time (32). This is an intriguing finding in light of the malignant course of the comorbid bipolar disorder and ADHD in children with the primary diagnosis of bipolar disorder.

Differential Diagnosis and Comorbidity with Conduct Disorder

Overlapping symptoms between pediatric mania and CD, especially impulsivity and hostility with involvement in high risk, antisocial, and/or aggressive behavior, pose a challenge in determining differential diagnosis vs. comorbidity.

There are subtle clues that help to make the differential diagnosis of pediatric bipolar disorder from CD. For example, while both manic children and children with CD may engage in shoplifting of expensive items, they differ in symptom presentation. Youths with CD often spend preparatory time in careful strategy planning, i.e., surveying traffic patterns and escape routes of the stores, in order to avoid being caught in action. Manic children engage in shoplifting typically under the spur of the moment, which coincides with the abrupt emergence of the disinhibition and grandiosity of the manic state, often appearing impervious to the possibility of being arrested by the police. Similarly, aggression in pediatric mania tends to be random, and emerges abruptly with the onset of irritability, whereas aggression in pediatric CD is typically predatory, organized, and goal directed (30), with insidious onset and progressive deterioration over time.

Accurate differential diagnosis of pediatric mania vs. pediatric CD has important clinical relevance and crucial impact on public health decision. Determining whether or not a child's shoplifting and fighting are secondary to the disinhibition of a manic state may guide the clinicians' decision to use or not to use pharmacological treatment, and/ or to direct the child to the mental health vs. the juvenile justice system.

While accurate differential diagnosis between pediatric bipolar disorder and CD is important, comorbidity of these two disorders is also well documented. Comorbidity of pediatric bipolar disorder with CD ranged from 41% to 74% in children with primary bipolar disorder, whereas it was 40% in children with primary CD (33). Kovacs and Pollock (34) reported 69% lifetime comorbidity and 54% episode comorbidity with CD in prepubertal children with bipolar disorder. Similarly, in a sample of 96 adolescent inpatients, 42% of the bipolar subgroup as opposed to only 27% of the entire sample was reported to have secondary CD (35).

Kovacs and Pollock (34) reported preliminary findings that differentiated bipolar children without comorbid CD ($n = 8$) from those with comorbid CD ($n = 18$). Pre-existing psychiatric condition was significantly different: Primary affective disorder was 38% versus 0% in the non-comorbid group vs. the comorbid group, respectively. Disruptive disorders (ADHD, CD) were 0% vs. 78% in the non-comorbid vs. comorbid groups, respectively. On follow-up, there was a trend for worse clinical outcome for the comorbid group, which had a somewhat higher number of psychiatric hospitalizations, more police contacts, and less "well time." Family history also differentiated the two groups. The non-comorbid group had a high rate of maternal mania and a relatively low rate of paternal substance abuse, whereas the comorbid group showed a trend for high rate of paternal substance abuse and a slightly increased rate of paternal antisocial personality disorder (ASPD). High rate of CD/ASPD (with and without mania) in relatives of youths with comorbid bipolar disorder and CD was also documented by Biederman et al. (36).

Overall, current evidence suggests that comorbid bipolar disorder may coexist in a substantial number of children with CD, confusing the clinical presentation, thus possibly contributing to reported failure to detect comorbid bipolar disorder in children with CD.

Differential Diagnosis and Comorbidity with Substance Use Disorder

Differential diagnosis between pediatric bipolar disorder and SUD is a task often encountered by clinicians. For example, one need to be aware that the cycling between the "highs" of amphetamine intoxication and the "lows" of the "crashes" of amphetamine withdrawal may simulate the rapid cycling of pediatric bipolar disorder (3). Violence may be secondary to cocaine intoxication as well as a manic state. Perceptual distortions may be present in both hallucinogen abuse and manic psychosis (37,38). A urine drug screen may help in the differential diagnosis, although many drugs of abuse may not have long enough half-life to be detected by urine screens.

While clinicians must make accurate differential diagnosis between pediatric bipolar disorder and SUD, it is important to recognize that there is a substantial and bidirectional overlap between the two disorders. It was reported that 39% of inpatient adolescents with primary bipolar disorder had comorbid SUD (26). Similarly, psychiatrically referred adolescent outpatients with primary SUD showed an increased risk for comorbid bipolar disorder, when compared to those without SUD (39). This bidirectional overlap has important clinical implications as to the importance of screening for both disorders when diagnosing youths with either bipolar disorder or CD.

Age of onset of bipolar disorder predicts risks for developing SUD. It was shown that youths with adolescents-onset BPD had a significantly higher risk for SUD than youths with child-onset BPD (39% vs. 8%, respectively) (40). Compared with those with child-onset BPD, youths with adolescent-onset BPD showed 8.8 times the risk for SUD (40). Of significance was the finding that this risk was independent from comorbid CD. Reasons for age of onset of BPD to be such a differential risk factor for comorbid SUD are unclear, except for the speculation that adolescence is a developmental phase prone to substance experimentation/abuse.

Mixed mania was also identified as risk factor for SUD, with a substantial number of SUD occurring coincidentally with mania. Thus, as documented in adult bipolar disorder, adolescents with bipolar disorder may resort to alcohol and drugs to self-medicate their irritability. In support of this speculation, Geller et al. (41) showed that lithium improved both SUD and bipolar symptoms.

Comorbidity with Anxiety Disorders

In contrast to comorbidity of pediatric bipolar disorder with externalizing disorders (ADHD, CD), comorbidity of pediatric bipolar disorder with anxiety disorders has been scarcely investigated in spite of its common occurrence. In adolescents with bipolar disorder, rates of comorbidity with anxiety disorders range from 32% (1) to 53% (42). In a clinical sample of 43 child and adolescent outpatients with bipolar disorder, a very high incidence of comorbidity with any anxiety disorder as well as with more than one anxiety disorders (76.5% and 41.9%, respectively) was shown (43). The most prevalent ones were obsessive compulsive disorder (44.2%), social phobia (39.5%), and panic disorder (PD) (25.6%).

This comorbidity is also bidirectional. In a community sample of high school students, those with any type of anxiety disorders were seven times more likely to have comorbid bipolar disorder than non-anxious students (44). Rao et al. (45) found that 50% of depressed adolescents with comorbid anxiety developed bipolar disorder, as compared to 0% of those without anxiety.

Specific interest in PD was the focus of some investigators. A high rate of 52% bipolar disorder was found in a sample of 26 children and adolescents with PD (46). Birmaher et al. (47) found that youths with PD were more likely to show comorbid bipolar disorder ($n=8$; 19.0%) than non-PD anxiety disorders ($n=22$; 5.4%) or non-anxious psychiatric disorders ($n=112$; 7.1%). Youths with both disorders had more psychotic symptoms and suicidal ideations than the two comparison groups. Of significance was the finding that youths with comorbid bipolar disorder and anxiety disorders reported emergence of mania secondary to antidepressants more often than those without comorbidity (43). Thus, clinicians must exercise cautious vigilance in considering antidepressant pharmacotherapy in youths with anxiety disorders to avoid triggering pharmacologic mania.

COURSE OF ILLNESS

Current evidence suggests that pediatric onset bipolar disorder is a severe, disabling, and chronic disorder, often characterized by an initial presentation of a major depressive disorder episode, and a chronic course marked by continuous morbidity with low recovery and high relapse rates, and a high occurrence of treatment resistance.

The predominance of MDD as initial clinical presentation in pediatric bipolar disorder is shown by studies documenting high rate of manic switches. In a prospective follow-up of 79 prepubertal children with MDD over a 2- to 5-year period, Geller et al. (48) found a rate of manic switch of 31.7%. In a 24-month follow-up of 58 adolescents who had been hospitalized for MDD, Strober et al. (49) reported a 28% rate of manic switching for depressed adolescents with psychosis.

Chronicity and severity of the course of illness in youths with bipolar disorder have been documented. In a 2-year prospective follow-up of 89 children and adolescents (mean age, 10.9 years) with bipolar disorder, Geller et al. (50) reported a 65.2%

recovery rate from mania, and a 55.2% relapse rate after recovery. Mean time to recovery was 36 weeks, and mean time to relapse was 28 weeks. Rate of recovery was predicted by an intact biological family, while risk of relapse was significantly associated with low level of maternal warmth. In a 5-year prospective follow-up of 54 adolescents initially hospitalized for bipolar disorder, the recovery rate was 96%, but there was also a high rate (46%) of relapse, and a high rate (20%) of suicide attempts (51). In a community sample of adolescents with bipolar disorder, it was found that 27% of these adolescents had recurrence of illness by age 24 years (2).

CONCLUSION

Pediatric bipolar disorder is a severe, chronic, and disabling illness that disrupts the child's psychosocial development including impairment of family, social, and academic functioning. Although its prevalence is unknown, it is estimated that a substantial number of psychiatrically referred children and adolescents is affected by the disorder.

Diagnosis of bipolar disorder in children and adolescents is a clinical challenge. Whether irritability or euphoria is the core mood symptom of pediatric bipolar disorder remains to be determined. Additionally, the non-episodic, continuous, and rapid cycling pattern, as well as a high rate of mixed mania, poses a unique diagnostic challenge, especially if clinicians rely on the presence of typical mood swings to make the diagnosis. Complexity in diagnosing pediatric bipolar is further compounded by its high comorbidity with other psychiatric disorders that frequently present a confusing overlap of symptoms with pediatric mania, especially ADHD in prepubertal children.

While resolution of these complex issues constitutes an on going challenge for researchers, an immediate task for clinicians is to combine the science provided by current evidence with the art of a keen diagnostic acumen to avoid the pitfalls of over- or under-diagnosing pediatric bipolar disorder. Accurate diagnosis is the first important step in providing early treatment intervention that may positively impact course of illness and improve overall functioning in the lives of these severely ill youths.

REFERENCES

1. Lewinsohn PM, Klein DN, Seeley JR. Bipolar disorders in a community sample of older adolescents—prevalence, phenomenology, comorbidity, and course. J Am Acad Child Adolesc Psychiatry 1995; 34:454–463.
2. Lewinsohn PM, Klein DN, Seeley JR. Bipolar disorder during adolescence and young adulthood in a community sample. Bipolar Disord 2000; 2:281–293.
3. Geller B, Luby J. Child and adolescent bipolar disorder: a review of the past 10 years. J Am Acad Child Adolesc Psychiatry 1997; 36(9):1168–1176.
4. Rice J, Reich T, Andreasen NC, et al. The familial transmission of bipolar illness. Arch Gen Psychiatry 1987; 44:441–447.
5. Weller RA, Weller EB, Tucker SG, et al. Mania in prepubertal children; has it been underdiagnosed? J Affect Disord 1986; 11:151–154.
6. Geller B, Zimerman B, Williams M, et al. DSM-IV mania symptoms in a prepubertal and early adolescent bipolar phenotype compared to attention-deficit hyperactive and normal controls. J Child Adolesc Psychopharmacol 2002; 12:11–25.

7. Wozniak J, Biederman J, Kiely K, et al. Mania-like symptoms suggestive of childhood onset bipolar disorder in clinically referred children. J Am Acad Child Adolesc Psychiatry 1995; 34:867–876.
8. Lish JD, Dime-Meenan S, Whybrow PC, et al. The National Depressive and Manic-Depressive Association (DMDA) survey of bipolar members. J Affect Disord 1994; 31:281–294.
9. Loranger A, Levine P. Age at onset of bipolar affective illness. Arch Gen Psychiatry 1978; 35:1345–1348.
10. American Psychiatric Association. Diagnostic and Statistic Manual for Mental Disorders. 4th ed. Washington, DC: American Psychiatric Press, 1994.
11. National Institute of Mental Health. National Institute of Mental Health Research Round Table on prepubertal bipolar disorder. J Am Acad Child Adolesc Psychiatry 2001; 40:871–878.
12. Leibenluft E, Charney DS, Towbin KE, et al. Defining clinical phenotypes of juvenile mania. Am J Psychiatry 2003; 160:430–437.
13. Geller B, Zimerman B, Williams M, et al. Phenomenology of prepubertal and early adolescent bipolar disorder: examples of elated mood, grandiose behaviors, decreased need for sleep, racing thoughts and hypersexuality. J Child Adolesc Psychopharmacol 2002; 12(1):3–9.
14. Wozniak J, Biederman J, Richards JA. Diagnostic and therapeutic dilemmas in the management of pediatric-onset bipolar disorder. J Clin Psychiatry 2001; 62(suppl 14):10–15.
15. Davis RE. Manic-depressive variant syndrome of childhood: a preliminary report. Am J Psychiatry 1979; 136(5):702–706.
16. Chang KD, Steiner H, Ketter TA. Psychiatric phenomenology of child and adolescent bipolar offspring. J Am Acad Child Adolesc Psychiatry 2000; 9(4):453–460.
17. Weckerly J. Pediatric bipolar mood disorder [review]. J Dev Pediatr 2002; 23:42–56.
18. Geller B, Williams M, Zimerman B, et al. Prepubertal and early adolescent bipolarity differentiate from ADHD by manic symptoms, grandiose delusions, ultra-rapid or ultradian cycling. J Affect Disord 1998; 51:81–91.
19. Gershon ES, Hamovit J, Guroff JJ, et al. A family study of schizoaffective, bipolar I, bipolar II, unipolar and normal control probands. Arch Gen Psychiatry 1982; 39:1157–1167.
20. Geller B, Zimerman B, Williams M, et al. Bipolar disorder at prospective follow-up of adults who had prepubertal major depressive disorder. Am J Psychiatry 2001; 158(1):125–127.
21. Pillai JJ, Friedman L, Stuve TA, et al. Increased presence of white matter hyperintensities in adolescent patients with bipolar disorder. Psychiatry Res 2002; 114(1):51–56.
22. Hirsfeld-Becker DR, Biederman J, Calltharp S, et al. Behavioral inhibition and disinhibition as hypothesized precursors to psychopathology: implications for pediatric bipolar disorder. Biol Psychiatry 2003; 53:985 999.
23. Fristad MA, Weller EB, Weller RA. The Mania Rating Scale: can it be used in children? A preliminary report. J Am Child Adolesc Psychiatry 1992; 31:252–257.
24. Biederman J, Wozniak J, Kiely K, et al. CBCL clinical scales discriminate prepubertal children with structured interview-derived diagnosis of mania from those with ADHD. J Am Child Adolesc Psychiatry 1995; 34(4):464–471.
25. Geller B, Zimerman B, Williams M, et al. Diagnostic characteristics of 93 cases of a prepubertal and early adolescent bipolar disorder phenotype by gender, puberty and comorbid attention deficit hyperactivity disorder. J Child Adolesc Psychopharmacol 2000; 10(3):157–164.
26. West SA, Strakowski SM, Sax KW, et al. Phenomenology and comorbidity of adolescents hospitalized for the treatment of acute mania. Biol Psychiatry 1996; 39:458–460.
27. Milberger S, Biederman J, Faraone SV, et al. Attention deficit hyperactivity disorder and comorbid disorders: issues of overlapping symptoms. Am J Psychiatry 1995; 152: 1793–1799.

28. Wozniak J, Biederman J, Mundy E, et al. A pilot family study of childhood-onset mania. J Am Child Adolesc Psychiatry 1995; 34(12):1577–1583.
29. Brent DA, Perper JA, Goldstein CE, et al. Risk factors for adolescent suicide: a comparison of adolescent suicide victims with suicidal inpatients. Arch Gen Psychiatry 1988; 45:581–588.
30. Wozniak J, Biederman J. A pharmacological approach to the quagmire of comorbidity in juvenile mania. J Am Child Adolesc Psychiatry 1996; 35(6):826–828.
31. Biederman J, Faraone S, Mick E, et al. Attention-deficit hyperactivity disorder and juvenile mania: an overlooked comorbidity? J Am Child Adolesc Psychiatry 1996; 35:997–1008.
32. Hazell PL, Carr V, Lewin TJ, et al. Manic symptoms in young males with ADHD predict functioning but not diagnosis after 6 years. J Am Child Adolesc Psychiatry 2003; 42: 552–560.
33. Kim EY, Miklowitz DJ. Childhood mania, attention deficit hyperactivity disorder and conduct disorder: a critical review of diagnostic dilemmas [review]. Bipolar Disord 2002; 4:215–225.
34. Kovacs M, Pollock M. Bipolar disorder and comorbid conduct disorder in childhood and adolescence. J Am Child Adolesc Psychiatry 1995; 34(6):715–723.
35. Kutcher SP, Marton P, Korenblum M. Relationship between psychiatric illness and conduct disorder in adolescents. Can J Psychiatry 1989; 34:526–529.
36. Biederman J, Faraone SV, Hatch M, et al. Conduct disorder with and without mania in a referred sample of ADHD children. J Affect Disord 1997; 44(2–3):177–188.
37. Horowitz HA. The use of lithium in the treatment of the drug-induced psychotic reaction. Dis Nerv Syst 1975; 36:159–163.
38. Horowitz HA. Lithium and the treatment of adolescent manic depressive illness. Dis Nerv Syst 1977; 38:480–483.
39. Wilens T, Biederman J, Abrantes A, et al. Clinical characteristics of psychiatrically referred adolescent outpatients with substance use disorders. J Am Child Adolesc Psychiatry 1997; 36:941–947.
40. Wilens TE, Biederman J, Millstein RB, et al. Risk for substance use disorders in youths with child- and adolescent-onset bipolar disorder. J Am Child Adolesc Psychiatry 1999; 38(6):680–685.
41. Geller B, Cooper TB, Sun K, et al. Double-blind and placebo-controlled study of lithium for adolescent bipolar disorders with secondary substance dependency. J Am Child Adolesc Psychiatry 1998; 37(2):171–178.
42. Bashir M, Russell J, Johnson G. Bipolar affective disorder in adolescence: a 10-year study. Aust N Z J Psychiatry 1987; 21:36–43.
43. Masi G, Toni C, Perugi G, et al. Anxiety disorders in children and adolescents with bipolar disorder: a neglected comorbidity. Can J Psychiatry 2001; 46:979–802.
44. Lewinsohn PM, Hops H, Roberts RE, et al. Adolescent psychopathology, I: prevalence and incidence of depression and other DSM-III-R disorders in high school students. J Abnorm Psychol 1993; 102:133–144.
45. Rao U, Ryan ND, Birmaher B, et al. Unipolar depression in adolescents. clinical outcome in adulthood. J Am Child Adolesc Psychiatry 1995; 34:566–578.
46. Biederman J, Faraone SV, Marrs A, et al. Panic disorder and agoraphobia in consecutively referred children and adolescents. J Am Child Adolesc Psychiatry 1977; 36:214–223.
47. Birmaher B, Kennah A, Brent D, et al. Is bipolar disorder specifically associated with panic disorder in youths? J Clin Psychiatry 2002; 63:414–419.
48. Geller B, Fox LW, Clark KA, et al. Rate and predictors of prepubertal bipolarity during follow-up of 6- to 12-years-old depressed children. J Am Child Adolesc Psychiatry 1994; 33(4):461–468.

49. Strober M, Lampert C, Schmidt S, et al. The course of major depressive disorder in adolescents: I. Recovery and risk of manic switching in a follow-up of psychotic and nonpsychotic subtypes. J Am Child Adolesc Psychiatry 1993; 32(1):34–42.
50. Geller B, Craney JL, Bolhofner K, et al. Two year prospective follow-up of children with a prepubertal and early adolescent bipolar phenotype. Am J Psychiatry 2002; 159:927–933.
51. Strober M, Schmidtlackner S, Freeman R, et al. Recovery and relapse in adolescents with bipolar affective illness—a 5-year naturalistic, prospective follow-up. J Am Child Adolesc Psychiatry 1995; 34(6):724–731.

7
Bipolar Disorders in Late Life

Peter Brieger and Andreas Marneros
Klinik und Poliklinik für Psychiatrie, Martin-Luther-Universität, Halle-Wittenberg, Germany

INTRODUCTION

Because of the demographic changes taking place in Western societies, late-life mental disorders have become and will remain of constantly growing importance for mental-health services (1,2). The category "late-onset mental disorder" (LOMD), as Berrios (3) pointed out, names a group of psychiatric conditions whose only common feature is their (putatively) higher incidence in old age. The concept is clear, but LOMD, per se, is of little help in the diagnosis of the conditions underlying the disorder. At the same time, recent research suggests that prevalence of bipolar disorders, in general, has been underestimated for a long time (4–7), and the knowledge of bipolar disorder in the elderly is, therefore, sparse and many questions remain open. There are several reasons for this:

- There is considerable heterogeneity as to when "late life" begins. Some studies on late-life mania or late-life bipolar disorders have used a threshold of 60 years (1,8,9), others, 65 years (10–12), and still others, even as early as 50 years (13). Obviously, this makes studies difficult to compare.
- Most studies rely on heterogeneous study samples. Often, they have not sufficiently distinguished between early-onset bipolar patients who have simply grown old and those with a late-onset, as well as failing to distinguish between onset and first medical contact (14).
- The assessment of affective syndromes in the elderly has several difficulties. There is considerable comorbidity with medical illnesses. Almost 80% of elderly bipolar patients suffer from a chronic medical disability (15), which may have an effect on subjective well-being and may have psychological or physiological consequences (16). Quite often, it is difficult to decide whether a manic syndrome in a patient is secondary to a general medical condition (17) or is primary. Here, a good psychiatric and medical examination, a family history, and most of all, longitudinal observation are important tools. It is not easy to use such complex assessments for research purposes.
- There still exists no good epidemiological data on the prevalence of "functional psychoses" in the elderly (2), which is especially true for late-life

bipolar disorders (18). For example, it has not yet been determined whether the finding of the Epidemiological Catchments Area (ECA) Study (19), which states that the lowest prevalence of all psychiatric disorders (with the exception of severe cognitive impairment) is found in people over 65 years of age, is an accurate finding or just a consequence of potential methodological errors.

- Our understanding of bipolar disorders has changed in recent years. Nowadays, the concept of a broad bipolar spectrum receives much attention (6,20,21) and has opened new perspectives for research, diagnosis, and treatment. Nevertheless, for late-life bipolar disorders, such spectrum concepts have not gained very much interest. There is no work on a "late-life bipolar spectrum." Therefore, most studies in late-life bipolar disorders have focused on (narrowly) defined bipolar I disorders according to DSM-IV (22). However, when one takes into account that the vast majority of bipolar disorders are not bipolar I, but rather belong to other forms (7), it can be assumed that the largest part of the field is still unknown. This is specifically true for bipolar II affective disorder (23), mixed states, or rapid cycling forms of bipolar illness (24). Late-onset bipolar schizoaffective disorder seems to be extremely rare (25).

CLASSIFICATION

One can distinguish between four subtypes of late-life bipolar disorders (Table 1):

1. Early-onset bipolars who continue to have episodes in old age: In most bipolar patients, age at onset of their disorder is early. First episodes often manifest before 30 years of age, if not in childhood or early adulthood (26) Although subjects with bipolar affective disorders suffer from a higher natural and unnatural (especially suicide) mortality than subjects from the general population (26,27), many of them do reach a late age. Because—quite different from what Schneider (28) had postulated—bipolar

Table 1 Bipolar Disorders in Late Life: Diagnostic Subgroups

Early-onset bipolar disorders	As bipolar disorders tend to be life-long illnesses, a relevant proportion of affected subjects will remain symptomatic in old age
Secondary mania syndromes	Various general medical or neurological conditions may cause manic syndromes. Owing to higher comorbidity rates, this is especially true for elderly patients
Late-onset bipolar disorders with an earlier "pseudounipolar" course	Some subjects develop (hypo)manic episodes only in old age, although they have had depressive episodes or temperamental abnormalities before. With such a development, their earlier illness course has to be "re-evaluated."
True late-onset bipolar disorders	Some bipolar disorders may manifest for the first time in old age with no prior antecedents

disorders are chronic conditions and do not necessarily have a good prognosis (26), their illness often continues to be of relevance until old age. Consequently, the natural course of bipolar disorders leads to elderly early-onset bipolar patients, who have had both depressive and (hypo)manic (or mixed) episodes before the age of 65 years.

2. Secondary manic syndromes: The term "secondary mania" refers to manic syndromes closely associated temporally with systemic medical or neurological conditions (17). Innumerable agents and conditions may cause manic syndromes in the elderly. Van Gerpen et al. (13) presented a list of more than 100 known causes of "secondary mania," which they grouped under the chapters "neurologic," "medications," "systemic," and "other." As elderly subjects are often multimorbid, and as they are more frequently exposed to these risk factors, they have a higher risk of developing secondary mania (17,29) than younger subjects.
3. Late-onset bipolar disorders with an earlier "pseudounipolar" course: These are patients who had no (hypo)manic or mixed episode before 65 years of age, and although they had indeed suffered from earlier depressive episodes, they only showed signs of manic or hypomanic symptoms after the age of 65 years. The diagnosis of a bipolar disorder is a longitudinal diagnosis. Jules Angst showed in a prospective cohort study (30) that new illness episodes manifested, at a constant risk, all during the course of a bipolar illness, even after the age of 70 years. This means that mania may even present after many years of a purely depressive course of an affective illness. Therefore, a small proportion of patients, who had been diagnosed as suffering from recurrent major depression, will turn bipolar even after the age of 65 years. These patients have only "revealed" themselves as suffering from a bipolar affective disorder after the age of 65 years, although, in retrospect, it is beyond doubt that their earlier depressive episodes were already part of the same illness. It is a basic problem of bipolar illness that a switch from unipolar to bipolar can occur at any time during life. A period of many years or even decades between depressive episodes and subsequent (hypo)-manic episodes is not unusual (31).
4. "True" late-onset bipolar illnesses: It is possible that a very small proportion of bipolar illnesses manifests for the first time after the age of 65 years, although research and clinical experience indicate that this group is the smallest of all four groups mentioned here. In such patients, a (hypo) manic or mixed episode occurs plus, possibly, a depressive episode, with no history of such episodes before the age of 65 years. It is not always easy to rule out the possibility that such patients suffer from "secondary mania." Furthermore, one must be careful that an earlier course of pseudounipolar depression or earlier undiagnosed hypomanic or mild mixed affective episodes have not simply been overseen. Still, in other patients, an earlier soft bipolar disorder such as a bipolar temperament (32,33) or cyclothymia (34), may be found. Again, all these considerations refer to bipolar I but not to other types of bipolar disorder.

Although the first type of late-life bipolar disorders can be recognized with sufficient validity, the others require considerable clinical and scientific skills. Most of all, a longitudinal view of the illness and its prior development is obligatory.

Shulman and Herrmann (29) have additionally outlined unipolar mania of late-life patients. The concept of "unipolar" mania is interesting. As with "pseudounipolar" or false unipolar depression, it is difficult to rule out the possibility that past or future depressive episodes have occurred or will occur. Most modern spectrum concepts do not describe clear-cut subtypes, but rather continua. They prefer a dimensional approach. Angst (35), Quitkin et al. (36), and others have observed that there are depression-prone and mania-prone subtypes of bipolar illness. Perhaps, "unipolar" mania lies on a continuum close to the mania-prone pole. It seems that "unipolar mania" is not a distinct subtype. Nevertheless, other researchers (37) have argued against this idea, leaving the question open.

CLINICAL PRESENTATION

Depression in the elderly population is a common condition (2), but mania in the elderly is relatively rare. Before one makes the diagnosis of a bipolar disorder (or mania) in an elderly person, secondary causes have to be carefully ruled out.

In the past, it was believed that mania in the elderly tends to present with "atypical" symptoms (Table 2). Some studies have found no relevant differences between the manic symptomatology of late-life mania patients and the presentation of younger manic patients (38,39). Another study observed lower activity, lower sexual interest, decreased initiating, and a lower tendency to make plans in elderly patients with mania (40). This is not a contradiction, as these differences are more of a quantitative rather than a qualitative nature and can be understood as consequences of the physiological aging process. Some authors have argued that mania in old age shows more mixed affective features (41), but, as yet, there is no good clinical evidence supporting such a hypothesis (29). Besides, the clinical heterogeneity and vagueness of the many concepts of "mixed states" in bipolar disorders (42) are particularly problematic for late-life bipolar disorders, where clinical features tend to "wear off" and become less clear-cut. Beyond the classical well-known psychopathology of mania, several studies have reported that late-life patients with mania show cognitive impairment (29,40,43), even in comparison to controls, which has also been supported by some longitudinal studies (8). Although cognitive impairment is a consistent finding in several studies of geriatric mania (29), the speculation that mania in late life is a forerunner of dementia has not been substantiated by outcome studies (11).

In non-geriatric bipolar patients, depression is far more common than mania or hypomania (21,44,45). One has to expect that to be true for late-life bipolar disorders as well. Nevertheless, we are not aware of specific studies on this topic. Late-life bipolar depression remains widely unstudied (29).

Table 2 Clinical Presentations that Have Been Reported to Differentiate Old-Age Mania from Mania in Younger Age

Lower activity
Lower sexual interest
Decreased initiating
Lower tendency to make plans
More mixed affective features? (no good clinical evidence)
Cognitive impairment

EPIDEMIOLOGY

Our knowledge of the epidemiology of bipolar disorders in late life is very limited (Table 3). A first report from the ECA Study found not a single case of bipolar disorder amongst 900 elderly community residents (46). Later reports corrected this number to a prevalence rate for bipolar disorder of 0.1% in subjects at an age of ≥65 years living in the community (18). Yet, one has to bear in mind that the diagnosis of mania in the elderly is not an easy one to make. It may be clouded by symptoms occurring due to medical conditions or cognitive dysfunction. Additionally, it had been thought to be a rather "exotic" condition for a while. Therefore, it may have been missed by standard diagnostic interviews, as it may have received insufficient attention or may have been overseen in the community. In psychogeriatric units, up to 12% of all treated patients suffer from bipolar disorders (47), whereas another study reported a frequency of 10% for bipolar disorders in nursing homes (48). Obviously, such data may not be generalized, as they stem from highly selected populations. They do not consider the subtyping, which we have outlined earlier, or the concept of a broad bipolar affective spectrum. Bipolar schizoaffective disorders with real late onset (after the age of 65 years) are unknown or extremely seldom (25).

Concerning the gender ratio, almost all studies have reported a 2:1—or even higher—female preponderance (9,12,29), a phenomenon which is in contrast to the general epidemiology of bipolar disorders (49,50). In a more recent study on the service use of elderly bipolar patients, the rather small sample ($N = 37$) consisted of almost 90% women (1). These preponderances may have been the effect of selection processes, as these results stem from clinical studies: it is well known that elderly

Table 3 Unresolved Questions of the Epidemiology of Old-Age Bipolar Disorders

Prevalence	Is the prevalence of bipolar disorders in old age as low as 0.1% as studies have indicated—or is this a methodological artifact?
Gender ratio	Most studies of old-age bipolar disorders report a female preponderance of at least 2:1. Nevertheless, such findings have not been controlled for "natural" demographic changes of the gender ratio (e.g., due to the shorter life expectancy of men) and for selection biases
Age at onset	Most studies of old-age bipolar disorders have reported a mean age at onset of the disorder of over 40 years, which is not compatible with the general understanding of bipolar disorders
Bipolar spectrum concept	The concept of a broad bipolar spectrum (including subthreshold and temperamental forms) has not gained much recognition in old-age psychiatry, although such a concept would change the epidemiology of old-age bipolar disorders fundamentally

women live more often on their own than elderly men. Therefore, they may (need to) access psychiatric services more easily. Furthermore, one has to be aware of the demographic effects on the gender ratio: elderly women live longer than elderly men. Thus, the female preponderance may have been a consequence of the age structure of the samples, as in samples of younger bipolar patients, the gender ratio is 1:1.

Age at onset is a difficult question in late-life bipolar patients. Although in younger samples of bipolar patients, the age at onset of the illness is between 20 and 30 years (26), most studies found that in hospitalized elderly bipolar patients, very few had developed mania before the age of 40 years (8,9,11). This lead Shulman to the question: "Where have all the young bipolars gone?" (29). Snowdon (9) spoke of the "paucity of early-onset cases." Owing to potential methodological shortcomings (retrospective assessment), one must view such results of age at onset in geriatric cases of bipolar illness with caution.

We are not aware of substantial data to indicate what proportion of late-life bipolar disorder or late-life mania patients belong to which of the four diagnostic categories we have outlined (Table 1). Nevertheless, in our experience, the proportion of "true" late-onset bipolar patients (i.e., patients who have had no earlier affective or subaffective episodes, who have no temperamental abnormalities, and who give no indication of a secondary mania) is small.

COURSE AND OUTCOME

There is no clear evidence that bipolar disorders after the age of 65 years have a different course or outcome than bipolar patients at an earlier age, when one considers the physiological aging effects (26,29). However, the question of whether "kindling" processes (51) occur, so that elderly bipolar affective patients exhibit a shortening of episodes or a shortening of the cycle between two episodes, is a controversial topic: methodological difficulties (52) may hamper such descriptive observations. At present, it is not justified to assume that late-life bipolar disorder patients suffer from shorter illness cycles than younger bipolar patients per se, as a recent analysis provided by the Zurich study has shown (30). Some investigations showed that in the later years (>75 years), an "inactivity" of the disorder could begin, which would mean no new episodes (25).

Three studies (1,8,11) have compared late-life bipolar patients to elderly patients with unipolar depression. Univocally—and anything but surprisingly—they found that bipolar patients had a worse course and outcome than unipolar patients. There was an indication that patients with bipolar disorders more frequently had a cognitive decline than unipolar patients did (8). Thirty-two percentage had experienced a decline of the Mini-Mental State Score to below 24, which is an indication of dementia, at least phenomenologically. Furthermore, in two prospective studies (8,11), the mortality rate of bipolar patients was high: in the study of Dhingra and Rabins (8), more than one-third of the bipolar subjects had died after 5–7 years, whereas in the study of Shulman et al. (11) the bipolar patients had a 2.4-fold mortality rate than the unipolar patients: 50% of the bipolar patients and 20% of the unipolar patients were deceased by the end of the follow-up (mean 5.6 years).

Retrospective and prospective studies of late-life bipolar disorders showed that a high proportion of these patients suffered from comorbid neurological and other medical diseases (11,29). In the study of Shulman et al. (11), 36% of bipolar patients, but only 8% of the unipolar patients, had a comorbid neurological disorder of different etiology (vascular, traumatic, degenerative). Two earlier studies had also reported high comorbidity rates for neurological disorders. In Snowdon's study (9) and Stone's study (12) 17% and 24% respectively, of the late-life bipolar patients suffered from such additional neurological illnesses. Hence, the question arises as to how many of these late-life bipolar patients suffered from a secondary manic syndrome.

Secondary mania (i.e., due to medical or organic conditions) differs from "primary" forms of late-life bipolar disorders concerning course and outcome: as organic factors and comorbid medical conditions make a specific and individual relevance influencing not only severity and treatment, but also prognosis, no general statement concerning course and outcome can be made (13). Nevertheless, one study (10), which did not look at diagnoses but at symptoms, reported that manic symptoms in the elderly were a predictor of a bad outcome—worse than initial depressive symptoms. The authors link this unfavorable consequence of manic symptoms to the results of delirium, as according to the authors' opinion, secondary manic symptoms seem to have an etiological relationship to delirium, which is known to be a predictor of bad outcome, including high mortality in general medical conditions (53).

FAMILY HISTORY

Several of the studies mentioned so far in patients with late-onset effective disorders have reported family-history rates for affective disorders (9,11,39). Regrettably, one has to agree with Shulman and Herrmann (29) that these studies "have produced inconsistent results based on inadequate methodologies." Up to 51% of patients with late-life bipolar disorders reported a positive family history in first-degree relatives (11). Amongst others, one has to be aware of the unusually long observation period of relatives of elderly subjects: there is a high natural prevalence of affective disorders in families of such subjects because these patients have lived a long life, may have large families, and also because the prevalence of affective disorders is high in the general population. Therefore, an age-matched control group is a mandatory prerequisite to come to a meaningful conclusion concerning family history in these patients. Tohen et al. (39) have reported that the lowest rates of familiality occur in patients with a very late-onset of mania, which indicates that such patients suffer from secondary mania more often.

NEUROIMAGING

It is not a surprise that neuroimaging has found various abnormalities in patients with late-life bipolar disorders (29,54), including subcortical hyperintensities (55). There are reports of a relationship between silent cerebral infarction and late-life mania (56,57). According to Fujikawa et al. (56), patients with late mania had higher rates of silent cerebral infarction than patients with late-life depression. Several studies have followed a "location" theory, which goes back to R. G. Robinson. According to this theory, major depression is associated with left frontal and left basal ganglia lesions, whereas mania is associated with right orbital frontal, basotemporal, basal ganglia, or thalamic lesions (58). Consequently, there are several reports of right-sided lesions in secondary manic patients (54,59). However, a recent meta-analysis with stringent methodology offered no support for the hypothesis that

Table 4 Biological Findings that Have Been Associated with Old-Age Bipolar Disorders

Increased rates of comorbid neurological disorders
Increased mortality
Subcortical hyperintensities or silent infarctions
Right orbital frontal, basotemporal, basal ganglia, or thalamic lesions
Increased rates of cognitive decline
High familiality of (bipolar) affective disorders

the risk of depression after stroke is affected by the location of the brain lesion (60), which consequently weakens and questions the argument for a similar mechanism for the development of organic mania. Overall, there is some indication for abnormalities in the neurobiology of old-age bipolar disorders (Table 4).

CONCLUSION

What is old-age bipolar disorder? We do not know enough to come to definite conclusions, but several aspects seem clear:

- Late-life bipolar disorders are not a homogenous disorder. Bipolar patients, who have grown old, or whose bipolar disorders were not previously diagnosed, can be found under this label, as well as patients with secondary mania (i.e., due to medical conditions) and a possibly rather small group of true late-onset bipolar disorders. Therefore, diagnosis must comprise a good longitudinal assessment of prior course, as well as a thorough search for organic factors.
- "True" late-life bipolar disorders do not seem to have a more unfavorable course and outcome than bipolar disorders in earlier age, when one considers physiological aging effects. The psychopathology of old age mania may be somewhat milder but is not fundamentally different from the general psychopathology of mania.
- Patients with late-life bipolar have higher mortality and seem to develop a cognitive decline more often. This may be a consequence of heterogeneous samples, with "endogenous" and organic cases. However, it is futile to try to distinguish between organic and non-organic cases, as clinical and diagnostic information may be insufficient.
- Secondary manias are not rare in elderly patients. It is important to make this diagnosis, as it has consequences for prognosis and treatment.
- Neurovascular lesions in the brain of late-life bipolar patients are frequently found. Again the reason is not clear. The theory that right-sided brain lesions enhance the risk of manic episodes needs further support.

Overall, late-life bipolar disorder is a disorder that has not received adequate attention. It could be expected that owing to the ongoing demographic changes—especially in Europe—more and more patients will be diagnosed as suffering from bipolar disorder in the future. Thus, scientifically speaking, late-life bipolar disorders are interesting illnesses in which one can study the interplay of biological, social, and psychological factors, psychopathology, course and outcome.

REFERENCES

1. Bartels SJ, Forester B, Miles KM, Joyce T. Mental health service use by elderly patients with bipolar disorder and unipolar major depression. Am J Geriatr Psychiatry 2000; 8:160–166.
2. Hybels C, Blazer D. Epidemiology and Geriatric Psychiatry. In: Tsuang MT, Tohen M, eds. Textbook in Psychiatric Epidemiology. 2nd ed. New York: Wiley-Liss, 2002:603–628.
3. Berrios GE. Late-onset mental disorders: a conceptual history. In: Marneros A, ed. Late-Onset Mental Disorders. The Potsdam Conference. London: Gaskell, 1999:1–23.
4. Akiskal HS. Classification, diagnosis and boundaries of bipolar disorders: A Review. In: Maj M, Sartorius N, Ibor J-JL, et al. eds. Bipolar Disorders (WPA Series, Vol. 5). Chichester: Wiley, 2002: 1–52.
5. Akiskal HS, Bourgeois ML, Angst J, Post R, Moller H, Hirschfeld R. Re-evaluating the prevalence of and diagnostic composition within the broad clinical spectrum of bipolar disorders. J Affect Disord 2000; 59(suppl 1):S5–S30.
6. Angst J, Gamma A, Benazzi F, Ajdacic V, Eich D, Rossler W. Toward a re-definition of subthreshold bipolarity: epidemiology and proposed criteria for bipolar-II, minor bipolar disorders and hypomania. J Affect Disord 2003; 73:133–146.
7. Angst J, Gamma A, Ajdacic V, Eich D, Pezawas L, Rössler W, eds. Recurrent brief depression as an indicator of severe mood disorders. In: Mixed States, Rapid Cycling and Atypical Bipolar Disorders. Cambridge: Cambridge University Press. In press
8. Dhingra U, Rabins PV. Mania in the elderly: a 5–7 year follow-up. J Am Geriatr Soc 1991; 39:581–583.
9. Snowdon J. A retrospective case-note study of bipolar disorder in old age. Br J Psychiatry, 1991; 158:485–490.
10. Berrios GE, Bakshi N. Manic and depressive symptoms in the elderly: their relationships to treatment outcome, cognition and motor symptoms. Psychopathology 1991; 24:31–38.
11. Shulman KI, Tohen M, Satlin A, Mallya G, Kalunian D. Mania compared with unipolar depression in old age. Am J Psychiatry 1992; 149:341–345.
12. Stone K. Mania in the elderly. Br J Psychiatry 1989; 155:220–224.
13. Van Gerpen MW, Johnson JE, Winstead DK. Mania in the geriatric patient population: a review of the literature. Am J Geriatr Psychiatry 1999; 7:188–202.
14. Almeida OP, Fenner S. Bipolar disorder: similarities and differences between patients will illness onset before and after 65 years of age. Int Psychogeriatr 2000; 14:311–322.
15. Sajatovic M, Popli A, Semple W. Ten-year use of hospital-based services by geriatric veterans with schizophrenia and bipolar disorder. Psychiatr Serv 1996; 47:961–965.
16. Brieger P. Comorbidity in bipolar disorder. In: Marneros A, Angst J, eds. Bipolar Disorders: 100 years After Manic-Depressive Insanity, Dordrecht. Boston London: Kluwer Academic Publishers, 2000:215–229.
17. Krauthammer C, Klerman GL. Secondary mania: manic syndromes associated with antecedent physical illness or drugs. Arch Gen Psychiatry 1978; 35:1333–1339.
18. Chen ST, Altshuler LL, Spar JE. Bipolar disorder in late life: a review. J Geriatr Psychiatry Neurol 1998; 11:29–35.
19. Robins LN, Regier DA. Psychiatric Disorders in America: The Epidemiologic Catchment Area Study. New York: Free Press, 1991.
20. Marneros A. Expanding the group of bipolar disorders. J Affect Disord 2001; 62:39–44.
21. Marneros A, Röttig S, Wenzel A, Blöink R, Brieger P. Schizoaffective mixed states. In: Marneros A, Goodwin FK eds. Mixed States, Rapid Cycling and Atypical Bipolar Disorder. Cambridge: Cambridge University Press, In press.
22. APA Diagnostic and Statistical Manual of Mental Disorders, 4th ed. Washington DC: American Psychiatric Association, 1994.
23. Benazzi F. Psychotic late-life depression: a 376-case study. Int Psychogeriatr 2000; 11:325–332.

24. Shulman KI. Atypical features of bipolarity in old age. In: Marneros A, Goodwin FK eds. Mixed States, Rapid Cycling and Atypical Bipolar Disorder Cambridge: Cambridge University Press, In press.
25. Marneros A. Late-onset schizoaffective disorders. In: Marneros A, ed. A. Late-Onset Mental Disorders. The Potsdam Conference. London: Gaskell, 1999:98–106.
26. Marneros A, Brieger P. The prognosis of bipolar disorder: a review. In: Maj M, Sartorius N, Ibor J-JL, et al. eds. Bipolar Disorders (WPA Series Vol. 5). Chichester: Wiley, 2002: 97–148.
27. Harris EC, Barraclough B. Excess mortality of mental disorder. Br J Psychiatry 1998; 173:11–53.
28. Schneider K. Klinische Psychopathologie. Stuttgart: Georg Thieme, 1946.
29. Shulman KI, Herrman N. Bipolar disorder in old age. In: Marneros A, Angst J, eds. Bipolar Disorders: 100 years After Manic-Depressive Insanity. Dordrecht, Boston London: Kluwer Academic Publishers, 2000:153–174.
30. Angst J, Gamma A, Sellaro R, Lavori PW, Zhang H. Recurrence of bipolar disorders and major depresssion. A life-long perspective. Eur Archiv Psychiatry Clin Neurosci 2003; 253:236–240.
31. Angst J, Felder W, Frey R, Stassen HH. The course of affective disorders. I. Change of diagnosis of monopolar, unipolar, and bipolar illness. Archiv Psychiatrie Nervenkrankh 1978; 226:57–64.
32. Akiskal HS, Brieger P, Mundt C, Angst J, Marneros A. Temperament und affektive Störungen. Die TEMPS-A Skala als Konvergenz europäischer und US-amerikanischer Konzepte [Temperament and affective disorders. The TEMPS-A Scale as a convergence of European and US-American concepts]. Nervenarzt 2002; 73:262–271.
33. Akiskal HS, Pinto O. Soft bipolar spectrum: footnotes to Kraepelin on the interface of hypomania, temperament and depression. In: Marneros A, Angst J, eds. Bipolar Disorders: 100 years After Manic-Depressive Insanity. Dordrecht, Boston: Kluwer Academic Publishers, 2000; 37–62.
34. Brieger P, Marneros A. Dysthymia and cyclothymia: origins and development. J Affect Disord 1997; 45:117–126.
35. Angst J. The course of affective disorders. II. Typology of bipolar manic-depressive illness. Archiv Psychiatrie Nervenkrankh 1978; 226:65–73.
36. Quitkin FM, Rabkin JG, Prien RF. Bipolar disorder: are there manic-prone and depressive-prone forms? J Clin Psychopharmacol 1986; 6:167–172.
37. Solomon DA, Leon AC, Endicott J, Coryell WH, Mueller TI, Posternak MA, Keller MB. Unipolar mania over the course of a 20-year follow-up study. Am J Psychiatry 2003; 160:2049–2051.
38. Broadhead J, Jacoby R. Mania in old age: a first prospective study. Int J Geriatr Psychiatry 1990; 5:215–222.
39. Tohen M, Shulman KI, Satlin A. First-episode mania in late life. Am J Psychiatry 1994; 151:130–132.
40. Young RC. Bipolar mood disorders in the elderly. Psychiatr Clin North Am 1997; 20:121–136.
41. Shulman K, Post F. Bipolar affective disorder in old age. Br J Psychiatry 1980; 136:26–32.
42. Marneros A. Origin and development of concepts of bipolar mixed states. J Affect Disord 2001; 67:229–240.
43. Young RC. Geriatric mania. Clin Geriatr Med 1992; 8:387–399.
44. Judd LL, Akiskal HS, Schettler PJ, Coryell W, Endicott J, Maser JD, Solomon DA, Leon AC, Keller MB. A prospective investigation of the natural history of the long-term weekly symptomatic status of bipolar II disorder. Arch Gen Psychiatry 2003; 60:261–269.
45. Judd LL, Akiskal HS, Schettler PJ, Endicott J, Maser J, Solomon DA, Leon AC, Rice JA, Keller MB. The long-term natural history of the weekly symptomatic status of bipolar I disorder. Arch Gen Psychiatry 2002; 59:530–537.

46. Kramer M, German PS, Anthony JC, Von Korff M, Skinner EA. Patterns of mental disorders among the elderly residents of eastern Baltimore. J Am Geriatr Soc 1985; 33:236–245.
47. Yassa R, Nair NP, Iskandar H. Late-onset bipolar disorder. Psychiatr Clin North Am 1988; 11:117–131.
48. Greenwald BS, Kremen N, Aupperle P. Tailoring adult psychiatric practices to the field of geriatrics. Psychiatr Q 1992; 63:343–366.
49. Tsuang MT, Tohen M. Textbook in Psychiatric Epidemiology. 2nd ed. New York: Wiley-Liss, 2002.
50. Marneros A, Angst J. Bipolar Disorders: 100 years After Manic-Depressive Insanity. Dordrecht, Boston, London: Kluwer Academic Publishers, 2000.
51. Post RM. Sensitization and kindling perspectives for the course of affective illness: toward a new treatment with the anticonvulsant carbamazepine. Pharmacopsychiatry 1990; 23:3–17.
52. Kessing LV. The effect of affective episodes in bipolar disorder. In: Maj M, Sartorius N, Ibor J J, Ibor L, et al., eds., Bipolar Disorders (WPA Series Vol. 5). Chichester: Wiley, 2002: 155–158.
53. McCusker J, Cole M, Abrahamowicz M, Primeau F, Belzile E. Delirium predicts 12-month mortality. Arch Intern Med 2002; 162:457–463.
54. Shulman K, Singh A. (1999) Comorbidity and bipolar disorder in old age. In: Tohen M, ed. Comorbidity in Affective Disorders. New York Basel: Marcel Dekker, 1999:249–261.
55. McDonald WM, Krishnan KR, Doraiswamy PM, Blazer DG. Occurrence of subcortical hyperintensities in elderly subjects with mania. Psychiatry Res 1991; 40:211–220.
56. Fujikawa T, Yamawaki S, Touhouda Y. Silent cerebral infarctions in patients with late-onset mania. Stroke 1995; 26:946–949.
57. Kobayashi S, Okada K, Yamashita K. Incidence of silent lacunar lesion in normal adults and its relation to cerebral blood flow and risk factors. Stroke 1991; 22:1379–1383.
58. Robinson RG. Mood disorders secondary to stroke. Semin Clin Neuropsychiatry 1997; 2:244–251.
59. Starkstein SE, Boston JD, Robinson RG. Mechanisms of mania after brain injury. 12 case reports and review of the literature. J Nerv Ment Dis 1988; 176:87–100.
60. Carson AJ, MacHale S, Allen K, Lawrie SM, Dennis M, House A, Sharpe M. Depression after stroke and lesion location: a systematic review. Lancet 2000; 356:122–126.

8
Clinical Course in Bipolar Disorder

Robert J. Boland
Department of Psychiatry and Human Behavior, Brown University and Miriam Hospital/LifeSpan, Providence, Rhode Island, U.S.A.

Martin B. Keller
Department of Psychiatry and Human Behavior, Brown University, Butler Hospital and Brown Affiliated Hospitals, Providence, Rhode Island, U.S.A.

INTRODUCTION

Since descriptions by Falret (1) and Kraepelin (2), we have recognized bipolar disorder as an illness defined by its changing course. Both described the disorder as a circular one, essentially alternating between the extreme highs and lows of mood. Kraepelin felt it was this circular course, with a return to normalcy, that differentiated this disorder from dementia praecox (i.e., schizophrenia). Work by Post (3) and others suggested that the course of bipolar disorder could worsen with time. It was found that an increasing number of manic episodes lead both to a further increase of future manic episodes and also a decrease in the period of normalcy between episodes. From this observation came the idea that the course of bipolar disorder was subject to a type of "kindling" phenomenon, analogous to that seen in epilepsy. In the 1960s, the work by Leonhard et al. (4) helped distinguish bipolar disorder from unipolar depression, in part due to perceived differences in the courses of the two disorders. Bipolar disorder was thought to occur earlier than unipolar depression and had more episodes over time.

The view of bipolar disorder, however, generally has continued to be one of the alternations of extremes, in a "burst" pattern (5), followed by periods of general quiescence. Less attention has been paid to what occurs between episodes of mania and major depression.

STUDYING THE COURSE OF BIPOLAR DISORDER

Many long-term studies exist that are designed to investigate the course of bipolar disorder. Such studies are, however, notoriously difficult to do, and various studies suffer from several problems, including recruitment biases, lack of standardized instruments, and lack of agreement on the definition of terms. The earliest studies of the course of bipolar disorder, including those by Wertham (6), Rennie (7), and Lundquist (8), though pioneering, had many limitations. These include a lack of rigorous diagnostic definitions and an inadequate demarcation of the boundaries between bipolar disorder and other disorder such as schizophrenia. As discussed by Marneros and Brieger (9), the modern era of long-term naturalistic studies of bipolar disorder began with the Zurich study (10). This was a prospective study of 220 patients with bipolar disorder who were followed for up to 28 years. It used a representative sample of the population, structured interviews, and operationalized definitions of disorders. Subsequent prospective long-term studies of interest include the Iowa-500 study (11), the Cologne Study (12), and the National Institute of Mental Health Collaborative Study of the Psychobiology of Depression, or Collaborative Depression Study (13).

This chapter will focus on data from the Collaborative Depression Study (CDS), which represents the most rigorous long-term investigation of the natural course of bipolar disorder to date. We will review knowledge about major course change points, which has been the traditional method of investigating a disease course. However, more recent data afford an in-depth look at the natural course of bipolar disorder, including the importance of minor and subsyndromal symptoms. We have only begun to appreciate the importance of these minor symptoms in the overall presentation of bipolar disorder and will review data about this in detail.

DEFINITION OF TERMS

Considerable confusion has resulted from the use of various terms to denote the difference change points during an affective illness. Similar terms such as "relapse" and "recurrence" have been used interchangeably and inconsistently in different studies. As a result, the MacArthur Foundations Research Network on the Psychobiology of Depression (14) recommended using the following terms:

1. Episode, defined by having a certain number of symptoms for a certain period of time.
2. Remission, defined by a period of time in which an individual no longer meets criteria for the disorder. In partial remission, an individual still has more than minimal symptoms. Full remission means the point at which an individual no longer meets criteria for the disorder and has no more than minimal symptoms.
3. Recovery, defined as a full remission that lasts for a defined period of time. Conceptually, it implies the end of an episode of an illness, not the illness per se.
4. Relapse, defined as a return of symptoms sufficient to satisfy full criteria for an episode. It occurs in an interval of time before what is defined as "recovery." Conceptually, this refers to the return of an episode, not a new episode.
5. Recurrence, defined as a return of full symptomatology occurring after the beginning of the recovery period. Conceptually, this represents the beginning of a new episode of an illness.

OVERVIEW OF THE CDS

The CDS was designed to study the natural course of unipolar and bipolar mood disorders. It is a prospective, long-term study of the psychopathology, treatment, and psychosocial functioning of persons with these disorders (13). The subjects were recruited from those seeking psychiatric treatment through inpatient and outpatient treatment facilities at five medical centers (in Boston, Chicago, Iowa City, New York, and St. Louis).

Nine-hundred-fifty-five subjects with various mood disorders entered the study. Subjects were recruited between the years of 1978 and 1981. These subjects were white, who spoke English, had an IQ of at least 70 and did not have an organic mental disorder or terminal illness. Diagnoses were based on the Schedule of Affective Disorder and Schizophrenia (SADS), using the Research Diagnostic Criteria (RDC) (15). Both bipolar I and II patients were recruited. Several subgroups, most notable the rapid cycling type of bipolar disorder and patients with mixed mania, were recruited into the study. The bipolar I group consisted of 146 patients, and the bipolar II consisted of 86 patients. Of the bipolar II group, 69 were defined as having definite bipolar II, in that their hypomanic episode lasted for at least 7 days. Seventeen patients had hypomanic symptoms for only 2 to 6 days and were classified as probable bipolar II. Eighty-nine patients were considered to have the rapid cycling type of bipolar disorder. DSM-IV criteria were used to define the rapid cycling group, and patients were included in this group if they had four or more mood disorders, each of at least 2 weeks' duration, during any 1-year period. The majority (almost 80%) of the rapid cycling group had met criteria for this disorder within the first year of the study. The mixed subgroup had manic or hypomanic and depressive symptoms intermixed throughout the day. The number of patients with mixed symptoms was small at the time of entry to the study (only seven out of the first 155 subjects). This number, however, increased with time. For some analyses, the mixed group was combined with the rapid cycling group.

Assessment tools at the time of intake included the SADS. At each 6-month follow-up, the subjects were given the Longitudinal Interval Follow-up Evaluation (LIFE) (16). Changes in psychopathology, measured to the week, were determined on a time line using the Psychiatric Status Rating (PSR). The PSR quantifies the severity of symptoms on a six-point scale (17) for major depression and mania and on a three-point scale for rating minor depression/dysthymia, hypomania, DSM-IV atypical depression, DSM-III adjustment disorder with depressed mood, and RDC cyclothymic personality.

Recovery was defined as having had at least 8 consecutive weeks with no more than two mild symptoms (as rated on the LIFE scale). A relapse was defined as having full RDC criteria for an episode of major depressive disorder, minor depression, mania, hypomania, or schizoaffective disorder after an 8-week period of recovery from an affective disorder (thus, the time to relapse could not be <9 weeks).

To characterize chronicity in patients, the investigators used two measures: the total percentage of time spent in a full-blown episode of major depression or mania and the total percentage of time spent with any affective symptoms at any level of severity. This method was previously used to evaluate chronicity in unipolar patients from the CDS group.

Though the investigators did not participate in decisions about treatment, they did collect information about the intensity and appropriateness of pharmacotherapy. Treatment for depressive and manic symptoms was rated for intensity. Algorithms were developed and updated over the years to describe the intensity of treatment in this cohort. However, it should be stressed that this is a naturalistic study that did not control for treatment as a variable.

Time to Recovery

Studies done before the use of lithium described a great range of times to recovery, varying from 2 months to more than 1 year (18). The generally accepted length of a manic episode is 2 to 5 months (9).

In the CDS, looking at 5-year follow-up data, 74% recovered (were free from both mania and major depression) within 6 months, 81% recovered within 1 year, 92% recovered within 2 years, and 94% recovered within 5 years (19). Recovery differed by group, and the nature of the index episode was the most important predictor of recovery. The most rapid recovery was found in subjects who had entered the study with an index episode of mania. The manic group had a median time to recovery of 5 weeks compared with a median of 9 weeks for the depressed group and 14 weeks for the combined mixed/cycling group. These differences were significant when comparing the manic and mixed/cycling group.

These differences in rates of recovery were most marked in the period just after entry into the study. However, on longer-term follow-up (5 years), patients with pure manic symptoms continued to recover faster than the other groups. At 5-year follow-up, the group with an index episode of mania had a median time to recovery of 6 weeks. This compared significantly with a recovery time of 11 weeks for the depressed and 17 weeks for the mixed/cycling group (19).

For those who were manic on entry in the study, several variables predicted the time to recovery. A longer duration of major depressive disorder before entry into the study predicted a longer time to recovery. The number of previous major affective episodes also predicted a more chronic outcome: 55% of the patients in their first episode of illness recovered by 6 months, whereas 73% of patients with one or two prior episodes and 90% of patients with three or more prior episodes recovered in that time.

For patients who were depressed at the time of entry into the study, a longer prior duration of illness also predicted a longer time to recovery. In this group, a diagnosis of "secondary" major depressive bipolar disorder in which their first affective episode was preceded by another RDC disorder (such as alcoholism or substance abuse) also predicted a longer time to recovery.

Relapse

Relapse was slowest for the manic group and similar for the depressive and mixed/cycling group (19). In the first 3 months, the cumulative probability of relapse was similar for all three groups. However, by 6 months, the manic group had a 20% cumulative probability of relapse compared with 33% for the depressed group and 36% for the mixed/cycling group. By 1 year, the manic group had a 48% probability of relapse, and the mixed/cycling group had a 57% chance of relapse. The depressed group had a time to relapse that was similar to the mixed/cycling group at 1-year follow-up. By 5 years, the manic group had an 81% chance of relapse compared with 91% for the mixed/cycling group. Relapse was also more severe in the mixed/cycling group: 59% of the mixed/cycling subjects relapsed into a major affective disorder compared with 38% of the pure manic subjects. The groups did not differ in their treatment received before relapse.

Recurrence

Bipolar disorder is considered a highly recurrent illness, and most long-term studies have supported this. The Zurich study, for example, found that following recovery from an episode, 82% of subjects experienced a recurrence during the study period, with a median number of nine episodes (18). In the Cologne study, the median number of episodes was five episodes over 25 years.

In the CDS, of the 206 patients studied, 176 had a symptom-free period of 4 months, 141 had a symptom-free period of 1 year, 106 had a symptom-free period of 2 years, and 79 had a symptom-free period of 3 years. In examining the first 4 years after recovery, a longer symptom-free period continued to be associated with sustained remission. However, after 4 years, the protection associated with longer symptom-free periods eventually dissipated. At 7 years after recovery, the cumulative likelihood of recurrence was 80% for all patients with bipolar and 66% for patients with bipolar disorder whose index episode was followed by at least 3 years without symptoms (20). Within 5 years of recovery, the likelihood of at least one recurrence was greater than 70% (19).

As the subjects were already in the index episode on entry into this study, some information about the index episode (such as the initial onset) was necessarily retrospective. The 5-year follow-up enabled an examination of the course of the next episode—thus allowing for a prospective analysis. Observations of this first prospective episode were consistent with observations of the index episode. It was found that the subjects who entered the study with a mixed/cycling episode had the lowest cumulative probability of recovery from a subsequent episode. During the first prospective episode, rates of recovery in all groups were similar for the first 6 months and then began to diverge, with 78% of the manic group (grouped by index episode) recovering, compared with 58% of the index mixed/cycling group. By 3 years, the recovery rate was 100% for the index manic group compared with 87% for the index mixed/cycling group (20). Of note is that the depressive group had a small sample size, which limited comparability with the other groups. However, the depressive group seemed comparable to the index manic group.

Previous authors had suggested a clustering of bipolar episodes (21). Reports of this have not been consistent. Angst et al. (22), for example, found no such evidence for clustering of episodes in the Zurich study. Similarly, the CDS found no evidence of clustering and in fact found the opposite effect in that episodes tended to increase over time without any early clustering effect. Bipolar patients who had prior episodes and prior hospitalizations were more likely, rather than less likely, to have both subsequent episodes and subsequent hospitalizations: this was a trend at 2 years and was statistically significant by 5 years of follow-up.

Chronicity

Rates of chronicity ("non-recovery" from an episode) are generally high across studies. The Zurich study found that 16% of patients showed chronicity, which they defined as an episode lasting at least 2 years (18). In the Cologne study, one-third of the patients suffered from persisting symptoms (12). Other shorter-term studies (23) have had similar results.

The CDS investigators examined several novel measures of chronicity, including recording the total percentage time that patients experienced either full or any affective symptoms. The results from this analysis are presented by subgroup.

Bipolar I Disorder

The CDS found that patients were symptomatically ill for an average of about half the time during the follow-up period (24). Only 12% of the time was spent in a full syndromal episode, the remainder of the time patients experienced either subsyndromal mania or depression (15%) or minor depression/dysthymia or hypomania (20%). Of the different affective states, depressive symptoms were the most common. Patients experienced three times more depressive episodes than manic and five times more than mixed/cycling episodes. Patients experienced a change in symptom status approximately six times a year, and a significant portion of these status changes involved changes in polarity—~3.5 times per year. About 60% of patient changed polarity once per year or less, 19% changed more than five times per year, 8% more than 10 times per year, and 4% changed polarity more than 20 times per year. Over 90% of patients experienced ≥1 week in a state of depression, 86% of patients experienced ≥1 week of mania, and about half the patients experienced ≥1 week of mixed symptoms. Most patients experienced all levels of the depressive spectrum and about half experienced all levels of the manic spectrum. In a 15-year follow-up of the cohort, 20% of patients had full-blown symptoms of either mania or depression during the entire 15 years of the follow-up (20).

Bipolar II Disorder

Using similar methodology, the CDS looked at patients with bipolar II disorder (25). It was found that, similar to bipolar I patients, the subjects were symptomatic for more than half the follow-up period. A significant time was spent in minor or subsyndromal states: patients spent ~15% of the time with subsyndromal symptoms, 25% of the time with minor depressive, dysthymic, or hypomanic symptoms, and 13% of the time in a major depressive episode. Patients spent < 1% of the time in a psychotic episode. As a whole, subsyndromal, minor depressive, and hypomanic episodes were three times more common than major depressive episodes. Depressive symptoms as a whole were much more common (almost 40-fold more common) than hypomanic symptoms and over 20 times more common than mixed/cycling symptoms.

Changes in symptom status were common, and patients experienced more than 42 status changes on average. Most experienced a symptom status change more than twice a year, and almost one-quarter of the patients experienced status changes more than five times a year. About one-third of all symptom status changes involved a shift in polarity: three-fourth of patients changed polarity about once a year.

Most patients experienced at least 1 week of depressive symptoms; almost one-half experienced at least 1 week with manic spectrum symptoms. Less than one-third had mixed/cycling symptoms. Approximately 80% of the patients spent at least 1 week's time in four out of the possible six symptomatic categories.

As some controversy exists as to the proper length of required for a hypomanic episode, the investigators looked separately at both short (2–6 days) and long duration (>7 days) hypomanic episodes. These two phenomena differed in one manner: patients with longer hypomanic episodes had more weeks with minor depressive symptoms.

Factors Influencing Course

Many studies of bipolar disorder have attempted to discover predictors of course and outcome. The results from such studies are varied, and these variations largely result from methodological differences. It is likely that little reliable data can be taken from shorter-term studies as only with the passing of years can meaningful patterns emerge.

Taken as a whole, the various long-term studies available have suggested some patterns. In summarizing data from available studies on the course of bipolar illness, Marneros and Brieger (9) suggested that the available data agree on several positive and negative predictors of course. Positive predictors likely include high premorbid functioning and good treatment compliance. Negative predictors include personality disorders, inter-episode impairment, chronicity, comorbid substance abuse, mood-incongruent features, and a tendency toward depressive symptoms. Negative life events are only weak predictors of course. The strongest predictor of future episodes is the number of past episodes, particularly if rapid cycling exists. Baseline variables, such as age, gender, and socioeconomic variables, are generally not helpful in predicting the course of illness.

Work done subsequently by the CDS generally confirms Marneros and Brieger's review. For bipolar I patients, the chronicity of symptoms was associated with four variables: poor social functioning, a longer intake episode, an intake episode that was depressive or mixed/cyclic only, and the presence of a comorbid drug disorder (24). For bipolar II patients, three variables were predictive of chronicity: longer duration of the intake episode, a family history of an affective disorder, and poor social functioning in the 5 years before intake (25). For both subtypes, other variables, most notable such baseline variables as gender, age, age of onset, and socioeconomic status, were not predictive of course.

Thus, the only baseline variable that seemed to have predictive value was family history. This is in keeping with previous data. Winokur et al. (26) reported that patients with a family history of mania were more likely to have multiple episodes of an affective illness and were more likely to have repeated hospitalization. In a subsequent evaluation, Winokur and Kadrmas (27) found that patients with multiple recurrences of bipolar disorder episodes were more likely to have a bipolar illness in primary relatives. The CDS found that a family history of mania predicted an increase of manic episodes at 5-year follow-up: 2.23 episodes over 5 years in those with a family history of mania versus 1.53 episodes for those without (28). A family history of any affective disorder, however, was not predictive of the number of episodes.

Course and Symptomatic Subtypes

Rapid cycling bipolar disorder is thought to be predictive of a poorer course. In the CDS, when compared with other types of bipolar disorder, rapid cycling was found to correlate with an earlier age of disease onset (29). Patients with rapid cycling were more likely than other bipolar patients to have depressive symptoms, and patients with rapid cycling were more likely to commit serious suicide attempts.

Among the symptomatic subtypes, one of the most striking findings was the difference between subjects entering the study with mixed episodes. The mixed group had a poorer overall outcome, which was evidenced by significant differences in all aspects of bipolar disorder's course and outcome: time to recovery, risk of relapse, and recurrence, all are worse with this form of the disorder (30). The response to treatment may also be poor for this subtype of mania, though more information is needed in this area. Given the risk of chronicity and recurrence of this disorder, there clearly needs to be an effort to better understand and treat this potentially virulent form of bipolar disorder.

Psychotic symptoms were common but brief: about half the patients had psychotic symptoms at some point during the follow-up but spent only about 2% of the follow-up weeks in a psychotic state (24). Psychotic symptoms were approximately equally divided between manic and depressive affective states. In the mixed/cycling group, having psychotic depression was associated with a slower time to recovery. Psychotic patients had a 37% probability of recovery by 6 months compared with 65% for the non-psychotic patients.

Course and Polarity Sequence

Several studies have suggested that the sequence of episodes correlates with the outcome (31,32). Specifically, episodes that begin with depression and then progress to mania appear too far worse than those that begin with a manic episode. However, most of these studies were short and did not allow for the prospective observation of multiple episodes across several years. An exception is Maj's group (33) in Naples Italy, who found that polarity switches before recovery from an episode were associated with a poorer course. This was particularly true if the index episode began with depression.

The CDS studied this as well (34). Of the patients who were manic at the time of entry, 30% developed depression after entry but before recovery. For patients still manic after 12 weeks, half the patients cycled to depression before recovery. A similar finding occurred in the depressed group. For those depressed at entry, 20% developed mania before recovery and 80% of these patients did not recover after cycling. Overall, it was found that episodes beginning with major depression were longer than those beginning with mania (34), and patients whose episodes began with depression had a higher overall morbidity of disease. It is notable that in the study, the polarity of the initial episode was generally stable over time: patients whose first prospective episode was manic were more likely to begin with mania during subsequent episodes; the same was true of depressive episodes, which supported the suggestion of earlier investigators that bipolar patients were either mania prone or depression prone (35).

Course and Comorbid Substance Abuse

Community-based studies suggest that the risk of comorbid substance abuse is high as 60–70%. Patients with comorbid alcoholism are less likely to recover from an episode of mania (36). Furthermore, the functional recovery is poorer than for those without comorbid substance dependence (20). Winokur et al. (37), in studying patient from the CDS cohort, suggested the course of bipolar illness differed depending on whether patients had primary or secondary alcoholism: patients with primary alcoholism had a more benign course of bipolar disorder than those with a secondary alcohol dependence, suggesting that patients in the first group likely had a more benign form of bipolar disorder that only manifested itself because of the added insult of alcoholism.

Treatment's Effect on Course

The treatment of bipolar disorder is intended, by definition, to alter the course of bipolar disorder. Data exists for the efficacy of several treatments in shortening the time to recovery as well as lengthening the time to recurrence. However, the data for both is not as convincing as one might wish. As these treatment issues are discussed in the chapters on treatment in this book, this subject will not be covered in any detail here. Furthermore, the naturalistic design of studies that investigate disease course is not suited to investigations of treatment: treatment in the CDS, for example, was not controlled, nor influenced during the study. However, such naturalistic long-term studies can offer some interesting clues regarding the effect of treatment on the course of bipolar disorder.

For the CDS, treatment was observed and rated as to levels of intensity. When treatment received was analyzed, it was found that ~75% of the bipolar subjects had both high intensity and sustained levels of treatment (24). Most of the remaining subjects received moderate levels of treatment. This is of interest: many naturalistic studies, including the CDS, have not found lithium (or other bipolar treatments) to have particularly robust effects on the length or episodes or the interval to recurrence. Inadequate treatment is often cited as the reason for this in naturalistic studies. However, arguing that point in the CDS cohort is more difficult in light of this treatment analysis.

Some concerns have been raised about whether antidepressant treatment is likely to precipitate rapid cycling bipolar disorder. The data from the CDS did not find that antidepressants (mostly tricyclic antidepressants) precipitated rapid cycling. Subjects who had rapid cycling during the study were no more likely than others to have been on an antidepressant before the episode (29). Furthermore, the resolution of rapid cycling symptoms was not associated with a decrease in antidepressant medication.

Concern also exists regarding the proper treatment of bipolar depression, given the lack of rigorous studies of this subject. It is notable that in the CDS, depressive symptoms were more common in patients who were receiving lithium carbonate alone than patients on a combination of lithium and an antidepressant. Though this is not proof of the efficacy of antidepressants in treating bipolar mania, it does lend some support to this common clinical practice. Furthermore, patient who switched from depression to mania were not more likely than other patients to be on antidepressants (34). Thus this study did not support the concern that antidepressants can switch a patient from depression into mania. Again, such conclusions are limited by the design of the study.

CONCLUSIONS AND FUTURE DIRECTIONS

The CDS both confirms and extends data from previous longitudinal studies. Some of the most interesting findings and areas for future research are described in this concluding section.

Bipolar Disorder as a Recurrent Illness

The CDS confirms the impression of most previous work that bipolar disorder is a highly recurrent illness. There was some suggestion by some investigators that bipolar disorder might "burn out" with age, but this does not seem to be the case. As to the nature of the recurrence, the CDS casts some doubt on theories of kindling. Though the overall finding that recurrence is best predicted by the number of previous episodes would seem supportive of kindling, there are other less complicated explanations for this finding. Some patients may simply have a more recurrent illness to begin with. A more convincing proof of kindling would be the observation that the disorder changes with succeeding episodes. For example, some earlier studies reported finding that episodes become lengthier, and the inter-episode period becomes shorter, in a manner similar to what is seen for epilepsy. Such a pattern was not found in the CDS cohort, and the episodes remained similar for an individual over time. Future research could focus on more direct testing of the kindling hypothesis. The most convincing evidence would be neuropathological evidence of disease progression; however, this gold standard is likely to remain elusive for some time.

Predictors of Course

The CDS is consistent with previous studies in suggesting that the strongest prognostic predictor is the number of previous episodes and the level of premorbid functioning. These findings have been reported in all major naturalistic studies (38). Beyond this variable, the search for useful predictors has been mixed. The symptomatic status of a patient, particularly predominance or depressive or mixed symptoms, seems to be a reliable predictor; this has been shown in the CDS and most other longitudinal studies. Rapid cycling also seems to predict a worse course, though the evidence for this is somewhat more equivocal. The reason for this can been seen in the unique nature of the CDS in its long length of follow-up: over time, many patients will experience most of the symptomatic states; thus, such symptomatic subtypes as rapid cycling and mixed mania become less stable over time. Family history is somewhat predictive, and this may be a clue regarding possible diagnostic subtypes of the disorder. Most demographic variables have been surprisingly unpredictive of course. This non-finding is consistent through most longitudinal studies, including the CDS. There may be a need for future research, targeting more varied populations. For example, the CDS cohort was Caucasian and English speaking. It is possible that studies concentrating on minorities and on low socioeconomic groups will uncover new relationships. The field of genetic research seems most promising in yielding new markers and predictors of disease. Current genetic findings remain preliminary and will surely involve challenging levels of complexity. However, some preliminary studies are promising: an example is the suggestion that there may be a subgroup of bipolar patients who are highly lithium responsive and that this characteristic might be heritable (39).

Disease Subtypes

Relevant to the discussion mentioned earlier are the nosological concerns. Though most agree that bipolar disorder is likely a heterogeneous disease, with wide differences across patients in disease expression and level of functioning, it is still difficult to agree on meaningful subtypes. Though the subtypes' rapid cycling, mixed mania, and seasonal bipolar disorder have been suggested and used at times, longitudinal data from the CDS and other studies suggest that these subtypes are not as stable as once thought. Perhaps, most intriguing from the CDS data is the observation that some patients have persistent depression symptoms and that these symptoms predict a poorer prognosis. Though some investigators have previously suggested the existence of a "depression-prone" bipolar subtype, this has not been rigorously confirmed in other studies. Given its prognostic significance, this is an important area of future research. As discussed earlier, genetic research is likely to play an important role in this line of investigation.

Importance of Minor and Subsyndromal Symptoms

Perhaps, the most unique finding of the CDS was its attention to minor symptoms and inter-episode phenomena. Prior studies tended to concentrate on the major episodes, and their methodology (e.g., counting the number of episodes per annum) made it difficult to study more minor syndromes. However, the CDS shows that patients are experiencing these more minor syndromes for much of their illness course. Furthermore, these more minor symptoms can still have a significant effect on functioning and on disease outcome. This is the first study to examine this subject in detail, and clearly more information is needed on this important subject.

REFERENCES

1. Falret JP. De la folie circulaire. Bull Acad Méd 1854; 19:382.
2. Kraepelin E. In: Translated by Barclay RM, Robertson GM, eds. Manic-Depressive Insanity and Paranoia. Edinburgh: E & S Livingstone, 1921.
3. Post RM. Sensitization and kindling perspectives for the course of affective illness: toward a new treatment with the anticonvulsant carbamazepine. Pharmacopsychiatry 1990; 23:3–17.
4. Leonhard K, Korff I, Shulz H. Die temperamente in den familien der monopolaren und bipolaren phasischen Psychosen. Psychiatr Neurol 1962; 143:416–434.
5. Winokur G. The Iowa 500: heterogeneity and course in manic-depressive illness (bipolar). Compr Psychiatry 1975; 16:125–131.
6. Wertham F. A group of benign psychoses: prolonged manic excitements. With a statistical study of age, duration and frequency in 2000 manic attacks. Am J Psychiatry 1929; 9: 17–78.
7. Rennie T. Prognosis in manic-depressive psychoses. Am J Psychiatry 1942; 98:801–814.
8. Lundquist G. Prognosis and course in manic-depressive psychoses: a follow-up study of 319 first admissions. Acta Psychiatr Scand 1945; 35(suppl):1–96.
9. Marneros A, Brieger P. Prognosis of bipolar disorder: a review. In: Maj M, Akiskal H, Lopez-Ibor JJ, Sartorious N, eds. Bipolar Disorder. West Sussex: John Wiley and Sons, 2002:97–148.
10. Angst J. Aur Atiologie und Nosologie Endogener Depressiver Psychosen. Springer: Berlin, 1966.
11. Tsuang MT, Woolson RF, Fleming JA. Long-term outcome of major psychoses. I. Schizophrenia and affective disorders compared with psychiatrically symptom-free surgical conditions. Arch Gen Psyhiatry 1979; 36:1295–1301.
12. Marneros A, Deister A, Rohde A. Psychopathological and social status of patients with affective, schizophrenia and schizoaffective disorders after long-term course. Acta Psychiatr Scand 1990; 82:352–358.
13. Katz M, Klerman GL. Introduction: overview of the clinical studies program. Am J Psychiatry 1979; 136:49–51.
14. Frank E, Prien RF, Jarrett RB, Keller MB, Kupfer DJ, Lavori PW, Rush AJ, Weissman MMl. Conceptualization and rationale for consensus definitions of terms in major depressive disorder: remission, recovery, relapse, and recurrence. Arch Gen Psychiatry 1991; 48:851–855.
15. Spitzer RL, Endicott J. Schedule for Affective Disorders and Schizophrenia (SADS). 3rd ed.. New York: Biometric Research, New York State Psychiatric Institute, 1979.
16. Shapiro RW, Keller MB. Longitudinal Interval Follow-up Evaluation (LIFE). Boston: Massachusetts General Hospital, 1979.
17. Keller MB, Lavori PW, Mueller TI, Endicott J, Coryell W, Hirschfeld RM, Shea T. Time to recovery, chronicity, and levels of psychopathology in major depression: a 5-year prospective follow-up of 431 subjects. Arch Gen Psychiatry 1992; 49:809–816.

18. Angst J, Sellaro R. Historical perspectives and natural history of bipolar disorder. Biol Psychiatry 2000; 48:445–457.
19. Keller MB, Lavori PW, Coryell W, Endicott J, Mueller TI. Bipolar I: a five-year prospective follow-up. J Nerv Ment Dis 1993; 181:238–245.
20. Coryell W, Turvey C, Endicott J, Leon AC, Mueller T, Solomon D, Keller M. Bipolar I affective disorder: predictors of outcome after 15 years. J Affect Disord 1998; 50:109–116.
21. Saran B. Lithium. Lancet 1969; 1:1208–1209.
22. Angst J, Grof P, Schou M. Lithium. Lancet 1969; 1:1097–1098.
23. Carlson GA, Kotin J, Davenport YB, Adland M. Follow-up of 53 bipolar manic-depressive patients. Br J Psychiatry 1974; 124:134–139.
24. Judd LL, Akiskal HS, Schettler PJ. The long-term natural history of the weekly symptomatic status of bipolar I disorder. Arch Gen Psychiatry 2002; 59:530–537.
25. Judd LL, Akiskal HS, Schettler PJ. A prospective investigation of the natural history of the long-term weekly symptomatic status of bipolar II disorder. Arch Gen Psychiatry 2003; 60:261–269.
26. Winokur G, Crowe R, Kadrmas A. A genetic approach to heterogeneity in psychoses: relationship of a family history of mania or depression to course in bipolar illness. Psychopathology 1986; 19:80–84.
27. Winokur G, Kadrmas A. A polyepisodic course in bipolar illness: possible clinical relationship. Compr Psychiatry 1989; 30:121–127.
28. Winokur G, Coryell W, Keller M, Endicott J, Akiskal H. A prospective follow-up of patients with bipolar and primary unipolar affective. Arch Gen Psychiatry 1993; 50: 457–465.
29. Coryell W, Solomon D, Turvey C, Keller M, Leon AC, Endicott J, Schettler P, Judd L, Mueller T. The long-term course of rapid-cycling bipolar disorder. Arch Gen Psychiatry 2003; 60:914–920.
30. Boland RJ, Keller MB. Mixed-state bipolar disorders: outcome data from the NIMH Collaborative Program on the Psychobiology of Depression. In: Goldberg JF, Harrow M, eds. Bipolar Disorders. Clinical Course and Outcome. Washington: American Psychiatric Press, 1999:115–128.
31. Faedda GL, Baldessarini RJ, Tohen M, Strakowski SM, Waternaux C. Episode sequence in bipolar disorder and response to lithium treatment. Am J Psychiatry 1991; 9:1237–1239.
32. Maj M, Pirozzi R, Magliano L, Bartoli L. Long-term outcome of lithium prophylaxis in bipolar disorder: A 5-year prospective study of 402 patients at a lithium clinic. Am J Psychiatry 1998; 155:30–35.
33. Maj M, Pirozzi R, Magliano L, Bartoli L. The prognostic significance of "switching" in patients with bipolar disorder: a 10-year prospective follow-up study. Am J Psychiatry 2002; 159:1711–1717.
34. Turvey C, Corylell W, Arndt S, Solomon DA, Leon AC, Endicott J, Mueller T, Keller M, Akiskal H. Polarity sequence, depression, and chronicity in bipolar I disorder. J Nerv Mental Dis 1999; 187:181–187.
35. Quitkin FM, Rabkin JG, Prien RF. Bipolar disorder: are there manic-prone and depressive-prone forms? J Clin Psychopharmacol 1986; 6:167–172.
36. Goldberg JF, Garno JL, Leon AC, Kocsis JH, Portera L. A history of substance abuse complicates remission from acute mania in bipolar disorder. J Clin Psychiatry 1999; 60: 733–740.
37. Winokur G, Coryell W, Akiskal H, Maser JD, Keller MB, Endicott J, Mueller T. Alcoholism in manic-depressive (bipolar) illness: familial illness, course of illness, and the primary–secondary distinction. Am J Psychiatry 1995; 152:365–372.
38. Turvey CL. The importance of natural course and depression in bipolar I disorder. In: Maj M, Akiskal H, Lopez-Ibor JJ, Sartorious N, eds. Bipolar Disorder. West Sussex: John Wiley and Sons, 2002:171–173.
39. Alda M, Grof E, Cavazzoni P, Duffy A, Martin R, Ravindran L, Grof P. Autosomal recessive inheritance of affective disorders in families of responders to lithium prophylaxis? J Affect Disord 1997; 44:153–157.

9

Recent Advances in Our Understanding of the Neurobiology of Bipolar Disorder

Jorge A. Quiroz, Jaskaran Singh, Carlos A. Zarate Jr., and Husseini K. Manji
Laboratory of Molecular Pathophysiology, National Institute of Mental Health, Bethesda, Maryland, U.S.A.

INTRODUCTION

Bipolar disorder (also known as manic-depressive illness) is a severe and often life-threatening illness (1) that has recently been recognized, by the Institute of Medicine, as a chronic condition that requires priority action (2). The costs associated with disability and premature death from major mood disorders represent an economic burden of tens of billions of dollars annually in the United States alone (3). Despite the devastating impact that bipolar disorder has on the lives of millions worldwide, there is still little known concerning its underlying etiology and neurobiology. This lack of knowledge regarding the cellular underpinnings of bipolar disorder has undoubtedly contributed to the lack of development of new treatments. Therefore, studies of the classic neurotransmitter systems, as well as studies of genetics, neuroendocrine systems, neuropeptides, circadian rhythms, intracellular signaling pathways, mitochondrial function, fatty acids, neurotrophic factors, and immune function (and the interplay of these systems), are critically needed to fully understand the pathophysiology of bipolar disorder. This chapter reviews the current relevant studies on the pathophysiology of bipolar disorder, and attempts to build a framework for the direction of future research.

MONOAMINERGIC NEUROTRANSMITTER SYSTEMS AND NEUROENDOCRINE ABNORMALITIES

The monoaminergic neurotransmitter systems have received the greatest attention in neurobiological studies of bipolar disorder. The interest in the monoaminergic systems in unipolar and bipolar disorders largely resulted from several clinical and preclinical observations that: (a) effective antidepressant drugs exert their primary biochemical effects by regulating intrasynaptic levels of serotonin and norepinephrine; (b) earlier antihypertensive drugs usually produced a depletion of intrasynaptic concentrations of serotonin and norepinephrine, frequently resulting in depressive episodes in susceptible patients; and (c) dopaminergic agonists and psychostimulants have been associated with precipitating manic episodes in susceptible patients.

In addition to these compelling pharmacological data, the biogenic amine neurotransmitter systems are distributed extensively in the limbic system, which is implicated in the regulation of sleep, appetite, arousal, sexual function, endocrine function, and emotional states such as fear and rage. The clinical symptomatology of bipolar disorder involves disruption of behavior, circadian rhythms, neurophysiology of sleep, and neuroendocrine and biochemical regulation within the brain (1,4). These complex illness manifestations are undoubtedly mediated by a network of interconnected neurotransmitter pathways; the monoamine neurotransmitter systems are ideally placed to mediate such complex behavioral effects, and thus represent attractive candidate systems underlying the pathophysiology of bipolar disorder (5). Clinical studies in the last 40 years have attempted to untangle the multiple biological factors that are presumed to be involved in the pathophysiology of bipolar disorder by using a variety of biochemical and neuroendocrine strategies. Assessments of cerebrospinal fluid (CSF) chemistry, neuroendocrine responses to pharmacological challenge, and neuroreceptor and transporter binding have demonstrated a number of abnormalities of the noradrenergic, serotonergic, and other neurotransmitter systems in bipolar disorder.

Noradrenergic System

Despite methodological difficulties in assessing central nervous system (CNS) noradrenergic (norepinephrine, NE) functions in humans, extensive investigation supports the presence of NE systems abnormalities in bipolar disorder (Table 1) (1,6).

Central and Peripheral Indices of Noradrenergic Function

Studies of peripheral NE activity have mainly found that urinary NE's major metabolite, 3-methoxy-4-hydroxyphenylglycol (MHPG), is decreased in bipolar depressed patients, whereas in longitudinal studies, MHPG excretion was shown to be higher in the manic compared with the depressed state (1,6–8). Similarly, in vivo studies have found plasma levels of NE and MHPG to be lower in bipolar than in unipolar depressed patients, and higher in bipolar patients when manic than when depressed. More importantly, CSF NE and MHPG have consistently been reported to be higher in mania than in depression.

For several reasons, it has been argued that the measurement of MHPG may be of limited value in assessing the noradrenergic system. Less than 20% of MHPG is derived from brain norepinephrine metabolism (9). Furthermore, because unconjugated MHPG is readily diffusible, there is a free exchange of this metabolite among plasma, CSF, and nerve tissues (including brain and spinal cord). On the other hand, measures of NE and its metabolites in CSF were thought to directly reflect intrasynaptic levels of NE. This assumption is, however, problematic since high correlations have been found between indices of NE function in plasma and CSF (10). In addition, standards for obtaining CSF such as elapsed time between needle insertion and sample collection have not been established, and sampling at a single point in time may not reflect the biochemical process of depression or mania, but rather a state-dependent fluctuation from a recent external or internal stress (1). The CSF MHPG levels, after correction for the plasma contribution of the metabolite, more accurately reflects its rate of formation in the CNS. Finally, Tsuji et al. (11) found

Table 1 A Summary of the Major Findings Supporting the Involvement of the Noradrenergic, Serotonergic, and Dopaminergic Systems in the Pathophysiology and Treatment of Bipolar Disorder

Noradrenergic
CSF, urinary NE and MHPG: mania > BPD depression; MDD > BPD depression
Plasma NE; basal levels: BPD depression < HV < MDD
Plasma NE: upon challenge: BPD depression > MDD > HV
CSF NE, correlated with dysphoric symptoms and severity in BPD
Effects of AMPT: reversal of antidepressant effects in unipolar patients, but produces "rebound hypomania" in lithium-treated BPD
Blunted growth hormone response to alpha 2 agonists and increases platelet alpha 2 binding density (BPD and MDD)
Agents which increase NE release/block reuptake are capable of triggering mania
Antidepressant and lithium reduce β-adrenergic receptor density and/or function (cAMP formation) in limbic and limbic-related areas of rat brain
Serotonergic
Reduced CSF 5-HIAA appears to be characteristic of suicidal, impulsive and aggressive patients, whether unipolar or bipolar
Reduced CSF 5-HIAA may be found in both depressive and manic states
Blunted neuroendocrine and temperature responses to various 5-HT agonists
Antidepressant efficacy of agents which increase intrasynaptic 5-HT
Agents which increase intrasynaptic 5-HT are capable of triggering manic episodes, albeit less so than catecholamine enhancing agents
Tryptophan depletion induces a rapid depressive relapse in Selective Serotonin Reuptake Inhibitors (SSRI)-treated patients (but not lithium treated)
Dopaminergic
Reduced CSF HVA in depressed patients
Blunted neuroendocrine and temperatures responses to DA agonists in MDD
Reduced internal jugular venoarterial HVA concentration gradients in MDD
Antidepressant efficacy of agents whose biochemical effects includes increasing intrasynaptic dopamine
ECT consistently enhances DA function
Depressogenic effects of AMPT and reserpine in susceptible individuals
Medications which block D2 receptors have antimanic efficacy
Lithium-treated euthymic bipolar patients show a rebound hypomania following AMPT
Depression is common in Parkinson's disease and there are reports of abolition of Parkinsonian symptoms during mania
Prominent anhedonia, amotivation, and psychomotor retardation in bipolar depression
Critical role of DA in reward, motivation and motoric circuits

Abbreviations: AMPT, α-methylparatyrosine; BPD, bipolar disorder; CSF, central system fluid; DA, dopamine; DST, dexamethasone suppression test; ECT, electroconvulsive therapy; HV, healthy volunteers; HVA, homovanillic acid; MDD, major depressive disorder (unipolar depression); MHPG, methoxy-hydroxy-phenyl-glycol; NE, norepinephrine; SSRIs, serotonin selective reuptake inhibitors; UP, unipolar; 5-HIAA, 5-hydroxyindoleacetic acid; 5-HT, serotonin. *Source*: From Ref. 305.

correlations among the CSF concentrations of MHPG and 3,4-dihydroxyphenylglycol (DHPG) in CSF and plasma but no significant correlations were found between the urinary levels and either plasma or CSF levels of these metabolites.

Post-Mortem Studies

Whereas numerous post-mortem studies have investigated the role of monoaminergic functioning in major depressive disorder and suicide, there is a dearth of studies examining the status of monoamine neurotransmitters in autopsy specimens from subjects specifically with bipolar disorder. Only one study has quantitated the levels of NE, serotonin (5-HT), dopamine (DA), and their respective major metabolites [MHPG, 5-hydroxyindoleacetic acid (5-HIAA), and homovanillic acid (HVA)] in post-mortem brains obtained from bipolar disorder patients (12). Compared with control subjects matched with respect to age, gender, post-mortem interval, and brain pH, NE turnover (MHPG/NE ratio) was markedly elevated in the frontal, temporal, and occipital cortex of patients with an antemortem diagnosis of bipolar disorder. In comparison, 5-HT and DA turnover (5-HIAA/5HT and HVA/DA ratios, respectively) were significantly reduced in temporal and occipital cortex, respectively. Post-mortem studies have shown an increased NE turnover in the cortex and in the thalamic areas of subjects with bipolar disorder (12,13). In a post-mortem study of the brains of 12 patients who had mood disorders compared with the brains of 12 non-psychiatric controls, the total number of neurons in the locus coeruleus (LC, the main noradrenergic nucleus of the brain) was higher in bipolar than in unipolar patients and this differences seen in both sides of the brain. The finding of an enlarged LC in bipolar disorder is consistent with a hypernormal pattern of bipolar disorder morphology comprising smaller sulcal and greater thalamic volumes, greater gray–white ratios, increased gyral complexity, and an enlarged amygdalae.

Tyrosine hydroxylase is the key enzyme in noradrenaline synthesis and can be detected using immunohistochemical analysis. The number of tyrosine hydroxylase-immunoreactive (TH-ir) neurons did not differ between bipolar and unipolar patients or between patients and controls in a post-mortem study of suicidal and non-suicidal depressed patients (14).

Other Studies

Other paradigms for studying NE receptor function suggest an altered sensitivity of α_2- and β_2-adrenergic receptors in mood disorders (6,8). Genetics studies show that a polymorphic variation of enzymes involved in amine metabolism [e.g., tyrosine hydroxylase, catechol-*O*-methyltransferase (COMT)] could confer different susceptibility to developing bipolar disorder symptoms (15–17).

The effects of catecholamine depletion have been investigated with α-methyl-paratyrosine (AMPT), an inhibitor of catecholamine synthesis, in patients with bipolar disorder. A group of patients who were in long-term remission with lithium therapy were given either AMPT or placebo. No changes in mood occurred during drug administration, however, 24–48 hr after receiving AMPT, patients had a transient relapse into hypomanic symptoms, suggesting that the mechanism of prevention of manic relapse by long-term lithium therapy may in part be dependent on stability of the catecholamine system (18).

Serotonergic System

There is a consistent body of data from CSF studies, neuroendocrine-challenge studies, serotonin receptor- and reuptake-site binding studies, pharmacologic studies, and most recently brain imaging studies, that there is a serotonergic neurotransmission dysfunction in patients with major depression (1,19,20) (Table 1). Overall, investigators have reported reduced levels of 5-HIAA in a subgroup of patients, especially those with impulsivity, aggression, and suicide attempts. In bipolar disorder patients, studies of CSF 5-HIAA in manic patients have generally produced variable and inconsistent results (1,21), i.e., baseline CSF 5-HIAA levels in manic patients, compared with non-depressed controls, have been reported as decreased in four studies, unchanged in nine studies, and increased in three studies. In contrast, most studies find no difference in the levels of CSF 5-HIAA between manic and depressed patients; of the four studies that examined CSF 5-HIAA accumulation following administration of probenecid (a competitive inhibitor that blocks the active transport of acid metabolites out of the brain and CSF) in manic patients, depressed patients, and controls, two studies reported that both manic and depressed patients have diminished CSF 5-HIAA formation compared with controls, and one study reported that manic patients have significantly lower CSF 5-HIAA accumulation than depressed patients and controls (1).

Studies have also reported decreased radioligand binding to the serotonin transporter (which takes up serotonin from the synaptic cleft) both in platelets and in the midbrain of depressed patients (19,20). Most recently, an intriguing preliminary positron emission tomography (PET) study reported decreases in 5-HT_{1A} receptor binding potential in raphe and hippocampus–amygdala in the brains of depressed patients, in particular, in both bipolar and unipolar depressed patients, with relatives with bipolar disorder (22). One factor that may contribute to the reduction in 5-HT_{1A} receptor binding in depression is increased cortisol secretion (known to occur in many depressed patients, see Section Hypothalamic–Pituitary–Adrenal Axis), since post-synaptic 5-HT_{1A} receptor mRNA expression is under tonic inhibition by corticosteroid receptor stimulation in some brain regions. These studies have identified an approximately 25% reduction in hippocampal 5-HT_{1A} receptor binding potential difference between depressed and healthy subjects in specific brain areas (23,24).

Pharmacological Probes and Depletion Studies

Neurotransmitter depletion models, specifically in this case tryptophan depletion to lower serotonin levels, permit a more direct strategy to clarify the involvement of serotonergic systems in mood disorders. In bipolar disorder, tryptophan depletion in lithium-treated euthymic patients did not result in a recurrence of symptoms (25). Thus, although lithium has often been postulated to exert many of its beneficial effects via an enhancement of serotonergic function, the tryptophan depletion studies suggest that other mechanisms may be more relevant.

Most recently, investigators have investigated the possibility that sensitivity to the negative mood and cognitive effects of reduced serotonin may represent an endophenotype for bipolar disorder, by studying unaffected relatives of bipolar disorder patients. In a double-blind, crossover design, unaffected relatives from multiple families with bipolar disorder and healthy control subjects underwent acute tryptophan depletion (ATD) (26). Unlike the control subjects, unaffected relatives experienced a lowering of mood during ATD but not with the placebo. Furthermore, unaffected relatives tended to show increased impulsivity in the ATD condition. Measurements obtained before ingestion of the amino acids drink indicated that, relative to control subjects, unaffected relatives showed reduced serotonin platelet concentrations, lower affinity for, and fewer binding sites of the serotonin transporter for imipramine; these differences were unaffected by ATD. Sobczak et al. (27) investigated the effects of ATD on cognitive performance in healthy first-degree relatives of bipolar patients (FH) and matched controls in a placebo-controlled, double-blind crossover design. Performances on planning, memory, and attention tasks were assessed at baseline and 5 hours after ATD. They found that speed of information processing on the planning task following ATD was impaired in the FH group but not in the healthy control group (similar to unaffected relatives in the Quintin et al. (26) study noted above). Furthermore, FH subjects with a bipolar disorder type I relative showed impairments in planning and memory, independent of ATD. In all subjects, ATD impaired long-term memory performance and speed of information processing. ATD did not affect short-term memory or focused and divided attention. Together, these results suggest that vulnerability to reduced tryptophan availability may represent an endophenotype for bipolar disorder, i.e., a biological abnormality that is a more immediate result of a genetic defect than a clinical syndrome.

Studies assessing the sensitivity of the serotonergic system by exploring changes in plasma levels of prolactin and cortisol after administration of D-fenfluramine in manic patients have shown contradictory results (28,29). D-Fenfluramine increases prolactin and cortisol, and therefore D-fenfluramine is considered to provide an index of overall activity of the central 5-HT system. More consistent results have been found after administration of sumatriptan (a 5-HT_{1D} agonist)—the growth hormone (GH) response is blunted in manic compared with depressed patients (30), revealing a sub-sensitivity of 5-HT function.

Post-mortem Studies

5-HT and DA turnover (5-HIAA/5HT and HVA/DA ratios, respectively) were significantly reduced in temporal and occipital cortices in the brains of patients with antemortem diagnoses of bipolar disorder (12). In addition, studies of 5-HT uptake sites using [^{1}H]citalopram have found reduced binding in the frontal cortex from bipolar depressed subjects compared with matched control subjects (31). The findings of reduced 5-HT turnover and uptake sites in bipolar disorder are consistent with results from post-mortem brains of patients with major depressive disorder and those who died by suicide. These results have led to the suggestion that decreased brain serotonergic transmission may be a shared feature of affective disorders and suicide and may be related to common symptomatology (i.e., depressed state) across these disorders (12). Post-mortem studies of cerebral 5-HT_{1A} receptor binding and mRNA expression in major depressive disorders and bipolar disorder suggest 5-HT_{1A} receptor dysfunction in mood disorders, but these data are limited to two studies involving small sample sizes (32).

Other Studies

Further evidence implicating the serotonergic system in the pathophysiology of bipolar disorder comes from polymorphism genotyping studies. In studying the allelic variation of the serotonin transporter-linked polymorphic region (5-HTTLPR), patients who were homozygotic for the long variant of the serotonergic receptor (*ll*) showed better mood amelioration after total sleep deprivation than those who were heterozygotic and homozygotic for the short variant (33). Additionally, an association between prophylactic response and the 5-HTTLPR has been described (34); in this study, the homozygotes for the short allele (*ss*) group showed poorer response to lithium prophylaxis. Finally, Mundo et al. (35) found that nearly two-thirds of bipolar patients with a history of antidepressant-induced mania had the *s* allele compared with 29% of bipolar subjects who had been exposed to antidepressants, but did not develop mania.

Dopaminergic System

In recent years, there has been an increasing appreciation that the original serotonergic and noradrenergic hypotheses do not fully explain the neurobiology of unipolar and bipolar disorders, or the mechanisms of action of effective treatments in such disorders. Surprisingly, the role of the dopaminergic (DA) system in the pathophysiology and treatment of bipolar disorder has not received greater study, yet it represents a prime candidate on a number of theoretical grounds (Table 1). The motor changes in bipolar disorder are perhaps the most defining characteristics of the illness, ranging from near catatonic immobility during depression to the profound hyperactivity of manic states (1,36). Similarly, loss of motivation is one of the central features of depression, and anhedonia and/or "hyperhedonic states" are among the most defining characteristics of bipolar depression and mania, respectively. The midbrain DA systems are known to play critical roles in regulating not only motor activity, but also motivational and reward circuits. It is clear that motivation and motor function are closely linked, and that motivational variables can influence motor output both qualitatively and quantitatively. Furthermore, there is considerable evidence that the mesolimbic DA pathway plays a crucial role in the selection and orchestration of goal-directed behaviors, particularly those elicited by incentive stimuli (37).

The strongest direct finding from clinical studies implicating DA in depression is reduced HVA (the major DA metabolite) in CSF, one of the most consistent biochemical findings in depression (1,6). There is also evidence for a decreased rate of CSF HVA accumulation in subgroups of depressed patients, including those with marked psychomotor retardation vs. agitation (38). Furthermore, depression occurs in up to 40% of patients with idiopathic Parkinson's disease (a neurological condition usually resulting from dopamine deficiency), and may precede motor symptoms. Some case reports have even reported the disappearance of Parkinson's disease symptoms during a manic episode (39,40).

Pharmacological Probes

The pharmacological data also support the idea that manipulating the dopaminergic system is capable of modulating mood disorders. DA agonists appear to be effective antidepressants and are able to precipitate mania in some patients with bipolar disorder (1,6). Recently, investigators used a catecholamine-depletion strategy—via use of the tyrosine hydroxylase inhibitor AMPT—in lithium-treated, euthymic bipolar disorder patients (18). Intriguingly, they did not observe any mood-lowering effects of AMPT, but observed a "rebound hypomania" in a significant percentage of the patients. Although preliminary, these results suggest a dysregulated signaling system wherein the adaptation to catecholamine depletion results in an over-compensation due to impaired homeostatic mechanisms. McTavish et al. (41) reported that a tyrosine-free mixture lowered both subjective and objective measures of the psychostimulant effects of methamphetamine in healthy volunteers, and lowered manic scores in acutely manic bipolar patients, suggesting that tyrosine availability to the brain attenuates pathological increases in dopamine neurotransmission following methamphetamine administration and (in the previous study) putatively in mania.

Neuroimaging Studies

In more recent neuroimaging studies, the concentration of the vesicular monoamine transporter protein (VMAT2), a stable pre-synaptic marker, was quantified with (+)

[(11)C] dihydrotetrabenazine (DTBZ) using PET (42). Sixteen bipolar I asymptomatic patients (nine men and seven women) who had a prior history of mania with psychosis and individually matched healthy subjects were studied. VMAT2 binding in the thalamus and ventral brainstem of the bipolar patients was higher than in the comparison subjects, suggesting greater concentrations of DA cells. In a follow-up study, the same research group attempted to assess the diagnostic specificity of the findings, by comparing VMAT2 concentrations between euthymic bipolar I patients, schizophrenic patients, and age-matched healthy volunteers (42). They found that VMAT2 binding in the thalamus was higher in bipolar I patients than in control subjects and in patients with schizophrenia. The authors interpreted the intriguing findings of increased VMAT2 expression in euthymic bipolar I patients as representing trait-related abnormalities in the concentration of monoaminergic synaptic terminals (such as DA). However, chronic lithium treatment has recently been demonstrated to increase VMAT protein in the rat frontal cortex (the only region examined) (43), raising the possibility that the PET human studies may have been confounded by treatment effects.

Yatham et al. (44) recently assessed pre-synaptic dopamine function in 13 antipsychotic- and mood-stabilizer-naive nonpsychotic first-episode manic patients by measuring [(18)F] 6-fluoro-L-dopa ([(18)F]DOPA) uptake in the striatum by PET. No significant differences in [(18)F]DOPA uptake rate constants in the striatum were found between the manic patients and the comparison subjects, however, treatment with valproate significantly reduced the [(18)F]DOPA uptake rate.

Cholinergic System

Much of the evidence supporting the involvement of the cholinergic system in mood disorders comes from neurochemical, behavioral, and physiologic studies in response to pharmacologic manipulations. These studies, carried out in the early 1970s, showed that the relative inferiority of noradrenergic compared with cholinergic tone was associated with depression, whereas the reverse was associated with mania (45). Studies with the central cholinesterase inhibitor physostigmine (administered intravenously), showed modulation of manic symptoms toward depression (46–48). Studying pupil size changes with cholinergic-agonists drugs in bipolar disorder patients have revealed a decreased cholinergic tone during mania. Severe manic patients required higher concentrations of pilocarpine in order to elicit a 50% reduction in pupil size. Consistently, improvements in mania after lithium or valproate treatments were closely correlated with decreases in pilocarpine requirements to elicit pupillary contraction (49,50). Therefore, lithium and valproate treatment may possibly potentiate brain cholinergic neurotransmission (51,52). However, the therapeutic responses observed with antidepressant and antimanic pharmacological agents have not been reliably associated with effects on the cholinergic system.

Gamma-Aminobutyric Acid

The majority of studies examining the role of gamma-aminobutyric acid (GABA) in patients with mood disorders have been conducted in patients with unipolar depression rather than in patients with bipolar disorder (53). Studies of CSF GABA in patients with bipolar disorder have been limited and generally inconclusive (54). The precise origin of plasma GABA in humans is difficult to prove, however, indirect evidence suggests that plasma GABA is an accurate reflection of brain GABA activity or function (53).

Low plasma GABA differentiates well patients from ill patients in about one-third of bipolar patients (53), and is also seen in euthymic unmedicated bipolar patients (55). Plasma GABA levels do not correlate with severity of symptoms for either depression or mania (i.e., levels are state independent); however, the key research in identifying whether the marker is familial and segregates with illness in families with affective disorders has not yet been done.

Petty et al. (53) reported that the plasma levels of GABA in bipolar disorder patients during both the manic and depressive phases were significantly lower than in healthy control subjects and similar to patients with unipolar depression. Based on their data, the investigators concluded that low plasma GABA is not specific to the depressed state, as it is also found in the manic phase of bipolar disorder. Because there is no correlation between the severity of depressive symptoms and levels of plasma GABA, and because low plasma GABA levels do not appear to normalize with clinical improvement (53,56,57), Petty et al. (53) have proposed that low plasma GABA may represent a trait-like marker for major depressive illness in a subset of patients.

As part of a multicenter, double-blind, randomized, acute-phase, placebo-controlled trial of divalproex in mania (58), plasma concentrations of GABA were measured before and after treatment. A preliminary analysis of these data revealed three interesting findings. First, there was no correlation demonstrated between baseline levels of plasma GABA (after a minimum 3-day washout) and severity of manic symptoms as determined by the Mania Rating Scale scores. Second, pretreatment levels of plasma GABA predicted response to divalproex but not to lithium or placebo. However, the correlation was such that patients with the higher levels of plasma GABA were more likely to respond to divalproex with improvement in their acute manic symptoms than patients with lower plasma GABA levels. And third, plasma levels of GABA decreased during treatment with divalproex compared with placebo (59).

The acute neurochemical effects of valproate on the GABA system are complex (60). Although acute administration of valproate leads to increased brain tissue levels of GABA, these changes are not strongly significant at clinically relevant doses (61). At lower doses, GABA concentrations in synaptosomes and nerve terminals are increased significantly by acute administration of valproate (62), and the activity of GABA transaminase (GABA-T, the GABA metabolizing enzyme), is decreased (60).

Using a localized spectral editing sequence, Sanacora et al. (63) recently reported the first in vivo magnetic resonance spectroscopy (MRS) study investigating the possibility of GABA system dysfunction in mood disorders. GABA levels were measured in the occipital cortex of medication-free depressed patients and healthy control subjects. The depressed patients demonstrated a highly significant (52%) reduction in occipital cortex GABA levels compared with the group of healthy controls. A follow-up study by the same group concluded that although low cortical GABA levels are present in patients with unipolar depression, they do not differ significantly from levels in healthy controls and in patients with bipolar depression.

Glutamate

Glutamate is the most abundant excitatory amino acid, and is the main excitatory neurotransmitter in mammalian hippocampal formation from the entorhinal cortex (perforant pathway) to the dentate gyrus [mossy fibers and the CA1–4 areas (Schaffer collaterals)] to the subiculum (64). In normal conditions, glutamate plays a prominent role in synaptic plasticity, learning, and memory (65–68). Glutamate can also be a potent neuronal excitotoxin under a variety of experimental conditions, triggering either rapid or delayed neurotoxicity (69–71). Glutamate-mediated excitotoxicity has been implicated in certain neurodegenerative disease, including amyotrophic lateral sclerosis (ALS), Alzheimer's disease, and Huntington's disease (71).

Glutamate's neurotransmitter actions occur at the pre-synaptic and post-synaptic level through stimulation of specific receptors that can be classified into two groups by structural characteristics (Fig. 1). These two receptor groups are directly related to the importance of glutamate in the neurobiology of bipolar disorder.

The first receptor group, named ionotropic glutamate receptors, are ion channels that, when stimulated, open the channel pore allowing sodium, potassium,

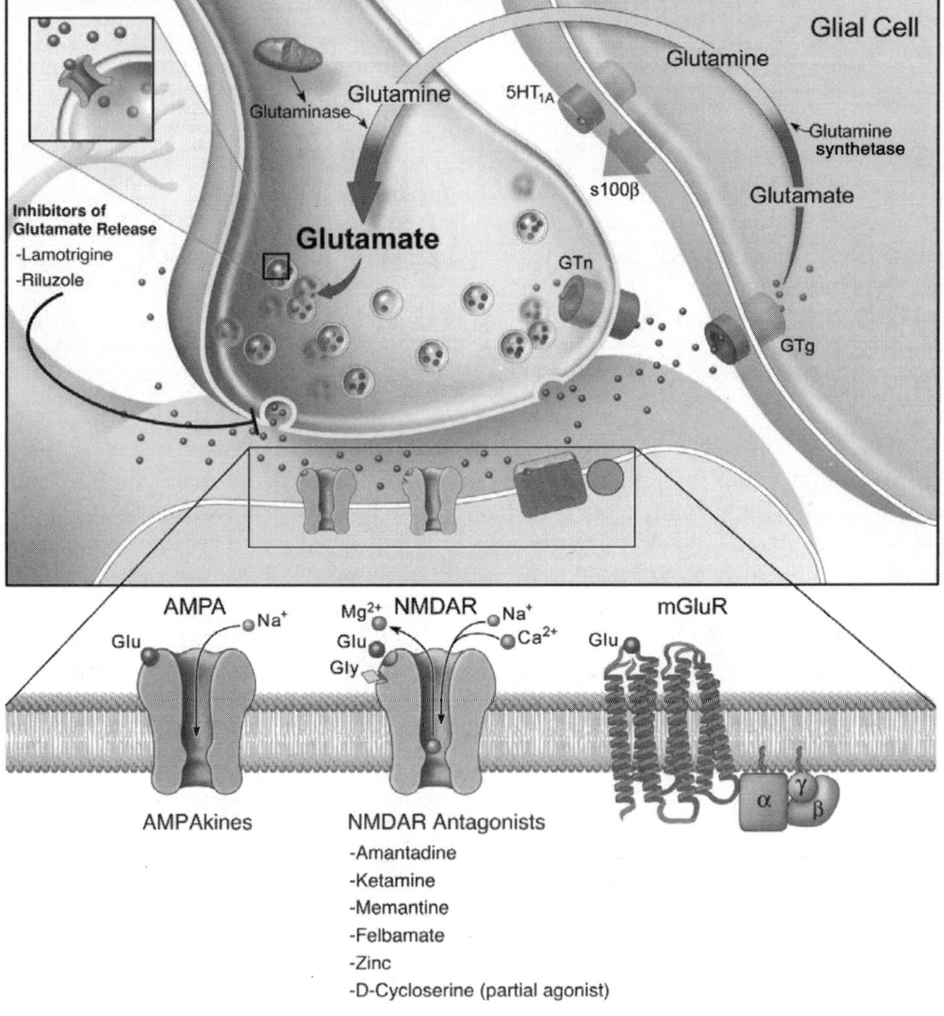

Figure 1 (*Caption on Facing Page*)

and calcium to flow freely into the cell. This opening of the pore changes the polarization of the neuronal surface and also activates intracellular signaling. Three different subgroups of ionotropic glutamate receptors have been identified by their pharmacological ability to bind different synthetic ligands. These three subgroups are *N*-methyl-D-aspartate (NMDA) receptors, α-amino-3-hydroxy-5-methyl-4-isoxazole propionic acid (AMPA) receptors, and kainate (KA) receptors. The latter two groups are often referred to together as the non-NMDA receptors. NMDA and AMPA receptors are found in high density in the cerebral cortex, hippocampus, striatum, septum, and amygdala. Importantly, it is believed that the large excesses of calcium (Ca^{2+}) entering cells via the NMDA receptor channel are the proximate cause of rapid cell death that occurs with anoxia, which is also referred to as excitotoxicity.

The second group of receptors, named metabotropic receptors, is G-protein-coupled receptors that exert their action directly through second messenger pathways. This second receptor group is responsible for modulating synaptic transmission and cell excitability through the activation of guanosine 5′-triphosphate (GTP) binding protein (G-protein)-linked receptors. They are classified into three different sub-groups: (a) sub-group I receptors, located in both the pre- and post-synaptic membranes, preferentially interact with the $G_{q/11}$ subunit of G-proteins, leading to activation of the enzyme phospholipase C (PLC), and through phosphoinositide hydrolysis activate the inositide triphosphate/calcium and diacylglycerol/protein

---

Figure 1 (*Facing page*) *The glutamatergic system as a target of novel medications.* Glutamate is synthesized in neurons from α-ketoglutarate through the tricarboxylic acid (TCA) cycle. After released, glutamate is re-uptaked by glutamate transporters, shown in glia (GTg) and a pre-synaptic neuron (GTn). In the glia, glutamate is catabolized to glutamine (through the enzyme glutamine synthetase), diffuses to the neurons and is then metabolized back to glutamate (through the enzyme glutaminase). The different glutamate receptors and the presumed antiglutamatergic drug site of action are presented in the figure. Glutamate (Glu) exerts its action at the pre-synaptic and post-synaptic level through the stimulation of specific receptors that can be classified by structural characteristics: the first group, "ionotropic glutamate receptors" are ion channels that when stimulated open the channel pore allowing sodium, potassium, and calcium to flow freely into the cell. This opening of the pore changes the polarization of the neuronal surface and activates intracellular signaling. NMDA and AMPA are ionotrophic glutamate receptors. Activation of these receptors allows the entry into the cell of primarily calcium and sodium respectively. The second group, "metabotropic receptors" (mGluR) are G-protein-coupled receptors, which directly act through second messenger pathways. *Riluzole* is a glutamate release inhibitor (acting through blockade of Na^{+} voltage dependent channels), a GABAA agonist and probably an AMPA and kainate antagonist. *Lamotrigine* has a number of biological effects including the inhibition of glutamate release (blockade of Na^{+} voltage dependent channels). *Memantine* is a non-competitive antagonist NMDA receptor. *Felbamate* is non-competitive NMDA receptor antagonist (in glycine NR1 and glutamate NR2B subunits), an AMPA receptor antagonist, an mGlu group I receptor antagonist and a glutamate release inhibitor (acting through blockade of Ca^{++} and Na^{+} voltage dependant channels). *Ketamine* is a high-affinity NMDA receptor antagonist. D-Cycloserine is a partial agonist at the NMDA receptor glycine (Gly) site. At high doses, *amantadine* reduces NMDA receptor function by approximately 50%, an effect attributed to its instability within the NMDA receptor channel. *Zinc* is a potent inhibitor of the NMDA receptor complex. *AMPAkines* allosterically produce positive modulation of AMPA receptors and have actively been studied in the treatment of schizophrenia. Studies have shown that the biarylpropylsulfonamide AMPA receptor potentiators (LY392098 and LY451616) have antidepressant effects in animal models of depression. *Source*: Modified and reproduced with permission from Ref. 302.

kinase C (PKC) cascades (discussed later); (b) the sub-group II, and (c) sub-group III receptors are located in the pre-synaptic membrane, and because of their coupling with Gi/o-proteins appear to negatively modulate glutamate and GABA neurotransmission output when activated.

Much pre-clinical evidence associates the glutamate neurotransmitter system with the pathophysiology of mood disorders. The acute effects of antidepressants in vitro and the chronic effects of antidepressants have been shown to modulate glutamatergic activity. On the other hand, NMDA antagonists have been shown to possess antidepressant-like properties in pre-clinical studies, as well as producing β-adrenoreceptor downregulation and modulation of serotonergic function. Evidence for abnormalities in glutamate function in humans has been found in plasma and CSF levels, brain imaging studies, and post-mortem studies (72). Thus, a number of glutamatergic plasticity-enhancing strategies may be of considerable utility in the treatment of mood disorders (Fig. 1).

Recently, Berman et al. (73) reported the first placebo-controlled, double-blind trial assessing the treatment effects of a single dose of the NMDA receptor–antagonist ketamine in patients with depression. The authors reported that patients with depression experienced significant improvement in depressive symptoms within a short period of time (72 hr) after taking ketamine but not after placebo. Additional evidence that glutamate modulation may be important in the pathophysiology of bipolar disorder comes from the clinical use of the anticonvulsant lamotrigine, a drug that inhibits the release of glutamate. In a double-blind, placebo-controlled study, lamotrigine was reported to be effective in acute bipolar I depression (74).

Recently, our investigative group conducted an open-label study with the agent riluzole, a pre-synaptic inhibitor of glutamate release, in patients with treatment-resistant major (unipolar) depression. A significant improvement was observed at the end of 6 weeks of riluzole treatment (75). In addition we found riluzole to be significantly helpful in an add-on study to lithium in treatment resistant bipolar depression subjects (312). Other agents, such as glutamatergic modulators including NMDA antagonists, and AMPA receptor potentiators, are under development and/or are currently being clinically tested (72).

Hypothalamic–Pituitary–Adrenal Axis

The hypothalamic–pituitary–adrenal (HPA) axis is the most intensely studied neuroendocrine axis in patients with major depression. Numerous reports document hypothalamus [e.g., corticotropin-releasing hormone (CRH)], pituitary [e.g., adrenocorticotropic hormone (ACTH)], and adrenal (e.g., glucocorticoid) hyperactivity in drug-free unipolar and bipolar depressed patients (4). Numerous studies have reported HPA axis hyperactivity in drug-free unipolar and bipolar depressed patients. Increased HPA activity has also been associated with mixed manic states, and less consistently with classic manic episodes (1,20). Depression is associated with disruption in HPA axis function, as shown by increased baseline HPA axis function (e.g., higher CRH in CSF), increased plasma ACTH and cortisol concentrations, and failure to suppress plasma ACTH and cortisol during the dexamethasone suppression test (DST) (19). In patients with severe depression, effective pharmacotherapeutic treatment is linked to normalization of the hyperactive HPA axis and resultant mood elevation (76).

The DST has also been studied in patients with bipolar disorder; approximately 25–60% of depressed bipolar patients are reported to have abnormal DST results, with some (but not all) studies reporting a normalization of the DST during the hypomanic, manic, or mixed phases of the illness. Cassidy et al. (77) reported disturbances in the HPA axis even during manic and mixed states; they found that dexamethasone levels were lower and cortisol levels were higher in mixed states, and appeared to be state, rather than trait, dependent.

The recent development of CRH (also known as CRF) antagonists for the treatment of depression will allow more direct clinical and experimental investigations into the role of CRH hypersecretion in the pathophysiology of depression. Discovered in 1981, CRH is a 41-amino acid-containing peptide that acts as the major physiological regulator of ACTH and β-endorphin secretion from the anterior pituitary (78), and as such, controls HPA axis activity. Within the hypothalamus, CRH-containing neurons project from the paraventricular nucleus to the median eminence (79). Activation of this CRH-containing neural circuit occurs in response to stress, resulting in an increase in synthesis and release of ACTH, β-endorphin, and other pro-opiomelanocortin products. CRH is also found in extrahypothalamic brain regions including the amygdala and the cortex.

The "hypersecretion of CRH" hypothesis of depression is supported by evidence showing elevated CRH concentrations in CSF, which have been documented in multiple studies of drug-free patients with major depression, as well as in suicide victims, although not all studies agree. Studying the number of CRH neurons and CRH RNA, Raadsheer et al. (80,81) reported that depressed patients had increased numbers of hypothalamic CRH neurons and CRH messenger RNA in post-mortem tissue when compared with control subjects. Concordantly, the increased CSF CRH concentration level found during depression was reduced during recovery after electroconvulsive therapy (ECT) (82) and treatment with fluoxetine (83). In addition, reduction of CRH concentrations has been reported in healthy volunteers following administration of desipramine (84). Furthermore, high or increasing CSF CRH concentrations, despite symptomatic improvement of major depression during antidepressant treatment, has been reported to be the harbinger of early relapse (85) as previously reported for DST non-suppression (discussed later). These findings, together with a vast literature documenting the depressogenic effects of CRH after direct CNS injection into laboratory animals, support the CRH hypersecretion hypothesis of depression.

The combined DEX/CRH test has been reported to be a more sensitive test of assessing HPA activity than the DST. In one study, the combined DEX/CRH test was administered in acutely manic patients over the course of 6 months (86). After CRH and dexamethasone pre-treatment, ACTH and cortisol release were significantly increased in both manic and depressed patients in comparison to a healthy control group. In the remitted manic patients, a significant decrease in hormonal release after DEX/CRH was evident when compared to the acute manic episode, but the degree of CRH-stimulated hormone secretion in remitted patients was still significantly larger than in normal controls. The investigators suggested that acute and remitted manic episodes are associated with a profound dysregulation of HPA-system activity (86). In a later study, Rybakowski and Twardowska (87) reported that in bipolar patients, the DEX/CRH test resulted in significantly higher cortisol levels in acutely depressed bipolar patients compared with unipolar depressed patients and healthy control subjects. In remitted patients, cortisol concentrations following DEX/CRH were significantly higher in bipolar than in unipolar patients.

Attenuated ACTH response to CRH has been observed in mood disorders, which is likely due, at least in part, to chronic hypersecretion of CRH from the nerve terminals in the median eminence. This hypersecretion results in downregulation of anterior pituitary CRH-receptor density, with resultant decreased pituitary responsivity to CRH, as has previously been demonstrated in laboratory animals. In a partial confirmation of this idea in humans, a post-mortem study of CRH-receptor density found decreased frontal cortex CRH-binding sites in suicide victims compared with controls (88).

Hormonal measures of the HPA axis show evidence of hyperactivity in depression, and structural changes have also been reported. Perhaps at least partly in response to the hypersecretion of CRH, the pituitary gland was reported to be enlarged in depressed patients in one study (89); this response was significantly correlated with post-dexamethasone cortisol concentrations (90). Another morphological change in depression, enlargement of the adrenal gland, has been reported in suicide victims (91) and in depressed patients using computed tomography (CT) (92,93). The adrenal gland enlargement in depressed patients, like other measures of HPA axis hyperactivity, diminishes after recovery from depression as assessed with magnetic resonance imaging (MRI) (94).

Hypothalamic–Pituitary–Thyroid Axis

Thyroid dysfunction has been implicated in the pathophysiology of both major depression and bipolar disorder. Evidence for thyroid dysfunction includes studies examining plasma levels of thyroid hormones, (a) assessed at the beginning of the illness, (b) in drug naive subjects, and (c) after pharmacological challenges. In addition, in both pre-clinical models and in bipolar patients, the effects of antibipolar medications on the thyroid axis, and importantly, the therapeutic effects after thyroid hormone supplementation, have been investigated.

A study in drug-naive bipolar patients showed thyroid hypofunction in 9% of the cases and some thyroid hyperfunction in an additional 9%. In this sample, bipolar II patients had higher mean thyroid-stimulating hormone (TSH) levels than bipolar I patients after thyrotropin-releasing hormone (TRH) stimulation (95). Coincidently, a blunted TRH stimulation occurred in 35% of unipolar patients and in 44% in bipolar depressed patients (96). Thyroid dysfunction appears to be present from early on in bipolar illness and independent of long-term exposure to the antithyroid medication lithium. In a first episode mania study, bipolar disorder-mixed patients had higher plasma TSH levels when compared with bipolar manic patients (97).

Particular research attention with regards to thyroid dysfunction has been focused on rapid cycling bipolar patients. In a small study, 6 of 10 rapid cycling patients were reported to have hypothyroidism, determined by TRH tests (98), although other studies have not found such an association. Recently, this sub-group of patients was reported to have a latent hypofunction of the hypothalamic–pituitary–thyroid (HPT) axis, that becomes manifest with a short-term lithium challenge (99). Carbamazepine use has also been demonstrated to alter thyroid function; chronic carbamazepine treatment was associated with increases in TRH levels in the CSF of patients with affective illness (100).

If TRH changes were compensatory and adaptive, then administering TRH to patients would be more likely to be associated with a positive antidepressant effect rather than exacerbation of the illness (if it were part of the primary pathophysiology). TRH administered intrathecally and parenterally led to sub-acute antidepressant effects (101). However, the positive effects of parenteral TRH could not be sustained longer than approximately 6 weeks in spite of repeated administration in two patients (102). Nonetheless, since TRH has a relatively rapid onset of action, such a manipulation raises the possibility that an appropriately delivered and targeted peptide could provide a bridging action until more chronic and sustained effects could be achieved with other manipulations.

Finally, although the role of thyroid potentiation and augmentation in major depression has been extensively studied, open-label studies have also indicated that adjunctive supraphysiological doses of thyroxine (T4) can improve depressive symptoms and stabilize the course of illness in bipolar and unipolar patients (103). Therefore, the therapeutic role of thyroid hormone interventions on the HPT axis is an area that deserves further research.

Other Neuropeptides

Recently, several neuropeptides (other than CRH) and their receptors have been investigated in mood disorder research. Somatostatin, a growth hormone release inhibitor, has been found to have lower CSF concentration levels in unipolar and bipolar depression (104) (as in several other conditions), and elevated levels during mania (105). Neuropeptide Y has also been found to be decreased in the CSF of unipolar depressed patients (106–108), but interestingly, neuropeptide Y mRNA expression has been found to be decreased in the prefrontal cortex of bipolar disorder patients when compared with controls (109,110). The role of substance P receptor (neurokinin 1) antagonists in major depression is still being clarified; initial studies suggested an antidepressant effect whereas a later study did not (111). Because research on these neuropeptides has been conducted primarily in major depression, it remains to be determined whether these findings extend to bipolar disorder. Thus, targeting CNS neuropeptide systems might result in a novel strategy to treat bipolar disorder patients in the future.

As has been reviewed, multiple neurotransmitter systems, and the neuropeptide and neuroendocrine systems, appear likely to have a role in bipolar disorder. Bipolar disorder arises from the complex interaction of multiple susceptibility (and protective) genes and environmental factors, and the phenotypic expression of the disease includes not only episodic and often profound mood disturbance, but also a constellation of cognitive, motor, autonomic, endocrine, and circadian sleep/wake abnormalities. Furthermore, whereas most antidepressants exert their initial effects by increasing the intrasynaptic levels of serotonin and/or norepinephrine, their clinical antidepressant effects, as well as the effect of mood stabilizer drugs, are observed only after chronic (days to weeks) administration, suggesting that a cascade of downstream effects are ultimately responsible for their therapeutic effects. These observations have led to the appreciation that although dysfunction within the monoaminergic neurotransmitter systems is likely to play important roles in mediating *some* facets of the pathophysiology of bipolar disorder, it likely represents the downstream effects of other, more primary abnormalities (112).

CIRCADIAN RHYTHMS IN THE PATHOPHYSIOLOGY AND TREATMENT OF BIPOLAR DISORDER

Almost all organisms have circadian (24 hr) cycles in a wide array of molecular, biochemical, physiological, and behavioral processes. These cycles are generated by endogenous circadian oscillators and adjusted by external cues, such as the 24 hour light/dark cycle (113,114). However, many cycles (or rhythms) can free run, meaning that the cycle will continue even when the organism does not have cues from the external environment (e.g., a light/dark cycle) (115). Evidence is accumulating that genes and their resultant gene products are major regulators of these free-running rhythms (113).

One of the core features of bipolar disorder is the cyclical expression of changing mood, behavioral, and neurovegetative states (116). Thus, a great deal of interest exists in the field regarding the foundation of this cyclic expression. Pre-clinical studies beginning in the fruit fly (*Drosophila*), and continuing with mice and other mammals, have begun to uncover the molecular underpinning of circadian cycles (117). The core clock mechanism appears to involve a transcriptional and/or translational feedback loop in which gene products are involved in negative feedback of themselves and other related genes (118–121).

Recent data have revealed that a human disorder, familial advanced sleep phase syndrome, is caused by a mutation in one of the clockwork genes (122). This finding suggests that regulation of the circadian clock could play a fundamental role in other human disorders, in particular in those where abnormalities in circadian rhythms have been identified (116). Lithium has been shown in numerous studies to modify the phase and period of circadian rhythms in a variety of species, ranging from unicellular organisms and insects to mice and humans (123–125). Most consistently, lithium lengthens the circadian period across species, including single cells, plants, invertebrates, and vertebrates (including primates) (123,126–131). A decreased activity of the *Drosophila* ortholog of glycogen synthase kinase-3 (sgg or shaggy) results in an increase in circadian period length (132), an effect that has been noted after treatment with lithium (123). Although there are many differences between the molecular components of circadian cycles in mammals and *Drosophila*, there are also many similarities. It is thus interesting to speculate that glycogen synthase kinase 3 (GSK-3) has a similar general action in the function of the mammalian circadian clock (116,133), and that this mechanism constitutes one of the putative mechanisms of action for lithium in bipolar patients.

It has long been recognized that a dysregulation of circadian rhythms is associated with the clinical manifestations of mood disorders (1). Thus, it is appropriate to examine the underlying biology of circadian function when describing the biological underpinnings of bipolar disorder (116,134). Pre-clinical progress in this area is moving rapidly. For example, there is recent evidence to demonstrate that the interaction between a central circadian pacemaker, the suprachiasmatic nucleus (SCN), and the sleep/wake cycle, likely determines variations in sleepiness, alertness, cognitive performance, and mood (135–137). Facilitation of these pathways is important for anticipatory behaviors that prepare the organism for appropriate adaptive responses including sleeping, eating, and the integrated corticolimbic response to the environment, in which mood regulation is intrinsic (138,139). Thus, factors that clearly play a role in both the neurovegetative profile and in other core features of both bipolar mania and depression are influenced by mammalian circadian cycles and the SCN.

In humans, circadian rhythms may be measured by sleep/wake cycles, control of body temperature, regulation of blood pressure and heart rate, and the release of many endocrine hormones (such as melatonin, growth hormone, cortisol, and others) (140). Using these measures, accumulating biochemical and phenotypic evidence strongly implicates a dysregulation of circadian physiology in a significant number of patients diagnosed with recurrent mood disorders. Many of these findings have been particularly evident in studies of bipolar patients who often show a phase advance of REM sleep and temperature relative to the sleep/wake cycle (141–147). Additional evidence of circadian dysregulation includes an elevation of nocturnal core temperature, as well as an increase in and a phase advance of nocturnal cortisol secretion (148–155). These findings that suggest a phase advance mean that the central pacemaker (SCN) is moving at a faster rate than other internal oscillators or external time cues (142,144,150,156–163).

Cycling of mood episodes can be dramatically altered pharmacologically as well as physiologically by shifting the sleep/wake cycle (142,164,165). A significant literature exists showing sleep deprivation as an effective treatment for bipolar and unipolar depression. On the whole, these studies demonstrate that one night of complete sleep deprivation transiently reverses depressive symptoms in approximately 50% of severely depressed patients (139,166). Unfortunately, the benefits of sleep deprivation are generally extinguished after a complete night of sleep (166).

In clinical practice, sleep deprivation is clearly associated with and is a precipitant of mania (1). However, most of the scientific evidence suggesting that sleep deprivation plays a role in the origin of mania comes from the previously described studies of sleep deprivation used as a therapy for the treatment of unipolar and bipolar depression (139,165,167–170). Notably, and again suggesting the importance of circadian maintenance in the disorder, 5–25% of bipolar patients undergoing sleep deprivation therapy cycle immediately into mania or hypomania (165,168). Converging evidence in molecular biology may implicate similar neurobiological targets in both medications used to treat mood disorders and in the therapeutic action of sleep deprivation. Second messenger systems that are targets for the action of mood stabilizers and antidepressants [such as phosphatidyl inositol, glycogen synthase kinase 3β (GSK-3β), cyclic AMP (cAMP), see Section Signaling Networks as Key Modulators of Long-Term Neuroplastic Events] may be integral to the physiological processes underlying the brain's response to sleep deprivation (133,171,172). In this regard, experiments in rats have demonstrated that brain-derived neurotrophic factor (BDNF), the TrkB BDNF receptor, and the gene promoter CREB (see later sections) are all upregulated during waking and/or in a rat model of sleep deprivation (173,174). These molecules are all upregulated by numerous other treatments for depression (175).

EVIDENCE OF HPA HYPERACTIVATION MODULATING NEURAL PLASTICITY

The term "neuroplasticity" includes diverse processes of vital importance by which the brain perceives, adapts to, and responds to a variety of internal and external stimuli. The evidence of neuroplasticity in the adult CNS has been characterized as including alterations of dendritic function, synaptic remodeling, long-term potentiation (LTP), axonal sprouting, neurite extension, synaptogenesis, and even neurogenesis. The potential hyperactivation of the HPA axis in mood disorders has been re-examined recently, largely due to the growing recognition of the specific brain areas in which atrophy, a neuroplastic event, may be present in many patients (see Section Impairments of Neuroplasticity and Cellular Resilience in Bipolar Disorder) (Fig. 2).

The relationship between HPA axis hyperactivity and atrophy has received support from data showing that chronic stress or glucocorticoid administration

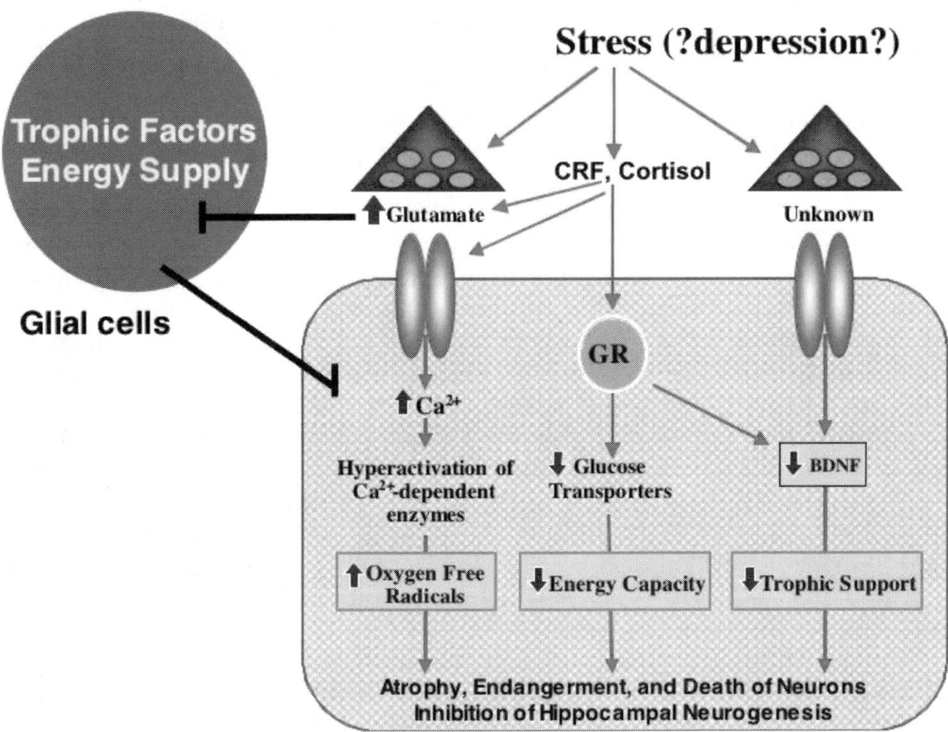

Figure 2 *Harmful effects of stress, hypothalamic pituitary adrenal (HPA) axis activation, and glutamate on neurons.* Depicted here are multiple mechanisms by which stress, and potentially affective episodes, may attenuate cellular resiliency, thereby resulting in atrophy, death, and endangerment of hippocampal neurons. Three primary mechanisms appear to be: (1) excessive NMDA and non-NMDA glutamatergic throughput; (2) downregulation of cell surface glucose transporters, which are involved in bringing glucose into the cell. Reduced levels of glucose transporters thus reduce the neuron's energetic reservoir, making them susceptible to energy failure when faced with excessive demands; (3) reduction in the levels of neurotrophic factors such as BDNF, which is essential for the neuron's normal trophic support and synaptic plasticity; and (4) a reduction in glial cells may contribute to impairments of neuronal structural plasticity by reducing the neuron's energy supply and reduced glial-mediated clearing of excessive synaptic glutamate. *Abbreviations*: NMDA, *N*-methyl-aspartate glutamate receptor; CRF, corticotropin release factor; GR, glucocorticoid receptor; BDNF, brain-derived neurotrophic factor. *Source*: Modified and reproduced with permission from Ref. 305.

has been demonstrated to produce atrophy and death of vulnerable hippocampal neurons in rodents and primates. MRI studies have also revealed reduced hippocampal volumes in patients with Cushing's disease and post-traumatic stress disorder (PTSD), which are other conditions associated with hypercortisolemia. One of the most consistent effects of stress on cellular morphology is atrophy of hippocampal neurons. This atrophy is observed in the CA3 pyramidal neurons, but not in other hippocampal cell groups (176,177) (i.e., CA1 pyramidal and dentate gyrus granule neurons). Atrophy of CA3 pyramidal neurons also occurs upon exposure to high levels of glucocorticoids, suggesting that activation of the HPA axis likely plays a major role in mediating stress-induced atrophy. In addition, long-term exposure to stress (i.e., for several months) has also been associated with true loss of hippocampal neurons in the CA3 pyramidal cell layer (178). Thus, it is possible that recurrent mood disorders, as in the case of bipolar disorder, may lower the threshold for cell death and/or atrophy in response to a variety of other physiological (e.g., normal aging) and pathological (e.g., ischemic) events, and thereby contribute to a variety of negative health-related effects (Fig. 2).

SIGNALING NETWORKS AS KEY MODULATORS OF LONG-TERM NEUROPLASTIC EVENTS

Recent research into the pathophysiology and treatment of mood disorders has moved from a focus on neurotransmitters and cell surface receptors to intracellular signaling cascades. Multicomponent cellular signaling pathways interact at various levels, thereby forming complex signaling networks that allow cells to receive internal and external cues, process those cues, and respond to information (179–181). These signaling networks (a) enable the integration of signals across multiple time scales, (b) enable the generation of distinct outputs depending on input strength and duration, and (c) regulate intricate feed-forward and feedback loops (Fig. 3) (179–181). Given their widespread and crucial role in the integration and fine-tuning of physiologic processes, it is not surprising that abnormalities in signaling pathways have now been identified in a variety of human diseases.

Signaling pathways also represent major targets for a number of hormones, including glucocorticoids, thyroid hormones, and gonadal steroids (182,183). These biochemical effects may play a role in mediating certain clinical manifestations of altered hormonal levels in mood disorder subjects (e.g., the frequent onset of bipolar disorder in puberty, triggering of episodes in the postpartum period, association of depression and potentially rapid cycling with hypothyroidism, and triggering of mood episodes in response to exogenous glucocorticoids).

Complex signaling networks may be especially important in the CNS, where they balance and integrate diverse neuronal signals and then transmit them to effectors, thereby forming the basis of a complex information processing network (179–181). The high degree of complexity generated by these signaling networks may be one mechanism by which neurons acquire the flexibility for generating the wide range of responses observed in the nervous system. These pathways are thus undoubtedly involved in regulating such diverse vegetative functions as mood, appetite, and wakefulness and are therefore likely to be involved in the pathophysiology of bipolar disorder (Fig. 3). We will now describe direct and indirect evidence supporting a role for signaling pathway abnormalities in the pathophysiology and treatment of bipolar disorder.

The Gs Protein/cAMP Generating Signaling Pathway

Several laboratories have reported abnormalities in G protein subunits in bipolar patients. Data from post-mortem brain studies have demonstrated increased levels of the stimulatory G protein ($G\alpha_s$), accompanied by increases in post-receptor stimulated adenylyl cyclase (AC) activity in bipolar disorder (184,185). These observations receive additional support from the demonstration of increased agonist-activated [^{35}S]GTPγS binding to G protein α-subunits in the frontal cortical membranes of bipolar disorder patients (186). Several studies have also found elevated $G\alpha_s$ protein levels and mRNA levels in peripheral circulating cells in bipolar disorder, although the dependency of these levels on clinical mood state remains unclear (52,185,187–190).

At present, there is no evidence to suggest that the alterations in the levels of Gα_s are due to a mutation in the Gα_s gene itself (191). There are numerous transcriptional and post-transcriptional mechanisms that regulate the levels of G protein subunits, and the elevated levels of Gα_s could potentially represent the indirect sequelae of alterations in any one of these other biochemical pathways (112,185,187,192).

There is a growing consensus that the ability of a simple monovalent cation like lithium to treat multiple aspects of an illness as complex as bipolar disorder originates from its primary effects on intracellular signaling pathways, rather than on any single neurotransmitter system per se (5,51,190). Although it appears that the lithium ion (at therapeutic concentrations) does not directly affect G protein function, there is considerable evidence that *chronic* lithium administration affects G protein function (5,51). It might be speculated that these G protein effects, which would theoretically attenuate excessive signaling through multiple pathways, likely contribute to lithium's long-term prophylactic efficacy in protecting susceptible individuals from spontaneous-, stress-, and drug (e.g., antidepressant, stimulant)-induced cyclic affective episodes.

The PKC Signaling Pathway

PKC is comprised of a family of closely related kinase sub-species, has a heterogeneous distribution in the brain (with particularly high levels in pre-synaptic nerve terminals), and together with other kinases, appears to play a critical role in the regulation of synaptic plasticity and various forms of learning and memory (193–196).

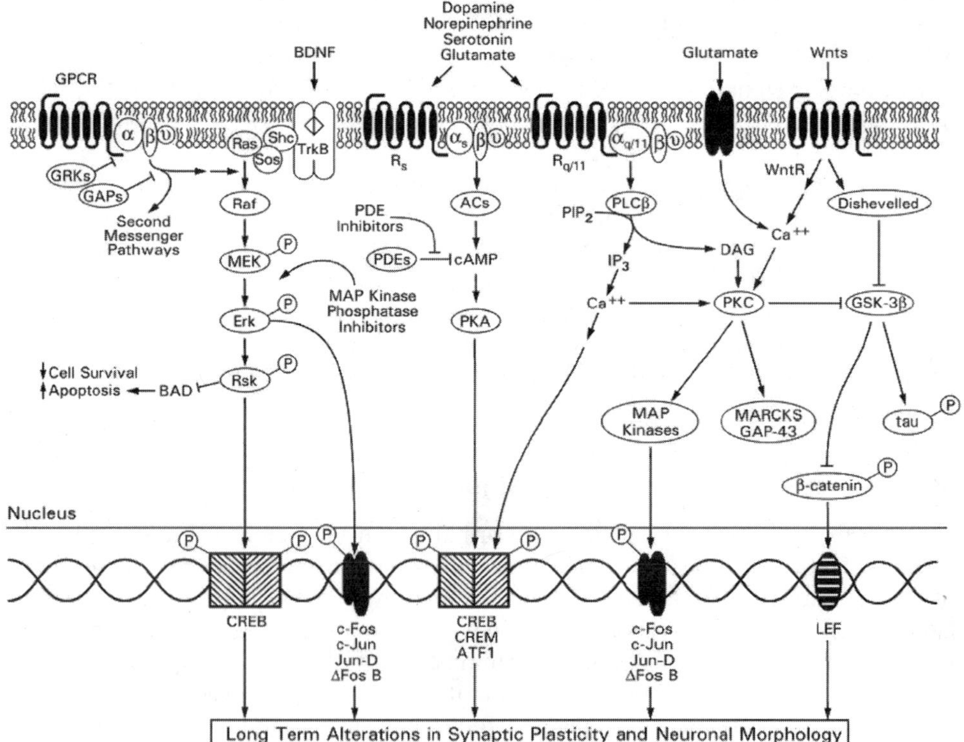

Figure 3 (*Caption on Facing Page*)

PKC is one of the major intracellular signal mediators generated after external stimulation of cells via a variety of neurotransmitter receptors (including muscarinic M1, M3, and M5 receptors, noradrenergic α_1 receptors, metabotropic glutamatergic receptors, and serotonergic $5HT_{2A}$ receptors), which induce the hydrolysis of various membrane phospholipids.

Figure 3 (*Facing page*) *Major intracellular signaling pathways in bipolar disorder*. The figure depicts some of the major intracellular signaling pathways involved in neural and behavioral plasticity. Cell surface receptors transduce extracellular signals such as neurotransmitters and neuropeptides into the interior of the cell. Most neurotransmitters and neuropeptides communicate with other cells by activating seven transmembrane spanning G protein-coupled receptors (GPCRs). As their name implies, GPCRs activate selected G proteins, which are composed of α and $\beta\gamma$ subunits. Two families of proteins turn off the GPCR signal, and may therefore represent attractive targets for new medication development. G protein-coupled receptor kinases (*GRKs*) phosphorylate GPCRs and thereby uncouple them from their respective G proteins. GTPase activating proteins (*GAPs*, also called RGS or regulators of G protein signaling proteins) accelerate the G protein turn off reaction (an intrinsic GTPase activity). Two major signaling cascades activated by GPCRs are the *cAMP* generating second messenger system, and the phosphoinositide (PI) system. cAMP activates protein kinase A (*PKA*), a pathway which has been implicated in the therapeutic effects of antidepressants. Among the potential targets for the development of new antidepressants are certain phosphodiesterases (*PDEs*). PDEs catalyze the breakdown of cAMP; thus, PDE inhibitors would be expected to sustain the cAMP signal, and may represent an antidepressant augmenting strategy. Activation of receptors coupled to PI hydrolysis results in the breakdown of phosphoinositide 4,5-biphosphate (PIP_2) into two second messengers—inositol 4,5-trisphosphate (IP_3) and diacylglycerol (*DAG*). IP_3 mobilizes Ca^{2+} from intracellular stores, whereas DAG is an endogenous activator of protein kinase C (*PKC*), which is also directly activated by Ca^{2+}. PKC, PKA, and other Ca^{2+}-dependent kinases directly or indirectly activate several important transcription factors, including *CREB*, *CREM*, *ATF-1*, *c-Fos*, *c-Jun*, *Jun-D*, and Δ*Fos B*. Endogenous growth factors such as brain-derived neurotrophic factor (*BDNF*) utilize different types of signaling pathways. BDNF binds to and activates its tyrosine kinase receptor (*TrkB*); this facilitates the recruitment of other proteins (*SHC*, *SOS*), which results in the activation of the ERK–MAP kinase cascade (via sequential activation of *Ras*, *Raf*, *MEK*, *Erk*, and *Rsk*). In addition to regulating several transcription factors, the ERK–MAP kinase cascade, via Rsk, downregulates *BAD*, a pro-apoptotic protein. Enhancement of the ERK–MAP kinase cascade may have effects similar to those of endogenous neurotrophic factors; one potential strategy is to utilize inhibitors of MAP kinase phosphatases (which would inhibit the turn-off reaction) as potential drugs with neurotrophic properties. In addition to utilizing GPCRs, many neurotransmitters (e.g., glutamate and GABA) produce their responses via ligand-gated ion channels. Although these responses are very rapid, they also bring about more stable changes via regulation of gene transcription. One pathway gaining increasing recent attention in adult mammalian neurobiology is the Wnt signaling pathway. *Wnts* are a group of glycoproteins active in development, but now known to play important roles in the mature brain. Binding of Wnts to the Wnt receptor (*WntR*) activates an intermediary protein, *Disheveled*, which regulates a glycogen synthase kinase (*GSK-3*β). GSK-3β exerts many cellular effects; it regulates cytoskeletal proteins, including *tau*, and also plays an important role in determining cell survival/cell death decisions. GSK-3β has recently been identified as a target for Li^+'s actions. GSK-3β also regulates phosphorylation of β-*catenin*, a protein that when dephosphorylated acts as a transcription factor at lymphoid enhancer factor (*LEF*) sites. *CREB*, cAMP response element binding protein; R_q and R_s, extracellular GPCRs coupled to stimulation or inhibition of adenylyl cyclases (*ACs*), respectively; *Rq/11*, GPCR coupled to activation of phospholipase C (*PLC*); *MARCKS*, myristoylated alanine-rich C kinase substrate, a protein associated with several neuroplastic events. *Source*: Modified and reproduced with permission from Ref. 302.

To date, there have only been a limited number of studies directly examining PKC in bipolar disorder (197). Although undoubtedly an over-simplification, particulate (or membrane) PKC is sometimes seen as the more active form of PKC, and thus examining the sub-cellular partitioning of this enzyme can be used as an index of the degree of activation. Friedman et al. (198) investigated PKC activity and PKC translocation in response to serotonin in platelets obtained from bipolar disorder patients before and during lithium treatment, and reported that the ratios of platelet membrane-bound to cytosolic PKC activities were elevated in the manic subjects. In addition, serotonin-elicited platelet PKC translocation was found to be enhanced in those subjects. Wang and Friedman (186) measured PKC isozyme levels, activity, and translocation in post-mortem brain tissue from bipolar disorder patients, and reported increased PKC activity and translocation in bipolar disorder brains compared with controls, effects which were accompanied by elevated levels of selected PKC isozymes in the cortices of the bipolar disorder patients.

Accumulated evidence from several investigative groups has clearly demonstrated that lithium, at therapeutically relevant concentrations, exerts significant effects on the PKC signaling cascade. Data suggest that chronic lithium attenuates PKC activity, and downregulate the expression of PKC isozymes α and ε in the frontal cortex and hippocampus of patients with bipolar disorder (112,199). Chronic lithium has also been demonstrated to dramatically reduce the hippocampal levels of a major PKC substrate, myristoylated alanine-rich C kinase substrate (MARCKS), which has a role in regulating long-term neuroplastic events.

Although these effects of lithium on PKC isozymes and MARCKS are striking, a major problem inherent in neuropharmacologic research is the difficulty in attributing therapeutic relevance to any observed biochemical finding. It is thus noteworthy that the structurally dissimilar antimanic agent valproate (VPA) produces very similar effects as lithium on PKC α and ε isozymes and MARCKS protein (112,199). Lithium and VPA appear to bring about their effects on the PKC signaling pathway by distinct mechanisms, consistent with clinical observations that some patients show preferential response to one or other of the agents, and that one often observes additive therapeutic effects in patients when the two agents are co-administered.

In view of the pivotal role of the PKC signaling pathway in the regulation of neuronal excitability, neurotransmitter release, and long-term synaptic events (197,200), we postulated that the attenuation of PKC activity may play a role in the antimanic effects of lithium and VPA. To test this idea, we piloted a study in seven bipolar manic patients treated with tamoxifen, a non-steroidal antiestrogen known to be a PKC inhibitor at higher concentrations (201); tamoxifen was found to possess antimanic efficacy in this study (202). Due to the small sample size, however, these study results have to be considered preliminary. In view of the preliminary data suggesting the involvement of the PKC signaling system in the pathophysiology of bipolar disorder, these results suggest that PKC inhibitors may be very useful agents in the treatment of mania, and warrant larger double-blind, placebo-controlled studies of tamoxifen and of novel selective PKC inhibitors.

Glycogen Synthase Kinase

The enzyme GSK-3 is a crucial kinase that functions as an intermediary in numerous intracellular signaling pathways, and recent research suggests the importance of this enzyme in bipolar disorder research (133,203). GSK-3—a constitutively active and a highly conserved enzyme in evolution—is found in two nearly identical isoforms (slight variations) in mammals, the α and β isoforms. This enzyme was first discovered (and named) based upon its ability to phosphorylate and thereby inactivate the enzyme glucogen synthase, which leads to a decrease in the synthesis of glycogen. GSK-3 is unique among kinases because it is generally constitutively active, and therefore most intracellular signals to GSK-3 inactivate this enzyme. Signals deactivating GSK-3 arise from insulin stimulation, numerous growth factors [e.g., phophoinositide (PI) 3-kinase], and developmental signals. A number of endogenous growth factors (e.g., nerve growth factor and BDNF) use the PI 3-kinase signaling cascade as a major effector system. Thus, growth factors may bring about many of their neurotrophic and neuroprotective effects at least partly by inhibiting GSK-3. GSK-3 phosphorylates—and thereby inactivates—many transcription factors, and modulates the function of cytoskeletal proteins such as the Alzheimer's disease protein tau (a previous name for GSK-3 was tau kinase). Inhibition of GSK-3 thus results in the release of this inhibition and the activation of multiple cellular targets.

Growing evidence suggests that GSK-3 plays an important role in regulating neuroplasticity and cellular resilience. Studies have suggested that changes in GSK-3 mediated mitogen-activated protein (MAP)-1B (a cytoskeletal protein) phosphorylation are associated with the loss and/or unbundling of stable axonal microtubules (204). Furthermore, GSK-3β inhibition results in the accumulation of synapsin I, a protein involved in synaptic vesicle docking and release of growth cone-like areas (205).

In addition to its putative role in regulating synapse formation and axonal growth, there is considerable excitement in the field regarding the role of GSK-3 in regulating cell death (apoptosis) in mature neuronal tissue, and regarding the development of GSK-3 inhibitors as novel therapeutic agents for bipolar disorder and classical neurodegenerative diseases. Although it was initially reported in 1993 that GSK-3 activity was required for β-amyloid-induced neurotoxicity in primary hippocampal neurons (206), this observation was not fully appreciated until further recent studies were done. These recent studies have demonstrated that GSK-3 may regulate cell death beyond its role in β-amyloid-induced toxicity. In one study, GSK-3 over-expression induced apoptosis in cultured cells, which was prevented by dominant negative mutants (207). Furthermore, the expression of FRAT-1, a protein that inhibits GSK-3, also rescued primary sympathetic neurons from PI 3-kinase inhibition-induced cell death (208).

Fatty Acids and Bipolar Disorder

Increased attention has been given to the role of fatty acids in mood disorders, particularly the omega-3 fatty acids (ω-3 FA) in the treatment of bipolar disorder. The predominant naturally occurring ω-3 FA are docosahexaenoic acid (DHA), eicosapentanoic acid (EPA), and linolenic acid. Omega-3 fatty acids appear to cross the blood–brain barrier easily and are incorporated as major components into neuronal membranes. Due to their highly folded chemical structure, ω-3 FA increase the fluidity of the membrane lipid bilayer, thereby changing transmembrane protein function. This is the proposed mechanism by which membrane phospholipids become more resistant to hydrolysis by phospholipases. Interest in a putative role for ω-3 FA in bipolar disorder comes from: (a) the observations about its efficacy in models of kindling (antikindling properties in rat models of epilepsy) (209); (b) the incorporation of ω-3 FA in the membrane (thereby suppressing the phosphatidylinositol-associated signal transduction pathway) (210,211); (c) the blockade of calcium influx through L-type calcium channels (212); and (d) downregulation and inhibition of various protein kinases (213,214). Mirnikjoo et al. (215) described a series of experiments showing that in vitro EPA and DHA significantly reduced the activity of cAMP-dependent protein kinase A (PKA), PKC, mitogen-activated protein kinase (MAPK), and calcium/calmodulin-dependent protein kinase II (CaMKII), effects that were not observed with similar fatty acids lacking an ω-3 double bond [e.g., arachidonic acid (AA)]. These pre-clinical observations, along with the absence of any documented drug interaction, the lack of toxicity, and the apparent safe use of ω-3 FA in pregnant women and children, were all factors that led to a clinical trial of ω-3 FA in mood disorders.

In double-blind studies in unipolar depression, patients receiving ω-3 FA had a significantly decreased score on the 21-item Hamilton Rating Scale for depression compared with the placebo group (216). However, the difference in response rates [50% decrease on the Montgomery–Asberg Depression Rating Scale (MADRS)] between groups did not reach statistical significance between patients receiving DHA or placebo (217). In bipolar disorder, a 4-month, double-blind, placebo-controlled study compared 9.6 g/day of ω-3 FA to olive oil (placebo), both given either alone or added to other medications, and found encouraging results (218). However, in a larger study including 121 bipolar patients who were depressed or rapid cycling, EPA 6 g/day was added to mood-stabilizing agents, in a double-blind, placebo-controlled trial for 4 months. No differences were found among groups receiving either EPA or placebo, in baseline to end-point scores for depressed or rapid cycling patients (219). These contradictory results prevent reaching any definitive conclusions regarding the efficacy of ω-3 FA in mood disorders.

In a parallel series of studies, the research group headed by Dr. S. Rapoport has used in vivo brain imaging methodologies to investigate the potential effects of mood-stabilizing agents on CNS fatty acids. This research group has shown that lithium and valproate produce selective reductions in the turnover rate of the phospholipid AA in the rat brain (220,221). In these studies, lithium produced a reduction in the AA turnover rate of 80%, accompanied by a reduction in the expression of the gene and protein of an AA-specific phospholipase A2 (cPLA2). Valproate decreased the turnover of AA by 33%, with no effect on cPLA2 protein levels, and was postulated to act directly on the incorporation of AA into brain phospholipids. Ongoing studies should delineate the facets of bipolar disorder that these membrane changes may modulate.

Neurotrophic Factors (BDNF) and Antiapoptotic Proteins (Bcl-2)

Activation of the HPA axis appears to play a critical role in mediating hippocampal atrophy, as previously discussed. In addition to directly causing neuronal atrophy, stress and glucocorticoids also appear to reduce cellular resilience, thereby making certain neurons more vulnerable to other insults, such as ischemia, hypoglycemia, and excitatory amino acid toxicity. The reduction in the resilience of hippocampal neurons may also reflect the tendency of various stressors to decrease the expression of BDNF in this region (222). BDNF and other neurotrophic factors are necessary for the survival and function of neurons, implying that a sustained reduction of these factors could affect neuronal viability. Increasing evidence suggests that neurotrophic factors inhibit cell death cascades by largely activating the MAP kinase signaling cascade, and upregulating major cell survival proteins such as bcl-2 (223).

Bcl-2 is now recognized as a significant neuroprotective protein, because overexpression of bcl-2 protects neurons against many different insults, including ischemia, the neurotoxic agent methyl-phenyl-tetrahydropyridine (MPTP), β-amyloid, free radicals, excessive glutamate, and growth factor deprivation (224). Increasing data suggest that bcl-2 is not only neuroprotective, but also exerts neurotrophic effects and promotes neurite sprouting, neurite outgrowth, and axonal regeneration (224). If enhanced bcl-2 expression appears capable of offsetting the potentially harmful consequences of stress-induced neuronal endangerment, then pharmacologically induced upregulation of bcl-2 may be considerably useful.

Overall, it is clear that the neurotrophic factor/MAP kinase/bcl-2 signaling cascade plays a critical role in cell survival in the CNS, and that there is a fine balance maintained between the levels and activities of cell survival and cell death factors. Modest changes in this signaling cascade or in the levels of the bcl-2 family of proteins (potentially due to genetic-, illness-, or insult-related factors) may therefore profoundly affect cellular viability. For example, pretreatment with pramipexole, a dopaminergic agonist agent used to treat Parkinson's disease, increased bcl-2 and inhibited methylphenylpyridinium-induced apoptosis in human neuroblastoma SH-SY5Y cells (225), and treatment of rats for 4 days with pramipexole markedly increased bcl-2 immunoreactivity in neuronal dendritic processes in both the cerebral cortex and hippocampus (226). Our group recently demonstrated the antidepressive efficacy of this agent in a double-blind, placebo-controlled study in bipolar II depressed patients taking therapeutic levels of lithium or valproate (227). These studies suggest that medications shown to affect the bcl-2 signaling cascade may be useful in the treatment of bipolar disorder.

ABNORMALITIES IN CALCIUM REGULATION AND MITOCHONDRIAL FUNCTION IN BIPOLAR DISORDER

Calcium Signaling Abnormalities

Calcium ions play a critical role in regulating the synthesis and release of neurotransmitters, neuronal excitability, and long-term neuroplastic events, and therefore it is not surprising that a number of studies have investigated intracellular Ca^{2+} in peripheral cells in bipolar disorder. Impaired regulation of Ca^{2+} cascades has been the most reproducible biological abnormality described in bipolar disorder research. For this reason, mechanisms involved in Ca^{2+} regulation have been postulated to underlie aspects of the pathophysiology of bipolar disorder. To date, approximately 15 studies have consistently revealed elevations in basal intracellular Ca^{2+} levels in platelets, lymphocytes, or neutrophils of patients with bipolar disorder. By contrast, there are only a few (four) negative studies. Although this may partly represent publication bias, the elevation in basal Ca^{2+} represents one of the most replicated findings in bipolar disorder research.

Increased platelet intracellular Ca^{2+} elevations have also been found in response to stimulation with thrombin, platelet activator factor (PAF), serotonin, dopamine, and thapsigargin. In lymphocytes, the same higher elevations were observed when the cells were stimulated with phytohemaglutinin, concavalin A, thrombin, and (as in platelets) thapsigargin and serotonin. There is, however, considerable evidence that a variety of circulating factors may influence the activity of blood cells and elements, and bipolar disorder patients are known to have numerous neurohormonal abnormalities (such as catecholamines and cortisol levels). Furthermore, many of these studies did not employ an extensive medication washout period, raising the possibility that the elevations in Ca^{2+} in circulating cells are simply secondary manifestations.

To investigate this potential confound, in an elegant series of studies, Epstein–Barr virus-immortalized B lymphoblasts (BLCL) were grown in culture (away from the patients' confounding circulating environment) for weeks. These studies found that even in the immortalized lymphoblasts, bipolar disorder patients showed elevated basal Ca^{2+} concentrations compared with healthy subjects or patients with other psychiatric disorders (228). In an extension of these studies, this research group investigated the components of the storage-operated Ca^{2+} entry (SOCE), and found a reduction in the mRNA expression of the TRPC7 (TRPM2) gene (whose gene product is implicated in SOCE functioning), in BLCLs from a sub-group of bipolar disorder I patients (229). These researchers concluded that reduced TRPC7 gene expression might be a trait associated with pathophysiological disturbances of Ca^{2+} homeostasis in a sub-group of bipolar I patients.

The regulation of free intracellular Ca^{2+} is a complex, multifaceted process, and the abnormalities observed in bipolar disorder could arise from abnormalities at a variety of levels (192). Ongoing studies should help delineate the specific regulatory sites at which the impairment in calcium occurs in bipolar patients.

Mitochondrial Function Abnormalities

It has been recently proposed that mitochondrial dysfunction may play an important role in the pathophysiology of bipolar disorder (230,231). Neuronal mitochondria participate not only in oxidative phosphorylation, and in networks with endoplasmic reticulum (ER), in regulating calcium homeostasis, but also in cellular resilience and neurotransmitter synaptic function (Fig. 4). Although bipolar disorder is not a classic mitochondrial disease, (a) pre-clinical work and clinical evidence reporting calcium dysregulation, (b) neuroimaging and post-mortem studies demonstrating cell loss and/or atrophy and white matter hyperintensities, as well as (c) the cellular effects of mood stabilizers on mitochondrial activity, all support the involvement of mitochondrial-ER network function in the pathophysiology and treatment of bipolar disorder.

MRS is a tool, which provides a non-invasive window into brain neurochemistry, and has been increasingly used in the study of neuropsychiatric disorders. In vivo brain MRS studies have reported abnormal levels of high-energy phosphate metabolism, most notably decreased phosphocreatine (PCr) and/or adenosine triphosphate (ATP) levels in bipolar patients (232–234). Kato et al. (235,236) and associates have conducted the most extensive series of studies investigating possible abnormalities in brain energy regulation in mood disorders. Consistent with the decreased PCr and ATP levels, data from this research group have also shown low pH levels (measured indirectly via ^{31}P MRS) in mood disorder patients compared with normal controls in the basal ganglia and the whole brain, observations that originally led to the postulate that bipolar disorder may be associated with mitochondrial dysfunction.

Additional evidence of dysregulated mitochondrial processes in bipolar disorder comes from an elegant series of recent gene microarray studies in post-mortem brain tissue. Konradi et al. (237) used gene arrays that analyzed mRNA expression in the hippocampus and found that the expression of only 43 genes, 42% of which coded for mitochondrial proteins, were decreased in bipolar disorder compared with schizophrenia. These genes included subunits of complexes I [nicotinamide adenine

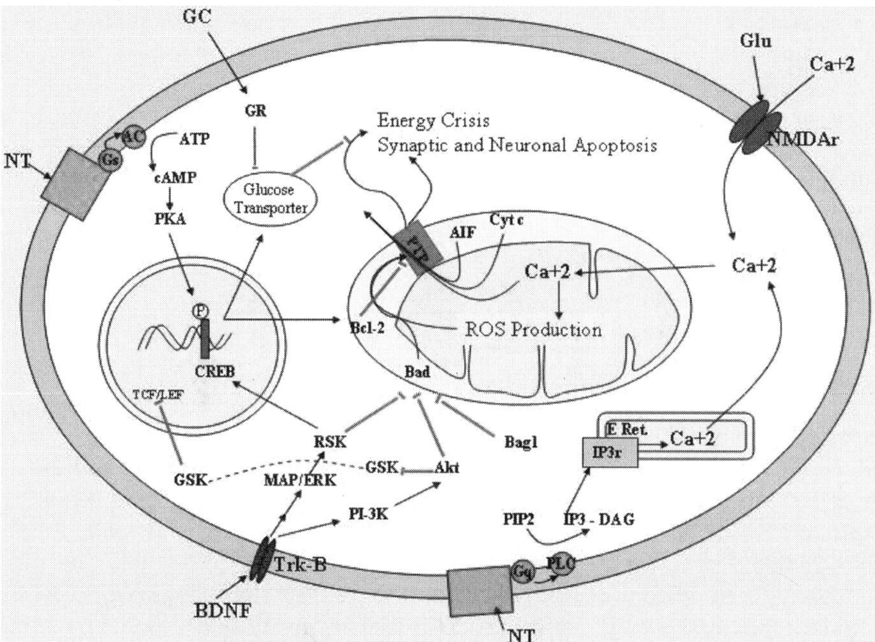

Figure 4 Intracellular signaling pathways relevant for the pathophysiology of bipolar disorder and its role in synaptic and neuronal apoptosis. *Abbreviations*: AC, adenylyl cyclase; AIF, apoptosis-inducing factor; Akt, protein kinase that inactivate GSK; ATP, adenosine triphosphate; Bad, pro-apoptotic protein regulated by RSK; Bag-1, bcl-2 binding antiapoptotic protein; Bcl-2, antiapoptotic protein B-cell leukemia/lymphoma; BDNF, brain-derived neurotrophic factor; Ca^{2+}, calcium; cAMP, cyclic adenosine monophosphate; CREB, cAMP response element binding protein; Cyt *c*, cytochrome *c*; DAG, diacylglycerol; E Ret, endoplasmic reticulum; GC, glucocorticoid; Glu, glutamate; GR, glucocorticoid receptor; Gs, protein G stimulatory of adenylyl cyclase; GSK, glycogen synthase kinase; Gq, protein G stimulatory of phospholipase C; IP3, inositol 4,5-trisphosphate; IP3r, inositol triphosphate receptor; MAP/ERK, mitogen-activated protein kinase (MAP) pathway also referred to as extracellular signal regulated kinase (ERK) pathway; NMDAr, *N*-methyl-D-aspartate receptor; NT, neurotransmitter and its G protein-coupled receptor; P, phosphate group; PIP2, phosphatidylinositol biphosphate; PI-3K, phosphatidylinositol 3-kinase; PKA, protein kinase A; PLC, phospholipase C; PTP, permeability transition pore; ROS, reactive oxidative species; RSK, kinase of ERK–MAP kinase cascade that downregulates Bad; TCF/LEF, transcription factors for specific genes; Trk-B, tyrosine kinase receptor. *Source*: Modified and reproduced with permission from Ref. 302.

dinucleotide dehydrogenase (NADH) in 1 gene], IV (cytochrome-*c* oxidase in 1 gene), and V (ATP synthase in 5 genes), which carry out oxidative phosphorylation in the mitochondrial inner membrane. Furthermore, in a post-mortem study, a decreased expression of the enzyme glutamic acid decarboxylase 67 (GAD-67) and of somatostatin (238) was reported in a subset of hippocampal interneurons in bipolar disorder patients. Although interpretation of the results of post-mortem brain studies requires caution due to the numerous potentially confounding factors (including antemortem medication history and/or substance abuse, post-mortem interval, and cause of death), other studies have been conducted to confirm these findings. For example, utilizing lymphoblastoid cell lines from bipolar patients and healthy controls, Washizuka et al. (239) reported a decreased expression level of NDUFV2 gene (a nuclear-encoded mitochondrial complex I subunit gene) in patients with bipolar I disorder.

Together, these observations indicate a particularly abnormal mitochondrial energy metabolism, and therefore agents capable of reversing the mitochondrial-driven impairments of cellular plasticity and resilience in bipolar disorder are actively being investigated.

IMPAIRMENTS OF NEUROPLASTICITY AND CELLULAR RESILIENCE IN BIPOLAR DISORDER

Structural and Functional Brain Imaging Studies

Evidence of volumetric brain changes suggestive of cell loss and atrophy has been observed in vivo in patients with bipolar disorder since the introduction of radiological imaging techniques in psychiatry. Limited initially by the spatial resolution of CT scans, descriptions in bipolar disorder were focused on reduced ventricular brain ratios (240–243), enlargement of third and lateral ventricles (244,245) and in one case, cortical atrophy (246). With the improved resolution of the MRI scan, measurements of discrete cortical areas and the sub-cortical nucleus showed that bipolar disorder patients, besides the ventricular changes described previously, also had other observable structural abnormalities. Studies in the literature showed that bipolar disorder patients have smaller left putamen volume when compared with controls, a reduction that correlated with the length of illness (247). Reduced thalamic areas (248), smaller pituitary volume (249) and smaller mean area of corpus callosum (250) have also been noted in bipolar disorder. When the cortex was studied, smaller temporal volumes (251) and reduced cortical gray matter (but not white matter) (252) were reported. Lastly, in unmedicated familial bipolar I patients compared with healthy controls, smaller volumes of bilateral dorsolateral prefrontal cortex, orbitofrontal cortex, inferior frontal cortex, anterior cingulate cortex, and right superior temporal gyrus have been found (253).

Importantly, the first description of surprising reductions in frontal lobe volumes in affective disorders, including a sub-group of bipolar disorder patients, was reported in 1997. Reductions of approximately 40% in mean gray matter volume in the subgenual prefrontal cortex region (located ventral to the genu of the corpus callosum) was demonstrated in bipolar disorder depressed patients and familial unipolar depressed patients (254). Additional studies suggest that these subgenual prefrontal cortex gray matter volume reductions may be particularly evident in populations with positive family histories of mood disorders (255).

Reductions in the volume of the hippocampus have also been observed in patients with a history of major depression, findings that may persist for decades after the depressive episodes have resolved (89,256–259). Interestingly, the loss of hippocampal volume appears to be correlated with the total lifetime duration of major depression but not with the age of the patients (257), leading to the suggestion that these changes may represent the sequelae of repeated and/or prolonged episodes of depression (176). Although not all studies have found volumetric changes in the hippocampus in bipolar disorder (260–262), a recent study of twins that were discordant for bipolar disorder showed that the right hippocampus was smaller in the bipolar vs. the non-bipolar twin (263). Hippocampal atrophy was also demonstrated in familial bipolar I patients (euthymic and medicated), specifically in the right posterior hippocampal tissue (264), adding new evidence implicating the involvement of this area in the pathophysiology of bipolar disorder.

However, the interpretation of causality between stress and hippocampal size cannot be guaranteed, as it has been shown in longitudinal studies with primates. In these primate studies, paternal half-siblings raised apart from one another by different mothers in the absence of fathers were randomized to one of three postnatal conditions that disrupted different aspects of early maternal care. Interestingly, adult hippocampal volumes did not differ with respect to the stressful postnatal conditions. Paternal half-siblings with small adult hippocampal volumes responded to the removal of all mothers after weaning with initially larger relative increases in cortisol levels. Plasma cortisol levels 3 and 7 days later, and measures of cortisol-negative feedback in adulthood were not, however, correlated with hippocampal size (265). Thus, these studies suggest that small hippocampi may also reflect an inherited characteristic of the brain and highlight the need for caution in attributing causality in the cross-sectional human morphometric studies of the hippocampus.

N-acetylaspartate (NAA) is one of the many neurochemical compounds that can be quantitatively assessed using MRS. NAA is the predominant resonance in the proton MRS spectrum of the normal adult human brain, and although the functional role of this amino acid has not been definitively determined (266), NAA is a putative neuronal marker, localized to mature neurons and not found in mature glial cells, CSF, or blood (267). A number of studies have now shown that initial abnormally low brain NAA measures may increase and even normalize with remission of CNS symptoms in disorders such as demyelinating disease, ALS, mitochondrial encephalopathies, and HIV dementia (267). NAA is synthesized within mitochondria, and inhibitors of the mitochondrial respiratory chain decrease NAA concentrations, effects that correlate with reductions in ATP and oxygen consumption (268).

Thus, NAA is now generally regarded as a measure of neuronal viability and function, rather than strictly as a marker for neuronal loss (267). In recent studies using high resolution spectroscopic imaging methods, Deicken et al. (269) reported a lower concentration of hippocampal NAA in familial bipolar I disorder. Similarly, Chang et al. (270) reported decreased NAA in children with familial bipolar disorder. Bertolino et al. (271) showed significant reductions of NAA and creatine–phosphocreatine bilaterally in the hippocampus of bipolar patients. Together, these studies add neurochemical evidence to the contention that mood disorders are associated with regional neuronal loss and/or reductions in neuronal viability and function.

Additional evidence that supports the findings on structural brain changes in bipolar disorder comes from functional brain imaging studies. Utilizing PET imaging, multiple abnormalities of regional cerebral blood flow and glucose metabolism in limbic and prefrontal cortex in mood disorders have been revealed. These abnormalities implicate limbic–thalamic–cortical and limbic–cortical–striatal–pallidal–thalamic circuits, involving the amygdala, orbital and medial prefrontal cortex, and anatomically related parts of the striatum and thalamus in the pathophysiology of mood disorders (272).

Post-Mortem Morphometric Findings

In addition to the accumulating neuroimaging evidence, several post-mortem brain studies are now providing direct evidence for reductions in regional CNS volume, cell number, and cell body size in bipolar disorder (Table 2). Baumann et al. (273)

Table 2 Post-Mortem Morphometric Brain Studies in Mood Disorders Demonstrating Cellular Atrophy and/or Loss

Reduced volume/cortical thickness
Cortical thickness rostral orbitofrontal cortex, MDD (282)
Laminar cortical thickness in layers III, V, and VI in subgenual anterior cingulate cortex (area 24) in BPD (306)
Volume of subgenual prefrontal cortex in familial MDD and BPD (275)
Volumes of nucleus accumbens (left), basal ganglia (bilateral) in MDD and BPD (273)
Parahippocampal cortex size (right) in suicide (307)
Reduced neuronal size and/or density
Pyramidal neuronal density, layers III and V in dorsolateral prefrontal cortex in BPD and MDD (283)
Neuronal size in layer V (–14%) and VI (–18%) in prefrontal cortex (area 9) in BPD (308)
Neuronal size in layer VI (–20%) in prefrontal cortex (area 9) in MDD (308)
Neuronal density and size in layer II–IV in rostral orbitofrontal cortex, in layer V/VI in caudal orbitofrontal cortex and in supra and infra granular layers in dorsolateral prefrontal cortex, in MDD (282)
Neuronal size in layer VI (–23%) in anterior cingulate cortex in MDD (309)
Neuronal density in layer III, V, and VI in subgenual anterior cingulated cortex (area 24) in BPD (306)
Layer specific interneurons in anterior cingulate cortex in BPD and MDD (311)
Non-pyramidal neuronal density in layer II (–27%) in anterior cingulate cortex in BPD (311)
Non-pyramidal neurons density in the CA2-region in BPD (278)
Reduced glia
Density/size of glia in dorsolateral prefrontal cortex and caudal orbitofrontal cortex in MDD and BPD layer specific (310)
Glial cell density in sub-layer IIIc (–19%) (and a trend to decrease in layer Va) in dorsolateral prefrontal cortex (area 9) in BPD (277)
Glial number in subgenual prefrontal cortex in familial MDD (–24%) and BPD (–41%) (275)
Glial cell density in layer V (–30%) in prefrontal cortex (area 9) in MDD (308)
Glial cell density in layer VI (–22%) in anterior cingulate cortex in MDD (309)
Glial cell counts, glial density, and glia-to-neuron ratios in amygdala in MDD (301)

Abbreviations: MDD, major depressive disorder; BPD, bipolar disorder. *Source*: Modified and reproduced with permission from Ref. 305.

reported reduced volumes of the left nucleus accumbens, the right putamen, and the bilateral external pallidum in post-mortem brain samples obtained from affectively ill patients compared with controls. Several recent post-mortem stereological studies of the prefrontal cortex have also demonstrated reduced regional volume, cell numbers, and/or sizes. Morphometric analysis of the density and size of cortical neurons in the dorsolateral prefrontal cortex and orbitofrontal cortex have revealed significant reductions in mood disorder patients as compared with control subjects (274), and the neuronal reductions were subtler than the corresponding glial alterations.

A reduction of 41% in glial cell number was reported in the subgenual prefrontal cortex in bipolar patients (275), consistent with neuroimaging data showing reductions in cortical gray matter volume found in the same brain region (276). In addition, a reduction of 19% in glial cell density in layer III of the dorsolateral prefrontal cortex in bipolar patients has been also reported (277). Overall, the layer-specific cellular changes observed in several distinct brain regions, including the prefrontal cortex, anterior cingulate cortex, and hippocampus (278) suggest that multiple neuronal circuits underlie the neuropathology of bipolar disorder (276,279).

Nevertheless, the marked reduction in glial cells in these regions has been particularly intriguing in view of the growing appreciation that glia play critical roles in regulating synaptic glutamate concentrations and CNS energy homeostasis, and in releasing trophic factors that participate in the development and maintenance of synaptic networks formed by neuronal and glial processes (275,280–284). Abnormalities of glial function could thus prove integral to the impairments of structural plasticity and overall pathophysiology of mood disorders.

Neurotrophic Properties of Mood Stabilizers and Antidepressants

There are several reports supporting the hypothesis that antidepressant treatment produces neurotrophic-like effects (222). Chronic administration of an atypical antidepressant, tianeptine, was reported to block the stress-induced atrophy of CA3 pyramidal neurons (285) and to block other stress-induced changes in brain structure and neurochemistry (286). Male tree shrews subjected to a chronic psychosocial stress paradigm were compared with non-stressed animals and found to have decreased NAA (287 or 267), decreased granule cell proliferation in the dentate gyrus of the hippocampus, and a reduction in hippocampal volume as measured in vivo by ^{1}H-MRS. All of these stress-induced effects were prevented or reversed in the animals treated concomitantly with tianeptine (286). The generalizability of these effects to other classes of antidepressants, however, is still unclear.

Elegant recent studies have demonstrated that another pathway involved in cell survival and plasticity, the cAMP–cAMP response element binding protein (CREB) cascade, is upregulated by antidepressant treatment (287). Upregulation of CREB, a gene promoter, and one of its major targets, BDNF, occurs in response to several different classes of antidepressant treatments, and occurs in a time frame consistent with the therapeutic action of antidepressants (288). Furthermore, chronic, but not acute, antidepressant treatments have been found to increase the number of new neurons in the dentate gyrus granule cell layer. These effects have been observed with different classes of antidepressants, but not with several other psychotropic medications investigated (288).

A role for the cAMP–CREB cascade and BDNF in the actions of antidepressant treatment is also supported by studies demonstrating that upregulation of these pathways has effects similar to antidepressant medications in animal behavioral models of depression such as the learned helplessness and forced swim test models (289–291). Remarkably, the antidepressant effect was observed as early as 3 days after a single infusion of BDNF in rat hippocampus and lasted for at least 10 days (291).

Several endogenous growth factors, including nerve growth factor (NGF) and BDNF, exert many of their neurotrophic effects via the extracellular signal-regulated kinase (ERK)/MAP kinase-signaling cascade. The net result of stimulating this cascade is an increase in the transcription and/or activity of a number of cell survival proteins, such as bcl-2 and BDNF. It is thus noteworthy that recent studies have demonstrated that chronic lithium and VPA robustly activate the ERK/MAP kinase cascade in cells of human neuronal origin and in rat frontal cortex and hippocampus (292,293). Consistent with ERK activation, both treatments produced a doubling of bcl-2 levels in the frontal cortex, an effect primarily due to a marked increase in the number of bcl-2 immunoreactive cells in layers II and III of the frontal cortex (294). The importance of neurons in layers II–IV of the frontal cortex in mood disorders has recently been emphasized—primate studies indicate that these areas are important for providing connections with other cortical regions, and that they are targets for sub-cortical input (282). Furthermore, chronic lithium also increases bcl-2 levels in the mouse hippocampus (295), and in cerebellar granule cells in culture (296), and VPA increases bcl-2 levels in human cells of neuronal origin (292).

Lithium, at therapeutically relevant concentrations, has been shown to exert neuroprotective effects in a variety of pre-clinical paradigms, consistent with the neurotrophic and neuroprotective effects of ERK/MAP kinase activation and bcl-2 upregulation. Consistently, VPA has been demonstrated to exert neuroprotective actions in cellular models as well, including glutamate toxicity, β-amyloid toxicity, and after exposure to other toxins (297–300).

HUMAN EVIDENCE FOR THE NEUROTROPHIC EFFECTS OF MOOD STABILIZERS

Although the body of preclinical data demonstrating neurotrophic and neuroprotective effects of mood stabilizers is striking, considerable caution must be exercised when extrapolating to the clinical situation with humans. In view of lithium and VPA's robust effects on the levels of the cytoprotective protein bcl-2 in the frontal cortex, Drevets et al. (254) re-analyzed older data demonstrating approximately 40% reductions in subgenual prefrontal cortex volumes in familial mood disorder subjects. Consistent with the neurotrophic and neuroprotective effects of lithium and VPA, Drevets (272) found that the patients treated with chronic lithium or VPA exhibited subgenual PFC volumes that were significantly larger than the volumes in non-lithium- or VPA-treated patients, and not significantly different from controls. It should be noted that, in contrast to mood stabilizers, chronic treatment of patients with selective serotonin reuptake inhibitors did not have any effect on gray matter volumes in this study.

In a more recent study, Drevets and colleagues (301) investigated glial cell densities in mood-disordered patients. Although the sample sizes were quite small, they made the intriguing observation that unipolar patients exhibited reduced glial cell densities, whereas only the bipolar patients who were not taking chronic lithium or VPA exhibited similar reductions. Considerable caution in extrapolating from these studies is warranted in view of their small sample sizes and cross-sectional nature.

To investigate the potential neurotrophic effects of lithium in humans more definitively, a longitudinal clinical study was undertaken using proton MRS to quantitate NAA levels (see Section Structural and Functional Brain Imaging Studies). It was found that chronic lithium increased NAA concentration in the human brain in vivo in both medication-free bipolar patients and in healthy controls (302). These findings provide intriguing indirect support for the contention that chronic lithium increases neuronal viability and function in the human brain. Furthermore, an approximate 0.97 correlation between lithium-induced NAA increases and regional voxel gray matter content was observed, thereby providing evidence for co-localization with the regional specific bcl-2 increases observed (e.g., gray vs. white matter) in the rodent brain cortices. These results suggest that chronic lithium may not only exert robust neuroprotective effects (as demonstrated in a variety of pre-clinical paradigms), but also exerts neurotrophic effects in humans (Fig. 5).

In follow-up studies to the NAA findings, it was hypothesized that, in addition to increasing functional neurochemical markers of neuronal viability, lithium-induced increases in bcl-2 would also lead to neuropil increases, and thus to increased brain gray matter volume in bipolar disorder patients. In this clinical research investigation, brain tissue volumes of bipolar patients were examined using high resolution three-dimensional MRI and validated quantitative brain tissue segmentation methodology to identify and quantify the various components by volume, including total brain white and gray matter content. Measurements were made at baseline (medication free, after a minimum 14-day washout) and then repeated after 4 weeks of lithium at therapeutic doses. The results showed that chronic lithium significantly increased total gray matter content in the human brains of patients with bipolar disorder (303). No significant changes were observed in brain

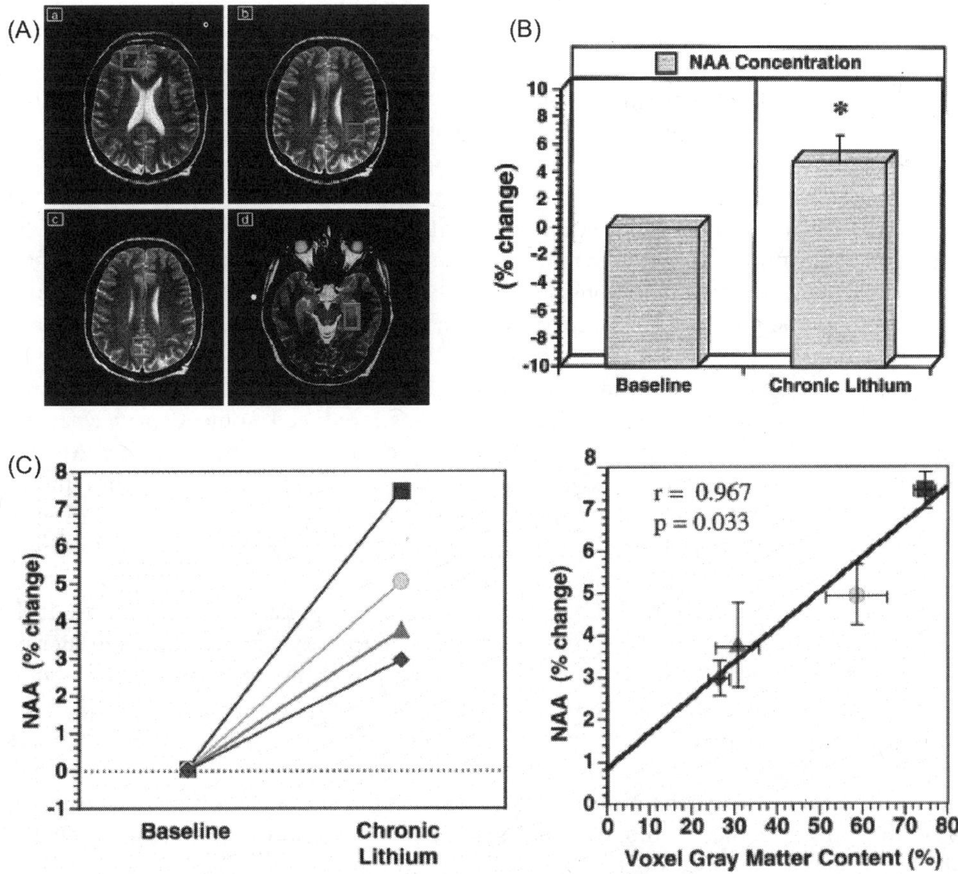

Figure 5 *Neurotrophic effect of lithium treatment measured by Magnetic Resonance Spectroscopy (MRS).* (A) Voxel placement for each region investigated with proton MRS. (a) Frontal lobe, (b) parietal lobe, (c) occipital lobe, and (d) temporal lobe. (B) Total brain *N*-acetyl-aspartate (NAA) concentration at baseline and after four weeks of lithium treatment. $^{*}p = 0.0217$ vs. baseline. (C) NAA increases on a regional basis (*left*) and it is positively correlates with percent voxel gray matter content (*right*). ■, Occipital; ●, temporal; ▲, frontal; and ◆, parietal. *Source*: Modified and reproduced with permission from Ref. 302.

white matter volume, or in quantitative measures of regional cerebral water content, thereby providing strong evidence that the observed increases in gray matter content are likely due to neurotrophic effects as opposed to any possible cell swelling and/or osmotic effects associated with lithium treatment. A more detailed sub-regional analysis of these brain imaging data is ongoing. Interestingly, the increased gray matter finding has recently been replicated in a cross-sectional MRI study; lithium-treated bipolar disorder patients had statistically higher cortical gray matter volumes when compared either to non-treated bipolar disorder patients or control subjects (304).

SUMMARY AND CONCLUSIONS

The pathophysiology of bipolar disorder must account for not only the profound changes in mood but also for a constellation of neurovegetative features derived from dysfunction in limbic related regions such as hippocampus, hypothalamus, and brainstem. The highly integrated monoamine and prominent neuropeptide pathways are known to originate and project heavily within these regions of the brain and it is thus not surprising that abnormalities have been noted in their function across clinical studies. But furthermore, we contend that for many refractory depression patients, new drugs simply mimicking many "traditional" drugs which directly or indirectly alter neurotransmitter levels and those which bind to cell surface receptors may be of limited benefit. This is because such strategies implicitly assume that the target circuits are functionally intact, and that altered synaptic activity will thus be transduced to modify the post-synaptic "throughput" of the system.

As discussed, there is a considerable body of evidence both conceptually and experimentally suggesting that impairments in neuroplasticity and cellular resilience may play an important role in the pathophysiology of bipolar disorder. The evidence presented here suggests that, in addition to neurochemical changes, many patients also have pronounced structural alterations (e.g., reduced spine density, neurite retraction, and overall neuropil reductions) in critical neuronal circuits. At this point, it is unclear if the regional cellular atrophy in mood disorders occurs due to the magnitude and duration of biochemical perturbations, an enhanced vulnerability to its deleterious effects (due to genetic factors and/or early life events), or a combination thereof. In this context, we have reviewed how stress can have a major impact on brain development, in particular by bringing about persistent changes in CRH-containing neurons, the HPA axis, the serotonergic system, the noradrenergic system, and the sympathetic nervous system. The possibility that these neurochemical alterations produce a state of neuroendangerment, which contributes to the subsequent development of morphological brain changes in adulthood, requires further investigation. Thus, optimal treatment may only be attained by providing both trophic and neurochemical support; the trophic support would be envisioned as enhancing and maintaining normal synaptic connectivity, thereby allowing the chemical signal to reinstate the optimal functioning of critical circuits necessary for normal affective functioning.

Emerging results from a variety of clinical and pre-clinical experimental and naturalistic paradigms suggest that a re-conceptualization about the pathophysiology, course, and optimal long-term treatment of recurrent mood disorders may be warranted. Optimal long-term treatment for these severe illnesses may require the early use of agents, which enhance neuroplasticity and cellular resilience. As we have extensively discussed above, there are a number of pharmacologic "plasticity enhancing" strategies that may be of considerable utility in the treatment of mood disorders. Among the most immediate ones are NMDA antagonists, glutamate release reducing agents, AMPA potentiators, cAMP phosphodiesterase inhibitors, and GR antagonists. An increasing number of strategies are being investigated to develop small molecule agents to regulate the activity of growth factors, MAP kinases cascades, and the bcl-2 family of proteins; this progress hold much promise for the development of novel therapeutics for the long-term treatment of severe, refractory bipolar disorder, and for improving the lives of millions who suffer from this condition.

REFERENCES

1. Goodwin FK, Jamison KR. Manic Depressive Illness. New York: Oxford University Press, Inc., 1990.
2. Institute of Medicine. Priority Areas for National Action: Transforming Health Care Quality. Washington, DC: The National Academies Press, 2003.
3. Simon GE. Social and economic burden of mood disorders. Biol Psychiatry 2003; 54(3):208–215.
4. Holsboer F. Neuroendocrinology of mood disorders. In: Kupfer DJ, ed. Psychopharmacology: The Fourth Generation of Progress. New York: Raven Press, 1995:957–969.
5. Manji HK, Lenox RH. The nature of bipolar disorder. J Clin Psychiatry 2000; 61(suppl 13): 42–57.
6. Manji H, Potter W. Monoaminergic mechanisms in bipolar disorder. In: Lt Y, Joffe RT, eds. Bipolar Disorder: Biological Models and Their Clinical Application. New York, NY: Marcel Dekker, 1997:235–254.
7. Bowden CL. Towards an integrated biological model of bipolar disorder. In: Lt Y, Joffe RT, eds. Bipolar Disorder: Biological Models and Their Clinical Application. New York, NY: Marcel Dekker, 1997:235–254.
8. Schatzberg AF, Schildkraut JJ. Recent studies on norepinephrine systems in mood disorders. In: Bloom FE, Kupfer DJ, eds. Psychopharmacology: The Fourth Generation of Progress. New York: Raven Press, 1995:957–969.
9. Kopin IJ, Jimerson DC, Markey SP, Ebert MH, Polinsky RJ. Disposition and metabolism of MHPG in humans: application to studies in depression. Pharmacopsychiatry 1984; 17(1):3–8.
10. Kopin IJ. Catecholamine metabolism: basic aspects and clinical significance. Pharmacol Rev 1985; 37(4):333–364.
11. Tsuji M, Yamane H, Yamada N, Iida H, Taga C, Myojin T. Studies on 3-methoxy-4-hydroxyphenylglycol (MHPG) and 3,4-dihydroxyphenylglycol (DHPG) levels in human urine, plasma and cerebrospinal fluids, and their significance in studies of depression. Jpn J Psychiatr Neurol 1986; 40(1):47–56.
12. Young LT, Warsh JJ, Kish SJ, Shannak K, Hornykeiwicz O. Reduced brain 5-HT and elevated NE turnover and metabolites in bipolar affective disorder. Biol Psychiatry 1994; 35(2):121–127.
13. Vawter MP, Freed WJ, Kleinman JE. Neuropathology of bipolar disorder. Biol Psychiatry 2000; 48(6):486–504.
14. Baumann B, Danos P, Diekmann S, Krell D, Bielau H, Geretsegger C, Wurthmann C, Bernstein HG, Bogerts B. Tyrosine hydroxylase immunoreactivity in the locus coeruleus is reduced in depressed non-suicidal patients but normal in depressed suicide patients. Eur Arch Psychiatr Clin Neurosci 1999; 249(4):212–219.
15. Kirov G, Murphy KC, Arranz MJ, Jones I, McCandles F, Kunugi H, Murray RM, McGuffin P, Collier DA, Owen MJ, Craddock N. Low activity allele of catechol-*O*-methyltransferase gene associated with rapid cycling bipolar disorder. Mol Psychiatry 1998; 3(4):342–345.

16. Rotondo A, Mazzanti C, Dell'Osso L, Rucci P, Sullivan P, Bouanani S, Gonnelli C, Goldman D, Cassano GB. Catechol *o*-methyltransferase, serotonin transporter, and tryptophan hydroxylase gene polymorphisms in bipolar disorder patients with and without comorbid panic disorder. Am J Psychiatry 2002; 159(1):23–29.
17. Serretti A, Macciardi F, Verga M, Cusin C, Pedrini S, Smeraldi E. Tyrosine hydroxylase gene associated with depressive symptomatology in mood disorder. Am J Med Genet 1998; 81(2):127–130.
18. Anand A, Darnell A, Miller HL, Berman RM, Cappiello A, Oren DA, Woods SW, Charney DS. Effect of catecholamine depletion on lithium-induced long-term remission of bipolar disorder. Biol Psychiatry 1999; 45(8):972–978.
19. Maes M, Meltzer H, D'Hondt P, Cosyns P, Blockx P. Effects on serotonin precursors on the negative feedback effects of glucocorticoids on hypothalamic–pituitary–adrenal axis function in depression. Psychoneuroendocrinology 1995; 20(2):149–167.
20. Garlow S, Mussellman D, Nemeroff C. The neurochemistry of mood disorders. In: Bunney BS, ed. Neurobiology of Mental Illness. New York, NY: Oxford University Press, 1999:348–364.
21. Shiah IS, Yatham LN. Serotonin in mania and in the mechanism of action of mood stabilizers: a review of clinical studies. Bipolar Disord 2000; 2(2):77–92.
22. Drevets WC, Frank E, Price JC, Kupfer DJ, Holt D, Greer PJ, Huang Y, Gautier C, Mathis C. PET imaging of serotonin 1A receptor binding in depression. Biol Psychiatry 1999; 46(10):1375–1387.
23. Sargent PA, Kjaer KH, Bench CJ, Rabiner EA, Messa C, Meyer J, Gunn RN, Grasby PM, Cowen PJ. Brain serotonin 1A receptor binding measured by positron emission tomography with [11C] WAY-100635: effects of depression and antidepressant treatment. Arch Gen Psychiatry 2000; 57(2):174–180.
24. Drevets WC, Frank E, Price JC, Kupfer DJ, Greer PJ, Mathis C. Serotonin type-1A receptor imaging in depression. Nucl Med Biol 2000; 27(5):499–507.
25. Hughes JH, Dunne F, Young AH. Effects of acute tryptophan depletion on mood and suicidal ideation in bipolar patients symptomatically stable on lithium. Br J Psychiatry 2000; 177:447–451.
26. Quintin P, Benkelfat C, Launay JM, Arnulf I, Pointereau-Bellenger A, Barbault S, Alvarez JC, Varoquaux O, Perez-Diaz F, Jouvent R, Leboyer M. Clinical and neurochemical effect of acute tryptophan depletion in unaffected relatives of patients with bipolar affective disorder. Biol Psychiatry 2001; 50(3):184–190.
27. Sobczak S, Riedel WJ, Booij I, Aan Het Rot M, Deutz NE, Honig A. Cognition following acute tryptophan depletion: difference between first-degree relatives of bipolar disorder patients and matched healthy control volunteers. Psychol Med 2002; 32(3):503–515.
28. Thakore JH, O'Keane V, Dinan TG. D-Fenfluramine-induced prolactin responses in mania: evidence for serotonergic subsensitivity. Am J Psychiatry 1996; 153(11):1460–1463.
29. Yatham LN. Prolactin and cortisol responses to fenfluramine challenge in mania. Biol Psychiatry 1996; 39(4):285–288.
30. Yatham LN, Zis AP, Lam RW, Tam E, Shiah IS. Sumatriptan-induced growth hormone release in patients with major depression, mania, and normal controls. Neuropsychopharmacology 1997; 17(4):258–263.
31. Dean B, Scarr E, Pavey G, Copolov D. Studies on serotonergic markers in the human hippocampus: changes in subjects with bipolar disorder. J Affect Disord 2003; 7(5)1:65–69.
32. Lopez JF, Chalmers DT, Little KY, Watson SJ. A.E. Bennett Research Award. Regulation of serotonin1A, glucocorticoid, and mineralocorticoid receptor in rat and human hippocampus: implications for the neurobiology of depression. Biol Psychiatry 1998; 43(8):547–573.
33. Benedetti F, Serretti A, Colombo C, Campori E, Barbini B, di Bella D, Smeraldi E. Influence of a functional polymorphism within the promoter of the serotonin transporter gene on the effects of total sleep deprivation in bipolar depression. Am J Psychiatry 1999; 156(9):1450–1452.

34. Serretti A, Lilli R, Mandelli L, Lorenzi C, Smeraldi E. Serotonin transporter gene associated with lithium prophylaxis in mood disorders. Pharmacogenomics J 2001; 1(1):71–77.
35. Mundo E, Walker M, Cate T, Macciardi F, Kennedy JL. The role of serotonin transporter protein gene in antidepressant-induced mania in bipolar disorder: preliminary findings. Arch Gen Psychiatry 2001; 58(6):539–544.
36. Parker G, Hadzi-Pavlovic D, Brodaty H, Boyce P, Mitchell P, Wilhelm K, Hickie I, Eyers K. Psychomotor disturbance in depression: defining the constructs. J Affect Disord 1993; 27(4):255–265.
37. Nestler EJ, Gould E, Manji H, Buncan M, Duman RS, Greshenfeld HK, Hen R, Koester S, Lederhendler I, Meaney M, Robbins T, Winsky L, Zalcman S. Preclinical models: status of basic research in depression. Biol Psychiatry 2002; 52(6):503–528.
38. Paul Willner, Jorgen Scheel-Kruger, eds. The Mesolimbic Dopamine System: From Motivation to Action. Chichester: Wiley, 1991:615–637.
39. Larmande P, Palisson E, Saikali I, Maillot F. Disappearance of akinesia in Parkinson disease during a manic attack. Rev Neurol (Paris) 1993; 149(10):557–558.
40. Scappa S, Teverbaugh P, Ananth J. Episodic tardive dyskinesia and Parkinsonism in bipolar disorder patients. Can J Psychiatry 1993; 38(10):633–634.
41. McTavish SF, McPherson MH, Harmer CJ, Clark L, Sharp T, Goodwin GM, Cowen PJ. Antidopaminergic effects of dietary tyrosine depletion in healthy subjects and patients with manic illness. Br J Psychiatry 2001; 179:356–360.
42. Zubieta JK, Huguelet P, Ohl LE, Koeppe RA, Kilbourn MR, Carr JM, Giordani BJ, Frey KA. High vesicular monoamine transporter binding in asymptomatic bipolar I disorder: sex differences and cognitive correlates. Am J Psychiatry 2000; 157(10):1619–1628.
43. Zucker M, Weizman A, Harel D, Rehavi M. Changes in vesicular monoamine transporter (VMAT2) and synaptophysin in rat substantia nigra and prefrontal cortex induced by psychotropic drugs. Neuropsychobiology 2001; 44(4):187–191.
44. Yatham LN, Liddle PF, Shiah IS, Lam RW, Ngan E, Scarrow G, Imperial M, Stoessl J, Sossi V, Ruth TJ. PET study of [(18)F]6-fluoro-L-dopa uptake in neuroleptic- and mood-stabilizer-naive first-episode nonpsychotic mania: effects of treatment with divalproex sodium. Am J Psychiatry 2002; 159(5):768–774.
45. Janowsky DS, Overstreet DH. The role of acetylcholine mechanisms in mood disorders. In: Kupfer DJ, ed. Psychopharmacology: The Fourth Generation of Progress. New York, NY: Raven Press, 1995:945–956.
46. Shopsin B, Janowsky D, Davis J, Gershon S. Rebound phenomena in manic patients following physostigmine. Preliminary observations. Neuropsychobiology 1975; 1(3):180–187.
47. Davis KL, Berger PA, Hollister LE, Defraites E. Physostigmine in mania. Arch Gen Psychiatry 1978; 35(1):119–122.
48. Khouzam HR, Kissmeyer PM. Physostigmine temporarily and dramatically reversing acute mania. Gen Hosp Psychiatry 1996; 18(3):203–204.
49. Sokolski KN, DeMet EM. Pupillary cholinergic sensitivity to pilocarpine increases in manic lithium responders. Biol Psychiatry 1999; 45(12):1580–1584.
50. Sokolski KN, DeMet EM. Cholinergic sensitivity predicts severity of mania. Psychiatr Res 2000; 95(3):195–200.
51. Jope RS. Anti-bipolar therapy: mechanism of action of lithium. Mol Psychiatry 1999; 4(2):117–128.
52. Lenox R, Manji H. Drugs for treatment of bipolar disorder: lithium. In: Nemeroff CB, ed. Textbook of Psychopharmacology. 2nd ed. Washington, DC: American Psychiatry Press, 1998:379–429.
53. Petty F, Kramer GL, Fulton M, Moeller FG, Rush AJ. Low plasma GABA is a trait-like marker for bipolar illness. Neuropsychopharmacology 1993; 9(2):125–132.
54. Berrettini WH, Nurnberger JI Jr, Hare TA, Simmons-Alling S, Gershon ES. CSF GABA in euthymic manic-depressive patients and controls. Biol Psychiatry 1986; 21(8–9):844–846.
55. Berrettini WH, Umberkoman-Wiita B, Nurnberger JI Jr, Vogel WH, Gershon ES, Post RM. Platelet GABA-transaminase in affective illness. Psychiatr Res 1982; 7(2):255–260.

56. Petty F, Kramer GL, Gullion CM, Rush AJ. Low plasma gamma-aminobutyric acid levels in male patients with depression. Biol Psychiatry 1992; 32(4):354–363.
57. Petty F. Plasma concentrations of gamma-aminobutyric acid (GABA) and mood disorders: a blood test for manic depressive disease? Clin Chem 1994; 40(2):296–302.
58. Bowden CL, Brugger AM, Swann AC, Calabrese JR, Janicak PG, Petty F, Dilsaver SC, Davis JM, Rush AJ, Small JG, et al. Efficacy of divalproex vs lithium and placebo in the treatment of mania. The Depakote Mania Study Group. JAMA 1994; 271(12):918–924.
59. Petty F, Rush AJ, Davis JM, Calabrese JR, Kimmel SE, Kramer GL, Small JG, Miller MJ, Swann AE, Orsulak PJ, Blake ME, Bowden CL. Plasma GABA predicts acute response to divalproex in mania. Biol Psychiatry 1996; 39(4):278–284.
60. Loscher W. Effects of the antiepileptic drug valproate on metabolism and function of inhibitory and excitatory amino acids in the brain. Neurochem Res 1993; 18(4):485–502.
61. Loscher W, Horstermann D. Differential effects of vigabatrin, gamma-acetylenic GABA, aminooxyacetic acid, and valproate on levels of various amino acids in rat brain regions and plasma. Naunyn Schmiedebergs Arch Pharmacol 1994; 349(3):270–278.
62. Loscher W, Vetter M. In vivo effects of aminooxyacetic acid and valproic acid on nerve terminal (synaptosomal) GABA levels in discrete brain areas of the rat. Correlation to pharmacological activities. Biochem Pharmacol 1985; 34(10):1747–1756.
63. Sanacora G, Mason GF, Rothman DL, Behar KL, Hyder F, Petroff OA, Berman RM, Charney DS, Krystal JH. Reduced cortical gamma-aminobutyric acid levels in depressed patients determined by proton magnetic resonance spectroscopy. Arch Gen Psychiatry 1999; 56(11):1043–1047.
64. Lopes da Silva FH, Witter MP, Boeijinga PH, Lohman AH. Anatomic organization and physiology of the limbic cortex. Physiol Rev 1990; 70(2):453–511.
65. Collingridge GL. Long-term potentiation. A question of reliability. Nature 1994; 371(6499):652–653.
66. Watkins J, Collingridge G. Phenylglycine derivatives as antagonists of metabotropic glutamate receptors. Trends Pharmacol Sci 1994; 15(9):333–342.
67. Collingridge GL, Bliss TV. Memories of NMDA receptors and LTP. Trends Neurosci 1995; 18(2):54–56.
68. Bannerman DM, Good MA, Butcher SP, Ramsay M, Morris RG. Distinct components of spatial learning revealed by prior training and NMDA receptor blockade. Nature 1995; 378(6553):182–186.
69. Whetsell WO Jr. Current concepts of excitotoxicity. J Neuropathol Exp Neurol 1996; 55(1):1–13.
70. Greene JG, Greenamyre JT. Bioenergetics and glutamate excitotoxicity. Prog Neurobiol 1996; 48(6):613–634.
71. Choi DW. Glutamate neurotoxicity and diseases of the nervous system. Neuron 1988; 1(8):623–634.
72. Zarate CA, Quiroz J, Payne J, Manji HK. Modulators of the glutamatergic system: implications for the development of improved therapeutics in mood disorders. Psychopharmacol Bull 2002; 36(4):35–83.
73. Berman RM, Cappiello A, Anand A, Oren DA, Heninger GR, Charney DS, Krystal JH. Antidepressant effects of ketamine in depressed patients. Biol Psychiatry 2000; 47(4): 351–354.
74. Calabrese JR, Bowden CL, Sachs GS, Ascher JA, Monaghan E, Rudd GD. A double-blind placebo-controlled study of lamotrigine monotherapy in outpatients with bipolar I depression. Lamictal 602 Study Group. J Clin Psychiatry 1999; 60(2):79–88.
75. Zarate CA Jr, Payne JL, Quiroz J, Sporn J, Denicoff KK, Luckenbaugh D, Charney DS, Manji HK. An open-label trial of riluzole in patients with treatment-resistant major depression. Am J Psychiatry 2004; 161(1):171–174.
76. Barden N, Reul JM, Holsboer F. Do antidepressants stabilize mood through actions on the hypothalamic–pituitary–adrenocortical system? Trends Neurosci 1995; 18(1):6–11.

77. Cassidy F, Ritchie JC, Carroll BJ. Plasma dexamethasone concentration and cortisol response during manic episodes. Biol Psychiatry 1998; 43(10):747–754.
78. Vale W, Spiess J, Rivier C, Rivier J. Characterization of a 41-residue ovine hypothalamic peptide that stimulates secretion of corticotropin and beta-endorphin. Science 1981; 213(4514):1394–1397.
79. Swanson LW, Sawchenko PE, Rivier J, Vale WW. Organization of ovine corticotropin-releasing factor immunoreactive cells and fibers in the rat brain: an immunohistochemical study. Neuroendocrinology 1983; 36(3):165–186.
80. Raadsheer FC, Hoogendijk WJ, Stam FC, Tilders FJ, Swaab DF. Increased numbers of corticotropin-releasing hormone expressing neurons in the hypothalamic paraventricular nucleus of depressed patients. Neuroendocrinology 1994; 60(4):436–444.
81. Raadsheer FC, van Heerikhuize JJ, Lucassen PJ, Hoogendijk WJ, Tilders FJ, Swaab DF. Corticotropin-releasing hormone mRNA levels in the paraventricular nucleus of patients with Alzheimer's disease and depression. Am J Psychiatry 1995; 152(9):1372–1376.
82. Nemeroff CB, Bissette G, Akil H, Fink M. Neuropeptide concentrations in the cerebrospinal fluid of depressed patients treated with electroconvulsive therapy. Corticotrophin-releasing factor, beta-endorphin and somatostatin. Br J Psychiatry 1991; 158:59–63.
83. De Bellis MD, Gold PW, Geracioti TD Jr, Listwak SJ, Kling MA. Association of fluoxetine treatment with reductions in CSF concentrations of corticotropin-releasing hormone and arginine vasopressin in patients with major depression. Am J Psychiatry 1993; 150(4):656–657.
84. Veith RC, Lewis N, Langohr JI, Murburg MM, Ashleigh EA, Castillo S, Peskind ER, Pascualy M, Bissette G, Nemeroff CB, et al. Effect of desipramine on cerebrospinal fluid concentrations of corticotropin-releasing factor in human subjects. Psychiatr Res 1993; 46(1):1–8.
85. Banki CM, Karmacsi L, Bissette G, Nemeroff CB. Cerebrospinal fluid neuropeptides in mood disorder and dementia. J Affect Disord 1992; 25(1):39–45.
86. Schmider J, Lammers CH, Gotthardt U, Dettling M, Holsboer F, Heuser IJ. Combined dexamethasone/corticotropin-releasing hormone test in acute and remitted manic patients, in acute depression, and in normal controls: I. Biol Psychiatry 1995; 38(12):797–802.
87. Rybakowski JK, Twardowska K. The dexamethasone/corticotropin-releasing hormone test in depression in bipolar and unipolar affective illness. J Psychiatr Res 1999; 33(5):363–370.
88. Nemeroff CB, Owens MJ, Bissette G, Andorn AC, Stanley M. Reduced corticotropin releasing factor binding sites in the frontal cortex of suicide victims. Arch Gen Psychiatry 1988; 45(6):577–579.
89. Krishnan KR, Doraiswamy PM, Figiel GS, Husain MM, Shah SA, Na C, Boyko OB, McDonald WM, Nemeroff CB, Ellinwood EH Jr. Hippocampal abnormalities in depression. J Neuropsychiatr Clin Neurosci 1991; 3(4):387–391.
90. Axelson DA, Doraiswamy PM, Boyko OB, Rodrigo Escalona P, McDonald WM, Ritchie JC, Patterson LJ, Ellinwood EH Jr, Nemeroff CB, Krishnan KR. In vivo assessment of pituitary volume with magnetic resonance imaging and systematic stereology: relationship to dexamethasone suppression test results in patients. Psychiatr Res 1992; 44(1):63–70.
91. Dorovini-Zis K, Zis AP. Increased adrenal weight in victims of violent suicide. Am J Psychiatry 1987; 144(9):1214–1215.
92. Amsterdam JD, Marinelli DL, Arger P, Winokur A. Assessment of adrenal gland volume by computed tomography in depressed patients and healthy volunteers: a pilot study. Psychiatr Res 1987; 21(3):189–197.
93. Nemeroff CB, Krishnan KR, Reed D, Leder R, Beam C, Dunnick NR. Adrenal gland enlargement in major depression. A computed tomographic study. Arch Gen Psychiatry 1992; 49(5):384–387.
94. Rubin E, Sackeim HA, Prohovnik I, Moeller JR, Schnur DB, Mukherjee S. Regional cerebral blood flow in mood disorders: IV. Comparison of mania and depression. Psychiatr Res 1995; 61(1):1–10.

95. Valle J, Ayuso-Gutierrez JL, Abril A, Ayuso-Mateos JL. Evaluation of thyroid function in lithium-naive bipolar patients. Eur Psychiatry 1999; 14(6):341–345.
96. Rush AJ, Giles DE, Schlesser MA, Orsulak PJ, Weissenburger JE, Fulton CL, Fairchild CJ, Roffwarg HP. Dexamethasone response, thyrotropin-releasing hormone stimulation, rapid eye movement latency, and subtypes of depression. Biol Psychiatry 1997; 41(9):915–928.
97. Zarate CA, Tohen M, Zarate SB. Thyroid function tests in first-episode bipolar disorder manic and mixed types. Biol Psychiatry 1997; 42(4):302–304.
98. Kusalic M. Grade II and grade III hypothyroidism in rapid-cycling bipolar patients. Neuropsychobiology 1992; 25(4):177–181.
99. Gyulai L, Bauer M, Bauer MS, Garcia-Espana F, Cnaan A, Whybrow PC. Thyroid hypofunction in patients with rapid-cycling bipolar disorder after lithium challenge. Biol Psychiatry 2003; 53(10):899–905.
100. Marangell LB, George MS, Bissette G, Pazzaglia P, Huggins T, Post RM. Carbamazepine increases cerebrospinal fluid thyrotropin-releasing hormone levels in affectively ill patients. Arch Gen Psychiatry 1994; 51(8):625–628.
101. Marangell LB, George MS, Callahan AM, Ketter TA, Pazzaglia PJ, L'Herrou TA, Leverich GS, Post RM. Effects of intrathecal thyrotropin-releasing hormone (protirelin) in refractory depressed patients. Arch Gen Psychiatry 1997; 54(3):214–222.
102. Callahan AM, Frye MA, Marangell LB, George MS, Ketter TA, L'Herrou T, Post RM. Comparative antidepressant effects of intravenous and intrathecal thyrotropin-releasing hormone: confounding effects of tolerance and implications for therapeutics. Biol Psychiatry 1997; 41(3):264–272.
103. Bauer M, Whybrow PC. Thyroid hormone, neural tissue and mood modulation. World J Biol Psychiatry 2001; 2(2):59–69.
104. Rubinow DR. Cerebrospinal fluid somatostatin and psychiatric illness. Biol Psychiatry 1986; 21(4):341–365.
105. Sharma RP, Bissette G, Janicak PG, Davis JM, Nemeroff CB. Elevation of CSF somatostatin concentrations in mania. Am J Psychiatry 1995; 152(12):1807–1809.
106. Widerlov E, Lindstrom LH, Wahlestedt C, Ekman R. Neuropeptide Y and peptide YY as possible cerebrospinal fluid markers for major depression and schizophrenia, respectively. J Psychiatr Res 1988; 22(1):69–79.
107. Gjerris A, Widerlov E, Werdelin L, Ekman R. Cerebrospinal fluid concentrations of neuropeptide Y in depressed patients and in controls. J Psychiatr Neurosci 1992; 17(1):23–27.
108. Heilig M, Zachrisson O, Thorsell A, Ehnvall A, Mottagui-Tabar S, Sjogren M, Asberg M, Ekman R, Wahlestedt C, Agren H. Decreased cerebrospinal fluid neuropeptide Y (NPY) in patients with treatment refractory unipolar major depression: preliminary evidence for association with preproNPY gene polymorphism. J Psychiatr Res 2004; 38(2):113–121.
109. Kuromitsu J, Yokoi A, Kawai T, Nagasu T, Aizawa T, Haga S, Ikeda K. Reduced neuropeptide Y mRNA levels in the frontal cortex of people with schizophrenia and bipolar disorder. Gene Expr Patterns 2001; 1(1):17–21.
110. Caberlotto L, Hurd YL. Reduced neuropeptide Y mRNA expression in the prefrontal cortex of subjects with bipolar disorder. Neuroreport 1999; 10(8):1747–1750.
111. Ranga K, Krishnan R. Clinical experience with substance P receptor (NK1) antagonists in depression. J Clin Psychiatry 2002; 63(suppl 11):25–29.
112. Manji HK, Lenox RH. Signaling: cellular insights into the pathophysiology of bipolar disorder. Biol Psychiatry 2000; 48(6):518–530.
113. Reppert SM. A clockwork explosion! Nature 1998; 21(1):1–4.
114. Dunlap JC. Molecular bases for circadian clocks. Cell 1999; 96(2):271–290.
115. Albrecht U, Oster H. The circadian clock and behavior. Behav Brain Res 2001; 125(1–2): 89–91.
116. Lenox RH, Gould TD, Manji HK. Endophenotypes in bipolar disorder. Am J Med Genet 2002; 114(4):391–406.
117. Chang DC, Reppert SM. The circadian clocks of mice and men. Neuron 2001; 29(3): 555–558.

118. King DP, Zhao Y, Sangoram AM, Wilsbacher LD, Tanaka M, Antoch MP, Steeves TD, Vitaterna MH, Kornhauser JM, Lowrey PL, Turek FW, Takahashi JS. Positional cloning of the mouse circadian clock gene. Cell 1997; 89(4):641–653.
119. Hogenesch JB, Gu YZ, Jain S, Bradfield CA. The basic-helix-loop-helix-PAS orphan MOP3 forms transcriptionally active complexes with circadian and hypoxia factors. Proc Natl Acad Sci USA 1998; 95(10):5474–5479.
120. Gekakis N, Staknis D, Nguyen HB, Davis FC, Wilsbacher LD, King DP, Takahashi JS, Weitz CJ. Role of the CLOCK protein in the mammalian circadian mechanism. Science 1998; 280(5369):1564–1569.
121. Reppert SM, Weaver DR. Molecular analysis of mammalian circadian rhythms. Annu Rev Physiol 2001; 63:647–676.
122. Toh KL, Jones CR, He Y, Eide EJ, Hinz WA, Virshup DM, Ptacek LJ, Fu YH. An hPer2 phosphorylation site mutation in familial advanced sleep phase syndrome. Science 2001; 291(5506):1040–1043.
123. Klemfuss H. Rhythms and the pharmacology of lithium. Pharmacol Ther 1992; 56(1):53–78.
124. Klemfuss H, Kripke DF. Light responsiveness of a circadian oscillator during lithium and potassium treatment. In: Labrecque G, ed. Annual Review of Chronopharmacology. Vol. 7. Oxford: Pergamon Press, 1990:5–8.
125. Healy D, Waterhouse JM. The circadian system and the therapeutics of the affective disorders. Pharmacol Ther 1995; 65(2):241–263.
126. Abe M, Herzog ED, Block GD. Lithium lengthens the circadian period of individual suprachiasmatic nucleus neurons. Neuroreport 2000; 11(14):3261–3264.
127. Klemfuss H, Kripke DF. Antimanic drugs stabilize hamster circadian rhythms. Psychiatr Res 1995; 57(3):215–222.
128. Kavaliers M. Period lengthening and disruption of socially facilitated circadian activity rhythms of goldfish by lithium. Physiol Behav 1981; 27(4):625–628.
129. Hofmann K, Gunderoth-Palmowski M, Wiedenmann G, Engelmann W. Further evidence for period lengthening effect of Li+ on circadian rhythms. Z Naturforsch [C] 1978; 33(3–4):231–234.
130. Weber U, Engelmann W, Mayer WE. Effects of tetraethylammoniumchloride (TEA), vanadate, and alkali ions on the lateral leaflet movement rhythm of *Desmodium motorium* (Houtt.) Merr. Chronobiol Int 1992; 9(4):269–277.
131. Welsh DK, Moore-Ede MC. Lithium lengthens circadian period in a diurnal primate, *Saimiri sciureus*. Biol Psychiatry 1990; 28(2):117–126.
132. Martinek S, Inonog S, Manoukian AS, Young MW. A role for the segment polarity gene shaggy/GSK-3 in the *Drosophila* circadian clock. Cell 2001; 105(6):769–779.
133. Gould TD, Manji HK. Signaling networks in the pathophysiology and treatment of mood disorders. J Psychosom Res 2002; 53(2):687–697.
134. Ikonomov OC, Manji HK. Molecular mechanisms underlying mood stabilization in manic-depressive illness: the phenotype challenge. Am J Psychiatry 1999; 156(10):1506–1514.
135. Dijk DJ, Duffy JF, Czeisler CA. Circadian and sleep/wake dependent aspects of subjective alertness and cognitive performance. J Sleep Res 1992; 1(2):112–117.
136. Boivin DB, Duffy JF, Kronauer RE, Czeisler CA. Dose–response relationships for resetting of human circadian clock by light. Nature 1996; 379(6565):540–542.
137. Hiddinga AE, Beersma DG, Van den Hoofdakker RH. Endogenous and exogenous components in the circadian variation of core body temperature in humans. J Sleep Res 1997; 6(3):156–163.
138. van de Wetering M, Cavallo R, Dooijes D, van Beest M, van Es J, Loureiro J, Ypma A, Hursh D, Jones T, Bejsovec A, Peifer M, Mortin M, Clevers H. Armadillo coactivates transcription driven by the product of the *Drosophila* segment polarity gene dTCF. Cell 1997; 88(6):789–799.
139. Wirz-Justice A, Van den Hoofdakker RH. Sleep deprivation in depression: what do we know, where do we go? Biol Psychiatry 1999; 46(4):445–453.

140. Miller JD, Morin LP, Schwartz WJ, Moore RY. New insights into the mammalian circadian clock. Sleep 1996; 19(8):641–667.
141. Atkinson M, Kripke DF, Wolf SR. Autorhythmometry in manic-depressives. Chronobiologia 1975; 2(4):325–335.
142. Wehr TA, Goodwin FK. Rapid cycling in manic-depressives induced by tricyclic antidepressants. Arch Gen Psychiatry 1979; 36(5):555–559.
143. Goodwin FK, Wirz-Justice A, Wehr TA. Evidence that the pathophysiology of depression and the mechanism of drug action of antidepressant drugs both involve alterations in circadian rhthyms. In: Racagni G, ed. Typical and Atypical Antidepressants: Clinical Practice. New York: Raven Press, 1982, 1982:5–8.
144. Kripke DF. Phase-advance theories for affective illness. In: Goodwin FK, ed. Circadian Rhythms in Psychiatry. Pacific Grove, CA: The Boxwood Press, 1983:41–69.
145. Schulz H, Lund R. On the origin of early REM episodes in the sleep of depressed patients: a comparison of three hypotheses. Psychiatr Res 1985; 16(1):65–77.
146. van den Hoofdakker RH, Beersma DG. On the explanation of short REM latencies in depression. Psychiatr Res 1985; 16(2):155–163.
147. Hallonquist JD, Goldberg MA, Brandes JS. Affective disorders and circadian rhythms. Can J Psychiatry 1986; 31(3):259–272.
148. Carroll BJ, Curtis GC, Mendels J. Neuroendocrine regulation in depression. II. Discrimination of depressed from nondepressed patients. Arch Gen Psychiatry 1976; 33(9): 1051–1058.
149. Branchey L, Weinberg U, Branchey M, Linkowski P, Mendlewicz J. Simultaneous study of 24-hour patterns of melatonin and cortisol secretion in depressed patients. Neuropsychobiology 1982; 8(5):225–232.
150. Linkowski P, Mendlewicz J, Kerkhofs M, Leclercq R, Golstein J, Brasseur M, Copinschi G, Van Cauter E. 24-Hour profiles of adrenocorticotropin, cortisol, and growth hormone in major depressive illness: effect of antidepressant treatment. J Clin Endocrinol Metab 1987; 65(1):141–152.
151. Linkowski P, Mendlewicz J, Leclercq R, Brasseur M, Hubain P, Golstein J, Copinschi G, Van Cauter E. The 24-hour profile of adrenocorticotropin and cortisol in major depressive illness. J Clin Endocrinol Metab 1985; 61(3):429–438.
152. von Zerssen D, Barthelmes H, Dirlich G, Doerr P, Emrich HM, von Lindern L, Lund R, Pirke KM. Circadian rhythms in endogenous depression. Psychiatr Res 1985; 16(1):51–63.
153. von Zerssen D, Doerr P, Emrich HM, Lund R, Pirke KM. Diurnal variation of mood and the cortisol rhythm in depression and normal states of mind. Eur Arch Psychiatr Neurol Sci 1987; 237(1):36–45.
154. Steiger A, von Bardeleben U, Herth T, Holsboer F. Sleep EEG and nocturnal secretion of cortisol and growth hormone in male patients with endogenous depression before treatment and after recovery. J Affect Disord 1989; 16(2–3):189–195.
155. Souetre E, Salvati E, Wehr TA, Sack DA, Krebs B, Darcourt G. Twenty-four-hour profiles of body temperature and plasma TSH in bipolar patients during depression and during remission and in normal control subjects. Am J Psychiatry 1988; 145(9):1133–1137.
156. Gillin JC, Duncan W, Pettigrew KD, Frankel BL, Snyder F. Successful separation of depressed, normal, and insomniac subjects by EEG sleep data. Arch Gen Psychiatry 1979; 36(1):85–90.
157. Kupfer DJ, Foster FG, Coble P, McPartland RJ, Ulrich RF. The application of EEG sleep for the differential diagnosis of affective disorders. Am J Psychiatry 1978; 135(1):69–74.
158. Gillin JC, Duncan WC, Murphy DL, Post RM, Wehr TA, Goodwin FK, Wyatt RJ, Bunney WE Jr. Age-related changes in sleep in depressed and normal subjects. Psychiatr Res 1981; 4(1):73–78.
159. Van Cauter E, Turek FW. Depression: a disorder of timekeeping? Perspect Biol Med 1986; 29(4):510–519.

160. Benca RM, Obermeyer WH, Thisted RA, Gillin JC. Sleep and psychiatric disorders. A meta-analysis. Arch Gen Psychiatry 1992; 49(8):651–668; discussion 669–670.
161. Teicher MH, Glod CA, Harper D, Magnus E, Brasher C, Wren F, Pahlavan K. Locomotor activity in depressed children and adolescents: I. Circadian dysregulation. J Am Acad Child Adolesc Psychiatry 1993; 32(4):760–769.
162. Monk TH, Buysse DJ, Frank E, Kupfer DJ, Dettling J, Ritenour AM. Nocturnal and circadian body temperatures of depressed outpatients during symptomatic and recovered states. Psychiatr Res 1994; 51(3):297–311.
163. Bicakova-Rocher A, Gorceix A, Reinberg A, Ashkenazi, II, Ticher A. Temperature rhythm of patients with major affective disorders: reduced circadian period length. Chronobiol Int 1996; 13(1):47–57.
164. Sack DA, Nurnberger J, Rosenthal NE, Ashburn E, Wehr TA. Potentiation of antidepressant medications by phase advance of the sleep–wake cycle. Am J Psychiatry 1985; 142(5):606–608.
165. Kasper S, Wehr TA. The role of sleep and wakefulness in the genesis of depression and mania. Encephale 1992; 18(spec no. 1):45–50.
166. Wu JC, Bunney WE. The biological basis of an antidepressant response to sleep deprivation and relapse: review and hypothesis. Am J Psychiatry 1990; 147(1):14–21.
167. Van den Hoofdakker RH. Total sleep deprivation: clinical and theoretical aspects. In: Praag HM, ed. Depression: Neurobiology, Psychopathological and Theoretical Advances: Chichester, John Wiley and Son, 1997:564–589.
168. Colombo C, Benedetti F, Barbini B, Campori E, Smeraldi E. Rate of switch from depression into mania after therapeutic sleep deprivation in bipolar depression. Psychiatr Res 1999; 86(3):267–270.
169. Szuba MP, Baxter LR Jr, Fairbanks LA, Guze BH, Schwartz JM. Effects of partial sleep deprivation on the diurnal variation of mood and motor activity in major depression. Biol Psychiatry 1991; 30(8):817–829.
170. Wehr TA, Sack DA, Rosenthal NE. Sleep reduction as a final common pathway in the genesis of mania. Am J Psychiatry 1987; 144(2):201–204.
171. Manji HK, Chen G. Post-receptor signaling pathways in the pathophysiology and treatment of mood disorders. Curr Psychiatr Rep 2000; 2(6):479–489.
172. Jope RS, Williams MB. Lithium and brain signal transduction systems. Biochem Pharmacol 1994; 47(3):429–441.
173. Cirelli C, Tononi G. Differential expression of plasticity-related genes in waking and sleep and their regulation by the noradrenergic system. J Neurosci 2000; 20(24):9187–9194.
174. Payne JL, Quiroz JA, Zarate CA, Manji HK. Timing is everything: does the robust upregulation of noradrenergically regulated plasticity genes underlie the rapid antidepressant effects of sleep deprivation? Biol Psychiatry 2002; 52(10):921–926.
175. Duman RS, Heninger GR, Nestler EJ. A molecular and cellular theory of depression. Arch Gen Psychiatry 1997; 54(7):597–606.
176. Sapolsky RM. Glucocorticoids and hippocampal atrophy in neuropsychiatric disorders. Arch Gen Psychiatry 2000; 57(10):925–935.
177. McEwen BS. Stress and hippocampal plasticity. Annu Rev Neurosci 1999; 22:105–122.
178. Sapolsky RM. Stress, glucocorticoids, and damage to the nervous system: the current state of confusion. Stress 1996; 1(1):1–19.
179. Bourne HR, Nicoll R. Molecular machines integrate coincident synaptic signals. Cell 1993; 72(suppl):65–75.
180. Bhalla US, Iyengar R. Emergent properties of networks of biological signaling pathways. Science 1999; 283(5400):381–387.
181. Weng G, Bhalla US, Iyengar R. Complexity in biological signaling systems. Science 1999; 284(5411):92–96.
182. Spiegel A. G Proteins, Receptors, and Disease. Totowa, NJ: Humana Press, 1998.
183. Manji HK. G proteins: implications for psychiatry. Am J Psychiatry 1992; 149(6): 746–760.

184. Young LT, Li PP, Kish SJ, Siu KP, Kamble A, Hornykiewicz O, Warsh JJ. Cerebral cortex Gs alpha protein levels and forskolin-stimulated cyclic AMP formation are increased in bipolar affective disorder. J Neurochem 1993; 61(3):890–898.
185. Warsh J, Young L, Li P. Guanine nucleotide binding (G) protein disturbances. In: Belmaker R, ed. Bipolar Affective Disorder in Bipolar Medications: Mechanisms of Action. Washington, DC: American Psychiatric Press, 2000:299–329.
186. Wang HY, Friedman E. Enhanced protein kinase C activity and translocation in bipolar affective disorder brains. Biol Psychiatry 1996; 40(7):568–575.
187. Manji HK, Chen G, Shimon H, Hsiao JK, Potter WZ, Belmaker RH. Guanine nucleotide-binding proteins in bipolar affective disorder. Effects of long-term lithium treatment. Arch Gen Psychiatry 1995; 52(2):135–144.
188. Mitchell PB, Manji HK, Chen G, Jolkovsky L, Smith-Jackson E, Denicoff K, Schmidt M, Potter WZ. High levels of Gs alpha in platelets of euthymic patients with bipolar affective disorder. Am J Psychiatry 1997; 154(2):218–223.
189. Spleiss O, van Calker D, Scharer L, Adamovic K, Berger M, Gebicke-Haerter PJ. Abnormal G protein alpha(s)—and alpha(i2)-subunit mRNA expression in bipolar affective disorder. Mol Psychiatry 1998; 3(6):512–520.
190. Wang HY, Friedman E. Effects of lithium on receptor-mediated activation of G proteins in rat brain cortical membranes. Neuropharmacology 1999; 38(3):403–414.
191. Ram A, Guedj F, Cravchik A, Weinstein L, Cao Q, Badner JA, Goldin LR, Grisaru N, Manji HK, Belmaker RH, Gershon ES, Gejman PV. No abnormality in the gene for the G protein stimulatory alpha subunit in patients with bipolar disorder. Arch Gen Psychiatry 1997; 54(1):44–48.
192. Li P, Andreopoulos S, Warsh J. Signal transduction abnormalities in bipolar affective disorder. In: Reith MEA, ed. Cerbral Signal Transduction. Humana Press, 2000:283–312.
193. Nishizuka Y. Intracellular signaling by hydrolysis of phospholipids and activation of protein kinase C. Science 1992; 258(5082):607–614.
194. Nishizuka Y. Protein kinase C and lipid signaling for sustained cellular responses. Faseb J 1995; 9(7):484–496.
195. Stabel S, Parker PJ. Protein kinase C. Pharmacol Ther 1991; 51(1):71–95.
196. Newton AC. Protein kinase C: structure, function, and regulation. J Biol Chem 1995; 270(48):28495–28498.
197. Hahn CG, Friedman E. Abnormalities in protein kinase C signaling and the pathophysiology of bipolar disorder. Bipolar Disord 1999; 1(2):81–86.
198. Friedman E, Hoau Yan W, Levinson D, Connell TA, Singh H. Altered platelet protein kinase C activity in bipolar affective disorder, manic episode. Biol Psychiatry 1993; 33(7):520–525.
199. Manji HK, Lenox RH. Ziskind-Somerfeld Research Award. Protein kinase C signaling in the brain: molecular transduction of mood stabilization in the treatment of manic–depressive illness. Biol Psychiatry 1999; 46(10):1328–1351.
200. Conn P, Sweatt J. Protein kinase C in the nervous system. In: Kuo J, ed. Protein Kinase C. New York: Oxford University Press, 1994:199–235.
201. Couldwell WT, Weiss MH, DeGiorgio CM, Weiner LP, Hinton DR, Ehresmann GR, Conti PS, Apuzzo ML. Clinical and radiographic response in a minority of patients with recurrent malignant gliomas treated with high-dose tamoxifen. Neurosurgery 1993; 32(3):485–489; discussion 489–490.
202. Bebchuk JM, Arfken CL, Dolan-Manji S, Murphy J, Hasanat K, Manji HK. A preliminary investigation of a protein kinase C inhibitor in the treatment of acute mania. Arch Gen Psychiatry 2000; 57(1):95–97.
203. Chen G, Huang LD, Jiang YM, Manji HK. The mood-stabilizing agent valproate inhibits the activity of glycogen synthase kinase-3. J Neurochem 1999; 72(3):1327–1330.
204. Lucas FR, Goold RG, Gordon-Weeks PR, Salinas PC. Inhibition of GSK-3beta leading to the loss of phosphorylated MAP-1B is an early event in axonal remodelling induced by WNT-7a or lithium. J Cell Sci 1998; 111(Pt 10):1351–1361.

205. Lucas FR, Salinas PC. WNT-7a induces axonal remodeling and increases synapsin I levels in cerebellar neurons. Dev Biol 1997; 192(1):31–44.
206. Takashima A, Noguchi K, Sato K, Hoshino T, Imahori K. Tau protein kinase I is essential for amyloid beta-protein-induced neurotoxicity. Proc Natl Acad Sci USA 1993; 90(16):7789–7793.
207. Pap M, Cooper GM. Role of glycogen synthase kinase-3 in the phosphatidylinositol 3-kinase/Akt cell survival pathway. J Biol Chem 1998; 273(32):19929–19932.
208. Crowder RJ, Freeman RS. Glycogen synthase kinase-3 beta activity is critical for neuronal death caused by inhibiting phosphatidylinositol 3-kinase or Akt but not for death caused by nerve growth factor withdrawal. J Biol Chem 2000; 275(44):34266–34271.
209. Yehuda S, Carasso RL, Mostofsky DI. Essential fatty acid preparation (SR-3) raises the seizure threshold in rats. Eur J Pharmacol 1994; 254(1–2):193–198.
210. Medini L, Colli S, Mosconi C, Tremoli E, Galli C. Diets rich in n-9, n-6 and n-3 fatty acids differentially affect the generation of inositol phosphates and of thromboxane by stimulated platelets, in the rabbit. Biochem Pharmacol 1990; 39(1):129–133.
211. Sperling RI, Benincaso AI, Knoell CT, Larkin JK, Austen KF, Robinson DR. Dietary omega-3 polyunsaturated fatty acids inhibit phosphoinositide formation and chemotaxis in neutrophils. J Clin Invest 1993; 91(2):651–660.
212. Pepe S, Bogdanov K, Hallaq H, Spurgeon H, Leaf A, Lakatta E. Omega 3 polyunsaturated fatty acid modulates dihydropyridine effects on L-type Ca^{2+} channels, cytosolic Ca^{2+}, and contraction in adult rat cardiac myocytes. Proc Natl Acad Sci USA 1994; 91(19):8832–8836.
213. Holian O, Nelson R. Action of long-chain fatty acids on protein kinase C activity: comparison of omega-6 and omega-3 fatty acids. Anticancer Res 1992; 12(3):975–980.
214. Slater SJ, Kelly MB, Taddeo FJ, Ho C, Rubin E, Stubbs CD. The modulation of protein kinase C activity by membrane lipid bilayer structure. J Biol Chem 1994; 269(7): 4866–4871.
215. Mirnikjoo B, Brown SE, Kim HF, Marangell LB, Sweatt JD, Weeber EJ. Protein kinase inhibition by omega-3 fatty acids. J Biol Chem 2001; 276(14):10888–10896.
216. Su KP, Huang SY, Chiu CC, Shen WW. Omega-3 fatty acids in major depressive disorder. A preliminary double-blind, placebo-controlled trial. Eur Neuropsychopharmacol 2003; 13(4):267–271.
217. Marangell LB, Martinez JM, Zboyan HA, Kertz B, Kim HF, Puryear LJ. A double-blind, placebo-controlled study of the omega-3 fatty acid docosahexaenoic acid in the treatment of major depression. Am J Psychiatry 2003; 160(5):996–998.
218. Stoll AL, Severus WE, Freeman MP, Rueter S, Zboyan HA, Diamond E, Cress KK, Marangell LB. Omega 3 fatty acids in bipolar disorder: a preliminary double-blind, placebo-controlled trial. Arch Gen Psychiatry 1999; 56(5):407–412.
219. Keck PE, Freeman MP, McElroy SL, Dhavale XX, Suppes T, Altshuler L, Frye M, Mintz J, Hwang S, Kupka R, Nolen W, Leverich G, Denicoff KD, Grunze H, Walden J, Post R. Double-blind, randomized, placebo-controlled trials of ethyl-eicosapentanoate in the treatment of bipolar depression and rapid cycling bipolar disorder. Submitted for publication.
220. Chang MC, Contreras MA, Rosenberger TA, Rintala JJ, Bell JM, Rapoport SI. Chronic valproate treatment decreases the in vivo turnover of arachidonic acid in brain phospholipids: a possible common effect of mood stabilizers. J Neurochem 2001; 77(3):796–803.
221. Chang MC, Grange E, Rabin O, Bell JM, Allen DD, Rapoport SI. Lithium decreases turnover of arachidonate in several brain phospholipids. Neurosci Lett 1996; 220(3):171–174.
222. Duman RS. Synaptic plasticity and mood disorders. Mol Psychiatry 2002; 7(suppl 1): S29–S34.
223. Manji HK, Chen G. PKC, MAP kinases and the bcl-2 family of proteins as long-term targets for mood stabilizers. Mol Psychiatry 2002; 7(suppl 1):S46–S56.

224. Manji HK, Moore GJ, Chen G. Lithium up-regulates the cytoprotective protein Bcl-2 in the CNS in vivo: a role for neurotrophic and neuroprotective effects in manic depressive illness. J Clin Psychiatry 2000; 61(suppl 9):82–96.
225. Kitamura Y, Kosaka T, Kakimura JI, Matsuoka Y, Kohno Y, Nomura Y, Taniguchi T. Protective effects of the antiparkinsonian drugs talipexole and pramipexole against 1-methyl-4-phenylpyridinium-induced apoptotic death in human neuroblastoma SH-SY5Y cells. Mol Pharmacol 1998; 54(6):1046–1054.
226. Takata K, Kitamura Y, Kakimura J, Kohno Y, Taniguchi T. Increase of bcl-2 protein in neuronal dendritic processes of cerebral cortex and hippocampus by the antiparkinsonian drugs, talipexole and pramipexole. Brain Res 2000; 872(1–2):236–241.
227. Zarate CA, Payne JL, Singh J, Quiroz JA, Luckenbaugh D, Denicoff KD, Charney DS, Manji HK. Pramipexole for bipolar II depression: a placebo-controlled proof of concept study. Biol Psychiatry 2004; 56(1):54–60.
228. Emamghoreishi M, Schlichter L, Li PP, Parikh S, Sen J, Kamble A, Warsh JJ. High intracellular calcium concentrations in transformed lymphoblasts from subjects with bipolar I disorder. Am J Psychiatry 1997; 154(7):976–982.
229. Yoon IS, Li PP, Siu KP, Kennedy JL, Macciardi F, Cooke RG, Parikh SV, Warsh JJ. Altered TRPC7 gene expression in bipolar-I disorder. Biol Psychiatry 2001; 50(8):620–626.
230. Kato T, Kato N. Mitochondrial dysfunction in bipolar disorder. Bipolar Disord 2000; 2(3 Pt 1):180–190.
231. Gray NA, Quiroz JA, Kato T, Manji HK. Critical roles for the mitochondrial-ER network in the pathophysiology and treatment of bipolar disorder. Submitted for publication.
232. Kato T, Shioiri T, Murashita J, Hamakawa H, Takahashi Y, Inubushi T, Takahashi S. Lateralized abnormality of high energy phosphate metabolism in the frontal lobes of patients with bipolar disorder detected by phase-encoded 31P-MRS. Psychol Med 1995; 25(3):557–566.
233. Deicken RF, Fein G, Weiner MW. Abnormal frontal lobe phosphorous metabolism in bipolar disorder. Am J Psychiatry 1995; 152(6):915–918.
234. Volz HP, Rzanny R, Riehemann S, May S, Hegewald H, Preussler B, Hubner G, Kaiser WA, Sauer H. 31P magnetic resonance spectroscopy in the frontal lobe of major depressed patients. Eur Arch Psychiatr Clin Neurosci 1998; 248(6):289–295.
235. Kato T, Murashita J, Kamiya A, Shioiri T, Kato N, Inubushi T. Decreased brain intracellular pH measured by 31P-MRS in bipolar disorder: a confirmation in drug-free patients and correlation with white matter hyperintensity. Eur Arch Psychiatr Clin Neurosci 1998; 248(6):301–306.
236. Hamakawa H, Murashita J, Yamada N, Inubushi T, Kato N, Kato T. Reduced intracellular pH in the basal ganglia and whole brain measured by 31P-MRS in bipolar disorder. Psychiatr Clin Neurosci 2004; 58(1):82–88.
237. Konradi C, Eaton M, MacDonald ML, Walsh J, Benes FM, Heckers S. Molecular evidence for mitochondrial dysfunction in bipolar disorder. Arch Gen Psychiatry 2004; 61(3):300–308.
238. Heckers S, Stone D, Walsh J, Shick J, Koul P, Benes FM. Differential hippocampal expression of glutamic acid decarboxylase 65 and 67 messenger RNA in bipolar disorder and schizophrenia. Arch Gen Psychiatry 2002; 59(6):521–529.
239. Washizuka S, Kakiuchi C, Mori K, Kunugi H, Tajima O, Akiyama T, Nanko S, Kato T. Association of mitochondrial complex I subunit gene NDUFV2 at 18p11 with bipolar disorder. Am J Med Genet 2003; 120B(1):72–78.
240. Andreasen NC, Swayze V II, Flaum M, Alliger R, Cohen G. Ventricular abnormalities in affective disorder: clinical and demographic correlates. Am J Psychiatry 1990; 147(7): 893–900.
241. Johnstone EC, Owens DG, Crow TJ, Colter N, Lawton CA, Jagoe R, Kreel L. Hypothyroidism as a correlate of lateral ventricular enlargement in manic-depressive and neurotic illness. Br J Psychiatry 1986; 148:317–321.

242. Nasrallah HA, McCalley-Whitters M, Jacoby CG. Cortical atrophy in schizophrenia and mania: a comparative CT study. J Clin Psychiatry 1982; 43(11):439–441.
243. Pearlson GD, Garbacz DJ, Tompkins RH, Ahn HS, Gutterman DF, Veroff AE, DePaulo JR. Clinical correlates of lateral ventricular enlargement in bipolar affective disorder. Am J Psychiatry 1984; 141(2):253–256.
244. Dewan MJ, Haldipur CV, Lane EE, Ispahani A, Boucher MF, Major LF. Bipolar affective disorder. I. Comprehensive quantitative computed tomography. Acta Psychiatr Scand 1988; 77(6):670–676.
245. Swayze VW II, Andreasen NC, Alliger RJ, Ehrhardt JC, Yuh WT. Structural brain abnormalities in bipolar affective disorder. Ventricular enlargement and focal signal hyperintensities. Arch Gen Psychiatry 1990; 47(11):1054–1059.
246. Tanaka Y, Hazama H, Fukuhara T, Tsutsui T. Computerized tomography of the brain in manic-depressive patients—a controlled study. Folia Psychiatr Neurol Jpn 1982; 36(2): 137–143.
247. Brambilla P, Harenski K, Nicoletti M, Mallinger AG, Frank E, Kupfer DJ, Keshavan MS, Soares JC. Differential effects of age on brain gray matter in bipolar patients and healthy individuals. Neuropsychobiology 2001; 43(4):242–247.
248. Dasari M, Friedman L, Jesberger J, Stuve TA, Findling RL, Swales TP, Schulz SC. A magnetic resonance imaging study of thalamic area in adolescent patients with either schizophrenia or bipolar disorder as compared to healthy controls. Psychiatr Res 1999; 91(3):155–162.
249. Sassi RB, Nicoletti M, Brambilla P, Harenski K, Mallinger AG, Frank E, Kupfer DJ, Keshavan MS, Soares JC. Decreased pituitary volume in patients with bipolar disorder. Biol Psychiatry 2001; 50(4):271–280.
250. Coffman JA, Bornstein RA, Olson SC, Schwarzkopf SB, Nasrallah HA. Cognitive impairment and cerebral structure by MRI in bipolar disorder. Biol Psychiatry 1990; 27(11):1188–1196.
251. Altshuler LL, Conrad A, Hauser P, Li XM, Guze BH, Denikoff K, Tourtellotte W, Post R. Reduction of temporal lobe volume in bipolar disorder: a preliminary report of magnetic resonance imaging. Arch Gen Psychiatry 1991; 48(5):482–483.
252. Lim KO, Rosenbloom MJ, Faustman WO, Sullivan EV, Pfefferbaum A. Cortical gray matter deficit in patients with bipolar disorder. Schizophr Res 1999; 40(3):219–227.
253. Davis KA, Yucel M, Cardenas VA, Deicken RH. Frontal and anterior cingulate cortex volume reduction in familial bipolar I disorder. In: Biological Psychiatry. San Francisco, CA, 2003.
254. Drevets WC, Price JL, Simpson JR Jr, Todd RD, Reich T, Vannier M, Raichle ME. Subgenual prefrontal cortex abnormalities in mood disorders. Nature 1997; 386(6627):824–827.
255. Hirayasu Y, Shenton ME, Salisbury DF, Kwon JS, Wible CG, Fischer IA, Yurgelun-Todd D, Zarate C, Kikinis R, Jolesz FA, McCarley RW. Subgenual cingulate cortex volume in first-episode psychosis. Am J Psychiatry 1999; 156(7):1091–1093.
256. Sheline YI, Wang PW, Gado MH, Csernansky JG, Vannier MW. Hippocampal atrophy in recurrent major depression. Proc Natl Acad Sci USA 1996; 93(9):3908–3913.
257. Sheline YI, Sanghavi M, Mintun MA, Gado MH. Depression duration but not age predicts hippocampal volume loss in medically healthy women with recurrent major depression. J Neurosci 1999; 19(12):5034–5043.
258. Bremner JD, Narayan M, Anderson ER, Staib LH, Miller HL, Charney DS. Hippocampal volume reduction in major depression. Am J Psychiatry 2000; 157(1):115–118.
259. Shah PJ, Ebmeier KP, Glabus MF, Goodwin GM. Cortical grey matter reductions associated with treatment-resistant chronic unipolar depression. Controlled magnetic resonance imaging study. Br J Psychiatry 1998; 172:527–532.
260. Altshuler LL, Bartzokis G, Grieder T, Curran J, Jimenez T, Leight K, Wilkins J, Gerner R, Mintz J. An MRI study of temporal lobe structures in men with bipolar disorder or schizophrenia. Biol Psychiatry 2000; 48(2):147–162.

261. Hauser P, Matochik J, Altshuler LL, Denicoff KD, Conrad A, Li X, Post RM. MRI-based measurements of temporal lobe and ventricular structures in patients with bipolar I and bipolar II disorders. J Affect Disord 2000; 60(1):25–32.
262. Brambilla P, Harenski K, Nicoletti M, Sassi RB, Mallinger AG, Frank E, Kupfer DJ, Keshavan MS, Soares JC. MRI investigation of temporal lobe structures in bipolar patients. J Psychiatr Res 2003; 37(4):287–295.
263. Noga JT, Vladar K, Torrey EF. A volumetric magnetic resonance imaging study of monozygotic twins discordant for bipolar disorder. Psychiatr Res 2001; 106(1):25–34.
264. Anzalone S, Pegues MP, Rogers LJ, Deicken RF. Reduced hippocampal volumes in familial bipolar I disorder. Biol Psychiatry 2002; 51(8s):69s–70s.
265. Lyons DM, Yang C, Sawyer-Glover AM, Moseley ME, Schatzberg AF. Early life stress and inherited variation in monkey hippocampal volumes. Arch Gen Psychiatry 2001; 58(12):1145–1151.
266. Baslow MH. Functions of *N*-acetyl-L-aspartate and *N*-acetyl-L-aspartylglutamate in the vertebrate brain: role in glial cell-specific signaling. J Neurochem 2000; 75(2):453–459.
267. Tsai G, Coyle JT. *N*-acetylaspartate in neuropsychiatric disorders. Prog Neurobiol 1995; 46(5):531–540.
268. Bates TE, Strangward M, Keelan J, Davey GP, Munro PM, Clark JB. Inhibition of *N*-acetylaspartate production: implications for 1H MRS studies in vivo. Neuroreport 1996; 7(8):1397–1400.
269. Deicken RF, Pegues MP, Anzalone S, Feiwell R, Soher B. Lower concentration of hippocampal *N*-acetylaspartate in familial bipolar I disorder. Am J Psychiatry 2003; 160(5):873–882.
270. Chang K, Adleman N, Dienes K, Barnea-Goraly N, Reiss A, Ketter T. Decreased *N*-acetylaspartate in children with familial bipolar disorder. Biol Psychiatry 2003; 53(11):1059–1065.
271. Bertolino A, Frye M, Callicott JH, Mattay VS, Rakow R, Shelton-Repella J, Post R, Weinberger DR. Neuronal pathology in the hippocampal area of patients with bipolar disorder: a study with proton magnetic resonance spectroscopic imaging. Biol Psychiatry 2003; 53(10):906–913.
272. Drevets WC. Neuroimaging studies of mood disorders. Biol Psychiatry 2000; 48(8):813–829.
273. Baumann B, Danos P, Krell D, Diekmann S, Leschinger A, Stauch R, Wurthmann C, Bernstein HG, Bogerts B. Reduced volume of limbic system-affiliated basal ganglia in mood disorders: preliminary data from a postmortem study. J Neuropsychiatr Clin Neurosci 1999; 11(1):71–78.
274. Rajkowska G. Cell pathology in bipolar disorder. Bipolar Disord 2002; 4(2):105–116.
275. Ongur D, Drevets WC, Price JL. Glial reduction in the subgenual prefrontal cortex in mood disorders. Proc Natl Acad Sci USA 1998; 95(22):13290–13295.
276. Manji HK, Quiroz JA, Sporn J, Payne JL, Denicoff K, Gray NA, Zarate CA Jr, Charney DS. Enhancing neuronal plasticity and cellular resilience to develop novel, improved therapeutics for difficult-to-treat depression. Biol Psychiatry 2003; 53:707–742.
277. Selemon L. Beyond gliosis: new roles for glia in response to antipsychotic drug treatment and disease. Biol Psychiatry 2002; 51(8S):98S.
278. Benes FM, Kwok EW, Vincent SL, Todtenkopf MS. A reduction of nonpyramidal cells in sector CA2 of schizophrenics and manic depressives. Biol Psychiatry 1998; 44(2):88–97.
279. Rajkowska G. Histopathology of the prefrontal cortex in major depression: what does it tell us about dysfunctional monoaminergic circuits? Prog Brain Res 2000; 126:397–412.
280. Coyle JT, Schwarcz R. Mind glue: implications of glial cell biology for psychiatry. Arch Gen Psychiatry 2000; 57(1):90–93.
281. Haydon PG. GLIA: listening and talking to the synapse. Nat Rev Neurosci 2001; 2(3): 185–193.
282. Rajkowska G, Miguel-Hidalgo JJ, Wei J, Dilley G, Pittman SD, Meltzer HY, Overholser JC, Roth BL, Stockmeier CA. Morphometric evidence for neuronal and glial prefrontal cell pathology in major depression. Biol Psychiatry 1999; 45(9):1085–1098.

283. Rajkowska G. Postmortem studies in mood disorders indicate altered numbers of neurons and glial cells. Biol Psychiatry 2000; 48(8):766–777.
284. Ullian EM, Sapperstein SK, Christopherson KS, Barres BA. Control of synapse number by glia. Science 2001; 291(5504):657–661.
285. Watanabe Y, Gould E, Daniels DC, Cameron H, McEwen BS. Tianeptine attenuates stress-induced morphological changes in the hippocampus. Eur J Pharmacol 1992; 222(1):157–162.
286. Czeh B, Michaelis T, Watanabe T, Frahm J, de Biurrun G, van Kampen M, Bartolomucci A, Fuchs E. Stress-induced changes in cerebral metabolites, hippocampal volume, and cell proliferation are prevented by antidepressant treatment with tianeptine. Proc Natl Acad Sci USA 2001; 98(22):12796–12801.
287. Thome J, Sakai N, Shin K, Steffen C, Zhang YJ, Impey S, Storm D, Duman RS. cAMP response element-mediated gene transcription is upregulated by chronic antidepressant treatment. J Neurosci 2000; 20(11):4030–4036.
288. Malberg JE, Eisch AJ, Nestler EJ, Duman RS. Chronic antidepressant treatment increases neurogenesis in adult rat hippocampus. J Neurosci 2000; 20(24):9104–9110.
289. Siuciak JA, Lewis DR, Wiegand SJ, Lindsay RM. Antidepressant-like effect of brain-derived neurotrophic factor (BDNF). Pharmacol Biochem Behav 1997; 56(1):131–137.
290. Chen AC, Shirayama Y, Shin KH, Neve RL, Duman RS. Expression of the cAMP response element binding protein (CREB) in hippocampus produces an antidepressant effect. Biol Psychiatry 2001; 49(9):753–762.
291. Shirayama Y, Chen AC, Nakagawa S, Russell DS, Duman RS. Brain-derived neurotrophic factor produces antidepressant effects in behavioral models of depression. J Neurosci 2002; 22(8):3251–3261.
292. Yuan PX, Huang LD, Jiang YM, Gutkind JS, Manji HK, Chen G. The mood stabilizer valproic acid activates mitogen-activated protein kinases and promotes neurite growth. J Biol Chem 2001; 276(34):31674–31683.
293. Chen G, Einat H, Yuan P, Manji H. Evidence for the involvement of the MAP/ERK signaling pathway in mood modulation. Biol Psychiatry 2002; 51(8S):126S.
294. Chen G, Zeng WZ, Yuan PX, Huang LD, Jiang YM, Zhao ZH, Manji HK. The mood-stabilizing agents lithium and valproate robustly increase the levels of the neuroprotective protein bcl-2 in the CNS. J Neurochem 1999; 72(2):879–882.
295. Manji HK, Moore GJ, Rajkowska G, Chen G. Neuroplasticity and cellular resilience in mood disorders. Millennium Article. Mol Psychiatry 2000; 5(6):578–593.
296. Chen RW, Chuang DM. Long term lithium treatment suppresses p53 and Bax expression but increases Bcl-2 expression. A prominent role in neuroprotection against excitotoxicity. J Biol Chem 1999; 274(10):6039–6042.
297. Bruno V, Sortino MA, Scapagnini U, Nicoletti F, Canonico PL. Antidegenerative effects of Mg(2+)-valproate in cultured cerebellar neurons. Funct Neurol 1995; 10(3):121–130.
298. Mark RJ, Ashford JW, Goodman Y, Mattson MP. Anticonvulsants attenuate amyloid beta-peptide neurotoxicity, Ca^{2+} deregulation, and cytoskeletal pathology. Neurobiol Aging 1995; 16(2):187–198.
299. Manji HK, Moore GJ, Chen G. Clinical and preclinical evidence for the neurotrophic effects of mood stabilizers: implications for the pathophysiology and treatment of manic-depressive illness. Biol Psychiatry 2000; 48(8):740–754.
300. Hashimoto R, Hough C, Nakazawa T, Yamamoto T, Chuang DM. Lithium protection against glutamate excitotoxicity in rat cerebral cortical neurons: involvement of NMDA receptor inhibition possibly by decreasing NR2B tyrosine phosphorylation. J Neurochem 2002; 80(4):589–597.
301. Bowley MP, Drevets WC, Ongur D, Price JL. Low glial numbers in the amygdala in major depressive disorder. Biol Psychiatry 2002; 52(5):404–412.
302. Moore GJ, Bebchuk JM, Hasanat K, Chen G, Seraji-Bozorgzad N, Wilds IB, Faulk MW, Koch S, Glitz DA, Jolkovsky L, Manji HK. Lithium increases *N*-acetyl-aspartate

in the human brain: in vivo evidence in support of bcl-2's neurotrophic effects? Biol Psychiatry 2000; 48(1):1–8.

303. Moore GJ, Bebchuk JM, Wilds IB, Chen G, Manji HK. Lithium-induced increase in human brain grey matter. Lancet 2000; 356(9237):1241–1242.
304. Sassi R, Nicoletti M, Brambilla P, Mallinger A, Frank E, Kupfer D, Keshavan M, Soares J. Increased gray matter volume in lithium-treated bipolar disorder patients. Neurosci Lett 2002; 329(2):243.
305. Manji, Duman. Impairments of neuroplasticity and cellular resilience in severe mood disorders: implication for the development of novel therapeutics. Psychopharmacol Bull spring 2001; 35(2):5–49.
306. Bouras C, Kovari E, Hof PR, Riederer BM, Giannakopoulos P. Anterior cingulate cortex pathology in schizophrenia and bipolar disorder. Acta Neuropathol (Berl) 2001; 102(4):373–379.
307. Altshuler LL, Casanova MF, Goldberg TE, Kleinman JE. The hippocampus and parahippocampus in schizophrenia, suicide, and control brains. Arch Gen Psychiatry 1990; 47(11):1029–1034.
308. Cotter D, Mackay D, Chana G, Beasley C, Landau S, Everall IP. Reduced neuronal size and glial cell density in area 9 of the dorsolateral prefrontal cortex in subjects with major depressive disorder. Cereb Cortex 2002; 12(4):386–394.
309. Cotter D, Mackay D, Landau S, Kerwin R, Everall I. Reduced glial cell density and neuronal size in the anterior cingulate cortex in major depressive disorder. Arch Gen Psychiatry 2001; 58(6):545–553.
310. Miguel-Hidalgo JJ, Rajkowska G. Morphological brain changes in depression: can antidepressants reverse them? CNS Drugs 2002; 16(6):361–372.
311. Benes FM, Vincent SL, Todtenkopf M. The density of pyramidal and nonpyramidal neurons in anterior cingulate cortex of schizophrenic and bipolar subjects. Biol Psychiatry 2001; 50(6):395–406.
312. Zarate CA, Quiroz JA, Singh JB, Denicoff KD, De Jesus G, Luckenbaugh DA, Charney DS, Manji HK. An open-label trial of the glutamate-modulating agent riluzole in combination with lithium for the treatment of bipolar depression. Biol Psychiatry 2005; 57(4):430–432.

10
Treatment of Mania

John Cookson
The Royal London Hospital, St. Clement's, London, U.K.

BENEFITS OF TREATMENT

Mania is a clearly defined condition that can present in different levels of severity varying from the mild (hypomanic) to the florid, raging, and psychotic. Only the mildest forms can be left untreated without risking harm to either the patient's welfare, relationships, and job, or to the well-being of those who are close to them (relatives, care givers, or staff). Severe forms constitute a psychiatric emergency, demanding immediate control including rapid tranquillization with medication. Treatment lessens the severity and shortens the duration of manic episodes, which in the pretreatment era was usually 3 to 12 months with a mean of 26 weeks. In one modern series, remission from mania occurred in 50% of manic episodes by 12 weeks (1). After the first episode of mania, the mean latency to recovery was 13.7 weeks and the median 5.4 weeks in terms of the DSM-defined syndrome of mania; 97% had recovered within two years, but only 35% had recovered in terms of personal and occupational functioning (2). The mean duration of hospitalization was 28 days.

Mania may immediately be followed by a phase of "post-manic" depression, which may be regarded as part of the same "cycle" of affective illness. Major depression ensued in 16% in one series treated with fluphenazine (3). Cognitive impairment particularly in attention and concentration may persist in some patients even when their mood has apparently recovered (4).

THE NEED FOR ADMISSION

While milder cases may be treated in outpatients or at home, mania requires admission most obviously when associated with aggressive behavior, but also when overspending, grandiosity, sexual indiscretion or substance abuse threatens health or safety.

The loss of insight, grandiosity, and hyperactivity often preclude voluntary admission. Compulsory admission should be considered before the situation deteriorates. When assessing the needs of the patient with mania, it is helpful to remember that the severity of their condition is often greater than it appears at interview with a doctor. Whatever the means of admission, the patient should always be reassured that admission will enable them to rest and have relief, for instance, from their excessive activities and personal conflicts, and from their "overexcitement."

MILIEU MANAGEMENT

The patient should be addressed tactfully, avoiding provocation or pressure. There should be stable external control, and administrative issues should be handled in a firm and nonnegotiable manner. Consistent limits should be set in order to prevent behavior that is dangerous or disruptive to the patient or others. All the staff should be consistent in this. The patient will often require either individual attention or nursing in a (locked) psychiatric intensive care setting to prevent them leaving the ward. The emphasis should be on calming the patient. Restrictions on visiting and time spent alone can help to reduce stimulation. When speaking with the patient, the voice should be lowered with slightly slower cadence than usual. Argument about the content of delusions should be avoided, although once responding to drug treatment, cognitive therapy challenging abnormal ideas may assist recovery.

A structured timetable may be helpful, and writing or coloring materials should be available if the patient can concentrate sufficiently to use them. Other reality-based diversionary activities should be provided.

Specific issues to be addressed are the alienation of family members, the progressive testing of limits by the patient, the overinvolvement with other patients and the tendency to dominate the ward. In 1974, Janowsky et al. (5) described these tendencies as "the manic game" and implied that the manic patient demands care without having to admit their need for it. Staff need to understand these maneuvers in order to avoid becoming too personally involved, for instance, in angry exchanges. Community meetings are helpful as they allow the responses of other patients to the manic person's behavior to be recognized and guided.

As the patient's condition improves, individual work should be aimed at identifying factors that may have contributed to the present episode, and helping the patient to tolerate feelings of depression or distress that may emerge. They may need help to reestablish personal and occupational relationships. Empathic meetings between a member of the ward team and relatives can prepare them to understand explanations that the patient's condition is a treatable illness that, in the longer term, needs their support and may benefit from prophylactic medication.

DRUG TREATMENT OF MANIA

When assessing the patient, enquiries should be made about their recent compliance with medication, as sudden discontinuation of lithium may have triggered the manic episode. It is usually prudent to cease any antidepressant medication they may have been taking.

A physical examination and tests of the blood and urine should, if possible, precede drug treatment or take place soon after the patient is sedated, in order to elucidate any physical illness, especially infection, and any causes of secondary mania (e.g., drugs), and to determine baseline renal, hepatic, and thyroid function. An ECG should be performed if high doses of medication are to be used.

Acute Tranquillization

Treatment of the severe and agitated patient begins with control by "acute" or "rapid" tranquillization. This requires an antipsychotic such as haloperidol (5–10 mg IM) or olanzapine (5–10 mg IM), either of which may be given intramuscularly, often in combination with a benzodiazepine such as lorazepam (1–2 mg IM). The more disturbed patient may be given an antipsychotic intramuscularly at hourly intervals three times, with additional benzodiazepines until they are calm. Larger single intramuscular doses are discouraged because they are excessive in some patients and because their effect may last for several days, obscuring the diagnosis, and making further management difficult; the patient may no longer appear very disturbed but is likely to deteriorate unless treatment is continued. Large doses of antipsychotic drugs have been associated with sudden deaths in disturbed young patients, probably through cardiac dysrhythmias. Formulary guidelines on doses of antipsychotics should not be exceeded without special precautions, including checking ECG and blood electrolytes; additional benzodiazepines should be used in preference. A comparative trial of intramuscular olanzapine (10 mg) vs. lorazepam (2 mg) found olanzapine more effective in reducing symptoms of agitation (6) in mania within 2 hour.

Once calmed the patient with mania then requires treatment over a period of 2 to 4 weeks to achieve further gradual improvement.

Treating Mania: Recommendations of Guidelines

Mania is one of the most insightless forms of mental disorder, and for treatment to be very useful it must be not only effective but also acceptable to the patient, easy to use, and not produce unpleasant side effects. Numerous guidelines exist for the management of bipolar disorder, perhaps reflecting the uncertainty that has prevailed about the efficacy and side effects of treatments (Table 1). There is now a convergence of views about the treatment of mania between North American (7,8), British (9), European (10), and Australasian guidelines (11). These now recommend that severe mania should be treated with an antipsychotic with or without lithium or valproate. Some include starting with valproate alone, using high doses (20–30 mg/kg) (12). Less severe mania should usually be treated initially with monotherapy with either an antipsychotic, preferably an atypical, or valproate or lithium; carbamazepine is an alternative.

Table 1 International Guidelines for Treatment of Mania

APA, 1994 (7)	"Mood Stabilizer" (lithium, valproate, or carbamazepine): antipsychotic or benzodiazepine only as "adjunct" for psychosis, agitation, and violence
APA, 2002 (8)	Severe mania: combination of lithium or valproate *plus* antipsychotic Mild mania: lithium or valproate *or* atypical antipsychotic
BAP (9)	Psychotic mania: antipsychotic (preferably atypical) Severe mania: antipsychotic (preferably atypical) *or* valproate Less ill: lithium, valproate, or carbamazepine
WFSBP (10)	Lithium or valproate or atypical antipsychotic with or without benzodiazepine or low potency classical antipsychotic
Aus-NZ (11)	"Mood stabilizer" (lithium, valproate, carbamazepine, or olanzapine) plus antipsychotic or benzodiazepine (or their combination)

Table 2 Consensus of Guidelines for Treatment of Mania

Severe mania	Antipsychotic preferably atypical, with or without valproate, lithium or carbamazepine
Mild mania	Antipsychotic, preferably atypical or lithium or valproate

The major change that has occurred since 1994 is that antipsychotics are no longer regarded as useful only for sedation or for psychosis but as being also antimanic. There has also been more reluctance to use the term "mood stabilizer" without specifying the drugs concerned. The notable remaining difference is that the revised American Guidelines of 2002 (8) favor starting with the combination of an antipsychotic with valproate or lithium, whereas other guidelines include options for monotherapy at the start. The consensus emerging from these official guidelines is summarized in Table 2.

Antipsychotic Drugs

Surveys of clinical practice have shown that antipsychotics are the most commonly used drugs in patients hospitalized with mania, whether in Britain, Scandinavia, other parts of Europe, or North America.

Classical Antipsychotic Drugs

Moderate or severe mania is usually most rapidly controlled by antipsychotic drugs. Phenothiazines (e.g., chlorpromazine) and thioxanthines (e.g., zuclopenthixol) are effective but the butyrophenone, haloperidol, is often particularly useful in a dose of 5–10 mg up to three times a day with an anticholinergic drug (to reduce extrapyramidal side effects). Haloperidol tends to produce initial sedation, which wears off after a day or so during continued treatment (13). If the patient remains very behaviorally disturbed, chlorpromazine may be more useful because, having antihistaminic properties, it is more sedative than haloperidol. However, many manic patients resent being made to feel drowsy and this limits the dose of chlorpromazine that they will accept. Chlorpromazine is hypotensive and should be used cautiously in the elderly.

Extrapyramidal side effects seem less of a problem with larger doses of haloperidol, but may emerge as the dose is reduced or a few days after it is discontinued. Anti-Parkinsonian medication should, therefore, be continued for up to 7 days after haloperidol is stopped.

Rapid improvement in mania occurs for 1 to 3 days after antipsychotic medication is commenced; the manic state tends then to improve more gradually over the next 2 weeks. There is no clear evidence that increasing the dose of haloperidol above 30 mg/day achieves greater improvement.

For manic patients whose failure to improve is due to poor compliance, depot antipsychotic medication including haloperidol or zuclopenthixol decanoates can be used. Zuclopenthixol acetate is a depot formulation, which has a duration of action of up to 3 days, and a more rapid onset of action than the decanoates; it is useful in disturbed patients who persistently refuse oral medication during the first few days of treatment.

Classical antipsychotics produce unpleasant extrapyramidal side effects such as akathisia, dystonia, and Parkinsonism that (although partially preventable by anticholinergic medication) are resented by patients and that limit their adherence to treatment. It is therefore very important to know whether the use of antipsychotics in mania is justified by evidence of efficacy and whether newer antipsychotics with fewer unpleasant acute side effects (atypical antipsychotics) are also effective in mania.

Atypical Antipsychotics

Atypical antipsychotics with proven efficacy in mania include olanzapine (15–20 mg/day), risperidone (up to 6 mg/day), quetiapine (600 mg/day), aripiprazole, and ziprasidone. Sulpiride and amisulpride are also used. Mild mania may be treated with atypical antipsychotic drugs or an older drug such as haloperidol 5–10 mg daily; valproate is an alternative. Lithium treatment may also be useful, but improvement takes up to 2 weeks to become apparent.

Assessing the Evidence

To prove that a drug is efficacious in a psychiatric condition, it is essential to show that it is superior to placebo, by conducting randomized double-blind placebo-controlled trials. The challenges of conducting such trials in mania have only been met in recent years, in the course of developing novel anticonvulsant and atypical antipsychotic treatments. These recent trials are therefore providing answers to questions that have long remained unresolved about the treatment of mania. Analysis of the results of these trials requires attention not only to the statistical significance of differences in special rating scales, but also to the size of the effect, and to the generalizability of results, which have been derived from highly selected patients in clinical trial centers, to other groups of patients with mania in routine practice. It is also important to consider how dropouts from the studies may have biased the interpretation of results.

High placebo response rates (with the exception of the Pope et al. study—Ref. 14) show how vital placebo-controlled studies are in identifying a drug's efficacy in a way that limits any potential bias. Table 3 lists the drugs that have been proved superior to placebo as monotherapy in such trials. To receive a license to market a drug for mania, most authorities, including the European Medicines Agency, require two trials performed at independent centers.

Table 3 Drugs Shown to be Superior to Placebo as Monotherapy in Mania in RCTs

Drug	Number of trials
Valproate	2
Lithium	4
Haloperidol	2
Olanzapine	2
Risperidone	3
Quetiapine	2
Ziprasidone	2
Aripiprazole	2
Carbamazepine	2

Lithium, Valproate, or Antipsychotics for Mania

The first drug to be proved efficacious in such trials was valproate (14,15). Although Table 3 shows that the drug with most trials (not all published) proving efficacy is lithium, this drug is not usually sufficiently rapid in onset to be useful as monotherapy (15). Although haloperidol has been the favorite drug of clinicians for treating mania (16,17), it is only in the course of comparative trials with risperidone (18) and quetiapine (19), that haloperidol has been proved conclusively to be efficacious. Most evidence for efficacy in mania now concerns the atypical antipsychotics, olanzapine, risperidone, quetiapine, ziprasidone, and aripiprazole. Questions arise about the relative efficacy of these atypical antipsychotics compared either with haloperidol or with valproate, and whether they should be used initially as monotherapy or combined with valproate or lithium. Also, since treatment often needs to commence with rapid tranquillization, and only two atypicals can be given intramuscularly (recently olanzapine and in some countries ziprasidone), haloperidol remains widely used despite its propensity to cause unpleasant extrapyramidal side effects.

Placebo-Controlled RCTs of Atypical Antipsychotics

The published trials (some as yet presented only in Posters at meetings) are summarized in Table 4, using a "Number-Needed-to-Treat" (NNT) analysis. NNT is calculated by dividing the difference in response rate between active drug and placebo into 100 and correcting to the next highest integer. It represents the number of patients who must be treated in order for one patient to achieve the defined response—usually a 50% reduction in score on a scale such as the 11-item Young Mania Rating Scale (YMRS)—as a result of the pharmacological effect of the drug. NNT thus provides a measure of the size of effect that can be expected of the drug in a clinical situation. For a drug to be useful monotherapy as a first-line treatment in a common and severe disorder such as mania, the NNT for 50% improvement in severity should be in the order of 2–4 (20).

Most studies were of 3 or 4 weeks duration and there was a placebo response rate of 19–43%, reflecting the effects of a variety of possible non-specific factors such as hospitalization, extra medication with benzodiazepines or chloral allowed during the first 10 days, and bias in the raters. Dropout rates for inefficacy ranged from 10% to 69% on placebo, and from 7% to 47% on active drug. Dropouts through adverse events (including suspected side effects) ranged from 1.5% to 10% on placebo, and from 0% to 11% on atypical antipsychotic; on haloperidol dropouts through lack of efficacy were 7% and 35% and through adverse events 3% and 10%. Total dropout rates ranged from 15% to 79% on placebo, from 11% to 58% on atypical antipsychotic, and were 10% and 45% on haloperidol and 32% on lithium.

Olanzapine. Olanzapine was the first of the atypical antipsychotics to be proved efficacious in mania in trials designed by Tohen et al. (21,22). Patients entering the studies had mean mania scores of 29 on the YMRS (maximum possible score 46). Patients with mixed mania could also be included. The starting doses in the two studies were 10 and 15 mg, and the mean modal doses were 14.9 and 16.4 mg/day. The commonest side effects were somnolence (22% more than placebo), dry mouth (15% more), dizziness (12% more), weakness (9% more), and weight gain.

Risperidone. In the trial of Hirschfeld et al. (23), risperidone was increased gradually over 4 days to a maximum of 6 mg/day. The NNT was 6 (95% confidence interval 4–13). Side effects on risperidone were somnolence (28% vs. 7% on placebo), hyperkinesias (Parkinsonism) in 16% vs. 5%.

Table 4 Monotherapy with Atypical Antipsychotics in Mania: Placebo-Controlled Parallel-Group Randomized Trials

Drug	Average dose/day (mg/day)	Numbers (N)	Duration (weeks)	Authors	Criterion of improvement	Dropouts (%)	Response (%)	Difference from placebo	Number needed to treat
Olanzapine	14.9	70	3	Tohen et al. (21)	50% reduction, YMRS	29	49	25	4 (3–10)
Placebo		64				51	24		
Olanzapine	16.4	55	4	Tohen et al. (22)	50% reduction, YMRS	38	65	22	5 (3–23)
Placebo		60				58	43		
Risperidone	4.1	134	3	Hirschfeld et. al. (23)	50% reduction, YMRS	44	43	19	6 (4–13)
Placebo		125				58	24		
Risperidone	5.6	146	3	Khanna et al. (24)	50% reduction, YMRS	11	73	37	3 (2–4)
Placebo		144				29	36		
Risperidone	4.2	154	3	Eerdekens et al. (18)	50% reduction YMRS	11	48	15	7 (4–26)
Placebo		140				15	33		
Haloperidol	8	144				10	47	14	8 (4–36)
Quetiapine	560	102	3 (extended to 12 weeks)	Brecher et al. (19)	50% reduction, YMRS	46	3/52: 42; 12/52: 60	3/52: 7; 12/52: 21	3/52: NSD (–16 to +5); 12/52: 5 (3–14)
Placebo		101				58	3/52: 35; 12/52: 39	3/52: 20; 12/52: 31	3/52: 5 (3–16); 12/52: 4 (3–6)
Haloperidol	5.2	99				45	3/52: 55; 12/52: 70		

(Continued)

Table 4 Monotherapy with Atypical Antipsychotics in Mania: Placebo-Controlled Parallel-Group Randomized Trials (*Continued*)

Drug	Average dose/day (mg/day)	Numbers (*N*)	Duration (weeks)	Authors	Criterion of improvement	Dropouts (%)	Response (%)	Difference from placebo	Number needed to treat
Quetiapine	586	107	3 (extended to 12 weeks)	Paulsson et al. (25)	50% reduction, YMRS	33	53.3	25.9	4 (3–8)
Placebo		95				64	27.4	25.9	4 (3–8)
Lithium		98				32	53.3		
Aripiprazole	27.9	125	3	Keck et al. (26)	50% reduction, YMRS	58	40	21	5 (4–10)
Placebo		123				79	19		
Ziprasidone	80–160	131	3	Keck et al. (27)	50% reduction, MRS	46	50	15	6 (4–152)
Placebo		66				56	35		
Ziprasidone	80–160	139		Segal et al. (28)	50% reduction, MRS	39	46	16.8	6 (4–33)
Placebo		66				46	29.2		

The study by Khanna et al. (24), conducted in India, was distinguished by relatively high YMRS scores on entry (about 10 points higher than in most other studies of atypical antipsychotics in mania), and by a high rate of study completion on risperidone with low dropout rates particularly for lack of efficacy. The mean modal dose in this study was higher (5.4 mg/day). The rate of response on risperidone was highest in this study and the NNT was impressively low at 3 (95% confidence interval 2–4). Extrapyramidal side effects occurred in 35% of those on risperidone, and 6% on placebo.

The study by Eerdekens et al. (18) had a slower dosing schedule reaching a maximum of 6 mg/day by day 5. This study also had a haloperidol comparator group with a mean modal dose of 8 mg/day (see below). Both active drugs were effective compared with placebo from day 7. By day 21, the NNT for 50% improvement was 7 (95% confidence interval 4–26) for risperidone and similar for haloperidol at 8 (95% confidence interval 4–36). Side effects on risperidone included extrapyramidal symptoms (17% compared with 40% on haloperidol).

In the studies of Khanna et al. (24) and of Eerdekens et al. (18), the improvement on active treatments was continuing to develop during the third week of treatment; the extension to 12 weeks in the Eerdekens study demonstrated further improvement in YMRS scores with active treatment up to 12 weeks, suggesting that the dose initially administered may not have been sufficient to achieve maximum improvement. On the other hand, in the study of Hirschfeld et al. (23), the improvement appeared to be complete within 2 to 3 weeks.

Risperidone had been described as worsening or precipitating mania in predisposed patients, mainly those with schizophrenia, schizoaffective disorder, or organic brain disease (29). No evidence of such exacerbation of mania was found in these placebo-controlled trials of risperidone.

Quetiapine. The two trials of monotherapy enrolled patients with relatively high scores on the YMRS (average 33 points); patients with mixed mania were excluded. Significant efficacy at 3 weeks was observed in one study and in the combined analysis. In the 12-week extension, both trials showed significant efficacy but the dropout rate on placebo was very high. Patients who responded to quetiapine were usually receiving 600 mg/day or more. The dose was increased toward this amount over 5 days and then to a maximum of 800 mg/day. The commonest side effects were somnolence, dry mouth, weight gain, and dizziness.

Ziprasidone and Aripiprazole. The results of trials of these drugs are also shown in Table 4. In common with most of the other trials, these had high dropout rates on placebo. The dropout rate on aripiprazole was somewhat higher than on other drugs. Number needed to treat was slightly higher with ziprasidone.

Placebo-Controlled Monotherapy Trials of Haloperidol in Mania

Two monotherapy studies have included haloperidol as an active comparator, the risperidone study of Eerdekens et al. (18), and the quetiapine study of Brecher et al. (19) (see Table 4).

In the study of Eerdekens et al (18), the haloperidol dose started at 4 mg/day and was adjusted to 2–12 mg/day by day 5. The timecourse of improvement was similar to that with risperidone, and by day 21, the NNT for 50% improvement was 8 (95% confidence interval 4–36). This is far larger than one would expect with the most commonly used antimanic drug of the previous decade; this might be either because the mean modal dose of haloperidol was only 8 mg/day, or because the patients in the trial were in some ways not typical of routine clinic patients and were more resistant to treatment.

A comparator group on haloperidol (up to 8 mg/day) was also included in the study by Brecher et al. (19) of quetiapine (up to 800 mg/day) and placebo, analyzed at 3 and 12 weeks. At 3 weeks, the response rate (50% reduction in YMRS score) on haloperidol, on a mean dose of only 5.2 mg/day, was 55% compared with 35% on placebo, giving an NNT of 5 (95% confidence interval 3–16). There were more dropouts on placebo than on haloperidol or quetiapine, so that the analysis using last observations carried forward was biased in favor of the active drugs, and especially so after 3 weeks when more patients on placebo or haloperidol than on quetiapine dropped out. By 12 weeks, the response rate on haloperidol was 70% and on placebo 39%, giving an NNT of 4 (3–6). Side effects in the form of extrapyramidal symptoms were much more common on haloperidol (59.6%) than on placebo (15.8%), as was akathisia (33.3% on haloperidol and 5.9% on placebo). Somnolence occurred more often with haloperidol (9.1%) than placebo (5%).

Patterns of Symptom Improvement: Sedative, Antipsychotic, or Antimanic?

It had been suggested that antipsychotics owe their effects in mania either to non-specific sedation (that is making the person drowsy or asleep), or to combating psychotic symptoms. However, this view fails to recognize that non-sedative dopamine-blocking drugs can improve mania (30). In all studies of olanzapine and risperidone and in the combined analysis of quetiapine studies, the improvement in mania occurred in patients with or without psychotic symptoms. When individual items of the mania rating scale were analyzed, drug treatment (with olanzapine, quetiapine, and probably the other atypicals) improved the whole range of symptoms (including elation, flight of ideas, grandiosity, sexual interest, irritability, aggression, and general appearance, as well as the items most sensitive to sedation: insomnia, overactivity, and pressure of speech).

These findings lead to the inevitable conclusion that the drugs are not just antipsychotic, and in some cases, sedative, but antimanic.

Depression in Mania

Depressive symptoms are very common during mania, and if amounting to a major depressive syndrome, the condition is classified as mixed mania according to DSM-IV. However, at least 12 forms of bipolar mixed states have been described and are likely to respond differently to treatments (31).

It has been suggested, but never proved, that classical antipsychotics may worsen or induce depression, apart from their obvious extrapyramidal side effects. In the trials of atypical antipsychotics, the changes in symptoms of depression have usually been monitored. Three drugs have been demonstrated to improve depressive symptoms alongside the improvement in mania; these are olanzapine, risperidone, and aripiprazole. Olanzapine improved depression scores more than placebo (21,22). In the study of Khanna et al. (24), depression scores were already low at the start, but improved further, the change being greater on risperidone than placebo even by day 3. In the study of Eerdekens et al. (18), MADRS depression scores, low at the start, fell more on risperidone than on placebo from week 1, and on haloperidol only at week 2.

In the study by Brecher et al. (19), depression scores (MADRS) improved by day 21 on both quetiapine and haloperidol, more than on placebo. In trials that permitted inclusion of mixed mania, it has been shown that this improves with treatment in the case of olanzapine (32).

Comparative RCTs of Antipsychotics in Mania Without Placebo

In a comparative trial in mania, in which additional lorazepam was permitted, risperidone showed similar efficacy to haloperidol or lithium (28).

In the largest randomized comparative study of haloperidol (33), it was compared with olanzapine over 6 and 12 weeks. Among patients on haloperidol (up to 15 mg/day, mean modal dose at sixth week 7 mg/day), the proportion responding (50% reduction in YMRS score) at 6 weeks was 74%; the proportion showing syndromal remission (according to DSM-IV) was 44%, a figure similar to that found in consecutive admissions for mania by Rifkin et al. (34). Improvement in mania scores (YMRS) was greater for haloperidol than for olanzapine at 6 weeks, but not different at 12 weeks. In patients with low levels of depressive symptoms at commencement on haloperidol, a total of 16.8% switched into depression within 12 weeks. However, as there was no placebo group, it is not known whether this represents the natural history of the patients' mood cycles, perhaps accelerated by effective treatment of mania, or some additional depressant effect of haloperidol. The switch rate among patients on olanzapine was lower at 6 weeks, but at 12 weeks, the difference was not significant.

In the study by Brecher et al. (19), the switch rates into depression over 12 weeks were similar for haloperidol (8.1%) and placebo (8.9%), and tended to be lower for quetiapine (2.9%).

Thus, both olanzapine and quetiapine show trends to produce a lower switch rate into depression than haloperidol. However, both drugs (in the doses used) seemed also to lead to slower improvement in mania than haloperidol.

Extrapyramidal symptoms occur to a much less extent with olanzapine or quetiapine than with haloperidol. In the largest comparative trial (33), treatment-emergent akathisia was observed in 40% on haloperidol and 10% on olanzapine, dystonia in 6.8% and 1.3%, and Parkinsonism in 54% and 13%, respectively.

Trials of Atypical Antipsychotic Vs. Valproate in Mania

A study comparing oral haloperidol (0.2 mg/kg/day) with high initial doses of valproate semisodium (20 mg/kg/day) in psychotic mania found similar timecourse of improvement with both the drugs (12). However, this finding may not be generalizable, as the response to haloperidol was unusually slow. There have been two studies comparing olanzapine with valproate (as valproate semisodium or divalproex) in mania (35,36). Sponsored by the two different pharmaceutical companies, and using slightly different dose regimes, they show consistent results. Both drugs appear effective improving mania. The improvement was slightly faster and slightly greater with olanzapine (average doses 17.4 and 14.7 mg/day) than with valproate (1401 and 2115 mg/day). Insomnia, overactivity, and flight of ideas improved significantly more with olanzapine in one study. Interestingly, this superiority of olanzapine over valproate was seen only in the non-psychotic group of manic patients (35). The drugs seemed equally effective in psychotic mania, as they did in mixed mania.

Apart from speed of action, which is greater with antipsychotics, there are differences in side effects. Olanzapine produced more somnolence (39% vs. 21% and 47% vs. 29%), dry mouth (34% vs. 6%), running nose (14% and 3%), edema (14% and 0%), increased appetite (12% vs. 2%), and weight gain, whereas valproate produced more gastrointestinal disturbance with nausea (29% vs. 10%). Other side effects of valproate and olanzapine occur but are too rare to have been detected in these trials.

Carbamazepine or Valproate in Mania

The first parallel-group placebo-controlled trial of carbamazepine was recently published (37); the earlier widespread use of carbamazepine was based on evidence from crossover studies and other trial designs. Valproate is effective in a proportion of manic patients including non-responders to antipsychotic drugs and lithium. Patients who respond to valproate do not necessarily respond to carbamazepine and vice versa. In the first large parallel-group placebo-controlled study (which included only patients who were unresponsive to or intolerant of lithium), 59% of patients on valproate improved compared to only 16% of those on placebo (14). Most of the improvement occurred within 1 to 4 days of achieving therapeutic levels.

A second and larger study comparing divalproex to lithium or placebo in a 3-week parallel-group double-blind study (15) is shown in Table 5. Half of the patients had been unresponsive to lithium previously. Valproate was as effective in rapid-cycling mania as in other manic patients, and equally effective in the patients previously judged responders or non-responders to lithium. However, few patients in the study returned to normal functioning within 3 weeks.

Mechanisms of Antimanic Actions of Drugs

It is thought that antipsychotics owe their antimanic effects mainly to blockade of receptors for dopamine, but additionally to some extent to blockade of noradrenaline at alpha-1 receptors (as in the case of haloperidol), and blockade of histamine at H-1 receptors (causing sedation as in the case of chlorpromazine) (17,38). Some atypical antipsychotics share all these actions as well as being potent blockers of serotonin receptors (e.g., olanzapine, quetiapine, and risperidone), but are selective for subtypes of dopamine receptors, and others block only subtypes of dopamine receptors (amisulpride). It cannot be assumed that drugs effective in schizophrenia will be effective in mania or vice versa.

Lithium reduces presynaptic release of dopamine transmission, as well as blocking D-1 receptors. Valproate too is thought to reduce dopamine turnover, perhaps by increasing the function of the inhibitory transmitter gamma-amino-butyric acid (GABA). An antikindling effect may underlie some of the actions of carbamazepine, but the pharmacological mechanism of action in mania is unclear. Thus, dopamine function is reduced through different mechanisms by antipsychotics and by lithium or valproate. It is therefore reasonable to assume that combinations of these drugs may have additive benefits to improve mania.

Monotherapy or Combination Treatment

Antipsychotic-Resistant Mania

A proportion of manic patients show only partial improvement or initial improvement followed by partial relapse with antipsychotic drugs. There is little evidence that increasing the dose will produce further improvement. Clozapine may prove to be useful in resistant mania as in resistant schizophrenia (39). However, at the present time, the main alternatives or adjuncts to the antipsychotic drugs are lithium and the anticonvulsants, valproate, and carbamazepine.

Current American guidelines (8) recommend a combination of lithium or valproate with an antipsychotic as the first-line treatment for "severe" mania, but a choice between lithium, valproate, and an atypical antipsychotic for "mild" mania.

Table 5 Placebo-Controlled Trials of Lithium, Valproate, and Carbamazepine: Dropout Rates and NNTs

Treatment	Average dose/day (mg/day)	Numbers (*N*)	Duration (weeks)	Authors	Criterion of improvement	Dropouts (%)	Response (%)	Difference from placebo	Number needed to treat
Divalproex		20	3	Pope et al. (14)	50% reduction MRS	41	45	36	3 (2–9)
Placebo		23				74	9		
Divalproex		63	3	Bowden et al. (15)	50% reduction SADS-M	36	48	23	5 (3–14)
Placebo		73				54	25	24	5 (3–22)
Lithium		35				44	49		
Carbamazepine, extended release	952	101	3	Weisler et al. (37)	50% reduction YMRS	52.9	41.5	19.1	5 (4–16)
Placebo		103					22.4		

Abbreviation: SADS-M, schizophrenia and affective disorders scale mania component.

It is noteworthy that no definition of severe mania is offered. Other guidelines, including the British (9), recommend a choice of either an antipsychotic or valproate for severe mania, an antipsychotic for psychotic mania, and for the "less ill" either lithium, valproate, or carbamazepine.

Clinical Trial Evidence for Combination Treatment

Evidence concerning the efficacy of combination treatment is complex. Although several studies have demonstrated an advantage of combining an antipsychotic with lithium or valproate over lithium or valproate alone, only one study has investigated the advantage of the combination over antipsychotic alone (40).

The majority of these studies involved a design in which patients, who had not responded to one drug administered for at least three weeks, had additional treatment with the combination of drugs using a placebo control for the added drug. In some studies, a proportion of patients commenced on the combination without previous treatment, and the control group received only the lithium, valproate, or carbamazepine with placebo instead of antipsychotic. Thus, there have been no studies of combination treatment in which a control group receives only placebo. It is therefore not possible to determine directly the size of effect of giving combination treatment to drug-free patients with mania over giving placebo alone, or to determine the size of advantage of combination therapy over monotherapy initiated in drug-free patients with mania.

The studies of combination treatment shown in Table 6 have proved that several antipsychotics provided additional efficacy when added to lithium or valproate compared with lithium or valproate alone. These are: haloperidol, risperidone, olanzapine, and quetiapine. A similar study with ziprasidone was negative.

Risperidone in combination with lithium or valproate was shown to be more effective than either lithium or valproate alone (41,42) and as efficacious as haloperidol in combination with either lithium or valproate (41), in patients with manic or mixed episodes. In combination with carbamazepine, risperidone did not provide significant additional efficacy perhaps because risperidone blood levels were reduced by about 50% in patients on carbamazepine (42). This was presumably because of its induction of liver enzymes that metabolize drugs. The advantage of risperidone over placebo was far more evident in those who had already been on a mood stabilizer for at least 2 weeks before randomization, than in those who started mood stabilizer shortly before starting risperidone or placebo. Response to risperidone was independent of the presence or absence of psychotic symptoms (42).

In the study of Sachs et al. (41), 63% of patients had already received lithium or valproate before randomization to risperidone or placebo, and might therefore be considered non-responders to the mood stabilizer; the rest commenced on lithium or valproate at the same time as being randomized to start on risperidone or placebo. The benefit of additional antipsychotic medication was much less apparent in the latter group. Significant improvement in response to either risperidone or haloperidol was limited to patients with pure mania and was not evident in those with mixed manic states, who comprised 21% of patients.

In combination studies with olanzapine, this drug was shown to provide additional efficacy when added in patients who had already received lithium or valproate for at least three weeks (43). The effect was statistically significant in the subgroup on valproate but only a trend in the smaller subgroup on lithium.

Conversely, the addition of valproate to classical antipsychotics (mainly haloperidol) has been shown to produce greater improvement than addition of placebo (40).

Table 6 Studies of Combination of Antipsychotic with Lithium, Valproate, or Carbamazepine

Authors	Treatment	Duration (weeks)	Extra drugs	Treatments	Mean modal dose (mg/day)	Numbers (*N*)	Inclusion criteria, criterion of response	Dropouts (%)	Response (%)	Difference from placebo (%)	Number needed to treat (95% (I)
Yatham et al. (42)	Combination with lithium, valproate, or carbamazepine	3	Benzodiazepines, LZP 4 mg/day for 7 days	Risperidone	4.0	69	Manic or mixed YMRS ≥ 20	36	59	18	6 (3–56)
				Placebo		73	50% less, Y-MRS	52	41		
Sachs et al. (41)	Combination with lithium or valproate	3	Benzodiazepines for sleep, LZP 4 mg/day for 7 days	Haloperidol	6.2	53	Manic or mixed YMRS ≥ 20,	53	50	20	5 (3–64)
				Placebo		51	CGI much or very much improved	49	30	23	5 (3–23)
				Risperidone	3.8	52		35	53		
Muller-Oerling-hausen et al. (40)	Combination with antipsychotics	3		Valproate		69	50% less, Y-MRS	10	70	24	5 (3–13)
				Placebo		67		16	46		
Tohen et al. (43)	Combination with lithium or valproate	6		Olanzapine		229	50% less, Y-MRS	32	68	23	5 (3–9)
				Placebo		115		31	45		
Sachs et al. (44)	Combination with lithium or valproate	3		Quetiapine		81	50% less, Y-MRS	38.5	54.3	21.7	5 (3–15)
				Placebo		89		51	32.6		
DelBello et al. (45)	Combination with lithium or valproate in adolescents	6		Quetiapine		15	50% less, Y-MRS	47	87	34	3 (2–29)
				Placebo		15		7	53		

Side Effects with Combinations of Lithium and Antipsychotics

Lithium can increase extrapyramidal (Parkinsonian) side effects in patients on antipsychotic drugs (46), and can itself produce cog-wheel rigidity in a small minority of patients (47). In contrast to antipsychotic-induced Parkinsonism, this does not improve with anticholinergic drugs. Cerebellar tremor and incoordination are signs of lithium toxicity, as are more severe forms of fine tremor and Parkinsonism.

Combinations of high levels of lithium with high doses of antipsychotics including haloperidol have been associated with severe neurological symptoms, hyperthermia, impaired consciousness, and irreversible brain damage (48,49). The conditions reported resemble both lithium toxicity and neuroleptic malignant syndrome. Antipsychotic drugs can increase intracellular lithium levels suggesting a possible mechanism for this interaction (50). Subsequent series have demonstrated the safety of combining haloperidol (up to 30 mg/day) with lithium at levels of up to 1 meq/L (51).

In practice, when combining lithium with antipsychotics, the blood levels should generally be maintained below 1 meq/L, staff should be advised to observe and report the development of neurological symptoms, and lithium should be temporarily discontinued if they develop. The combination of antipsychotics and lithium in bipolar patients can also lead to troublesome somnambulism requiring dosage reduction.

Many patients who fail to improve when taking carbamazepine alone do so when lithium is added (52). This combination may—as with antipsychotics—increase the risk of lithium neurotoxicity (53).

ECT in Mania

The earlier reports of the use of ECT in mania showed that about two-thirds of the patients responded. More recently, in a retrospective study, 78% of patients treated with ECT had shown marked improvement compared to 62% on lithium (54). In a double-blind trial, ECT was superior to lithium during the first 8 weeks especially for severe mania and for mixed states (55). In some countries, clinicians reserve ECT for only the most severe and drug-resistant manic patients, whereas in other countries it is regarded as generally helpful in mania and used often.

The use of lithium during ECT is discussed above; neurotoxic complications have been reported. The use of ECT for patients on lithium has been associated with acute organic brain syndrome or prolonged confusional states, but a small retrospective case–control study did not find a higher frequency of adverse effects of ECT in patients on lithium (56).

In the United States, lithium is generally withheld prior to electroconvulsive therapy to reduce the risk of arrhythmia. The ECT Handbook (57) advises stopping lithium 36 to 48 hours before ECT and holding it until after the final ECT treatment, to avoid delirium or prolonged seizures. Many clinicians withhold solely the dose of lithium immediately proceeding an ECT session, and some simply continue routine lithium dosing.

TREATING SUBTYPES OF MANIA

Mania with Psychotic Features

Earlier guidelines regard psychotic features as being an indication for us of "neuroleptic" or antipsychotic drugs. However, psychosis has not been identified as a predictor of differential response to any of the treatments. Rather, psychosis is often an indicator of severity of mania, and antipsychotics are recommended particularly for their ability to control severe mania rapidly.

Treatment of Mixed Mania

The description "mixed state" has been used in more than a dozen ways, each of which carries different implications about treatment (58).

Studies of the atypical antipsychotics olanzapine (59), risperidone, and aripiprazole showed that in patients with coexisting depressive symptoms, these improved as the manic state did.

Lithium is less favored than valproate, and atypical antipsychotic drugs are recommended in preference to older drugs. Some guidelines caution that typical antipsychotics may worsen depression, although evidence for this is rarely cited. Carbamazepine has been recommended for dysphoric mania, a form of mixed state (60,61). ECT is recommended in some, as is clozapine for refractory patients.

Treatment of Mania with Rapid Cycling

Most authorities emphasize the importance of discontinuing antidepressants particularly tricyclic drugs and drugs of abuse, and of checking thyroid function. There is agreement that such patients can be refractory to treatment, particularly with lithium. Depot formulations of classical antipsychotics have been used and recently atypical antipsychotics are suggested, although some believe that combinations of "mood stabilizers" may also be required.

In studies of olanzapine mania improved to a similar extent in those with rapid cycling. There is no mention of rapid cycling in any of the placebo-controlled studies of risperidone. However, open studies suggest risperidone may be of benefit, usually as augmentation to lithium or valproate (see Chapter 20).

Management on Recovery from Mania

Although lack of insight is characteristic of mania and is often the last symptom to improve, on recovery from an episode of mania, most people will have begun to acknowledge that they have been ill. A therapeutic alliance between the patient and the treatment team should be developing. At this time, efforts should be made to improve their understanding of their condition, by means of psychoeducation about bipolar illness and about treatments available. They should be encouraged to recognize the early features of mania (such as racing thoughts, insomnia, irritability, or comments from others about their mood). They should have a plan of what steps to take in the event of a recurrence of such symptoms. In particular, they should have access to antipsychotic medication, which they might usefully take in order to avert the development of another manic episode. The possibility of prophylactic treatment should also be discussed, including lithium. This approach can increased the time to first manic recurrence and improve social functioning and employment (62).

CONCLUSION

Mania can affect people of all social and occupational groups and is usually a phase in a recurring bipolar illness. Manic episodes are very disruptive to family life and employment, and there is a high rate of divorce and successful suicide in bipolar patients. Treatment will often minimize or allow such disruptions to be avoided, and reduce the suicide risk. There is overwhelming evidence for the value of antipsychotic medication in mania. Lithium and valproate are also useful. "NNT" analysis shows that only a minority of episodes of mania, severe enough to enter clinical trials, respond to monotherapy; but combinations of an antipsychotic with another antimanic drug (lithium or valproate) provide additional efficacy, and for some patients, carbamazepine is a useful alternative. Sufferers from these conditions are now able to choose from a range of treatments. Doctors and relatives should encourage patients with bipolar disorder to make these choices, and doctors should advise them on how, by providing them with sufficient information. Treatment of a manic episode is often the opportunity to begin the process of forging a therapeutic alliance, to commence psychoeducation with the patient and care givers, and to start further treatment with the aim of averting future episodes.

REFERENCES

1. Kupfer DJ, Frank E, Grochocinski VJ, Luther JF, Houck PR, Swartz HA, Mallinger AG. Stabilization in the treatment of mania, depression and mixed states. Acta Neuropsychiatr 2000; 12:112–116.
2. Tohen M, Zarate CA, Hennen J, Khalsa H-MK, Strakowski SM, Gebre-Medhin P, Salvatore P, Baldessarini RJ. The McLean–Harvard First-Episode Mania Study: prediction of recovery and first recurrence. Am J Psychiatry 2003; 160:2099–2107.
3. Zarate CA, Tohen M. Double-blind comparison of the continued use of antipsychotic treatment versus its discontinuation in remitted manic patients. Am J Psychiatry 2004; 161:169–171.
4. Clark L, Iverson SD, Goodwin GM. Sustained attention deficit in bipolar disorder. Br J Psychiatry 2002; 180:313–319.
5. Janowsky DS, El-Yousef MK, Davis JM. Interpersonal manoeuvres of manic patients. Am J Psychiatry 1974; 131:250–255.
6. Meehan K, Zhang F, David S, Tohen M, Janicak P, Small J, Koch K, Rizk R, Walker D, Tran P, Breier A. A Double-blind, randomized comparison of the efficacy and safety of intramuscular injections of olanzapine, lorazepam, or placebo in treating acutely agitated patients diagnosed with bipolar mania. J Clin Psychopharmacol 2001; 21:389–397.
7. American Psychiatric Association. Practice guideline for the treatment of patients with bipolar disorder. American Psychiatric Association. Am J Psychiatry 1994; 151(12 suppl):1–36.
8. Hirschfeld RMA, Bowden CL, Gitlin MJ, Keck PE, Suppes T, Thase ME. Practice guideline for the treatment of patients with bipolar disorder (revision). Am J Psychiatry 2002; 159:1–50.
9. Goodwin GM. Evidence-based guidelines for treating bipolar disorder: recommendations from the British Association for Psychopharmacology. J Psychopharmacol 2003; 17(2):149–173; discussion 147.
10. Grunze H, Kasper S, Goodwin G, Bowden C, Baldwin D, Licht RW, et al. The World Federation of Societies of Biological Psychiatry (WFSBP) Guidelines for the biological treatment of bipolar disorders, Part II: Treatment of mania. World J Biol Psychiatry 2003; 4:5–13.
11. Royal Australian and New Zealand College of Psychiatrists Clinical Practice Guidelines Team for Bipolar Disorder. Australian and New Zealand clinical practice guidelines for the treatment of bipolar disorder. Aust N Z J Psychiatry 2004; 38:280–305.
12. Keck PE, McElroy SL, Tugrul KC, Bennett JA. Valproate oral loading in the treatment of acute mania. J Clin Psychiatry 1993; 54:305–308.

13. Cookson JC, Moult PJA, Wiles D, Besser GM. The relationship between prolactin levels and clinical ratings in manic patients treated with oral and intravenous test doses of haloperidol. Psychol Med 1983; 13:279–285.
14. Pope HG, McElroy SL, Keck PE, Hudson JI. Valproate in the treatment of acute mania: a placebo-controlled study. Arch Gen Psychiatry 1991; 48:62–68.
15. Bowden C, Brugger AM, Swann AC, et al. Efficacy of divalproex vs. lithium and placebo in the treatment of mania. J Am Med Assoc 1994; 271:918–924.
16. Chou JC, Zito JM, Vitrai J, et al. Neuroleptics in acute mania: a pharmacoepidemiologic study. Ann Pharmacother 1996; 30:1396–1398.
17. Cookson JC. Use of antipsychotic drugs and lithium in mania. Br J Psychiatry 2001; 178(suppl 41):s148–s156.
18. Eerdekens M, Karcher K, Grossman F, Kramer M. Risperidone monotherapy in acute bipolar mania. Poster presented at World Psychiatric Association, 2003.
19. Brecher M, Huizar K, ElBaghdady A. Quetiapine monotherapy for acute mania associated with bipolar disorder. Poster presented at the Fifth Annual International Conference on Bipolar Disorder, Pittsburgh, Pennsylvania, U.S.A., June 12–14, 2003.
20. Cookson JC, Taylor D, Katona C. Placebo effects, evaluating evidence, and combining psychotherapy (Chapter 5). In: Use of Drugs in Psychiatry: The Evidence From Psychopharmacology. London: Gaskell Press, 2002:117–131.
21. Tohen M, Sanger TM, McElroy SL, Tollefson GD, Chengappa KN, Daniel DG, Petty F, Centorrino F, Wang R, Grundy SL, Greaney MG, Jacobs TG, David SR, Toma V. Olanzapine versus placebo in the treatment of acute mania. Olanzapine HGEH Study Group. Am J Psychiatry 1999; 156:702–709.
22. Tohen M, Jacobs TG, Grundy SL, McElroy SL, Banov MC, Janicak PG, Sanger T, Risser R, Zhang F, Toma V, Francis J, Tollefson GD, Breier A. Efficacy of olanzapine in acute bipolar mania: a double-blind, placebo-controlled study. The Olanzapine HGGW Study Group. Arch Gen Psychiatry 2000; 57:841–849.
23. Hirschfeld R, Keck PE, Karcher K, Kramer M, Grossman F. Rapid antimanic effect of risperidone monotherapy: a 3-week multicentre, double-blind, placebo-controlled trial. Poster presented at the 41st Annual Meeting of the American College of Neuropsychopharmacology (ACNP), December 8–12, 2002.
24. Khanna S, Vieta E, Lyons B, Grossman F, van Kammen D, Kramer M. Risperidone in the treatment of acute bipolar mania: a double-blind, placebo-controlled study of 290 patients. Poster presented at 16th Congress of the European College of Neuropsychopharmacology (ECNP), Prague, September 2003.
25. Paulsson B, Huizar K. Quetiapine monotherapy versus placebo for acute bipolar mania (STAMP 2) (abstract). Bipolar Disord 2003; 5:74.
26. Keck PE, Marcus R, Tourkodimitris S, Ali M, Liebeskind A, Saha A, Ingenito G. The Aripiprazole Study Group. A placebo-controlled, double-blind study of the efficacy and safety of aripiprazole in patients with acute mania. Am J Psychiatry 2003; 160: 1651–1658.
27. Keck PE, Versiani M, Potkin S, West SA, Giller E, Ice K. The Ziprasidone in Mania Study Group. Ziprasidone in the treatment of acute bipolar mania: a three-week, placebo-controlled, double-blind, randomised trial. Am J Psychiatry 2003; 160:741–748.
28. Segal S, Riesenberg RA, Ice K, English P. Ziprasidone in mania: a 21-day randomized, double-blind, placebo-controlled trial. Poster presentation ECNP Prague, 2003.
29. Aubrey AM, Simon AE, Bertsky C. Possible induction of mania and hypomania by olanzapine or risperidone: a critical review of reported cases. J Clin Psychiatry 2000; 61: 649–655.
30. Cookson JC, Silverstone T, Wells B. A double-blind comparative clinical trial of pimozide and chlorpromazine in mania: a test of the dopamine hypothesis. Acta Psychiatr Scand 1981; 64:381–397.
31. Cookson JC, Ghalib S. The treatment of bipolar mixed states. In: Marneros A, Goodwin FK. Cambridge England: Cambridge University Press.

32. Baker RW, Tohen M, Risser RC, Stauffer VL, Breier A, Tollefson GD. Depression during mania: treatment response to olanzapine or placebo. Poster Presentation, Stanley Foundation Conference on Bipolar Disorder, Amsterdam, 2000.
33. Tohen M, Goldberg JF, Gonzalez-Pinto AM, Azorin JM, Vieta E, Hardy-Bayle MC, Lawson WP, Emsley RA, Baker RW, Risser RC, Namjoshi MA, Evans AR, Breier A. A 12-week double-blind comparison of olanzapine versus haloperidol in the treatment of acute mania. Arch Gen Psychiatry 2003; 60:1218–1226.
34. Rifkin A, Doddi S, Karajgi B, et al. Dosage of haloperidol for mania. Br J Psychiatry 1994; 165:113–116.
35. Tohen M, Baker RW, Altshuler LL, Zarate CA, Suppes T, Ketter TA, Milton DR, Risser R, Gilmore JA, Breier A, Tollefson GA. Olanzapine versus divalproex in the treatment of acute mania. Am J Psychiatry 2002; 159:1011–1017.
36. Zajecka JM, Weisler R, Sachs G, Swann AC, Wozniak P, Sommerville KW. A comparison of the efficacy, safety, and tolerability of divalproex sodium and olanzapine in the treatment of bipolar disorder. J Clin Psychiatry 2002; 63:1148–1155.
37. Weisler RH, Kalali AH, Ketter TA, SPD417 Study Group. A multicenter, randomized, double-blind, placebo-controlled trial of extended-release carbamazepine capsules as monotherapy for bipolar disorder patients with manic or mixed episodes. J Clin Psychiatry 2004; 65:478–484.
38. Peroutka SJ, Snyder SH. Relationship of neuroleptic drug effects at brain dopamine, serotonin, alpha-adrenergic, and histamine receptors to clinical potency. Am J Psychiatry 1980; 137:1518–1522.
39. Suppes T, Webb A, Paul B, Carmody T, Kraemer H, Rush AJ. Clinical outcome in a randomised 1-year trial of clozapine versus treatment as usual for patients with treatment-resistant illness and a history of mania. Am J Psychiatry 1999; 156:1164–1169.
40. Muller-Oerlinghausen B, Retzow A, Henn FA, Giedke H, Walden J. Valproate as an adjunct to neuroleptic medication for the treatment of acute episodes of mania: a prospective, randomized, double-blind, placebo-controlled, multicentre study. J Clin Psychopharmacol 2000; 20:195–203.
41. Sachs GS, Grossman F, Ghaemi SN, Okamoto A, Bowden CL. Combination of a mood stabilizer with risperidone or haloperidol for treatment of acute mania: a double-blind, placebo-controlled comparison of efficacy and safety. Am J Psychiatry 2002; 159: 1146–1154.
42. Yatham LN, Grossman F, Augustyns I, Vieta E, Ravindran A. Mood stabilisers plus risperidone or placebo Mood stabilisers plus risperidone or placebo in the treatment of acute mania in the treatment of acute mania: international, double-blind, randomised controlled trial. Br J Psychiatry 2003; 182:141–147.
43. Tohen M, Chengappa KN, Suppes T, Zarate C-A Jr, Calabrese JR, Bowden CL, Sachs GS, Kupfer DJ, Baker RW, Risser RC, Keeter EL, Feldman PD, Tollefson GD, Breier A. Efficacy of olanzapine in combination with valproate or lithium in the treatment of mania in patients partially nonresponsive to valproate or lithium monotherapy. Arch Gen Psychiatry 2002; 59:62–69.
44. Sachs G, Chengappa KNR, Suppes T, Mullen JA, Brecher M, Devine NA, Sweitzer DE. Quetiapine with lithium or divalproex for the treatment of bipolar mania: a randomized, double-blind, placebo-controlled study. Bipolar Disord 2004; 6:213–223.
45. DelBello MP, Schwiers ML, Rosenberg HL, Strakowski SM. A double-blind, randomized, placebo-controlled study of quetiapine as adjunctive treatment for adolescent mania. J Am Acad Child Adolesc Psychiatry 2002; 41:1216–1223.
46. Tyrer P, Alexander MS, Regan A, Lee I. An extrapyramidal syndrome after lithium therapy. Br J Psychiatry 1980; 136:191–194.
47. Asnis GM, Asnis D, Dunner DL, Fieve RR. Cogwheel rigidity during chronic lithium therapy. Am J Psychiatry 1979; 136:1225–1226.
48. Cohen WJ, Cohen NH. Lithium carbonate, haloperidol, and irreversible brain damage. J Am Med Assoc 1974; 230:1283–1287.

49. Loudon JB, Waring H. Toxic reactions to lithium and haloperidol. Lancet 1976; 2:1088.
50. Von Knorring L. Possible mechanisms for the presumed interaction between lithium and neuroleptics. Human Psychopharmacol 1990; 5:287–292.
51. Johnson DAW, Lowe MR, Batchelor DH. Combined lithium-neuroleptic therapy for manic-depressive illness. Human Psychopharmacol 1990; 5(suppl):262–297.
52. Kramlinger KG, Post RM. Addition of lithium carbonate to carbamazepine: antimanic efficacy in treatment-resistant mania. Acta Psychiatr Scand 1989; 79:378–385.
53. Shukla S, Godwin CD, Long LE, Miller MG. Lithium–carbamazepine neurotoxicity and risk factors. Am J Psychiatry 1984; 141:1604–1606.
54. Black DW, Winokur G, Nasrallah A. Treatment of mania: a naturalistic study of electroconvulsive therapy versus lithium in 438 patients. J Clin Psychiatry 1987; 48:132–139.
55. Small JG, Klapper MH, Kellams JJ, Miller MJ, Milstein V, Sharpley PH, Small IF. Electroconvulsive treatment compared with lithium in the management of manic states. Arch Gen Psychiatry 1988; 45:727–732.
56. Jha AK, Stein GS, Fenwick P. Negative interaction between lithium and electroconvulsion therapy. A case-controlled study. Br J Psychiatry 1996; 168:241–243.
57. Kellner CH, Pritchett JT, Beale MD, Coffey CE. Handbook of ECT. Washington: American Psychiatric Press, 1997.
58. Cookson JC, Ghalib S. The treatment of bipolar mixed states. In: Marneros A, Goodwin FK, eds. Mixed States, Rapid Cycling and Atypical Bipolar. Cambridge, England: Cambridge University Press, 2004.
59. Sanger TM, Tohen M, Vieta E, Dunner DL, Bowden CL, Calabrese JR, Feldman PD, Jacobs TG, Breier A. Olanzapine in the acute treatment of bipolar I disorder with a history of rapid cycling. Affect Disord 2003; 73:155–161.
60. Post RM, Uhde TW, Roy-Byrne PP, Joffe RT. Correlates of antimanic responses to carbamazepine. Psychiatry Res 1987; 21.
61. Post RM, Rubinow DR, Uhde TW, Roy-Byrne PP, Linnoila M, Rosoff A, Cowdry R. Dysphoric mania: clinical and biological correlates. Arch Gen Psychiatry 1989; 46: 353–358.
62. Perry A, Tarrier N, Morriss R, McCarthy E, et al. Randomised controlled trial of efficacy of teaching patients with bipolar disorder to identify early symptoms of relapse and obtain treatment. Br Med J 1999; 318:149–153.

11
Bipolar Depression

Robert M. A. Hirschfeld and L. A. Vornik
Department of Psychiatry and Behavioral Sciences, University of Texas Medical Branch, Galveston, Texas, U.S.A.

INTRODUCTION: PHENOMENOLOGY, DIAGNOSIS, AND CLINICAL COURSE

The notion that bipolar and unipolar depression might be distinct illnesses was first proposed in the middle of the 20th century. Before this time, manic-depressive illness was considered to encompass a broad range of psychopathology, including recurrent unipolar depression. We now recognize that there are substantial differences between depression arising from bipolar disorder and with depression arising from unipolar disorder.

Up to one-third of all patients seeking treatment for depression suffer from bipolar disorder. This includes patients within the bipolar spectrum of bipolar I, bipolar II, and cyclothymia. Unfortunately, many patients with bipolar depression are treated as though they had unipolar depression, sometimes with disastrous results—for example, if the antidepressant precipitates a switch into mania. Thus, recognition of bipolarity is critical to patient care.

The overwhelming majority of clinical and research attention on bipolar disorder has focused on the stabilization of acute mania and its management over the long-term. Much less clinical and research attention has been focused on the diagnosis and management of bipolar depression. This is unfortunate, because many bipolar patients report that their depression episodes are actually more painful, debilitating, and protracted than their manic episodes.

This chapter will overview the phenomenology, diagnosis, and clinical course of bipolar depression and will review various treatment approaches including pharmacotherapy, alternative treatments, and psychosocial interventions. This chapter will also address special issues specific to the treatment of bipolar depression and conclude with clinical recommendations for effective treatment.

The presenting clinical picture of an episode of depression in a bipolar patient often provides few clues of bipolarity. However, bipolar depression is more likely to have an earlier age of onset and a more rapid onset than unipolar depression (1). Anergia and psychotic features are more frequent in bipolar depression (2), but other symptoms generally do not differ in frequency from unipolar depression.

Nevertheless, bipolar depression is often more severe than unipolar depression and is usually more difficult to treat.

Differences in the clinical picture of depression exist among bipolar subtypes. Depressed patients with bipolar I have less anxiety and are more likely to have psychotic features. Patients with bipolar II are more likely to have fatigue, hypersomnia, decreased appetite, decreased interest, and more anxiety symptoms (3).

The presenting picture of bipolar depression is not distinct and provides few clues of bipolarity. The first symptom of bipolar disorder in approximately half of the patients is depression (4). A remarkable finding that is consistent through many surveys of patients with bipolar disorder is that patients have to wait for an average of 10 years from their first symptoms to first medication (4–6). About 70% of patients with bipolar disorder have been misdiagnosed before receiving a correct diagnosis. The most frequent incorrect diagnosis is usually unipolar depression (6). It is imperative that clinicians ask about a history of bipolarity in all patients evaluated for depression (6). A history of mood swings; substance abuse, or poor impulse control suggests that bipolarity may be present.

The sequence order of bipolar episodes is helpful in predicting prognosis. Episodes that begin with mania (i.e., mania, followed by depression) have a much better prognosis than those beginning with depression and switching into mania. Depressive and mixed episodes appear to have equal prognosis (7). Patients with multiple switching within episodes and with long depressive episodes tend to have a poorer prognosis (8).

BIPOLAR DEPRESSION: TREATMENT ACUTE PHARMACOTHERAPY

Lithium

For many years, lithium was considered to be the standard treatment for bipolar depression. Improvement rates of 80% have been reported in nine placebo-controlled studies, conducted mostly in the 1970s (9). Response rates for lithium were equivalent to those for tricyclic antidepressants (TCAs) (10). A recent study of outpatients with bipolar depression compared the efficacy of lithium monotherapy with combined lithium and paroxetine and combined lithium and imipramine. Overall, the combination therapies were not superior to lithium monotherapy. However, at blood levels of lithium < 0.8 mEq/L, both the paroxetine and impramine combinations were superior to lithium monotherapy (11). The disadvantages of lithium in the acute treatment of bipolar depression are its slow onset of action (usually between 1 and 2 months) and the side-effect profile, such as weight gain, tremor, gastrointestinal disturbances, and lethargy.

Recent studies have also demonstrated the effectiveness of lithium as maintenance treatment in reducing depressive morbidity in both bipolar I and II (12).

Antiepilectic Drugs

Lamotrigine

There have been two monotherapy placebo-controlled, double-blind trials.

In the first, bipolar I patients with a major depressive episode received fixed doses of lamotrigine 50 mg or 200 mg per day versus placebo for 7 weeks (13). The titration schedule started with 25 mg of lamotrigine for the first 2 weeks, 50 mg in the third week, and then increases in the 200-mg arm to 100 mg in the fourth week and 200 mg in the fifth week. There was a non-significant trend ($p = 0.084$) at end point for the lamotrigine 200-mg group on the change from baseline on the 17-item Hamilton-D (HAM-D), the primary efficacy variable. However, there was a significant drug/placebo difference for the 200-mg dose. There were no significant differences on these measures for the lamotrigine 50-mg group. Lamotrigine separated from placebo on the Montgomery-Åsberg Depression Rating Scale (MADRS) at week 3 and throughout the rest of the study (Fig. 1). The only side effect with significantly higher rates than placebo was headache. There were no differences among the three groups on rash. Treatment-emergent manic and hypomanic episodes were low and did not differ between the active groups and the placebo.

Another study examined bipolar I or II patients with a depressed episode (14). This 10-week placebo-controlled study allowed flexible dosing between 100 mg and 400 mg of lamotrigine. The bipolar I subjects in this study separated from placebo on the MADRS total score. The bipolar II subjects did not separate because of lower baseline MADRS score in the bipolar II lamotrigine arm vs. the Bipolar II placebo arm (26.4 vs. 28.3).

Taken together, these studies suggest that lamotrigine has an important role in the acute treatment of bipolar depression. Results suggest efficacy for bipolar I depression, beginning at week 3 with a favorable, benign tolerability profile for monotherapy. A slow titration is essential to reduce risk of serious rash.

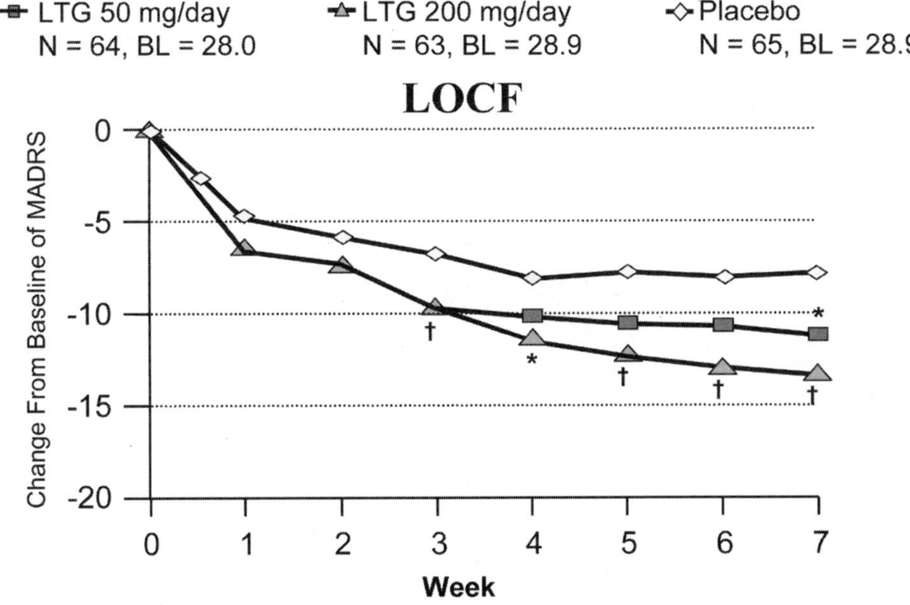

* p < 0.1; † p < 0.05

LOCF = Last Observation Carried Forward

Figure 1 Change from baseline in MADRS LOCF scores during the 7-week study of lamotrigine vs. placebo in the acute treatment of bipolar I depression. *Source*: From Ref. 13.

Divalproex and Sodium Valproate

A pilot placebo-controlled double-blind study was conducted to evaluate the efficacy of divalproex vs. placebo in the treatment of bipolar depression (15). Patients with bipolar I or II disorder with depression were treated in this flexible dose study beginning at 250 mg qhs with a mean maximum daily dose of divalproex of 1391 mg per day. Forty-three percentage (9/21) of the divalproex-treated patients met criteria for recovery, whereas 27% (6/22) of the placebo patients met these criteria ($p < 0.4$). The endpoint HAM-D total score did not differ between placebo and divalproex. However, there were significant differences in favor of divalproex at several points during the study. The study was not powered to test adequately the utility of divalproex in the treatment of bipolar depression, but these results certainly would support further research on the utility of divalproex monotherapy in the treatment of bipolar depression.

Atypical Antipsychotics

Olanzapine and Olanzapine/Fluoxetine Combination

The utility of olanzapine, either as monotherapy or in combination with fluoxetine, was evaluated in a very large placebo-controlled clinical trial (16). The study involved bipolar I depressed patients with an MADRS score of at least 20. Patients were randomized to olanzapine monotherapy (370), olanzapine/fluoxetine combination (OFC) (86), or placebo (377) for 8 weeks. The mean modal dose of olanzapine in the monotherapy arm was 9.7 mg per day. In the OFC, the olanzapine dose was 7.4 mg per day and fluoxetine 39.3 mg per day. Both olanzapine monotherapy and OFC separated from placebo at week 1 and both continued to demonstrate significance throughout the study (Fig. 2). Remission rate for OFC was 49%, 33% for

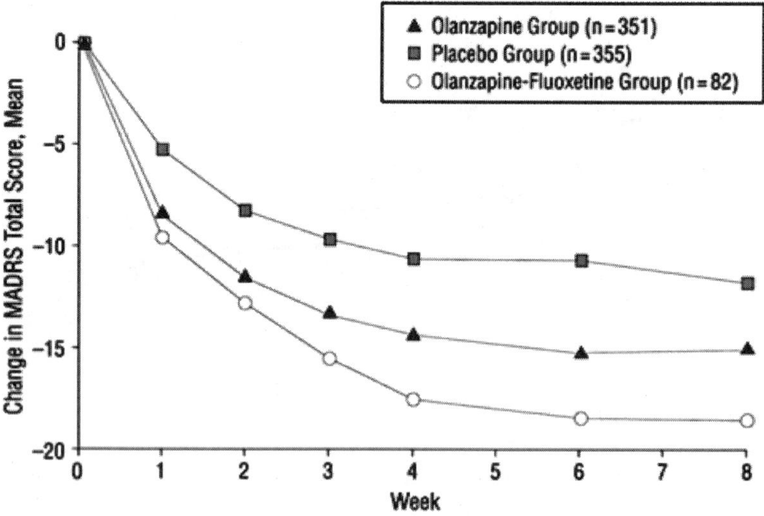

Figure 2 Least squares mean change in MADRS total scores during the 8-week study of olanzapine and OFC vs. placebo. Improvement in MADRS scores with use of olanzapine and the OFC was significantly greater than with use of placebo throughout the study ($p < 0.001$). Improvement in MADRS scores with use of OFC was significantly greater than with use of olanzapine at weeks 4–8 ($p < 0.02$). *Source*: From Ref. 16.

olanzapine monotherapy, and 25% for placebo. OFC remission rates were significantly higher than both placebo and monotherapy, and monotherapy was significantly higher than placebo.

An analysis of the baseline to endpoint change in the individual MADRS items revealed eight out of the 10 differences were different for OFC versus placebo (concentration difficulties and suicidal thoughts were the two exceptions). However, for olanzapine monotherapy, only three out of the 10 items separated from placebo—inner tension, reduced sleep, and reduced appetite. Changes in these symptoms may be attributed to the sedating and appetite-stimulating side effects of olanzapine. Therefore, the antidepressant qualities of olanzapine monotherapy are not as clearly demonstrated or evident as they are for OFC.

Treatment-emergent mania was low in all groups with no significant differences between placebo and the active agents. In general, the side effect profile was similar for olanzapine and OFC and included somnolence, weight gain, increased appetite, and asphenia.

Patients completing the 8-week acute treatment phase entered a 6-month open-label extension with either olanzapine or OFC. Of the patients who were in remission upon entering the open-label phase, 62% remained free of relapse over the 6 months of the trial. Of the patients to relapse, median time to relapse was 194 days.

Quetiapine

The efficacy of quetiapine in the treatment of depression in bipolar I or II patients was tested in an 8-week, 3-arm (quetiapine 600 mg per day, quetiapine 300 mg per day, and placebo) study (17). Of the 542 patients who were randomized, approximately two-thirds were bipolar I and one-third bipolar II. Approximately 20% were rapid cycling and the rest non-rapid cycling. Titration was rapid with target doses of 300 mg per day, by day 4 or 600 mg per day by week 1.

Both doses of quetiapine separated from placebo (Fig. 3) by week 1 and continued throughout the 8 weeks of the study. The effect size was 0.75 for the 600 mg dose and 0.64 for the 300 mg dose (mixed-model analysis). Remission rates (MADRS ≤ 12) were $> 50\%$ for both doses and 37% for placebo ($p < 0.001$). An analysis of the 10 individual MADRS items revealed separation from placebo on eight of the 10 items for both groups (with the exception of reduced appetite and lassitude). Both doses were effective in both rapid cycling and non-rapid cycling patients.

Treatment-emergent mania was low in all groups without significant differences. Sedation, somnolence, and dizziness were the major side effects.

This study strongly supports the efficacy of quetiapine monotherapy in the treatment of both bipolar I and bipolar II depression. Concerns about sedation and somnolence might lead the clinician to consider a slower titration or lower maximum dose.

Antidepressants

Tricyclic Antidepressants

Literature is sparse on controlled studies of TCAs for bipolar depression (18). TCAs are more effective in the treatment of unipolar depression than in bipolar depression. The risk of switching patients from bipolar depression to mania and of shortening cycle lengths makes TCAs unattractive choices for the treatment of bipolar depression.

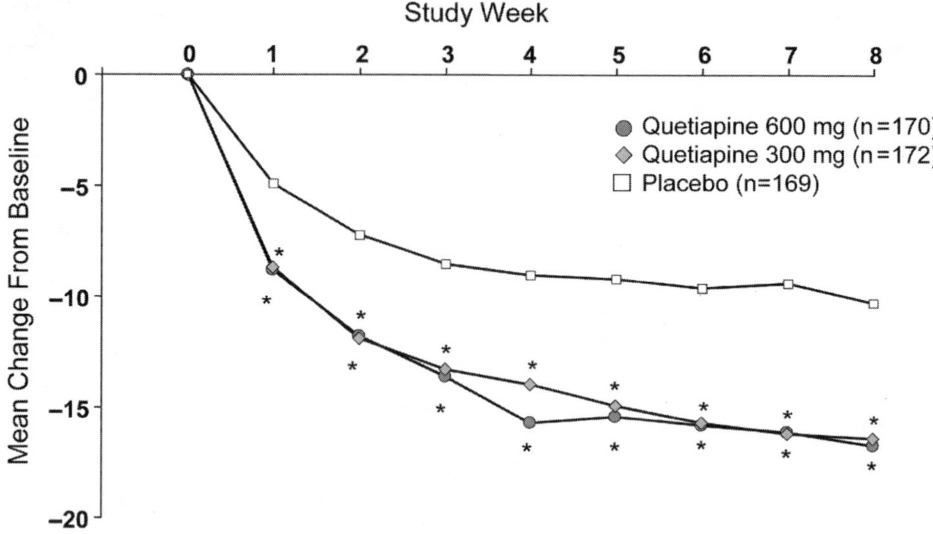

* p<0.001 (vs. placebo)

Figure 3 Change from baseline to final assessment in MADRS LOCF scores during the 8-week study of quetiapine vs. placebo. *Source*: From Ref. 17.

Monoamine Oxidase Inhibitors

Monoamine oxidase inhibitors (MAOIs) are more effective in the treatment of bipolar depression than in unipolar depression. This may be due in part to the superior efficacy of MAOIs in treating patients with anergy and reversed neurovegetative symptoms of hypersomnia and hyperphasia (19–21). Patients who respond often have marked improvements.

Newer Generation Antidepressants

There are surprisingly few studies of the use of selective serotonin reuptake inhibitors (SSRIs) and other newer generation antidepressants in bipolar depression.

Paroxetine

Paroxetine is the most well studied of the SSRIs. Three double-blind, controlled studies of paroxetine were conducted versus placebo, imipramine, venlafaxine, and combined lithium and divalproex (11,22,23). In the one large multicenter study of paroxetine plus lithium versus imipramine plus lithium versus lithium monotherapy, there were no differences between the treatment groups (11). The other studies were not powered to establish significant drug–drug or drug–placebo differences.

A double-blind, randomized study by Young et al. (22) compared the efficacy of adding paroxetine (36 mg/day) to divalproex sodium with adding a second mood stabilizer to divalproex in 27 patients with bipolar depression types I and II. Patients treated with the combination of paroxetine and divalproex did not differ in efficacy from those treated with the add-on lithium. However, paroxetine was significantly better tolerated than the combination of two mood stabilizers, suggesting that adding paroxetine to a mood stabilizer may have clinical utility than adding a second mood stabilizer (22).

Vieta et al. (23) administered paroxetine or venlafaxine to 60 patients in a 6-week, single-blind, randomized trial. All patients experienced breakthrough depression while being treated with a mood stabilizer and were in a current depressive episode of bipolar disorder. Although significant improvements were observed in patients treated with both paroxetine and venlafaxine, there were no differences between the groups. One patient switched into mania while on paroxetine, and four patients switched while on venlafaxine.

Citalopram

Citalopram, added to lithium, divalproex, and/or carbamazepine, was studied in 45 patients on an open-label basis (24). Sixty-four percentage of the patients responded within 8 weeks. In general, the patients tolerated the citalopram well.

Despite the lack of evidence of efficacy from large, placebo-controlled, randomized, double-blind clinical trials, SSRIs are used widely in the treatment of bipolar depression. Many clinicians believe that they are effective and have a lower switch rate than TCAs and MAOIs (25).

Bupropion

Several open-label studies and case reports have suggested that bupropion is effective in the treatment of bipolar depression, with a significantly lower switch rate than other antidepressants (26). A study by Sachs et al. (27) found a substantially lower switch rate in bipolar patients treated with bupropion (10%) vs. desipramine (50%), with equal response rates between the two groups. However, the results of other studies have suggested that bupropion-treated patients do not have lower switch rates than patients treated with other antidepressants (28).

Venlafaxine

Venlafaxine has been studied in the treatment of bipolar depression in several studies. In a previously mentioned study (23), patients were randomized to paroxetine (starting at 20 mg/day) or venlafaxine (at 75 mg/day) for 6 weeks. The mean daily dose of venlafaxine was 179 mg/day and of paroxetine 32 mg/day. There were no differences between the treatment groups on reduction of the HAM-D score (the mean HAM-D change for paroxetine was −6.9 and for venlafaxine −9.0). Response rates were 43% for paroxetine and 48% for venlafaxine. Patients on venlafaxine experienced increased rates of dry mouth and insomnia, whereas those on paroxetine had more nausea and headache. Thirteen percentage of the venlafaxine patients switched to hypomania or mania, whereas 3% of the paroxetine patients did so.

In another study, patients with breakthrough major depressive episodes who were on ongoing adequately dosed mood stabilizers were randomized to bupropion, sertraline, or venlafaxine (29). The primary question in the study was switch rate into mania or hypomania on these antidepressants as a group. Therefore, individual response rate for each drug was not analyzed. However, an acute clinical response rate to these antidepressants as a group was 50% on CGI-Depression for Bipolar Illness. In the 1-year continuation phase, the response rate of much or very much improved was 44%. In the acute 10-week phase, 9% of trials were associated with switched into mania or hypomania, and another 9% with a week of more of hypomania alone (with no to minimal dysfunction).

Another study compared venlafaxine XR with lamotrigine when added to a mood stabilizer in the treatment of bipolar I and II patients with major depression for 8 weeks. Mean HAM-D-17 and CGI-I rating scores improved significantly from baseline to endpoint in both treatment groups. However, there were no differences in reduction in scores between the two agents. Response and remission rates were also equivalent (30).

Other Medications

Benzodiazepines

Benzodiazepines may be useful adjunctively in the treatment of patients with bipolar depression but should not be used as first-line agents. For example, benzodiazepines are useful in treating patients with significant anxiety symptoms or syndromes. Benzodiazepines' augmentation may also be useful for managing aggression and impulsivity.

PSYCHOSOCIAL TREATMENTS

Bipolar disorder can have devastating effects on personal, occupational, and family life. Treatments that address these problems can be extremely helpful. Several psychotherapies and other psychosocial treatments have been developed or adapted for bipolar disorder. Among these are behavioral family management (31), a psychoeducational approach (32), and a modified cognitive behavioral package (33).

These psychosocial approaches have several features in common. They include educational components on the nature and course of bipolar disorder and communication components that enhance the communication between patients and family members. This enhanced communication helps patients resolve interpersonal problems resulting from the disorder. The psychosocial approaches also focus on current issues, not on early life experience and aim to help patients to manage their illness more effectively and to foster early identification of signs of relapse and recurrence.

A unique psychosocial issue for the management of bipolar disorder is attendance to regularization of body and social rhythms. Changes in social rhythms, especially abrupt ones, can trigger or exacerbate episodes. Disruptions in sleep or a highly stimulating environment can also have harmful consequences. Thus, it is imperative to successful treatment that bipolar patients learn to understand and manage their illness. Psychosocial interventions may help patients accomplish this task.

ELECTROCONVULSIVE THERAPY

Electroconvulsive therapy (ECT) may be the most effective available antidepressant treatment. Although there are no data yet confirming the effectiveness of ECT for the treatment of bipolar depression, ECT is particularly effective in patients with psychotic depression, which is more prevalent among bipolar patients. Therefore, ECT should be seriously considered in bipolar patients with depression, particularly psychotic or treatment-resistant depression. Switching into mania can occur following ECT treatment of bipolar depressed patients. However, continuation with ECT will treat mania as well (34).

SPECIAL ISSUES

A substantial problem in the pharmacotherapy of bipolar depression is the risk of precipitating mania or hypomania (i.e., "switching"). Data from a number of studies in the 1970s and 1980s suggest that MAOIs and TCAs—when used without concurrent mood stabilizers—are very likely to induce switching in patients with bipolar depression (35,36). However, some findings from longitudinal studies do not support this. In a six-decade record review of patients treated at the Burghölzli in Zurich, Angst (37) concluded that there is no evidence for treatment-induced switching. Although the evidence is modest, many clinicians believe that the newer agents, particularly bupropion and the SSRIs, are less likely to induce switches than the TCAs or MAOIs.

Another concern in the pharmacotherapy of bipolar depression is the induction of rapid cycling with antidepressant treatment. This is more likely to occur in women, particularly those with an early age of onset of their bipolar depression (38). Concurrently administered mood stabilizers may not prevent or alleviate antidepressant-induced rapid cycling. Discontinuation of antidepressants will often stop the cycling, however.

Antidepressants may reduce cycle length (i.e., the period of time from the beginning of one episode of illness to the beginning of the next) in bipolar patients. Wehr et al. (39) found dramatic decreases in the cycle lengths of bipolar depressed patients treated with TCAs.

CONCLUSIONS AND RECOMMENDATIONS

Over the years, most clinical and research attention in bipolar disorder has been concentrated on the management of acute bipolar mania. Considerably less attention was devoted to the management of bipolar depression. This is unfortunate, as recent survey results reveal that bipolar depression causes more severe symptoms and greater psychosocial impairment than mania. Specifically, patients diagnosed with bipolar disorder experience symptoms of depression for a significantly greater proportion of time than symptoms of mania. Likewise, depression accounts for significantly more disruptive days than mania. The psychosocial impairment in terms of work/school, social/leisure, and family life associated with depression is also significantly greater than that associated with mania. Depression symptoms are also cited significantly more often than mania as causing patients to feel ashamed of work, feeling upset, and being disinterested in work. Furthermore, patients are more likely to have consulted a physician while suffering from depression compared with mania (40). Bipolar depression is also under-recognized, with patients often receiving a diagnosis of unipolar depression. At the same time, a recent study has shown that patients with bipolar depression report significantly more disruption in work, social, and family life than patients with unipolar depression (40). Therefore, the successful treatment of bipolar disorder requires improved recognition of bipolar depression and effective treatment.

Among the treatment options for bipolar depression available today, several agents should be considered for first-line treatment of bipolar I depression: lithium, lamotrigine, OFC, and quetiapine. These recommendations result from new data emerging since the publication of the APA Practice Guideline for the Treatment of Patients with Bipolar Disorder in 2002 (41). Monotherapy with antidepressants is not recommended because of the risk of manic switching and destabilization induced by antidepressants in bipolar patients. In severe bipolar depression, an antidepressant may be started simultaneously with a mood stabilizer (42). In patients who fail to respond to the initial combination therapy of a mood stabilizer and an SSRI, combination of a different mood stabilizer with an MAOI is appropriate. In patients with severe bipolar depression with psychotic features, or in patients at risk of suicide, when a rapid response is necessary, ECT should be seriously considered.

REFERENCES

1. Winokur G, Coryell W, Endicott J, et al. Further distinctions between manic-depressive illness (bipolar disorder) and primary depressive disorder (unipolar depression). Am J Psychiatry 1993; 150(8):1176–1181.
2. Andreasen NC, Grove WM, Endicott J, et al. The phenomenology of depression. Psychiatr Psychobiol 1988; 3:1–10.
3. Andreasen NC, Grove WM. The classification of depression: traditional vs. mathematical approaches. Am J Psychiatry 1982; 139(1):45–52.
4. Suppes T, Leverich GS, Keck PE Jr, et al. The Stanley Foundation Bipolar Treatment Outcome Network. II. Demographics and illness characteristics of the first 261 patients. J Affect Disord 2001; 67:45–59.
5. Lish JD, Dime-Meenan S, Whybrow PC, et al. The National Depressive and Manic–Depressive Association (DMDA) survey of bipolar members. J Affect Disord 1994; 1: 281–294.
6. Hirschfeld RMA, Lewis L, Vornik LA. Perceptions and impact of bipolar disorder: how far have we really come? Results of the National Depressive and Manic-Depressive Association 2000 Survey of Individuals with Bipolar Disorder. J Clin Psychiatry 2003; 64:161–174.
7. Hlastala SA, Frank E, Mallinger AG, et al. Bipolar depression: an underestimated treatment challenge. Depress Anxiety 1997; 5(2):73–83.
8. Turvey CL, Coryell WH, Solomon DA, et al. Long-term prognosis of bipolar I disorder. Acta Psychiatr Scand 1999; 99(2):110–119.
9. Zornberg GL, Pope HG Jr. Treatment of depression in bipolar disorder: new directions for research. J Clin Psychopharmacol 1993; 13(6):397–408.
10. Hirschfeld RMA, Clayton PJ, Cohen I, et al., and the American Psychiatric Association. Practice guidelines for the treatment of patients with bipolar disorder. Am J Psychiatry 1984; 151(suppl 12):1–36.
11. Nemeroff CB, Evans DL, Gyulai L, et al. Double-blind, placebo-controlled comparison of imipramine and paroxetine in the treatment of bipolar depression. Am J Psychiatry 2001; 158:906–912.
12. Tondo L, Baldessarini RJ, Hennen J, et al. Lithium maintenance treatment of depression and mania in bipolar I and bipolar II disorders. Am J Psychiatry 1998; 155(5):638–645.
13. Calabrese JR, Bowden CL, Sachs GS, et al. A double-blind placebo-controlled study of lamotrigine monotherapy in outpatients with bipolar I depression. Lamictal 602 Study Group. J Clin Psychiatry 1999; 60(2):79–88.
14. Bowden CL. Novel treatments for bipolar disorder. Expert Opin Invest Drugs 2001; 10:661–671.
15. Sachs G, Altshuler L, Ketter T, et al. Divalproex sodium vs. placebo for the treatment of bipolar depression. Poster presented at the American College of Neuropsychopharmacology, Waikoloa, Hawaii, Dec 10–14, 2001.
16. Tohen M, Vieta E, Calabrese J, et al. Efficacy of olanzapine and olanzapine–fluoxetine combination in the treatment of bipolar I depression. Arch Gen Psychiatry 2003; 60(11):1079–1088.

17. Calabrese JR, Macfadden W, McCoy R, et al. Double-blind, placebo-controlled study of quetiapine in bipolar depression. Poster presented at the 157th Annual Meeting of the American Psychiatric Association, New York, NY, May 1–6, 2004.
18. Goodwin FK, Jamison KR. Manic–Depressive Illness. New York: Oxford University Press, 1990.
19. Himmelhoch JM, Fuchs CZ, Symons BJ. A double-blind study of tranylcypromine treatment of major anergic depression. J Nerv Ment Dis 1982; 170(10):628–634.
20. Himmelhoch JM, Thase ME, Mallinger AG, et al. Tranylcypromine vs. imipramine in anergic bipolar depression. Am J Psychiatry 1991; 148(7):910–916.
21. Thase ME, Mallinger AG, McKnight D, et al. Treatment of imipramine-resistant recurrent depression, IV: a double-blind crossover study of tranylcypromine for anergic bipolar depression. Am J Psychiatry 1992; 149(2):195–198.
22. Young, LT, Joffe RT, Robb JC, et al. Double-blind comparison of addition of a second mood stabilizer vs. an antidepressant to an initial mood stabilizer for treatment of patients with bipolar depression. Am J Psychiatry 2000; 157:124–126.
23. Vieta E, Martinez-Aran A, Goikolea JM, et al. A randomized trial comparing paroxetine and venlafaxine in the treatment of bipolar depressed patients taking mood stabilizers. J Clin Psychiatry 2002; 63:508–512.
24. Kupfer DJ, Chengappa KN, Gelenberg AJ, et al. Citalopram as adjunctive therapy in bipolar depression. J Clin Psychiatry 2001; 62:985–990.
25. Boerlin HL, Gitlin MJ, Zoellner LA, et al. Bipolar depression and antidepressant-induced mania: a naturalistic study. J Clin Psychiatry 1998; 59(7):374–379.
26. Haykal RF, Akiskal HS. Bupropion as a promising approach to rapid cycling bipolar II patients. J Clin Psychiatry 1990; 51(11):450–455.
27. Sachs GS, Lafer B, Stoll AL, et al. A double-blind trial of bupropion vs. desipramine for bipolar depression. J Clin Psychiatry 1994; 55(9):391–393.
28. Fogelson DL, Bystritsky A, Pasnau R. Bupropion in the treatment of bipolar disorders: the same old story? J Clin Psychiatry 1992; 53(12):443–446.
29. Post RM, Leverich GS, Nolen WA, et al. A re-evaluation of the role of antidepressants in the treatment of bipolar depression: data from the Stanley Foundation Bipolar Network. Bipolar Disord 2003; 5(6):396–406.
30. McIntyre RS, Mancini DA, Fulton KA, et al. Double-blind, acute depression study comparing venlafaxine XR and lamotrigine when added to mood stabilizer in the treatment of bipolar depression. Poster presented at the XXIVth Congress of the Collegium Internationale Neuro-Psychopharmacologicum (CINP), Paris, France, Jun 20–24, 2004.
31. Miklowitz DJ, Goldstein MJ. Behavioral family treatment for patients with bipolar affective disorder. Behav Modif 1990; 14(4):457–489.
32. Miller IW, Keitner GI, Epstein NB, et al. Families of bipolar patients: dysfunction, course of illness, and pilot treatment study. In: Proceedings of the 22nd Meeting of the Society for Psychotherapy Research. Pittsburgh: Society for Psychotherapy Research, 1991.
33. Basco MR, Rush AJ. Cognitive-Behavioral Therapy for Bipolar Disorder. New York: Guildford Press, 1996.
34. Small JG, Milstein V, Small IF. Electroconvulsive therapy for mania. Psychiatr Clin North Am 1991; 14(4):887–903.
35. Wehr TA, Goodwin FK. Can antidepressants cause mania and worsen the course of affective illness?. Am J Psychiatry 1987; 144(11):1403–1411.
36. Wehr TA, Goodwin FK. Do antidepressants cause mania? Psychopharmacol Bull 1987; 23(1):61–65.
37. Angst J. Switch from depression to mania: a record study over decades between 1920 and 1982. Psychopathology 1985; 18:140–154.
38. Altshuler LL, Post RM, Leverich GS, et al. Antidepressant-induced mania and cycle acceleration: a controversy revisited. Am J Psychiatry 1995; 152(8):1130–1138.

39. Wehr TA, Sack DA, Rosenthal NE, et al. Rapid cycling affective disorder: contributing factors and treatment responses in 51 patients. Am J Psychiatry 1988; 145(2):179–184.
40. Hirschfeld RM. Bipolar depression: the real challenge. Eur Neuropsychopharmacol 2004; 14(suppl 2):S83–S88.
41. American Psychiatric Association. Practice guideline for the treatment of patients with bipolar disorder (revision). Am J Psychiatry 2002; 159(suppl 4):1–50.
42. Yatham LN, Calabrese JR, Kusumakar V. Bipolar depression: criteria for treatment selection, definition of refractoriness, and treatment options. Bipolar Disord 2003; 5(2): 85–97.

12
The Treatment of Mixed States

Eduard Vieta and Jose Sanchez-Moreno
Bipolar Disorders Program, Hospital Clinic, University of Barcelona, Barcelona, Spain

INTRODUCTION

One of the main criticisms to the concept of bipolarity is the existence of mixed states (1,2). Indeed, if there are only two opposite poles, mixed states should not exist. The American Psychiatric Association classification of mental disorders does not address this contradiction, allowing for mixed bipolar states that actually involve the full manic and depressive syndrome.

Kraepelin (3) was the first to emphasize the clinical relevance of mixed states. He described six subtypes of mixed states: depression with racing thoughts, excited depression, depressive-anxious mania, improductive mania, inhibited mania, and manic stupor, all of them of as a result of different combinations of mood, cognitive, and psychomotor symptoms (Table 1). Unfortunately, these useful descriptions were hardly used by clinicians and mixed states remained a source of misdiagnosis for many years.

In recent years, there has been greater awareness about the importance of mixed states. Several authors have contributed to this fact, including Himmelhoch, Akiskal, Marneros, McElroy, Perugi, Bauer, Benazzi, and many others, for whom the DSM and the ICD definitions are very disappointing. Their contribution, together with the development of clinical trials enrolling mixed patients, have led to a further knowledge about how to diagnose and treat these patients, who suffer from one of the most stressing and life-threatening psychiatric conditions.

The prevalence of mixed states may range between 14% and 67%, depending on the definition (Table 2). Akiskal described a number of symptoms as more characteristics of a mixed state during a manic episode (Table 3).

Mixed states may be more frequent in women (4) and in patients with alcohol or neuropsychiatric comorbidity (5). Mixed patients have more past depressive episodes (6), higher risk of suicide (7), and family history is more often depressive than manic (8). These authors, along with Akiskal, have emphasized the relationship between mixed states and pre-morbid temperament. Mixed bipolar patients would be more likely to have depressive temperament than pure manics (4,9).

For some reason, that may have to do with educational or cultural issues, or even with differences about antidepressant use across the oceans, drug trials

Table 1 Mixed States According to Kraepelin

	Mood	Cognition	Behavior
Pure mania	M	M	M
Depressive or anxious mania	D	M	M
Agitated depression	D	D	M
Mania with poverty of thought	M	D	M
Classical depression	D	D	D
Manic stupor	M	D	D
Depression with racing thoughts	D	M	D
Inhibited Mania	M	M	D

D, Depression; M, Mania.

conducted in North America are more likely to enroll mixed patients than trials conducted in Europe or Asia. Generally, mixed manic patients are more likely to score lower in mania rating scales and to provide informed consent to participate in drug trials, because they have more illness awareness during the episode (insight is more related to depressive symptoms than to manic symptoms).

The first published trial on the treatment of mixed states was carried out as early as 1759. Indeed, 100 years before the description of Falret and Baillarger, a Spanish physician, Piquer, described a case report on a patient who suffered from "a melancholic-manic affect." Piquer described his condition as "an illness in which, at some point, there was a predominant mood, and suddenly the opposite, but always as a result of insanity, not nature." His patient was Ferdinand the VI, king of Spain, and the treasure of the full description of his illness and treatment was recently rediscovered and published by Vieta and Barcia (10). Table 4 shows the treatments assayed in this very special mixed bipolar patient around 1759. Of course, many things have changed since then, and a good number of evidence-based treatment options are available now for this condition.

Table 2 Rates of Mixed States

Study	Patients (N)	Percentage
Winokur et al. (17)	61	16
Kotin and Goodwin (1972)	20	65
Himmelhoch et al. (5)	84	31
Akiskal and Puzantian (5)	60	25
Nunn (1979)	112	36
Prien et al. (21)	103	67
Post et al. (1989)	48	46
Dell'Osso et al. (8)	108	45
McElroy et al. (1995)	71	40
Cassidy et al. (1998)	273	14
Akiskal et al. (4)	104	37
Dilsaver et al. (1999)	105	40
Total	1149	43

Table 3 Discriminatory "Depressive" Symptoms in Dysphoric Mania

Depressed mood
Irritability
Mood lability
Anhedonia
Hopelessness/helplessness
Suicidal ideation and/or attempt
Guilt
Fatigue

TREATMENT OF MIXED STATES: GENERAL RULES

The first and crucial step in the treatment of mixed states is to make a correct diagnosis. As mentioned, there are a number of mixed subtypes and it is reasonable to think that treatment may differ according to subtype. However, little evidence is available about how to treat mixed states other than dysphoric mania. Hence, the only controlled data available so far come from sub-analyses of randomized controlled trials in mania that enrolled a variable number of mixed patients fulfilling standardized criteria for mania and scoring over a certain threshold in a mania scale, with no specific requirements with regards to the intensity of depressive symptoms. Unfortunately, there is no trial dealing specifically with the treatment of mixed states. Therefore, most of the information provided in this chapter has been obtained from trials that were not powered to seek for differences between treatment approaches in mixed bipolar patients.

As mentioned, the first steps in the treatment of mixed states are making a correct diagnosis and screening for comorbidities that are more frequent in these patients. Several studies suggest that mixed bipolar patients have higher prevalence rates of substance abuse (5), physical comorbidities (11), and suicidal behavior (12), which are all them very relevant aspects for treatment choice. Mixed states are difficult to treat, and recovery from an index-mixed episode takes usually longer than recovery from a manic or depressive episode (13,14).

Table 4 Treatments Assayed for Bipolar Disorder During the 18th Century in His Majesty Ferdinand VI of Spain

Donkey milk
Turtle soup with frogs, calf, and snakes
Enemas
Lime tea with cherries
Mother-of-pearl dust
Fumaria
Head baths
Deer antler jelly with tender vipers
Violet
Diet
Borage potion
Pimpernel
Agrimony

As general rules, there is some consensus about discontinuing antidepressants during mixed states, because they have been described to worsen them (15,16), and benzodiazepines may be used if there is prominent anxiety or insomnia, which is quite common (17). Very simple, but supportive psychotherapy may be useful to help the patient to understand what is happening. Formal psychotherapy, however, such as cognitive-behavioral therapy or psychoeducation, should only be delivered once the patient has achieved remission from acute symptoms (18).

The American Psychiatric Association guidelines for the treatment of bipolar disorder recommend to treat severe mixed episodes with the combination of lithium or divalproate plus an antipsychotic, and among these atypicals are preferred (19). For milder episodes, monotherapy with lithium, divalproate, or olanzapine may be enough (19). Other drugs, such as carbamazepine, oxcarbazepine, or clozapine, may be used in treatment resistant patients (19), and electroconvulsive therapy (ECT) is also an option. We will review the data that supported these statements and more recent data that may shed more light into the treatment of this condition.

LITHIUM

Lithium has been reported to be more effective in pure mania than in depressive mania (20–22). Neither lithium nor the combination of lithium and imipramine were effective in the prevention of mixed episodes (23). However, lithium may still play a role in the treatment of mixed states, especially in combination with atypical antipsychotics.

ANTICONVULSANTS

In a divalproate comparative mania trial vs. lithium and placebo, the presence of concomitant depressive symptoms was associated with response to divalproate but not to lithium (22). This finding has not been consistently replicated, but still divalproate may be a good choice for manic patients with dysphoric features. For example, Calabrese and Delucchi (24) found that among rapid cyclers, those with mixed episodes were more likely to respond to divalproate, both acutely and prophylactically. Carbamazepine has also been suggested to be a good option in these patients (25,26), but controlled data are not available. The same happens with oxcarbazepine. Other anticonvulsants, such as lamotrigine, have failed to show acute antimanic properties (27) and, in fact, mixed states were a predictor of non-response in the long-term trials (Calabrese, personal communication). Topiramate has been reported to be helpful in open studies, but controlled studies in mania were negative, although they excluded explicitly mixed patients (28).

ANTIPSYCHOTICS

The first-generation antipsychotics are clearly efficacious in the treatment of manic symptoms, but may be less efficacious than the second generation in the treatment of depressive symptoms during mania, according to some authors (29). This statement, however, has not been confirmed in controlled trials, but what those trials did suggest was that there was a higher switch rate to depression with haloperidol, as compared with olanzapine (30).

Most of the available data on the treatment of mixed states come from randomized controlled mania trials with atypical antipsychotics, and depending on the proportion of mixed patients in the trials, specific subanalyses may be performed. For instance, olanzapine has a large number of trials and some of them enrolled a substantial proportion of mixed manics, whereas the quetiapine mania trials excluded mixed patients and, therefore, little evidence is available about the efficacy of quetiapine in mixed states. We shall discuss the available evidence on these drugs individually.

For clozapine, only open studies are available, suggesting that it may be effective for the treatment of mixed states (31). Due to safety concerns and limited evidence, clozapine should not be used as a first-line treatment in this condition, even though clinical experience suggests that it may be quite effective. For treatment-refractory cases, however, it remains as a valuable option.

Risperidone trials only enrolled a very limited number of mixed patients. Some trials excluded them (32), and others, perhaps because they were conducted in Asian or European countries, or perhaps because of higher severity, were only able to enroll few patients with this condition (33). Only one trial, comparing risperidone plus lithium or divalproate vs. lithium or divalproate alone and haloperidol plus lithium and divalproate, included slightly more than 20% mixed patients (34), but there were no significant differences among the three groups at the endpoint. A large, observational study enrolling more than 500 bipolar patients, 31 of whom were mixed, reported risperidone plus mood stabilizers to be effective in this condition (35), but this was not a controlled study. The average risperidone dose in mixed manic patients may be around 4 mg/day (36).

At least two out of eight olanzapine mania trials enrolled enough mixed patients to allow for statistical subanalyses of the data. The second placebo-controlled study (37) enrolled 43% mixed patients. Improvement in the Young Mania Rating Scale (YMRS) was similar for pure and mixed patients treated with olanzapine (15 vs. 14 points), but probably due to limited sample size differences between olanzapine and placebo did not reach statistical significance in mixed patients. However, looking at patients scoring 20 or more in the Hamilton Depression Rating Scale (HDRS), the olanzapine-treated patients improved significantly more than the patients who received placebo. Further analyses from the two placebo-controlled trials suggest that olanzapine may be useful for the treatment of mixed mania (38). The second olanzapine study that enrolled a significant number of mixed manics (52%, more than 150 patients) compared olanzapine plus lithium or divalproate with lithium or divalproate alone (39). This study did show a statistical advantage for olanzapine-treated patients versus placebo in patients taking mood stabilizers. Open studies have also reported good results with olanzapine in mixed patients (40,41).

Quetiapine has been quite extensively studied in mania, but most trials excluded mixed patients. Only a small controlled trial of adjunctive quetiapine in adolescents taking divalproate provided some information, such as significant improvements in both mania and depression rating scales (42). Zarate et al. (43) reported preliminary good results as well in a retrospective study. Finally, quetiapine might be useful for the long-term treatment of mixed states in rapid cyclers if the results of a small, observational study are replicated (44).

Ziprasidone has been assessed in a few placebo-controlled mania trials. Pooled data from those suggest that it may be effective in the treatment of mixed mania, as 101 mixed patients on ziprasidone monotherapy improved significantly more than 50 on placebo (45).

The aripiprazole monotherapy trials enrolled a good number of mixed patients, allowing for statistical sub-analyses of pooled data. Pooling the three datasets, there is a significant advantage of aripiprazole over placebo in the treatment of mixed mania (46). There are no data available as yet for combination therapy with this drug.

There are no published studies with amisulpride in the treatment of mania or mixed states. A recent uncontrolled study with only 20 patients, including three mixed manics, reported significant improvements in both mania and depression rating scales (47), but this is indeed very little evidence about how this drug works in this population.

ELECTROCONVULSIVE THERAPY

ECT has been reported to be an effective treatment for various mixed states, including mixed mania, mixed depression, and agitated depression (16,48–50). Baseline ratings of depression during mania were the strongest predictor of response to ECT, rather than lithium, in a randomized, controlled trial (51).

As a summary, Table 5 provides a simple classification of currently available treatments for mixed states according to scientific evidence. Hopefully, further research will make this table obsolete soon. Beyond clinical trials, experience also tells us that combination therapy is more likely to be successful than monotherapy. In the near future, we hope that different combination of the compounds that are mentioned in the table, and other that may come, will be assessed in randomized trials specifically addressed to mixed bipolar patients, and different mixed presentations.

CONCLUSIONS

Bipolar mixed states remain a nosological dilemma, a diagnostic challenge, and a neglected area of therapeutic research. Only dysphoric mania has been reasonably addressed in clinical trials, but very little is known about the treatment of other

Table 5 Current Evidence on the Treatment of Mixed States

Positive controlled data for both monotherapy and combination
Divalproate
Olanzapine
Limited positive controlled data
Ziprasidone
Aripiprazole
ECT
Limited data
Lithium
Carbamazepine
Clozapine
Risperidone
Quetiapine
Negative data
Lamotrigine
Topiramate
Imipramine

mixed states. There is some indirect evidence that mixed mania may be more responsive to anticonvulsants than to lithium. Divalproate, and to a lesser extent carbamazepine, may be used either in monotherapy or as adjuncts to lithium. Use of other anticonvulsants, such as gabapentin, lamotrigine, leviteracetam, oxcarbazepine, tiagabine, topiramate, or zonisamide is not supported by controlled data as yet. The use of antidepressants is largely discouraged, as they may worsen this condition. Atypical antipsychotics, on the other hand, may be effective and safe either in monotherapy or in combination with lithium or valproate. Only the trials with olanzapine, aripiprazole, and ziprasidone enrolled a substantial number of patients to allow for statistical sub-analyses on this population. Risperidone, quetiapine, and clozapine have also been studied in randomized clinical trials but the number of patients enrolled was quite small. Both evidence and clinical experience point at combination therapy of an atypical antipsychotic and an anticonvulsant or lithium as first-line therapy for mixed states. A good alternative is ECT.

REFERENCES

1. Court JH. Manic-depressive psychosis: an alternative conceptual model. Br J Psychiatry 1968; 114:1523–1530.
2. Whybrow PC, Mendels J. Toward a biology of depression: some suggestions from neurophysiology. Am J Psychiatry 1969; 125:1491–1500.
3. Kraepelin E. Manic-Depressive Insanity and Paranoia. Edinburgh: E & S Livingstone, 1921; reprinted in Carlson ET, ed. Dementia Praecox and Paraphrenia Together with Manic-Depressive Insanity and Paranoia, Classics of Medicine Library. Birmingham, 1989.
4. Akiskal HS, Hantouche EG, Bourgeois ML, Azorin JM, Sechter D, Allilaire JF, Lancrenon S, Fraud JP, Chatenet-Duchene L. Gender, temperament, and the clinical picture in dysphoric mixed mania: findings from a French national study (EPIMAN). J Affect Disord 1998; 50:175–186.
5. Himmelhoch JM, Mulla D, Neil JF, Detre TP, Kupfer DJ. Incidence and significance of mixed affective states in a bipolar population. Arch Gen Psychiatry 1976; 33:1062–1066.
6. Perugi G, Micheli C, Akiskal HS, Madaro D, Socci C, Quilici C, Musetti L. Polarity of the first episode, clinical characteristics, and course of manic depressive illness: a systematic retrospective investigation of 320 bipolar I patients. Compr Psychiatry 2000; 41:13–18.
7. Goldberg JF, Garno JL, Leon AC, Kocsis JH, Portera L. Association of recurrent suicidal ideation with nonremission from acute mixed mania. Am J Psychiatry 1998; 155:1753–1755.
8. Dell'Osso L, Placidi GF, Nassi R, Freer P, Cassano GB, Akiskal HS. The manic-depressive mixed state: familial, temperamental and psychopathologic characteristics in 108 female inpatients. Eur Arch Psychiatry Clin Neurosci 1991; 240:234–249.
9. Hantouche EG, Allilaire JP, Bourgeois ML, Azorin JM, Sechter D, Chatenet-Duchene L, Lancrenon S, Akiskal HS. The feasibility of self-assessment of dysphoric mania in the French national EPIMAN study. J Affect Disord 2001; 67:97–103.
10. Vieta E, Barcia D. El Trastorno Bipolar en el Siglo XVIII. Barcelona: MRA Ediciones, 1999.
11. Himmelhoch JM, Garfinkel ME. Sources of lithium resistance in mixed mania. Psychopharmacol Bull 1986; 22:613–620.
12. Dilsaver SC, Chen YW, Swann AC, Shoaib AM, Krajewski KJ. Suicidality in patients with pure and depressive mania. Am J Psychiatry 1994; 151:1312–1315.
13. Keller MB, Lavori PW, Coryell W, Andreasen NC, Endicott J, Clayton PJ, Klerman GL, Hirschfeld RM. Differential outcome of pure manic, mixed/cycling, and pure depressive episodes in patients with bipolar illness. JAMA 1986; 255:3138–3142.

14. Kupfer DJ. Models of bipolar disease and their clinical implications. Biol Psychiatry 2000; 48:428–429.
15. Akiskal HS, Mallya G. Criteria for the "soft" bipolar spectrum: treatment implications. Psychopharmacol Bull 1987; 23:68–73.
16. Koukopoulos A, Faedda G, Proietti R, D'Amico S, de Pisa E, Simonetto C. Un syndrome depressif mixte. Encephale 1992; 18 Spec No 1:19–21.
17. Winokur G, Clayton P, Reich T. Manic-Depressive Illness. St Louis, MO: C.V. Mosby Company, 1969.
18. Vieta E, Colom F. Psychological interventions in bipolar disorder: from wishful thinking to an evidence-based approach. Acta Psychiatr Scand Suppl 2004; 422:34–38.
19. American Psychiatric Association. Practice guideline for the treatment of patients with bipolar disorder (revision). Am J Psychiatry 2002; 159(suppl 4):1–50.
20. Secunda SK, Swann A, Katz MM, Koslow SH, Croughan J, Chang S. Diagnosis and treatment of mixed mania. Am J Psychiatry 1987; 144:96–98.
21. Prien RF, Himmelhoch JM, Kupfer DJ. Treatment of mixed mania. J Affect Disord 1988; 15:9–15.
22. Swann AC, Bowden CL, Morris D, Calabrese JR, Petty F, Small J, Dilsaver SC, Davis JM. Depression during mania. Treatment response to lithium or divalproex. Arch Gen Psychiatry 1997; 54:37–42.
23. Prien RF, Gelenberg AJ. Alternatives to lithium for preventive treatment of bipolar disorder. Am J Psychiatry 1989; 146:840–848.
24. Calabrese JR, Delucchi GA. Spectrum of efficacy of valproate in 55 patients with rapid-cycling bipolar disorder. Am J Psychiatry 1990; 147:431–434.
25. Post RM, Uhde TW, Roy-Byrne PP, Joffe RT. Correlates of antimanic response to carbamazepine. Psychiatry Res 1987; 21:71–83.
26. Ballenger JC. The clinical use of carbamazepine in affective disorders. J Clin Psychiatr Suppl 1988; 49:13–19.
27. Bowden CL. Acute and maintenance treatment with mood stabilizers. Int J Neuropsychopharmacol 2003; 6:269–275.
28. Vieta E, Torrent C, Garcia-Ribas G, Gilabert A, Garcia-Pares G, Rodriguez A, Cadevall J, Garcia-Castrillon J, Lusilla P, Arrufat F. Use of topiramate in treatment-resistant bipolar spectrum disorders. J Clin Psychopharmacol 2002; 22:431–435.
29. Yatham LN. Acute and maintenance treatment of bipolar mania: the role of atypical antipsychotics. Bipolar Disord 2003; 2(suppl 5):7–19.
30. Tohen M, Goldberg JF, Gonzalez-Pinto Arrillaga AM, Azorin JM, Vieta E, Hardy-Bayle MC, Lawson WB, Emsley RA, Zhang F, Baker RW, Risser RC, Namjoshi MA, Evans AR, Breier A. A 12-week, double-blind comparison of olanzapine vs. haloperidol in the treatment of acute mania. Arch Gen Psychiatry 2003; 60:1218–1226.
31. Suppes T, McElroy SL, Gilbert J, Dessain EC, Cole JO. Clozapine in the treatment of dysphoric mania. Biol Psychiatry 1992; 32:270–280.
32. Hirschfeld RM, Keck PE Jr, Kramer M, Karcher K, Canuso C, Eerdekens M, Grossman F. Rapid antimanic effect of risperidone monotherapy: a 3-week multicenter, double-blind, placebo-controlled trial. Am J Psychiatry 2004; 161:1057–1065.
33. Khanna S, Vieta E, Lyons B, Grossman F, Eerdekens M, Kramer M. Risperidone in the treatment of acute bipolar mania: a double-blind, placebo-controlled study of 290 patients. Br J Psychiatry. In press.
34. Sachs GS, Grossman F, Ghaemi SN, Okamoto A, Bowden CL. Combination of a mood stabilizer with risperidone or haloperidol for treatment of acute mania: a double-blind, placebo-controlled comparison of efficacy and safety. Am J Psychiatry 2002; 159: 1146–1154.
35. Vieta E, Goikolea JM, Corbella B, Benabarre A, Reinares M, Martinez G, Fernandez A, Colom F, Martinez-Aran A, Torrent C, Group for the Study of Risperidone in Affective Disorders (GSRAD). Risperidone safety and efficacy in the treatment of bipolar

and schizoaffective disorders: results from a 6-month, multicenter, open study. J Clin Psychiatry 2001; 62:818–825.
36. Benabarre A, Vieta E, Colom F, Martinez A, Reinares M, Corbella B. Treatment of mixed mania with risperidone and mood stabilizers. Can J Psychiatry 2001; 46:866–867.
37. Tohen M, Jacobs TG, Grundy SL, McElroy SL, Banov MC, Janicak PG, Sanger T, Risser R, Zhang F, Toma V, Francis J, Tollefson GD, Breier A. Efficacy of olanzapine in acute bipolar mania: a double-blind, placebo-controlled study. The Olanzipine HGGW Study Group. Arch Gen Psychiatry 2000; 57:841–849.
38. Baldessarini RJ, Hennen J, Wilson M, Calabrese J, Chengappa R, Keck PE Jr, McElroy SL, Sachs G, Vieta E, Welge JA, Yatham LN, Zarate CA Jr, Baker RW, Tohen M. Olanzapine vs. placebo in acute mania: treatment responses in subgroups. J Clin Psychopharmacol 2003; 23:370–376.
39. Tohen M, Chengappa KN, Suppes T, Zarate CA Jr, Calabrese JR, Bowden CL, Sachs GS, Kupfer DJ, Baker RW, Risser RC, Keeter EL, Feldman PD, Tollefson GD, Breier A. Efficacy of olanzapine in combination with valproate or lithium in the treatment of mania in patients partially nonresponsive to valproate or lithium monotherapy. Arch Gen Psychiatry 2002; 59:62–69.
40. Vieta E, Reinares M, Corbella B, Benabarre A, Gilaberte I, Colom F, Martinez-Aran A, Gasto C, Tohen M. Olanzapine as long-term adjunctive therapy in treatment-resistant bipolar disorder. J Clin Psychopharmacol 2001; 21:469–473.
41. Gonzalez-Pinto A, Tohen M, Lalaguna B, Perez-Heredia JL, Fernandez-Corres B, Gutierrez M, Mico JA. Treatment of bipolar I rapid cycling patients during dysphoric mania with olanzapine. J Clin Psychopharmacol 2002; 22:450–454.
42. Delbello MP, Schwiers ML, Rosenberg HL, Strakowski SM. A double-blind, randomized, placebo-controlled study of quetiapine as adjunctive treatment for adolescent mania. J Am Acad Child Adolesc Psychiatry 2002; 41:1216–1223.
43. Zarate CA Jr, Rothschild A, Fletcher KE, Madrid A, Zapatel J. Clinical predictors of acute response with quetiapine in psychotic mood disorders. J Clin Psychiatry 2000; 1:185–189.
44. Vieta E, Parramon G, Padrell E, Nieto E, Martinez-Aran A, Corbella B, Colom F, Reinares M, Goikolea JM, Torrent C. Quetiapine in the treatment of rapid cycling bipolar disorder. Bipolar Disord 2002; 4:335–340.
45. Potkin SG, Keck P, Giller E, Ice K, Warrington L, Mandel FS. Ziprasidone in bipolar mania: Efficacy across patient subgroups. 157th Annual Meeting of the American Psychiatric Association, New York, NY, U.S.A., May 1–6, 2004.
46. Jody D, McQuade RD, Carson WH, Iwamoto T, Abou-Gharbia N, Hardy SA, Archibald DG. Efficacy of Aripiprazole in Subpopulations of Bipolar Disorder. 157th Annual Meeting of the American Psychiatric Association, New York, NY, U.S.A., May 1–6, 2004.
47. Vieta E, Ros S, Goikolea JM, Benabarre A, Popova E, Comes M, Capapey J, Sanchez-Moreno J. Amisulpride in the treatment of mania. J Clin Psychiatry. In press.
48. Dilsaver SC, Swann AC, Shoaib AM, Bowers TC, Halle MT. Depressive mania associated with nonresponse to antimanic agents. Am J Psychiatry 1993; 150:1548–1551.
49. Evans DL, Nemeroff ChB. The dexamethasone suppression test in mixed bipolar disorder. Am J Psychiatry 1983; 140:615–617.
50. Ciapparelli A, Dell'Osso L, Tundo A, Pini S, Chiavacci MC, Di Sacco I, Cassano GB. Electroconvulsive therapy in medication-nonresponsive patients with mixed mania and bipolar depression. J Clin Psychiatry 2001; 62:552–555.
51. Small JG, Klapper MH, Kellams JJ, Miller MJ, Milstein V, Sharpley PH, Small IF. Electroconvulsive treatment compared with lithium in the management of manic states. Arch Gen Psychiatry 1988; 45:727–732.
52. Kotin J, Goodwin FK. Depression during mania: clinical observations and theoretical implications. Am J Psychiatry 1972; 129:679–686.

53. Akiskal HS, Puzantian VR. Psychotic forms of depression and mania. Psychiatr Clin North Am 1979; 2:419–439.
54. Nunn CM. Mixed affective states and the natural history of manic-depressive psychosis. Br J Psychiatry 1979; 134:153–156.
55. Post RM, Rubinow DR, Uhde TW, Roy-Byrne PP, Linnoila M, Rosoff A, Cowdry R. Dysphoric mania. Clinical and biological correlates. Arch Gen Psychiatry 1989; 46: 353–358.
56. McElroy SL, Strakowski SM, Keck PE Jr, Tugrul KL, West SA, Lonczak HS. Differences and similarities in mixed and pure mania. Compr Psychiatry 1995; 36:187–194.
57. Cassidy F, Murry E, Forest K, Carroll BJ. Signs and symptoms of mania in pure and mixed episodes. J Affect Disord 1998; 50:187–201.
58. Dilsaver SC, Chen YR, Shoaib AM, Swann AC. Phenomenology of mania: evidence for distinct depressed, dysphoric, and euphoric presentations. Am J Psychiatry 1999; 156: 426–430.

13
Rapid Cycling

Andreas Erfurth
Department of General Psychiatry, Medical University of Vienna, Vienna, Austria

Giulio Perugi
Department of Psychiatry, University of Pisa, Pisa, Italy

DEFINITION

Bipolar disorders are characterized by elevated morbidity and mortality (1–3). Although pharmacotherapy can positively influence the course of the disease, recurrence has been estimated in a range between 10% and 30% in the case of perfect compliance to prophylactic therapy (4). In some patients, the course of the disease assumes characteristics of elevated cyclicity with a—sometimes increasing—number of both depressive and manic episodes.

The classic definition of rapid cycling has been proposed in 1974 by Dunner and Fieve (5). Bipolar disorder with rapid cycling is present when four or more episodes of mania, hypomania, or major depression were identified during the last 12 months. The same criterion is used by the Diagnostic and Statistical Manual of Mental Disorders of the American Psychiatric Association (DSM-IV-TR™)"... At least four episodes of a mood disturbance in the previous 12 months that meet criteria for a Major Depression, Manic, Mixed, or Hypomanic Episode" adding "Episodes are demarcated either by partial or full remission for at least 2 months or a switch to an episode of opposite polarity (e.g., Major Depressive Episode to Manic Episode)" (6).

In the DSM-IV-TR, rapid cycling is considered to be a specific course of the affective illness rather than a distinct subtype of the disorder (6). According to the medium duration of a cycle (e.g., the time between the beginning of an episode and the beginning of a new episode of the same polarity), rapid cycling can be divided into: (a) the *classical type*, with a duration of cycles between 3 days and 12 weeks; (b) the *ultra-rapid type*, with cycles of less than 3 days; (c) the *ultra–ultra-rapid* or *rapid ultradian type*, with cycles of 24 hours or less (7). The ultradian type has been proposed as separate subtype (8) due to its possibly specific epidemiological and clinical characteristics (9–16).

Unfortunately, the ultra-rapid and the ultra–ultra-rapid type are difficult or impossible to distinguish from some mixed states and some bipolar disorders in adolescence or associated with substance abuse, which are characterized by marked instability of mood and/or volition and by considerable emotional reactivity. It is most probable that the distribution and the demarcation of the three subtypes of rapid cycling in different publications strongly influences the outcome of clinical research, including data on treatment response.

Moreover, rapid cycling can be distinguished by the presence or absence of precipitating factors and thus classified as (a) spontaneous or (b) related to external—sometimes unrecognizable—factors such as pharmaceutical interventions, drugs of abuse, pregnancy, and various physical and mental disorders including thyroid dysfunction (7,17–19). Finally, it is possible to distinguish between cases of rapid cycling (a) with early (<20 years of age) or (b) tardive onset (>40 years of age) (7).

EPIDEMIOLOGICAL AND CLINICAL CHARACTERISTICS

Ten to twenty percent of bipolar patients develop rapid cycling; 70–90% of rapid cyclers are women (5,17,19–29). While some studies were not able to show this prevalence in women (30–32), a meta-analysis on 2000 patients confirmed the prevalence in women (72% vs. 28%; i.e., a ratio of approximately 3:1) (29). Probably some of the difference in the results can be explained by a high number of ultra-rapid or ultradian cases in those samples with a 1:1 ratio (as men are more represented in the ultra-rapid group). Hypothyroidism, higher use of antidepressant drugs and the role of female sexual hormones have been suggested to explain the high prevalence of women in rapid cycling bipolar disorder (28).

Rapid cycling is somehow rare in unipolar affective disorders; if rapid cycling is present in these patients, it is often associated with a positive family history for bipolar disorder (33). Most patients who at one time of their disease exhibit rapid cycling have also periods where they are free from any cycling (22,27,31). Rapid cycling per se probably does not affect the ratio of well being vs. time spent in an affective episode, while it seems quite evident that those rapid cyclers who directly switch from one episode into another episode of opposite polarity have an unfavorable course of their bipolar disorder as compared to patients with clear remission between episodes (34–36).

Patients with episodes of major depression exhibiting characteristics of pre-morbid cyclothymic temperament show a high risk of developing manic, particularly hypomanic episodes, and are probably particularly vulnerable to develop rapid cycling early in their life (20,37). Hyperthymic bipolars, particularly females, more often show the tardive onset type of rapid cycling (21).

As already mentioned, ultra-rapid and ultradian cyclicity can often be observed in youth and adolescence. In a report on 90 bipolar I patients (age 5–17), approximately half of them showed an elevated number of episodes with no or few free intervals (38). In another sample of 26 patients between 7 and 18 years, the duration of episodes was quite brief in 80% of the observed cases; in this study, rapid cycling was often associated with hyperactivity, mixed states, suicidality, and psychotic features (39). A further study on 60 bipolar children and adolescents confirmed that ultra-rapid and ultradian cases represent the most common phenotype in this age group (40).

In summary, the fact that ultradian rapid cycling is most common in young bipolar I patients (the male vs. female ratio being 1:1) suggests that factors linked to the evolution in childhood can be hold responsible for this prevalence. After puberty, the prevalence of rapid cycling reaches the same prevalence as in bipolar adults

(41). In adults, the classical forms prevail; they are more typically seen in women and are mostly of the bipolar II rather than bipolar I type (19,29).

In rapid cyclers the manic-depressive cycle usually begins with a depressive episode followed by mania/hypomania and finally by euthymia (D–M–E) (17,20,22). In some (20,22), but not all (26,27,31) studies, this pattern (D–M–E) was shown to be stable during the follow-up. In a recent study that examined the clinical characteristics and the course of bipolar patients in relationship to the depressive episodes followed by mania or euthymia, no differences were found in the length of the depressive episodes or the predisposition to cycling (42).

In the majority of studies, cases of rapid cycling are constituted by bipolar II patients with an onset of the disease after the 40th year of life (and starting with a depressive episode) (20,26,27,37,43–45). In these "classical" forms, substance abuse and mixed states are very rare and the episodes tend to have a clear demarcation from each other.

The results of two recent studies have confirmed these observations. In a study with 320 bipolar patients (43), those who began their disease with a depressive episode had an elevated risk of developing rapid cycling; while those who first presented with a mixed state had a higher risk to become chronic, with prevalence of mixed states and absence of rapid cycling. In this clinical population, mixed states and rapid cycling seamed to represent two different evolutions of bipolar disorder (43). In the second study (with a follow-up of 13.3 years), the risk of developing rapid cycling (observed in 15.6% of patients) was higher in bipolar II (30.3%) than in bipolar I disorder (6.0%). Premorbid cyclothymia was associated with rapid cycling, as was late onset and onset of the bipolar disease with a depressive episode (37).

As to other clinical characteristics, rapid cycling has been associated with comorbidity with other axis I disturbances, particularly with anxiety disorders and substance abuse (18). It remains unclear whether alcohol or drug abuse is linked to the induction of rapid cycling (19). While both substance abuse and ultradian cycling seem to be associated with early onset of the disease and male gender, further studies are needed to examine the role of substance abuse in rapid cycling. In this context, it has been suggested that the association of rapid cycling and female bipolar II disorder might be linked to the lack of comorbidity (46): in a study on 110 rapid cyclers who had recently abused or were dependent on alcohol, cannabis, or cocaine (or crack), most patients were male bipolar I cyclers (47). Finally, rapid cycling clearly shows an increased risk of suicide (3).

FAMILY HISTORY, GENETICS, AND RAPID CYCLING

Family history studies (48,49) have examined the risk of rapid cycling within bipolar families. Studies on molecular genetics have found an association of rapid cycling with the low activity catecholamine-*O*-methyltransferase allele (50,51).

THE ROLE OF ANTIDEPRESSANTS AND OF OTHER TREATMENTS

According to Kukopulos et al. (21), the prevalence of rapid cycling increased after the introduction of antidepressants in the 1960s. Indeed, it was observed that antidepressant drugs are able to induce switching from depression into hypomania/mania

(20–22,26,31,43). Possibly women have a higher risk to develop such a switch after antidepressant treatment (20,28).

It has been hypothesized that antidepressants might induce (and maintain) bipolar rapid cycling (26,27,43) by their capacity of increasing biogenic amines within the synaptic cleft (29). The prevalence of rapid cycling induced by antidepressants has been described as being within a wide range (of up to 50% of bipolar patients) (22,23); this prevalence can be considerably reduced by adding one or more mood stabilizers to the antidepressant.

It has been suggested that switching (and thus induction of rapid cycling) might be linked to noradrenergic function more than to serotoninergic function. Tricyclics and older monoamine oxidase inhibitors probably do not differ in their risk of inducing switches (22). It is unclear whether selective serotonin reuptake inhibitors have a lower risk of switching than tricyclics (19,31). In summary, data are not sufficient to demonstrate that antidepressants differ in their risk of inducing switches into hypomania or mania and thus in their risk of inducing rapid cycling.

It is an interesting question whether typical antipsychotics used for the treatment of manic episodes could cause switching into depression (52). Anyway, there are no data to support the hypothesis that typical antipsychotics might precipitate or cause rapid cycling. Modern atypical antipsychotics do not cause rapid cycling; they are widely used in the treatment of acute mania and as mood stabilizers including in patients with rapid cycling (52).

Lithium and the antiepileptic mood stabilizers do also not show any risk of inducing rapid cycling (52). (This includes the long-term use of lithium with its risk of iatrogenic hypothyroidism.)

THYROID FUNCTION AND RAPID CYCLING

In patients with rapid cycling, low thyroid hormone levels have been observed as well as elevated TSH values and other signs of hypothyroidism (25,53,54). Based on these observations, it has been suggested that hypothyroidism is a risk factor for the development of rapid cycling (25). In particular, a higher frequency of hypothyroidism was described in rapid cycling women (53), but it has also been hypothesized that the higher prevalence of women between rapid cyclers could increase the presence of hypothyroidism (without a real association between these two factors) (25). Indeed, several studies do not confirm a relationship between rapid cycling and thyroid function (22,25–27,30,31,55–57). Finally, in a study on patients receiving long-term treatment with lithium salts, the prevalence of rapid cycling was not increased in women with sub-clinic hypothyroidism (55).

RAPID CYCLING AND THE FEMALE REPRODUCTIVE CYCLE

Price and DiMarzio (58) first observed that female rapid cyclers more frequently exhibit a premenstrual syndrome than controls. This type of course seems to be more frequent post-partum (5,21); also estrogen replacement therapy has been linked to female rapid cycling (7). Other studies, however, showed that the female manic-depressive cycles were independent from the menstrual cycle (26), also suggesting that menopause is not linked to the risk of developing rapid cycling (22,25). A careful, prospective study on 25 premenopausal bipolar rapid cyclers did not show an influence of the menstrual cycle on mood oscillations (59). In conclusion, while an effect of the female reproductive cycle on the genesis of rapid cycling can not be excluded at present, this factor does not seem to be very strong.

RAPID CYCLING AND BIOLOGICAL RHYTHMS

It seems plausible that biological rhythms (60) play a role in the induction and the maintenance of rapid cycling: particularly sleep and sleep–wake manipulations (such as sleep deprivation) seem to be linked to changes in the course of affective disorders and thus the risk of switching and subsequent development of rapid cycling (61–69). This shows the importance of psychoeducative interventions such as the interpersonal and social rhythm therapy in order to manage "the chaos of bipolar disorder" (70). While biological factors of rapid mood rhythms remain somewhat unclear (71–75), the stabilization of social zeitgebers and biological rhythms are of crucial importance for the prophylaxis of rapid cycling in bipolar disorder (76–84).

PHARMACOLOGICAL TREATMENT OF RAPID CYCLING

The first treatment intervention for rapid cycling should always be the assessment (and treatment) of possibly underlying medical conditions such as hypothyroidism or alcohol and drug abuse. Furthermore, a careful evaluation of medication history can yield important information on a possible correlation between drug treatment (85–89) and consecutive rapid cycling.

Lithium Salts

Rapid cycling seems to be quite resistant to the treatment with lithium salts. This resistance was first described by Dunner and Fieve (5): 82% of rapid cyclers were lithium non-responders as compared to 41% of the non-rapid cycling patients.

Since this pivotal publication, several studies have shown the limitations of lithium salts in the treatment of rapid cycling (and of mixed states) (87,89,90): lithium seems to lack success particularly in patients with a pattern of depression–mania–euthymia (20,21): it is possible, though, that renunciation of antidepressant drugs could increase the effects of lithium on rapid cycling.

Valproate

Valproate seems to be more efficacious than lithium in the treatment of bipolar rapid cycling (19,91) showing considerable effects also in patients with ultra-rapid and ultradian cycling.

Carbamazepine and New Antiepileptics

Also carbamazepine has been associated with a favorable response in rapid cyclers (23): similarly to patients with mixed states, neurological comorbidity, mental retardation, or brain injury, carbamazepine seems superior to lithium in this group of patients. Further controlled data are needed (as for the possible treatment of rapid cyclers with other antiepileptic drugs such as oxcarbazepine, topiramate (92), or gabapentin).

In the group of the new antiepileptics, lamotrigine is the only substance that has shown efficacy in rapid cycling in a double-blind, placebo-controlled prophylaxis study: lamotrigine at present can be considered the first-line treatment for mood stabilization during bipolar depression and for the prophylaxis of bipolar rapid cycling (93) (particularly in those cases with a depression–mania–euthymia pattern—which are known to be highly lithium resistant).

Other Strategies

While the effects of hypothyroidism on the induction of rapid cycling seem somewhat unclear (25,55), levothyroxine seems to be an important option in the treatment of (intractable) rapid cycling (94).

Also electroconvulsive therapy has been described as successful treatment of intractable rapid cycling (95,96) and should be studied further.

The most promising new strategy for the treatment of rapid cycling remains the use of atypical antipsychotics (52). Particularly olanzapine has been shown to have highly beneficial effects on rapid cycling both as monotherapy (97) and as add-on-strategy (98) to other mood stabilizers.

CONCLUSIONS

Within bipolar disorders, the rapid cycling pattern is associated with female gender, age over 40, the bipolar II subtype and cyclothymic temperamental characteristics. Ultra-rapid and ultradian forms probably represent a distinct clinical and epidemiological group (probably placed on top of mixed states).

There is not enough evidence to suggest that rapid cycling is a distinct diagnosis; rapid cycling can thus be considered a variant form of bipolar disorders.

Careful treatment of bipolar depression seems to be crucial factor for the prophylaxis of rapid cycling (99). There is no conclusive evidence to support the use of one group of antidepressants over an other (100–103).

The use of mood stabilizers such as valproate (19,91) and lamotrigine (93) are of great importance in the prophylaxis and treatment of rapid cycling. Atypical antipsychotics will probably have an increasing role in the prophylaxis of rapid cycling (104–106), olanzapine has been shown to have beneficial effects in several controlled studies (97,98). ECT and levothyroxine are important options in treatment-resistant cases of rapid cycling.

In conclusion, diagnosis and treatment for rapid cycling should be further refined (107,108) to reduce the overall morbidity and mortality (108,109) of patients with this stable (110) course modifier.

REFERENCES

1. NIMH/NIH Consensus Development Conference Statement: mood disorders, pharmacologic prevention of recurrences. Am J Psychiatry 1985; 142:469–476.
2. Paykel ES, Priest RG. Recognition and management of depression in general practice: consensus statement. Br Med J 1992; 305:1198–2002.

3. Harris EC, Barraclough B. Suicide as an outcome for mental disorders. Br J Psychiatry 1997; 170:205–228.
4. Hirschfeld RMA. Clinical importance of long-term antidepressant treatment. Br J Psychiatry 2001; 179(suppl 42):4–8.
5. Dunner DC, Fieve RR. Clinical factors in lithium carbonate prophylaxis failure. Arch Gen Psychiatry 1974; 30:229–233.
6. American Psychiatric Association. Diagnostic and Statistical Manual of Mental Disorders, 4th revision, text revision (DSM-IV-TR™). American Psychiatric Press, 2000.
7. Alarcon RD. Rapid cycling affective disorders: a clinical review. Compr Psychiatry 1985; 26:522–540.
8. Kramliger KG, Post RM. Ultra-rapid and ultradian cycling in bipolar affective illness. Br J Psychiatry 1996; 168:314–323.
9. Bunney WE, Hartmann EL. Study of the patient with 48-hour manic-depressive cycles: Part I. Arch Gen Psychiatry 1965; 12:611–625.
10. Jenner FA, Gjessing LR, Cox JR, Davies-Gones A, Hullin RP, Hanna SM. A manic-depressive psychotic with a persistent forty-eight hour cycle. Br J Psychiatry 1967; 113:895–910.
11. Doerr P, von Zerssen D, Fischler M, Schulz H. Relationship between mood changes and adrenal cortical activity in a patient with 48-hour unipolar-depressive cycles. J Affect Disord 1979; 1:93–104.
12. Paschalis C, Pavlou A, Papadimitriou A. A stepped forty-eight hour manic-depressive cycle. Br J Psychiatry 1980; 137:332–336.
13. Trikkas G, Varsou E, Markianos E, Karandreas N, Stefanis C. Clinical and biological correlates of a 48-hour cycling manic-depressive patient. In: Stefanis CN, ed. Recent Advances in Depression. Oxford: Pergamon Press, 1983:109–116.
14. Juckel G, Hegerl U, Mavrogiorgou P, Gallinat J, Mager T, Tigges P, Dresel S, Schröter A, Stotz G, Meller I, Greil W, Möller HJ. Clinical and biological findings in a case with 48-hour bipolar ultra-rapid cycling before and during valproate treatment. J Clin Psychiatry 2000; 61:585–593.
15. Voderholzer U, Weske G, Ecker S, Riemann D, Gann H, Berger M. Neurobiological findings before and during successful lithium therapy of a patient with 48-hour rapid-cycling bipolar disorder. Neuropsychobiology 2002; 45(suppl 1):13–19.
16. Zis A, Goodwin F. Major affective disorder as a recurrent illness. Arch Gen Psychiatry 1979; 36:835–839.
17. Kilzieh N, Akiskal HS. Rapid-cycling bipolar disorder: an overview of recent research and clinical experience. Psychiatr Clin N Am 1999; 22:585–607.
18. McElroy SL, Altshuler LL, Suppes T, Keck PE Jr, Frye MA, Denicoff KD, Nolen WA, Kupka RW, Leverich GS, Rochussen JR, Rush AJ, Post RM. Axis I psychiatric comorbidity and its relationship to historical illness variables in 288 patients with bipolar disorder. Am J Psychiatry 2001; 158:420–426.
19. Calabrese JR, Shelton MD, Rapport DJ, Kujawa M, Kimmel SE, Caban S. Current research on rapid cycling bipolar disorder and its treatment. J Affect Disord 2001; 67:241–255.
20. Kukopulos A, Reginaldi D, Laddomada P, Floris G, Serra G, Tondo L. Course of the manic-depressive cycle and changes caused by treatment. Pharmakopsychiatr Neuropsychopharmakol 1980; 13:156–167.
21. Kukopulos A, Caliari B, Tundo A, Minnai G, Floris G, Reginaldi D, Tondo L. Rapid cyclers, temperament and antidepressants. Compr Psychiatry 1983; 24:249–258.
22. Wehr TA, Sack DA, Rosenthal NE, Cowdry RW. Rapid cycling affective disorder: contributing factors and treatment responses in 51 patients. Am J Psychiatry 1988; 145:179–184.
23. Goodwin FK, Jamison KR. Manic-Depressive Illness. New York: Oxford University Press, 1990.

24. Wolpert EA, Goldberg JF, Harrow M. Rapid cycling in unipolar and bipolar affective disorders. Am J Psychiatry 1990; 147:725–728.
25. Bauer M, Whybrow P, Winokur A. Rapid cycling bipolar affective disorder. I. Association with grade I hypothyroidism. Arch Gen Psychiatry 1990; 47:427–432.
26. Bauer MS, Calabrese J, Dunner DL, Post R, Whybrow PC, Gyulai L, Tay LK, Younkin SR, Bynum D, Lavori P, Price RA. Multisite data reanalysis of the validity of rapid cycling as a course modifier for bipolar disorder in DSM-IV. Am J Psychiatry 1994; 151:506–515.
27. Coryell W, Endicott J, Keller M. Rapidly cycling affective disorder: demographics, diagnosis, family history and course. Arch Gen Psychiatry 1992; 49:126–131.
28. Leibenluft E. Women with bipolar illness: clinical and research issues. Am J Psychiatry 1996; 153:163–173.
29. Tondo L, Baldessarini LU. Rapid cycling in women and men with bipolar manic-depressive disorders. Am J Psychiatry 1998; 155:1434–1436.
30. Joffe R, Kutcer S, MacDonald C. Thyroid function and bipolar affective disorder. Psychiatry Res 1987; 21:117–121.
31. Maj M, Magliano L, Pirozzi R, Marasco C, Guarneri M. Validity of rapid cycling as a course specifier for bipolar disorder. Am J Psychiatry 1994; 151:1015–1019.
32. Grunze H, Amann B, Dittmann S, Walden J. Clinical relevance and treatment possibilities of bipolar rapid cycling. Neuropsychobiology 2002; 45(suppl 1):20–26.
33. Tay LK, Dunner DL. A report of three patients with "rapid cycling" unipolar depression. Compr Psychiatry 1992; 33:253–255.
34. Maj M, Pirozzi R, Formicola AMR, Tortorella A. Reliability and validity of four alternative definitions of rapid cycling bipolar disorder. Am J Psychiatry 1999; 156:1421–1424.
35. Turvey CL, Coryell WH, Solomon DA, Leon AC, Endicott J, Keller MB, Akiskal H. Long-term prognosis of bipolar I disorder. Acta Psychiatr Scand 1999; 99:110–119.
36. Maj M, Pirozzi R, Magliano L, Bartoli L. The prognostic significance of "switching" in patients with bipolar disorder: a 10-year prospective follow-up study. Am J Psychiatry 2002; 159:1711–1717.
37. Baldessarini LU, Tondo L, Floris G, Hennen J. Effects of rapid cycling on response to lithium maintenance treatment in 360 bipolar I and bipolar II disorder patients. J Affect Dis 2000; 61:13–22.
38. Findling RL, Gracious BL, McNamara NK, Youngstrom EA, Demeter CA, Branicky LA, Calabrese JR. Rapid, continuous cycling and psychiatric co-morbidity in pediatric bipolar I disorder. Bipolar Disord 2001; 3:202–210.
39. Geller B, Sun K, Zimerman B, Luby J, Frazier J, Williams M. Complex and rapid-cycling in bipolar children and adolescents: a preliminary study. J Affect Disord 1995; 34:259–268.
40. Geller B, Williams M, Zimerman B, Frazier J, Beringer L, Warner K. Prepubertal and early adolescent bipolarity differentiate from ADHD by manic symptoms; grandiose delusions; ultra-rapid or ultradian cycling. J Affect Disord 1998; 51:81–91.
41. Geller B, Cook EH. Ultradian rapid cycling in prepubertal and early adolescent bipolarity is not in transmission disequilibrium with Val/Met COMT alleles. Biol Psychiatry 2000; 47:605–609.
42. Gitlin M, Boerlin H, Fairbanks L, Hammen C. The effect of previous mood states on switch rates: a naturalistic study. Bipolar Disord 2003; 5:150–152.
43. Perugi G, Micheli C, Akiskal HS, Madaro D, Socci C, Quilici C, Musetti L. Polarity of the first episode, clinical characteristics, and course of manic depressive illness: a systematic retrospective investigation of 320 bipolar I patients. Compr Psychiatry 2000; 41:13–18.
44. Suppes T, Dennehy EB. Evidence-based long-term treatment of bipolar II disorder. J Clin Psychiatry 2002; 63(suppl 10):29–33.

45. Judd LL, Paulus MJ, Schettler PJ, Akiskal HS, Endicott J, Leon AC, Maser JD, Mueller T, Solomon DA, Keller MB. Does incomplet recovery from first lifetime major depressive episode herald a chronic course of illness? Am J Psychiatry 2000; 157: 1501–1504.
46. Calabrese JR, Shelton MD, Bowden CL, Rapport DJ, Suppes T, Shirley ER, Kimmel SE, Caban SJ. Bipolar rapid cycling: focus on depression as its hallmark. J Clin Psychiatry 2001; 62:34–41.
47. Shelton MD, Rapport DJ, Youngstrom E, Packer K, Sak-Jackson K, Bilali S, Elhaj O, Findling R, Calabrese JR. Substance use disorders and their response to treatment in dual diagnosis bipolar disorder. Presented at the 2003 Meeting of the International Conference on Bipolar Disorders, Pittsburgh, PA, U.S.A.
48. Lish JD, Gyulai L, Resnick SM, Kirtland A, Amsterdam JD, Whybrow PC, Price RA. A family history study of rapid-cycling bipolar disorder. Psychiatry Res 1993; 48:37–45.
49. Nurnberger J, Guroff J, Hamovit J, Berrettini W, Gershon E. A family study of rapid-cycling bipolar illness. J Affect Disord 1988; 15:87–91.
50. Kirov G, Murphy KC, Arranz MJ, Jones I, McCandles F, Cunugi H, Murray RM, McGuffin P, Collier DA, Owen MJ, Craddock N. Low activity allele of catechola-mine-*O*-methyltransferase gene associated with rapid cycling bipolar disorder. Mol Psychiatry 1998; 3:342–345.
51. Papolos DF, Veit S, Faedda GL, Saito T, Lachman HM. Ultra–ultra rapid cycling bipolar disorder is associated with the low activity catecholamine-*O*-methyltransferase allele. Mol Psychiatry 1998; 3:346–349.
52. Yatham LN, Calabrese JR, Kusumakar V. Bipolar depression: criteria for treatment selection, definition of refractoriness, and treatment options. Bipolar Disord 2003; 5: 85–97.
53. Cowdry R, Wehr T, Zis A, Goodwin F. Thyroid abnormalities associated with rapid cycling bipolar illness. Arch Gen Psychiatry 1983; 40:414–420.
54. Kusalic M. Grade II and grade III hypothyroidism in rapid cycling bipolar patients. Neuropsychobiology 1992; 25:177–181.
55. Oomen HA, Schipperijn AJ, Drexhage HA. The prevalence of affective disorder and in particular of a rapid cycling of bipolar disorder in patients with abnormal thyroid function tests. Clin Endocrinol 1996; 45:215–223.
56. Post RM, Kramlinger KG, Joffe RT, Roy-Byrne P, Rosoff A, Frye MA, Huggins T. Rapid cycling bipolar affective disorder: lack of relation to hypothyroidism. Psychiatry Res 1997; 72:1–7.
57. Kupka RW, Nolen WA, Post RM, McElroy SL, Altshuler LL, Denicoff KD, Frye MA, Keck PE Jr, Leverich GS, Rush JA, Suppes T, Pollio C, Drexhage HA. High rate of autoimmune thyroiditis in bipolar disorder: lack of association with lithium exposure. Biol Psychiatry 2002; 51:305–311.
58. Price WA, DiMarzio L. Premenstrual tension syndrome in rapid cycling bipolar affective disorder. J Clin Psychiatry 1986; 47:415–417.
59. Leibenluft E, Ashman BS, Feldman-Naim S, Yonkers KA. Lack of relationship between menstrual cycle phase and mood in a sample of women with rapid cycling bipolar disorder. Biol Psychiatry 1999; 46:577–580.
60. Linkowski P, Mendlewicz J, Leclercq R, Brasseur M, Hubain Ph, Goldstein J, Copinchi G, van Cauter E. The 24-hour profile of adrenocorticotropin and cortisol in major depressive illness. J Clin Endocrinol Metab 1985; 61:429–438.
61. Mendlewicz J, Sevy S, DeMaertelaer V. REM sleep latency and morbidity risk of affective disorders in depressive illness. Neuropsychobiology 1989; 22:14–17.
62. Soldatos C, Paparrigopoulos T. Sleep patterns in depression. WPA Teach Bull 1996; 2:4–5.
63. Riemann D, Voderholzer U, Berger M. Sleep and sleep–wake manipulations in bipolar depression. Neuropsychobiology 2002; 45(suppl 1):7–12.

64. Berger M, Vollmann J, Hohagen F, Koning A, Lohner H, Voderholzer U, Riemann D. Sleep deprivation combined with consecutive sleep phase advance as a fast-acting therapy in depression: An open pilot trial in medicated and unmedicated patients. Am J Psychiatry 1997; 154:870–872.
65. Christodoulou GN, Malliaras DE, Lykouras EP, Papadimitriou GN, Stefanis CN. Possible prophylactic effect of sleep deprivation. Am J Psychiatry 1978; 135:375–376.
66. Wu JC, Bunney WE. The biological basis of an antidepressant response to sleep deprivation and relapse: review and hypothesis. Am J Psychiatry 1990; 147:14–21.
67. Papadimitriou GN, Christodoulou GN, Katsouyanni K, Stefanis CN. Therapy and prevention of affective disorders by sleep deprivation. J Affect Disord 1993; 27:107–116.
68. Leibenluft E, Albert PS, Rosenthal NE, Wehr TA. Relationship between sleep and mood in patients with rapid-cycling bipolar disorder. Psychiatry Res 1996; 63:161–168.
69. Feldman-Naim S, Turner EH, Leibenluft E. Diurnal variation in the direction of mood switches in patients with rapid-cycling bipolar disorder. J Clin Psychiatry 1997; 58: 79–84.
70. Frank E, Swartz HA, Kupfer DJ. Interpersonal and social rhythm therapy: managing the chaos of bipolar disorder. Biol Psychiatry 2000; 48:593–604.
71. Illnerova H, Vanecek J. Two-oscillator structure of the pacemaker controlling the circadian rhythm of *N*-acetyltransferase in the rat pineal gland. J Compr Physiol 1982; 145:539–548.
72. Wehr TA, Moul DE, Barbato G, Giesen HA, Seidel SA, Barker C, Bender C. Conservation of photoperiod-responsive mechanisms in humans. Am J Physiol 1993; 265: 846–857.
73. Dilsaver SC, Greden GF. Antidepressant withdrawal-induced activation (hypomania and mania): is withdrawal-induced cholinergic overdrive causally significant? J Clin Psychopharmacol 1984; 4:174–175.
74. Ko GN, Leckman JF, Heninger JR. Induction of rapid mood cycling during L-DOPA treatment in a bipolar patient. Am J Psychiatry 1981; 138:1624–1625.
75. Joyce PR, Fergusson DM, Woolard G, Abbott RM, Horwood LJ, Upton J. Urinary catecholamines and plasma hormones predict mood state in rapid cycling bipolar affective disorder. J Affect Disord 1995; 33:233–243.
76. Ehlers CL, Frank E, Kupfer DJ. Social zeitgebers and biological rhythms. Arch Gen Psychiatry 1988; 45:948–952.
77. Leibenluft E, Clark CH, Myers FS. The reproducibility of depressive and hypomanic symptoms across repeated episodes in patients with rapid-cycling bipolar disorder. J Affect Disord 1995; 33:83–88.
78. Ashman SB, Monk TH, Kupfer DJ, Clark CH, Myers FS, Frank E, Leibenluft E. Relationship between social rhythms and mood in patients with rapid cycling bipolar disorder. Psychiatry Res 1999; 86:1–8.
79. Paykel ES, Tanner J. Life-events, depressive relapse and maintenance treatment. Psychol Med 1976; 6:481–485.
80. Post RM. Transduction of psychosocial stress into the neurobiology of recurrent affective disorder. Am J Psychiatry 1992; 149:999–1010.
81. Papadimitriou GN, Dikeos DG, Daskalopoulou EG, Stefanis CN. Affective disorders and self-esteem: a clinical study. XXI CINP Congress 1998; Book of Abstracts, p. 294.
82. Post RM, Rubinow DR, Ballenger JC. Conditioning and sensitization in the longitudinal course of affective illness. Br J Psychiatry 1986; 149:191–201.
83. Sklar AD, Harris RF. Effects of parent loss: interaction with family size and sibling order. Am J Psychiatry 1985; 142:708–714.
84. Cutler NR, Post RM. Life course of illness in untreated manic-depressive patients. Compr Psychiatry 1982; 23:101–115.
85. Wehr TA, Goodwin FK. Rapid cycling in manic-depressives induced by tricyclic antidepressants. Arch Gen Psychiatry 1979; 36:555–559.

86. Wehr TA, Goodwin FK. Can antidepressants cause mania and worsen the course of affective illness? Am J Psychiatry 1987; 144:1403–1411.
87. Prien R, Kupfer D, Mansky P, Small J, Tuason V, Voss C, Johnson W. Drug therapy in the prevention of recurrences in unipolar and bipolar affective disorders: report of the NIMH Collaborative Study Group comparing lithium carbonate, imipramine, and a lithium carbonate–imipramine combination. Arch Gen Psychiatry 1984; 41:1096–1104.
88. Altshuler L, Post RM, Leverich GS, Mikalauskas K, Roogg A, Ackerman L. Antidepressant-induced manic and cyclic acceleration: a controversy revisited. Am J Psychiatry 1995; 152:1130–1138.
89. Calabrese JR, Rapport DJ, Kimmel SE, Shelton MD. Controlled trials in bipolar I depression: focus on switch rates and efficacy. Eur Neuropsychopharmacol 1999; 9 (suppl 4):109–112.
90. Ghaemi SN. On defining "mood stabilizer." Bipolar Disord 2001; 3:154–158.
91. Erfurth A, Michael N, Grunze H, Walden J. Treatment of mixed affective states and of rapid cycling: therapeutic options beyond lithium. Nervenheilkunde 2001; 20(suppl 2): S39–S40.
92. Erfurth A, Kuhn G. Topiramate monotherapy in the maintenance treatment of bipolar I disorder: effects on mood, weight and serum lipids. Neuropsychobiology 2000; 42(suppl 1):50–51.
93. Calabrese JR, Suppes T, Bowden CL et al. A double-blind, placebo-controlled, prophylaxis study of lamotrigine in rapid cycling bipolar disorder. Lamictal 614 Study Group. Clin Psychiatry 2000; 61:841–850.
94. Stancer HC, Persad E. Treatment of intractable rapid-cycling manic-depressive disorder with levothyroxine. Arch Gen Psychiatry 1982; 39:311–312.
95. Kho KH. Treatment of rapid cycling bipolar disorder in the acute and maintenance phase with ECT. J ECT 2002; 18:159–161.
96. Berman E, Wolpert EA. Intractable manic-depressive psychosis with rapid cycling in an 18-year-old woman successfully treated with electroconvulsive therapy. J Nerv Ment Dis 1987; 175:236–239.
97. Vieta E, Calabrese R, Hennen J, et al. Comparison of rapid-cycling and non-rapid-cycling bipolar I manic patients during treatment with olanzapine: analysis of pooled data. J Clin Psychiatry 2004; 65:1420–1428.
98. Tohen M, Chengappa KN, Suppes T, et al. Efficacy of olanzapine in combination with valproate or lithium in the treatment of mania in patients partially nonresponsive to valproate or lithium monotherapy. Arch Gen Psychiatry 2002; 59:62–69.
99. Thase ME, Sachs GS. Bipolar depression: pharmacotherapy and related therapeutic strategies. Biol Psychiatry 2000; 48:558–572.
100. Extein I, Potter WZ, Wehr TA. Rapid mood cycles after a noradrenergic but not a serotonergic antidepressant. Am J Psychiatry 1979; 136:1602–1603.
101. Peet M. Induction of mania with selective serotonin re-uptake inhibitors and tricyclic antidepressants. Br J Psychiatry 1994; 164:549–550.
102. Haykal RF, Akiskal HS. Bupropion as a promising approach to rapid cycling bipolar II patients. J Clin Psychiatry 1990; 51:450–455.
103. Kupfer DJ, Carpenter LL, Frank E. Possible role of antidepressants in precipitating mania and hypomania in recurrent depression. Am J Psychiatry 1988; 145:804–808.
104. Thase ME. What role do atypical antipsychotic drugs have in treatment-resistant depression? J Clin Psychiatry 2002; 63:95–103.
105. Vieta E. Atypical antipsychotics in the treatment of mood disorders. Curr Opin Psychiatry 2003; 16:23–27.
106. Suppes T, Ozcan ME. Carmody T. Response to clozapine of rapid cycling vs. non-cycling patients with a history of mania. Bipolar Disord 2004; 6:329–332.
107. Mackin P, Young AH. Rapid cycling bipolar disorder: historical overview and focus on emerging treatments. Bipolar Disord 2004; 6:523–529.

108. Schneck CD, Miklowitz DJ, Calabrese JR, et al. Phenomenology of rapid-cycling bipolar disorder: data from the first 500 participants in the Systematic Treatment Enhancement Program. Am J Psychiatry 2004; 161:1902–1908.
109. Coryell W, Solomon D, Turvey C, et al. The long-term course of rapid-cycling bipolar disorder. Arch Gen Psychiatry 2003; 60:914–920.
110. Koukopoulos A, Sani G, Koukopoulos AE, et al. Duration and stability of the rapid-cycling course: a long-term personal follow-up of 109 patients. J Affect Disord 2003; 73:75–85.

14
Long-Term Mood Stabilization

Zubin Bhagwagar and Guy M. Goodwin
University Department of Psychiatry, Warneford Hospital, Oxford, U.K.

Because it is a serious, chronic, and disabling condition, the long-term treatment of bipolar disorder is of critical importance. Indeed, bipolar disorder has been calculated to have a greater impact as a disability than schizophrenia, diabetes mellitus, or HIV (1). Estimates of its prevalence range from 1.5% to 5% depending on the definitions used (2,3). The lifetime risk of suicide in patients with a diagnosis of bipolar disorder ranges from 8% to 20% (4,5) and in a sample of nearly 10,000 patients with recurrent affective disorder (primarily bipolar), approximately 19% of deaths were attributable to suicide (4).

RECURRENCE IN BIPOLAR DISORDER

Kraepelin (6) first highlighted, in a systematic manner, the pattern of fluctuations of symptoms in mania and depression and described it as a cyclical illness. This has probably led to the common conceptualization of the illness as episodic: It is only relatively recently that there has been an understanding of the chronicity of bipolar disorder. The common presence of subsyndromal symptoms mean that the "episodic" nature of the illness is often questionable and that adequate long-term prophylaxis is crucial and necessary for optimal management of the condition.

Weekly evaluations of the illness profile have suggested that the primary burden of the illness in the long term lies in the depressive pole. Symptoms in the depressive spectrum predominate over manic (3:1) or mixed (5:1) symptoms (7). Its chronicity is emphasized in the same study since patients with a diagnosis of bipolar disorder type I were symptomatically ill 47% of weeks throughout a mean follow-up duration of nearly 13 years. Syndromal relapse is also a major problem, however. While the natural course of the illness has been described as being variable, it is clear that more than 90% of individuals who experience a manic episode will go on to develop future episodes (8). Despite continuous maintenance treatment, survival analysis indicated a 5-year risk of relapse into mania or depression of 73% and of those who relapsed, two-thirds had multiple relapses.

WHAT IS A MOOD STABILIZER?

The long-term prophylaxis of a patient with bipolar disorder traditionally rests with the small group of medicines designated "mood stabilizers." However, there is little or no consensus agreement on the definition of this term (9,10). The ideal mood stabilizer would be an agent that prevents new episodes of either pole of the illness, as proven in a long-term relapse prevention or maintenance study. Unfortunately, the term has been uncritically granted to some anticonvulsants in advance of adequate evidence. Moreover, in practice, most agents may be more efficacious in the prevention of one pole of illness than the other.

Accordingly, a more realistic definition of a mood stabilizer is any medicine that decreases the frequency or severity of episodes at one pole of the illness without worsening the other pole of the illness. This definition demands clinical trials for every putative mood stabilizer with sufficient power to define the risks of relapse to depression and mania, whereas, when we have trials at all, they more usually conflate both outcomes. Furthermore, the concept of partial mood stabilization implicitly accepts the likely need for treatment with combinations of individually less than ideal agents.

It has recently been suggested that a more conservative "two by two" definition be met before an agent is accepted as a mood stabilizer (11). Thus, a mood stabilizer would be expected to treat both acute mania and depression and prevent further manic or depressive symptoms/episodes. Based on this rather stringent definition, it has been shown that probably only lithium meets the criteria to be called a mood stabilizer. No other medicine currently meets these criteria even when a relaxation of the criteria was attempted.

In practice, the value of the term mood stabilizer will depend upon how it is to be used, and how it influences practice. The risk of a too liberal definition is polypharmacy, with many poorly characterized medicines adopted for long-term use—this is a major current concern in North America. The risk of a conservative definition may be under-treatment—lithium or nothing. We favor a more liberal definition, supported by monotherapy data, but also a recognition of the need for trials of combination treatment in their own right.

PHARMACOLOGICAL TREATMENT

Pharmacological treatments have been the mainstay of the long-term management of bipolar disorder. However, there is a dearth of well-conducted randomized controlled trials (RCTs) in this field. Interpretation of the early data is also confounded by the short duration of trials, the lack of placebo control, inclusion of schizoaffective or unipolar depressed patients, and the rebound illness associated with the rapid withdrawal of lithium. Nevertheless, recent renewed interest in maintenance indications for new medicines has produced a new body of evidence for the efficacy of a several agents and promises to revive thinking on how to treat patients long term.

Lithium

Lithium has long been the gold standard treatment for the prophylaxis of bipolar disorder. The initial data on the efficacy of lithium were obtained when trial designs and protocols were of a different standard to what is expected today. As already indicated, this led to doubts about the strength of the evidence. Nevertheless as a testimony to its reputation, lithium has been almost routinely used as an active comparator in trials of newer agents yielding, perhaps inadvertently, high-quality data on its clinical efficacy.

The Evidence to 2000

At least 10 placebo-controlled trials in the 1970s and 1980s were taken to have established the efficacy of lithium in the prevention of manic and depressive episodes (12–21). While there are considerable and significant differences between these trials in study design, end points, number of patients, duration of follow-up, and psychiatric status at entry, almost all seem to suggest the superiority of lithium over placebo in the prevention of episodes of depression or mania. Some studies did not distinguish the primary outcome but suggested that lithium seemed to be more effective than placebo in the overall prevention of episodes of relapse (12–16). Two studies where manic relapses were specifically defined as the primary outcome measure showed that lithium was more effective than placebo (17,19). Of the studies that made a specific mention of depressive relapses as the outcome measure (17–19), all but one (19) suggested that lithium was superior to placebo in the prevention of depressive episodes.

A drawback of these trials was the random assignment of abrupt lithium discontinuation. Only two trials studied participants stabilized on lithium regimens before random assignment to treatment with gradual withdrawal (and studied a homogenous group of patients). Prien et al. (16) studied 205 patients with mania randomly assigned to lithium (0.5–1.4 meq/L) or placebo with follow-up for 2 years and found relapse rates of 41% in the lithium group vs. 81% in the placebo group. It was not clear, however, whether lithium was more effective against depressive or manic relapses. Another study examined a much smaller cohort ($N = 22$) of patients with bipolar disorder type II randomly assigned to treatment regimens using lithium carbonate, imipramine hydrochloride, lithium carbonate plus imipramine, or placebo with a 2-year follow-up (20). Lithium seemed to prevent relapses in general compared with placebo (20% vs. 67%), with effectiveness being demonstrated for the manic (0% vs. 17% relapse), and depressive (20% vs. 50%) poles of the illness.

Recent Evidence (2000 Onward)

The first of the new trials was designed primarily to study the efficacy of divalproex, as prophylactic therapy for bipolar disorder (22). Although the placebo arm failed to separate from the active arms—event rates were low, and the study allowed recruitment of some patients who had minor or questionable bipolar I disorder—it is nevertheless a seminal study. It was a randomized, double-blind, parallel-group multicenter study of treatment outcomes conducted over a 52-week maintenance period. Patients who met the recovery criteria within 3 months of the onset of an index manic episode ($N = 372$) were randomized to maintenance treatment with divalproex, lithium, or placebo in a 2:1:1 ratio. While failing on the hard primary outcome of admission to hospital, secondary analysis and trial experience helped to shape the design of future studies. For example, a lower threshold for relapse has allowed easier recruitment, higher event rates and hence greater assay sensitivity in subsequent studies.

Hence, two successful trials designed to study the efficacy of the novel anticonvulsant lamotrigine in the management of bipolar depression also used lithium as an active comparator (23,24). In a trial examining the efficacy of lamotrigine in the prevention of recurrence in patients following a depressive episode, patients stabilized on open-label treatment ($N = 463$) were randomly assigned to lamotrigine (50, 200, or 400 mg/day; $N = 221$), lithium (0.8–1.1 meq/L; $N = 121$), or placebo ($N = 121$) monotherapy for up to 18 months (24). Time to intervention for any mood episode was statistically superior ($p = 0.029$) for lithium compared with placebo with median survival times 170 and 93 days, respectively. Lithium was statistically superior to placebo at prolonging the time to intervention for a manic or hypomanic episode ($p = 0.026$) with median survival times of 86 and 72, respectively. Lithium was also superior to placebo with regards to survival in the study ($p = 0.022$) with median survival times of 86 and 46, respectively. However, lithium was not different from placebo in preventing episodes of depression ($p = 0.209$; median survival times of 46 and 47 days, respectively). Tremor, somnolence, diarrhea, and headache were the commonest reported side effects in the lithium group, who received doses of that ensured relatively high lithium levels (target 0.8 mmol/L).

The second study examining the efficacy of lamotrigine in the prophylaxis of bipolar disorder studied a smaller group of patients with an index episode of mania (23). Similar to the previous study, after an 8- to 16-week open-label phase during which treatment with lamotrigine was initiated and other psychotropic medicine regimens were discontinued, patients ($N = 175$) were randomized to lamotrigine (100–400 mg daily), lithium (0.8–1.1 meq/L), or placebo as double-blind maintenance treatment for as long as 18 months. Lithium was superior to placebo in prolonging the time to intervention for any mood episode (lithium vs. placebo, $p = 0.003$; median survival times 292 vs. 85 days, respectively). Lithium was superior to placebo in prolonging the time to a manic, hypomanic, or mixed episode ($p = 0.006$; median survival for lithium was not estimable as the probability of survival for patients on lithium was above 50% throughout the trial, placebo mean survival 203 days). However, lithium was not superior to placebo for the prevention of a depressive episode ($p = 0.17$; median survival time for lithium was not estimable as the probability of survival for patients on lithium was above 50% throughout the trial, placebo mean survival time 269 days).

The new data have allowed a new meta-analysis of long-term lithium therapy for the prophylaxis of bipolar disorder (25). Five RCTs (770 participants) were included and lithium was shown to be more effective than placebo in preventing all relapses (random effects relative risk = 0.65, 95% CI = 0.50–0.84) and manic relapses (relative risk = 0.62, 95% CI = 0.40–0.95). The protective effect of lithium on depressive relapses was smaller and was less robust (relative risk = 0.72, 95% CI = 0.49–1.07).

Taken together, these data conclusively show that lithium is superior to placebo in the maintenance of euthymia. This effect seems to be driven by clear efficacy against the recurrence of manic episodes while the data suggest that lithium may not be as effective in the prophylaxis of depressive episodes.

Olanzapine

There is now good evidence that several atypical antipsychotics are effective in the treatment of acute mania (26–32). In parallel, there has been a drive to use these agents in the long-term prophylaxis of bipolar disorder because their improved tolerance, largely due to fewer motor side effects, increases the scope for the use of antipsychotics in a range of disorders. Olanzapine has been the best studied in this regard, although most of the data are not yet fully in the public domain. For example, a 47-week, randomized, double-blind study has compared flexibly dosed olanzapine (5–20 mg/day) to divalproex (500–2500 mg/day) for the treatment of manic or mixed episodes of bipolar disorder ($N = 251$) (33). This study had a high dropout rate with nearly 85% patients withdrawing from both groups by the end of the trial. The improvement with olanzapine on the Young Mania Rating Scale was superior to that with valproate in the early phase of the trial (from weeks 2 to 15) but there was no difference between the two treatments subsequently. Further studies have compared olanzapine with placebo in a relapse prevention design and olanzapine with lithium in acute responders to a combination of both agents. The preliminary presentations suggest olanzapine has a similar profile to lithium—with greater efficacy against manic relapse.

Therefore together with the clear evidence that olanzapine is effective in the acute management of manic illness, data supporting its use in the prophylaxis of bipolar disorder are also emerging.

Valproate

Despite evidence for its efficacy in acute mania (34), the long-term study described above failed to find a difference between valproate and placebo on the primary outcome (22). Secondary analyses of this trial have been given a positive interpretation. Thus, divalproex was superior to placebo in terms of lower rates of discontinuation for either a recurrent mood episode or depressive episode. Divalproex was superior to lithium in longer duration of successful prophylaxis in the study and less deterioration in depressive symptoms and Global Assessment Scale scores.

The modest evidence base supporting the use of valproate remains at odds with its widespread preference to lithium as a first line long-term treatment in North America.

Lamotrigine

The two placebo-controlled RCTs of lamotrigine in the long-term management of bipolar disorder provide good evidence for its efficacy and how it compares with lithium (23,24). Following an index episode of mania or hypomania, lamotrigine was superior to placebo in the time to intervention for any mood episode ($p = 0.02$; median time for survival 85 vs. 58 days, respectively) with no significant differences between lamotrigine and lithium ($p = 0.46$; median time for survival 85 vs. 101 days, respectively). Following an index episode of depression, lamotrigine was significantly superior to placebo in the time to intervention of any mood episode ($p = 0.029$; median survival time 256 days for lamotrigine 200 mg/day vs. 93 days, respectively), with, again, no difference between lamotrigine and lithium. Thus, the main strength of lamotrigine seemed to lie in its efficacy in preventing depressive relapses while lithium has the complementary property of showing slightly more of an effect against relapse to mania.

The use of lamotrigine is made more uncertain by the limited data favoring efficacy in acute bipolar depression, and the practical problems of the slow taper in of therapeutic doses, made necessary by the risk of serious rash. Lamotrigine also has pharmacokinetic interactions with valproate (the lamotrigine dose should be halved) and carbamazepine (when the dose may be doubled).

Other Medicines

Carbamazepine has been used longer than any other except lithium in the management of bipolar disorder, but without the same body of evidence. The trials supporting the efficacy of carbamazepine in acute mania are confounded by small numbers, diagnostic heterogeneity (inclusion of patients with schizoaffective disorder), adjunctive treatments like lithium, and short duration. In maintenance treatment of bipolar disorder, carbamazepine is not as effective as lithium (35–39).

Antidepressants have also often been used as maintenance treatment for the prophylaxis of episodes of depression, but with little high-quality trial data to support their use. In a 2-year follow-up study, 117 bipolar patients received lithium carbonate, imipramine hydrochloride, and both (40). Lithium carbonate and the combination treatment were superior to imipramine in preventing manic recurrences and were as effective as imipramine in preventing depressive episodes. Similar results were seen with another trial with a smaller number of patients (20). Hence, the main concern with the long-term use of antidepressants during the treatment of bipolar disorder has been the induction of switch to the manic pole of the illness, especially when used without the cover of a mood-stabilizing agent (41). Indeed, the use of antidepressants as monotherapy in the prophylaxis of bipolar I disorder is not recommended (42).

There is a complete absence of long-term double-blind RCTs of medicines such as topiramate and gabapentin in the prophylaxis of bipolar disorder, despite their frequent designation as "mood stabilizers."

Combining Medicines

Cancer chemotherapy has been transformed in the last 40 years not by new medicines, but by the use of individually ineffective and toxic medicines *in combination*. Clinical trials have established the efficacy and tolerability of the successful regimens. Psychiatry still awaits the results of the first randomized trials to prove that combinations are also truly effective in treating bipolar disorder. Combinations are the standard approach after monotherapy has been seen to fail. A logical combination therapy would appear to require two (or even more?) largely antimanic agents when mania is the primary problem and an antidepressant and/or lamotrigine with an antimanic agent when depression is the main problem (42). However, we need pragmatic trials to establish just how effective such an approach is.

SUICIDE PREVENTION IN BIPOLAR DISORDER

The lifetime risk of suicide in patients with a diagnosis of bipolar disorder ranges from 8% to 20% (4,5). It reflects the major burden of illness caused by the depressive component in bipolar disorders. Suicide rates, averaging 0.4% per year in men and women diagnosed with bipolar disorder, are more than 20-fold higher than in the general population (43). Suicide and self-harm may occur early in the illness course and in association with severe depressive and mixed phases of illness.

Individual RCTs have been under-powered to investigate suicide rates. Hence, most of our understanding of the issue comes from naturalistic studies. There has been a strong suggestion that patients on lithium tend to have lower rates of suicide either compared with themselves off lithium or with other patients who are not on lithium. Based on a literature synthesis, risks for all suicidal acts/100 person-years averaged 3.10 without lithium versus 0.210 during treatment versus approximately 0.315 for the general population (44). The corresponding rates were 4.65 versus 0.312 for suicide attempts and 0.942 versus 0.174 for completed suicides. Subjects with bipolar versus various recurrent major affective disorders showed similar benefits (95% versus 91% sparing of all suicidal acts). A meta-analysis also suggests that suicide rates on versus off lithium are significantly different and this effect seemed independent of treatment discontinuation (45). Among 5647 patients studied, suicide was much less frequent during lithium treatment (0.159 vs. 0.875 deaths/100 patient-years), and the computed risk ratio in studies with rates on/off lithium was 8.85.

A recent population-based sample of 20,638 health plan members in two North American states with a diagnosis of bipolar disorder compared suicide attempts or suicide deaths in bipolar patients on olanzapine or divalproex treatment (46). After adjusting for age, sex, health plan, year of diagnosis, comorbid medical and psychiatric conditions, and concomitant use of other psychotropic agents risk of dying by suicide was 2.7 times higher during treatment with divalproex than during treatment with lithium. The corresponding hazard ratios for non-fatal attempts for attempts resulting in hospitalization (1.7) and attempts diagnosed in the emergency department (1.8) were also significantly in favor of lithium treatment.

It would be premature to take these data as conclusive. Naturalistic studies are subject to a range of inherent and uncorrectable biases. At best they can generate hypotheses, not prove or disprove them. They should be the prelude to systematic review of individually inconclusive RCTs or the conduct of trials of sufficient power to prove that one treatment is superior to another in reducing key outcomes like suicide.

It is possible to study suicidality as an outcome in RCTs. Data from a multicenter, randomized, international, 2-year study comparing the risk for suicidal behavior in patients treated with clozapine versus olanzapine in 980 patients with schizophrenia or schizoaffective disorder has been reported (47). Suicidal behavior was significantly less in patients treated with clozapine versus olanzapine and fewer clozapine-treated patients attempting suicide, or requiring rescue interventions to prevent suicide.

It is tempting to suppose that we can achieve a reduction of mortality—mainly the risk of suicide—with adequate treatment. Indeed, it must be a primary objective for any medical intervention. For the moment, the best evidence in bipolar disorder supports a strategy based on the use of lithium.

PSYCHOLOGICAL INTERVENTIONS

While it is a widely accepted consensus that pharmacological interventions are necessary for the treatment of bipolar disorder, it is equally clear that they are not sufficient for the management of the patient. The added utility of psychological interventions to complement treatment with medicines is now widely accepted as good, not just ideal, practice. Their nature and objectives—maintaining periods of euthymia in conjunction with medication—mean they are best delivered in periods of remission.

Improving Treatment Adherence

In a large-scale pharmacy study of over 1500 patients, Johnson and McFarland (48) reported that the median duration of continuous use of lithium after it was first prescribed was only 76 days (48). A study of patient treatment adherence found that about 50% of individuals stopped their medication at least once against medical advice in the preceding 2 years (49). Reported non-adherence rates for long-term prophylactic pharmacotherapy range from 20% to 66% with a median prevalence of 41% (50). Individuals who had been non-adherent with medication were significantly more likely to be concerned by missing highs and by the hassle associated with taking medication. Even in the 47-week study of olanzapine and valproate described above, 85% of patients withdrew from the trial in both groups (33).

In fact, non-adherence with medication regimes is a major issue in all chronic disorders when largely asymptomatic patients are often obliged to accept indefinite treatment to prevent possible bad outcomes. Some way of increasing adherence (also known as compliance, or even concordance) needs to be implemented early to ensure an optimal outcome (51). Exactly what is best to achieve this is uncertain. A pilot study of concordance therapy (CCT)—combining education, coaching, and motivational interviewing—showed that statistically significant improvements in attitudes towards lithium were associated with improvements in self-reported adherence (52). These results were also supported by laboratory results demonstrating statistically significant increases in serum plasma lithium levels.

Improved adherence may be a non-specific effect of other psychological treatments. A study of cognitive therapy specifically designed to prevent relapses for bipolar affective disorder showed encouraging results when used in conjunction with mood stabilizers, part of the effect being associated with improved adherence (53). Cognitive therapy resulted in significantly fewer bipolar episodes, days in a bipolar episode, and number of admissions for this type of episode with significantly higher social functioning.

A study of combination family-focused therapy (FFT) with pharmacotherapy during a post-episode interval showed that patients undergoing FFT had fewer relapses and longer survival intervals than patients undergoing routine crisis management and pharmacotherapy (54). Patients undergoing FFT also showed better medication adherence during the 2 years than patients undergoing CM.

Psychoeducation

The effect of "psychoeducation" as it is often called has been shown to decrease relapse rates in bipolar I patients who were largely adherent to treatment (55). The action of psychoeducation thus seems to go beyond enhancement of adherence. It suggests a model composed of three components—lifestyle regularity and healthy habits, early detection of prodromal signs followed by prompt medical intervention, and treatment compliance.

Specific Therapies

The principles of interpersonal and social rhythm therapy (IPSRT), a treatment that is specifically designed for patients with bipolar disorder, derive from a psychochronobiological theory of affective illness and the relationship between stressful life events and bipolar episodes (56–58). It has been hypothesized that social *zeitgebers* (personal relationships, social demands, or tasks that entrain biological rhythms) and *zeitstörers* (time disturbers) may serve as the link between the biological and psychosocial processes that place an individual at risk for developing mood symptoms (see Ref. 59 for review).

In an initial report based on 39 subjects with bipolar I disorder, it was shown that life events (regardless of severity of threat) characterized by a high degree of social disruption were associated with the onset of manic but not depressive episodes (60). This observation was confirmed in a follow-up study showing that life events associated with a high degree of social disruption occurring in the 8 weeks before the onset of an episode were more frequently associated with the onset of manic episodes relative to bipolar cycling, bipolar depressed, or unipolar depressive episodes (61). Subsequent therapeutic intervention has not demonstrated a high specificity for IPSRT and the same may also be true for CBT.

It is difficult to decide whether enhanced care results from relatively non-specific increases in patient understanding and non-specific intervention, or whether very specific issues are critical. Most of the treatment approaches have many different components, but education, self-monitoring, and an emphasis on patient initiative tend to be common to all. How far simple improvements in good, but everyday, practice can achieve treatment enhancement remains to be demonstrated.

WHEN TO START LONG-TERM TREATMENT AND FOR WHOM

Since lithium was first introduced into clinical practice, the policy of when to start it has been a conservative one. Patients have been offered treatment after two episodes in 3 years or three episodes in 5 years. In consequence, the emphasis has been on patients with an established and poor illness course. Attitudes to this strategy have changed recently and most clinicians would endorse a more radical effort to treat from earlier in the illness course (42). This has not been shaped by evidence but by the application of logic: bipolar disorder tends to follow an increasingly recurrent course. If recurrence can be prevented from as early as possible, the course may be more benign. To achieve this objective is also likely to be difficult without a serious effort to enhance patient care through the essentially educational approaches described above as psychological interventions.

The patients who we are most keen to see start early treatment will have severe bipolar I disorder. We remain most unsure what strategies to adopt for less severe bipolar II and bipolar spectrum disorders, simply because almost all the existing data are from RCTs in bipolar I patients. Accordingly, policy tends to be extrapolated to the minor bipolar conditions, rather than being generated from primary evidence.

CONCLUSIONS

Bipolar disorder remains an under-researched, poorly resourced, and often undiagnosed condition. Long-term treatment to stabilize mood has long been a primary objective of clinical management. Moreover, there is probably no single agent that meets the strict definition of a mood stabilizer. The only medicine that perhaps comes close to satisfying the more conservative criteria is lithium, which has been shown to be efficacious in preventing the recurrence of either pole of illness, but with a greater effect against mania. Atypical antipsychotics, specifically olanzapine may have a comparable profile of action. Lamotrigine is perhaps the single well-characterized agent for the prevention of relapses of bipolar depression. Valproate and carbamazepine have been widely used, but have a limited evidence base. The use of these medicines in combination is almost the rule in everyday practice, but lacks coherent data to support a combining strategy.

The risk of suicide remains throughout the illness course. Evidence is accumulating that long-term treatment, particularly with lithium, may reduce the risk of suicide.

The use of psychoeducational and cognitive techniques to complement pharmacotherapy gives better results in the long term and needs to be an accepted part of the management of the illness.

REFERENCES

1. Murray CL, Lopez AD. The Global Burden of Disease. Cambridge, MA: Harvard University Press, 1996.
2. Angst J. The emerging epidemiology of hypomania and bipolar II disorder. J Affect Disord 1998; 50(2–3):143–151.
3. Kessler RC, McGonagle KA, Zhao S, Nelson CB, Hughes M, Eshleman S, Wittchen HU, Kendler KS. Lifetime and 12-month prevalence of DSM-III-R psychiatric disorders in the United States. Results from the National Comorbidity Survey. Arch Gen Psychiatry 1994; 51(1):8–19.
4. Goodwin F, Jamieson K. Manic-Depressive Illness. New York: Oxford University Press, 1990.
5. Bostwick JM, Pankratz VS. Affective disorders and suicide risk: a reexamination. Am J Psychiatry 2000; 157(12):1925–1932.
6. Kraepelin E. Manic Depressive Insanity and Paranoia (trans. by Barclay RM from the 8th edition of Lehrbuch der Psychiatrie, Vols. III and IV). Edinburgh: Livingstone, 1921.
7. Judd LL, Akiskal HS, Schettler PJ, Endicott J, Maser J, Solomon DA, Leon AC, Rice JA, Keller MB. The long-term natural history of the weekly symptomatic status of bipolar I disorder. Arch Gen Psychiatry 2002; 59(6):530–537.
8. Gitlin MJ, Swendsen J, Heller TL, Hammen C. Relapse and impairment in bipolar disorder. Am J Psychiatry 1995; 152(11):1635–1640.
9. Calabrese JR, Rapport DJ. Mood stabilizers and the evolution of maintenance study designs in bipolar I disorder. J Clin Psychiatry 1999; 60(suppl 5):5–13; discussion 14–15.
10. Ketter TA, Calabrese JR. Stabilization of mood from below versus above baseline in bipolar disorder: a new nomenclature. J Clin Psychiatry 2002; 63(2):146–151.
11. Bauer MS, Mitchner L. What is a "mood stabilizer?" An evidence-based response. Am J Psychiatry 2004; 161(1):3–18.
12. Baastrup PC, Poulsen JC, Schou M, Thomsen K, Amdisen A. Prophylactic lithium: double blind discontinuation in manic-depressive and recurrent-depressive disorders. Lancet 1970; 2(7668):326–330.
13. Coppen A, Noguera R, Bailey J, Burns BH, Swani MS, Hare EH, Gardner R, Maggs R. Prophylactic lithium in affective disorders. Controlled trial. Lancet 1971; 2(7719):275–279.
14. Cundall RL, Brooks PW, Murray LG. A controlled evaluation of lithium prophylaxis in affective disorders. Psychol Med 1972; 2(3):308–311.
15. Prien RF, Klett CJ, Caffey EM Jr. Lithium carbonate and imipramine in prevention of affective episodes. A comparison in recurrent affective illness. Arch Gen Psychiatry 1973; 29(3):420–425.
16. Prien RF, Caffey EM Jr, Klett CJ. Prophylactic efficacy of lithium carbonate in manic-depressive illness. Report of the Veterans Administration and National Institute of Mental Health collaborative study group. Arch Gen Psychiatry 1973; 28(3):337–341.

17. Stallone F, Shelley E, Mendlewicz J, Fieve RR. The use of lithium in affective disorders. 3. A double-blind study of prophylaxis in bipolar illness. Am J Psychiatry 1973; 130(9):1006–1010.
18. Fieve RR, Kumbaraci T, Dunner DL. Lithium prophylaxis of depression in bipolar I, bipolar II, and unipolar patients. Am J Psychiatry 1976; 133(8):925–929.
19. Dunner DL, Stallone F, Fieve RR. Lithium carbonate and affective disorders. V: A double-blind study of prophylaxis of depression in bipolar illness. Arch Gen Psychiatry 1976; 33(1):117–120.
20. Kane JM, Quitkin FM, Rifkin A, Ramos-Lorenzi JR, Nayak DD, Howard A. Lithium carbonate and imipramine in the prophylaxis of unipolar and bipolar II illness: a prospective, placebo-controlled comparison. Arch Gen Psychiatry 1982; 39(9): 1065–1069.
21. Gelenberg AJ, Kane JM, Keller MB, Lavori P, Rosenbaum JF, Cole K, Lavelle J. Comparison of standard and low serum levels of lithium for maintenance treatment of bipolar disorder. N Engl J Med 1989; 321(22):1489–1493.
22. Bowden CL, Calabrese JR, McElroy SL, Gyulai L, Wassef A, Petty F, Pope HGJ, Chou JCY, Keck PEJ, Rhodes LJ, Swann AC, Hirschfeld RMA, Wozniak PJ. A randomized, placebo-controlled 12-month trial of divalproex and lithium in treatment of outpatients with bipolar I disorder. Arch Gen Psychiatry 2000; 57:481–489.
23. Bowden CL, Calabrese JR, Sachs G, Yatham LN, Asghar SA, Hompland M, Montgomery P, Earl N, Smoot TM, DeVeaugh-Geiss J. A placebo-controlled 18-month trial of lamotrigine and lithium maintenance treatment in recently manic or hypomanic patients with bipolar I disorder. Arch Gen Psychiatry 2003; 60(4):364–392.
24. Calabrese JR, Bowden CL, Sachs G, Yatham LN, Behnke K, Mehtonen OP, Montgomery P, Ascher J, Paska W, Earl N, DeVeaugh-Geiss J. A placebo-controlled 18-month trial of lamotrigine and lithium maintenance treatment in recently depressed patients with bipolar I disorder. J Clin Psychiatry 2003; 64(9):1013–1024.
25. Geddes JR, Burgess S, Hawton K, Jamison K, Goodwin GM. Long-term lithium therapy for bipolar disorder: systematic review and meta-analysis of randomized controlled trials. Am J Psychiatry 2004; 161(2):217–222.
26. Tohen M, Sanger TM, McElroy SL, Tollefson GD, Chengappa KNR, Daniel DG, Petty F, Centorrino F, Wang R, Grundy SL, Greaney MG, Jacobs TG, David SR, Toma V, Keck PE, Russell J, Sussman N, Janicak PG, Levine R, Nemeroff CB, Risby ED, Gelenberg AJ, Risch SC, Altshuler L, Swann AC, Fawcett J. Olanzapine versus placebo in the treatment of acute mania. Am J Psychiatry 1999; 156:702–709.
27. Tohen M, Jacobs TG, Grundy SL, McElroy SL, Banov MC, Janicak PG, Sanger T, Risser R, Zhang F, Toma V, Francis J, Tollefson GD, Breier A. Efficacy of olanzapine in acute bipolar mania: a double-blind, placebo-controlled study. The Olanzipine HGGW Study Group. Arch Gen Psychiatry 2000; 57(9):841–849.
28. Tohen M, Baker RW, Altshuler LL, Zarate CA, Suppes T, Ketter TA, Milton DR, Risser R, Gilmore JA, Breier A, Tollefson GA. Olanzapine versus divalproex in the treatment of acute mania. Am J Psychiatry 2002; 159(6):1011–1017.
29. Tohen M, Goldberg JF, Gonzalez-Pinto Arrillaga AM, Azorin JM, Vieta E, Hardy-Bayle MC, Lawson WB, Emsley RA, Zhang F, Baker RW, Risser RC, Namjoshi MA, Evans AR, Breier A. A 12-week, double-blind comparison of olanzapine vs haloperidol in the treatment of acute mania. Arch Gen Psychiatry 2003; 60(12):1218–1226.
30. Sachs GS, Grossman F, Ghaemi SN, Okamoto A, Bowden CL. Combination of a mood stabilizer with risperidone or haloperidol for treatment of acute mania: a double-blind, placebo-controlled comparison of efficacy and safety. Am J Psychiatry 2002; 159(7): 1146–1154.
31. Altamura AC, Salvadori D, Madaro D, Santini A, Mundo E. Efficacy and tolerability of quetiapine in the treatment of bipolar disorder: preliminary evidence from a 12-month open-label study. J Affect Disord 2003; 76(1–3):267–271.

32. Keck PE Jr, Marcus R, Tourkodimitris S, Ali M, Liebeskind A, Saha A, Ingenito G. A placebo-controlled, double-blind study of the efficacy and safety of aripiprazole in patients with acute bipolar mania. Am J Psychiatry 2003; 160(9):1651–1658.
33. Tohen M, Ketter TA, Zarate CA, Suppes T, Frye M, Altshuler L, Zajecka J, Schuh LM, Risser RC, Brown E, Baker RW. Olanzapine versus divalproex sodium for the treatment of acute mania and maintenance of remission: a 47-week study. Am J Psychiatry 2003; 160(7):1263–1271.
34. Bowden CL, Brugger AM, Swann AC, Calabrese JR, Janicak PG, Petty F, Dilsaver SC, Davis JM, Rush AJ, Small JG, Garza-Trevino ES, Risch SC, Goodnick PJ, Morris DD. Efficacy of divalproex vs lithium and placebo in the treatment of mania. J Am Med Assoc 1994; 271:918–924.
35. Greil W, Ludwig-Mayerhofer W, Erazo N, Schochlin C, Schmidt S, Engel RR, Czernik A, Giedke H, Muller-Oerlinghausen B, Osterheider M, Rudolf GA, Sauer H, Tegeler J, Wetterling T. Lithium versus carbamazepine in the maintenance treatment of bipolar disorders—a randomised study. J Affect Disord 1997; 43(2):151–161.
36. Greil W, Kleindienst N. Lithium versus carbamazepine in the maintenance treatment of bipolar II disorder and bipolar disorder not otherwise specified. Int Clin Psychopharmacol 1999; 14(5):283–285.
37. Greil W, Kleindienst N. The comparative prophylactic efficacy of lithium and carbamazepine in patients with bipolar I disorder. Int Clin Psychopharmacol 1999; 14(5):277–281.
38. Hartong EG, Moleman P, Hoogduin CA, Broekman TG, Nolen WA. Prophylactic efficacy of lithium versus carbamazepine in treatment-naive bipolar patients. J Clin Psychiatry 2003; 64(2):144–151.
39. Okuma T, Inanaga K, Otsuki S, Sarai-K, Takahashi R, Hazama H, Mori A, Watanabe S. A preliminary double-blind study on the efficacy of carbamazepine in prophylaxis of manic depressive illness. Psychopharmacology 1981; 73:95–96.
40. Prien RF, Kupfer DJ, Mansky PA, Small JG, Tuason VB, Voss CB, Johnson WE. Drug therapy in the prevention of recurrences in unipolar and bipolar affective disorders. Report of the NIMH Collaborative Study Group comparing lithium carbonate, imipramine, and a lithium carbonate–imipramine combination. Arch Gen Psychiatry 1984; 41(11):1096–1104.
41. Post RM, Leverich GS, Nolen WA, Kupka RW, Altshuler LL, Frye MA, Suppes T, McElroy S, Keck P, Grunze H, Walden J. A re-evaluation of the role of antidepressants in the treatment of bipolar depression: data from the Stanley Foundation Bipolar Network. Bipolar Disord 2003; 5(6):396–406.
42. Goodwin GM. Evidence-based guidelines for treating bipolar disorder: recommendations from the British Association for Psychopharmacology. J Psychopharmacol 2003; 17(2):149–173; discussion 147.
43. Tondo L, Isacsson G, Baldessarini R. Suicidal behaviour in bipolar disorder: risk and prevention. CNS Drugs 2003; 17(7):491–511.
44. Baldessarini RJ, Tondo L, Hennen J. Lithium treatment and suicide risk in major affective disorders: update and new findings. J Clin Psychiatry 2003; 64(suppl 5):44–52.
45. Tondo L, Hennen J, Baldessarini RJ. Lower suicide risk with long-term lithium treatment in major affective illness: a meta-analysis. Acta Psychiatr Scand 2001; 104(3): 163–172.
46. Goodwin FK, Fireman B, Simon GE, Hunkeler EM, Lee J, Revicki D. Suicide risk in bipolar disorder during treatment with lithium and divalproex. J Am Med Assoc 2003; 290(11):1467–1473.
47. Meltzer HY, Alphs L, Green AI, Altamura AC, Anand R, Bertoldi A, Bourgeois M, Chouinard G, Islam MZ, Kane J, Krishnan R, Lindenmayer JP, Potkin S. Clozapine treatment for suicidality in schizophrenia: International Suicide Prevention Trial (InterSePT). Arch Gen Psychiatry 2003; 60(1):82–91.
48. Johnson RE, McFarland BH. Lithium use and discontinuation in a health maintenance organization. Am J Psychiatry 1996; 153(8):993–1000.

49. Jamison KR, Gerner RH, Goodwin FK. Patient and physician attitudes toward lithium: relationship to compliance. Arch Gen Psychiatry 1979; 36(8 Spec No):866–869.
50. Lingam R, Scott J. Treatment non-adherence in affective disorders. Acta Psychiatr Scand 2002; 105(3):164–172.
51. Fava GA, Bartolucci G, Rafanelli C, Mangelli L. Cognitive-behavioral management of patients with bipolar disorder who relapsed while on lithium prophylaxis. J Clin Psychiatry 2001; 62(7):556–559.
52. Scott J, Tacchi MJ. A pilot study of concordance therapy for individuals with bipolar disorders who are non-adherent with lithium prophylaxis. Bipolar Disord 2002; 4(6): 386–392.
53. Lam DH, Watkins ER, Hayward P, Bright J, Wright K, Kerr N, Parr-Davis G, Sham P. A randomized controlled study of cognitive therapy for relapse prevention for bipolar affective disorder: outcome of the first year. Arch Gen Psychiatry 2003; 60(2):145–152.
54. Miklowitz DJ, George EL, Richards JA, Simoneau TL, Suddath RL. A randomized study of family-focused psychoeducation and pharmacotherapy in the outpatient management of bipolar disorder. Arch Gen Psychiatry 2003; 60(9):904–912.
55. Colom F, Vieta E, Martinez-Aran A, Reinares M, Goikolea JM, Benabarre A, Torrent C, Comes M, Corbella B, Parramon G, Corominas J. A Randomized trial on the efficacy of group psychoeducation in the prophylaxis of recurrences in bipolar patients whose disease is in remission. Arch Gen Psychiatry 2003; 60(4):364–402.
56. Ehlers CL, Frank E, Kupfer DJ. Social zeitgebers and biological rhythms. A unified approach to understanding the etiology of depression. Arch Gen Psychiatry 1988; 45(10):948–952.
57. Monk TH, Flaherty JF, Frank E, Hoskinson K, Kupfer DJ. The social rhythm metric. An instrument to quantify the daily rhythms of life. J Nerv Ment Dis 1990; 178(2):120–126.
58. Monk TH, Kupfer DJ, Frank E, Ritenour AM. The social rhythm metric (SRM): measuring daily social rhythms over 12 weeks. Psychiatr Res 1991; 36(2):195–207.
59. Frank E, Swartz HA, Kupfer DJ. Interpersonal and social rhythm therapy: managing the chaos of bipolar disorder. Biol Psychiatry 2000; 48(6):593–604.
60. Malkoff-Schwartz S, Frank E, Anderson B, Sherrill JT, Siegel L, Patterson D, Kupfer DJ. Stressful life events and social rhythm disruption in the onset of manic and depressive bipolar episodes: a preliminary investigation. Arch Gen Psychiatry 1998; 55(8):702–707.
61. Malkoff-Schwartz S, Frank E, Anderson BP, Hlastala SA, Luther JF, Sherrill JT, Houck PR, Kupfer DJ. Social rhythm disruption and stressful life events in the onset of bipolar and unipolar episodes. Psychol Med 2000; 30(5):1005–1016.

15
Schizoaffective Disorder

Julio Bobes, Maria-Teresa Bascaran, Maria-Paz Garcia-Portilla, Pilar-Alejandra Saiz, and Manuel Bousoño
Departamento de Psiquiatria, Facultad de Medicina, Universidad de Oviedo, Oviedo, Spain

Gerardo Florez
Centro Asistencial "As Burgas," Ourense, Spain

Celso Arango
Servicio de Psiquiatria, Hospital General "Gregorio Maranon," Madrid, Spain

THE SCHIZOAFFECTIVE DILEMMA

As Tsuang and Marneros (1) pointed out, almost 20 years ago patients with schizoaffective disorder present a conceptual problem to theorists, a therapeutic problem to clinicians, and a diagnostic problem to researchers. That was the case since it was described in 1933, and that has been the case for the last 20 years. In fact, the DSM-III-R recognized that the schizoaffective disorder represents one of the most confused and arguable concepts in the psychiatric nosology. In this chapter, we will try to present the current knowledge about this uncertain disorder, focusing on practical approaches for its treatment.

Historical Overview

As many other issues in modern psychiatry, the origins of this confusing disorder can be tracked down to Kraepelin and his major division between "Dementia Praecox" and "Manic-Depressive Insanity." This division was based mainly in the course of the illness, although Kraepelin (2) also considered the presenting symptoms as a basic tool for diagnosis. This division, a clear landmark in psychiatry, made cross-sectional diagnosis a difficult task for psychiatrists; this is why when Bleuler (3) defined the term "schizophrenia," searching for a loss of psychological integration, it was accepted with great enthusiasm. Bleuler (1924) recognized the occurrence of affective symptoms in patients diagnosed with schizophrenia and psychotic symptoms in patients with an affective disorder. However, Bleuler ultimately concluded that schizophrenia was usually the illness in question and did not describe this group of patients with both types of symptoms as a group. In 1933, Kasanin (4) introduced the concept of "acute schizoaffective psychoses." Kasanin applied this term to patients characterized by: being young, sudden onset with marked emotional turmoil, good pre-morbid adjustment, presence of precipitating events, few symptoms of withdrawal or passivity, distortion of the outside world, and relatively short course with complete recovery.

Since Kasanin's contribution, the term "schizoaffective disorder" has been widely used, with considerable differences in meaning and application, in general to classify patients who present with features of both schizophrenia and affective illness and hence do not qualify for typical diagnosis of any of the two major conditions (5,6). Authors such as Kant, Langfeldt, and Vaillant have described conditions, which have in common a sudden onset, presence of confusion or disorientation, and a good recovery. In addition, terms as "cycloid psychosis," "psychogenic," or "reactive psychosis," and the French nomenclature "bouffée délirante" have been used synonymously with schizoaffective psychosis despite the fact that there are very important differences between these psychoses and the phenomenology that characterizes the schizoaffective disorder as nowadays conceptualized. The reason for the use of the different terms as schizoaffective disorder may lie in Kasanin's original description, which differs substantially from the modern definition in use (more based on a mixture of psychotic and affective symptoms than on the good prognosis or lack of defectual symptoms).

Marneros et al. in differentiating between the two disorders described "cases-in-between," in which both diagnoses can be made with equally strong arguments. The author identified concurrent and sequential forms and his definition was very similar to the actual one (7).

Diagnostic Criteria and Clinical Features

Currently used diagnostic tools for schizoaffective disorder are heavily influenced by the research diagnostic criteria (RDC) developed by Robert Spitzer et al. (8). In the RDC, in order to make a schizoaffective disorder diagnosis the following clinical features were needed:

- Detection of any of Kurt Schneider's first-rank psychotic symptoms (9).
- These psychotic symptoms persisted for at least a week without mood symptoms. If the psychotic symptoms persisted for more than a week a "mainly schizophrenic" subtype was diagnosed, if not, the diagnosis was of a "mainly affective" subtype schizoaffective disorder. Within the latter subtype, there were two types: schizoaffective mania and schizoaffective depression.
- Mood and psychotic symptoms overlapped during the course of the episode. This means that the essential features of the disorder must occur within a single uninterrupted period of illness.

Schizoaffective disorder was defined as the acute co-occurrence of a full mood syndrome plus a set of schizophrenia nuclear symptoms. These criteria were included in DSM-III-R and then passed into DSM-IV and DSM-IV-TR (10–12). The differences are that in the DSM criteria, psychotic symptoms have to persist at least 2 weeks in the absence of "prominent" mood symptoms, and that the mood syndrome could not have been "brief" when compared with the psychotic syndrome. The consequence of the 2 weeks period is that DSM did not consider the "mainly schizophrenic"–"mainly affective" subtypes included in the RDC criteria. This makes that almost all DSM schizoaffective disorder diagnoses are "mainly schizophrenic" subtypes for the RDC criteria. DSM-IV points out that the total duration of the psychotic disorder is a summation of the time that the patient has exhibited active psychotic symptoms and residual symptoms of psychosis, including negative symptoms. The time that the patient has been taking antipsychotic medication, with or without active or residual psychotic symptoms is also included. Finally, schizoaffective mania was converted into schizoaffective disorder bipolar type. Another important issue is that the sequential forms of schizoaffective disorder, described in classical definitions, are lost since the presence of concurrence psychotic and affective symptoms has to be present at some time. These changes illustrate how the number and type of diagnosis in which psychotic symptoms are included are highly dependent upon the set of classification procedures used by the different classification systems (13).

These criteria have provided psychiatrists a way to identify schizoaffective disorders; however, many limitations remain inherent to the concept of the disease:

- It has been clearly proved that Kurt Schneider's first-rank symptoms, or any other psychotic symptoms, are not pathognomonic for schizophrenia and can be found in mood disorders (14,15). But the same happens with affective symptoms, such as depressive symptoms, which are common traits of all endogenous psychosis (16).
- It has not been defined what the exact meanings of "prominent" (in some investigations it has been operationally defined as "one-third or more") or "brief" are.
- The predictive utility of the 2-week period has not been strongly validated.
- These criteria are defined in an episodic way. Course criteria are not included. This means that if the patient presents a further episode that fulfills the criteria for schizophrenia or an affective disorder, the diagnosis has to be changed. We also have to add that the distinction of depressive symptoms, and negative symptoms is a difficult one when it has to be done cross-sectionally because of their similarity. Longitudinally follow-up has been recommended to make this distinction, as negative symptoms tend to persist whereas depressive symptoms tend to remit (17).

In relation with the clinical features of the schizoaffective disorder, it has to be highlighted, that most of the studies conducted on this topic have revealed that there is not a characteristic symptom profile for schizoaffective disorder when compared with schizophrenia and mood disorders (18).

The diagnosis is further complicated when the psychotic and affective symptoms appear in children and adolescents. The high rate of positive psychotic symptoms that appear in child and adolescent affective disorders, such as major depression and mania, may lead to diagnostic confusion. Many diagnoses of schizoaffective or schizophrenia psychosis in this population end up being affective disorders later in life.

Concepts of Schizoaffective Disorder

Several concepts for schizoaffective disorder have been developed by authors like Brockington et al. (19) and Lapensée (20), the starting point for these concepts is the assumption that schizophrenia and mood disorders are distinct at some fundamental level (e.g., different genotypes). These concepts are the following:

1. Schizoaffective disorder is a variant of schizophrenia.
2. Schizoaffective disorder is a variant of mood disorder.

3. Schizoaffective disorder represents a heterogeneous combination of schizophrenia and mood disorder symptoms. This does not mean that both diseases are present, the detected incidence for schizoaffective disorder is simply too high for such a casual coincidence (19).
4. Schizoaffective disorder is another type of psychosis distinct from schizophrenia or mood disorder.
5. Schizoaffective disorder is part of a *continuum* of a share genetic vulnerability for psychotic disorders. From worst to best prognosis, this *continuum* would be as follows: schizophrenia—schizoaffective disorder—psychotic mood disorder—non-psychotic mood disorder.
6. Schizoaffective disorder represents a combination of all the previous concepts.

Family and outcome studies have been conducted trying to find which one of these concepts fits better with the results obtained. The pattern of inheritance and the outcome (episodic vs. chronic) have been chosen as discriminating variables because of the non-specificity of psychiatric symptoms and psychiatric treatments. All these studies have to be interpreted with caution because of the already-mentioned diagnostic difficulties.

In general, family studies have found elevated rates of both schizophrenia and mood disorders in first relatives of schizoaffective patients. The risk for a first-degree relative to have schizophrenia or mood disorders was higher than the risk of having a schizoaffective disorder (which was higher than in the general population) (21–24). For example, in a recent twin study conducted by Cardno et al. (25), the schizoaffective disorder shared a familial liability with both schizophrenia and manic syndromes. These results support concept number 3 and are consistent with a genetic heterogeneity. These results do not support concept number 4, the risk for first-degree relatives of developing a schizoaffective disorder should be higher than the risk of developing schizophrenia or mood disorders in order to support this concept. Similar conclusions can be obtained to discard concepts 1 and 2. The exact nature of that genetic heterogeneity is not known, but some authors have suggested that schizophrenia and mood disorders share some susceptibility genes. It is quite clear nowadays that both, schizophrenia and mood disorders, are genetically and etiologically heterogeneous themselves (26). This would mean that schizoaffective disorder represents a group of patients with high overlap of these shared genes (25).

Outcome studies have shown a similar picture, with schizoaffective disorder in between schizophrenia and mood disorders, which means that schizoaffective disorder has a better long-term outcome (measuring different outcome variables such as social and vocational functioning, hospitalizations, symptom stability) when compared with schizophrenia, but a worse outcome when compared with mood disorders (27). One example is the Roscommon Family Study (28), in this study, the functional status of schizoaffective disorder, measured with the *level of functioning scale*, was just in the middle between schizophrenia and mood disorders. Another example is the Cologne Longitudinal Study (29). The authors of this study indicated that 49.5% of the patients with schizoaffective disorder had a negative outcome compared with the 93.2% and the 35.8% of negative outcomes in the schizophrenia group and in the mood disorders group, respectively; similar conclusions were drawn from the study conducted at the University of Illinois (30). Obviously, and taking into account the definition and diagnostic heterogeneity of the schizoaffective disorder, not all the variables measured by the studies conducted to investigate this topic have followed this rule of "thumb," with some of them being more close to schizophrenia and others to mood disorders (31). But, in general, we can conclude that, at the present stage, outcome studies have also validated concept number 3, without excluding concept number 5.

These longitudinal studies have been able to identify prognostic factors for schizoaffective disorder. These are the factors that have been identified as poor outcome predictors (32,33): persistence of psychotic symptoms in the absence of affective symptoms, high rate of relapses, poor pre-morbid adjustment, high presence of typically schizophrenia symptoms, chronic course, and chronicity at detection.

Epidemiology

Little is known about the epidemiology of schizoaffective disorder, mainly because of its diagnostic and classification difficulties.

In the data obtained from the Epidemiologic Catchment Area Study—a study that used the *Diagnostic Interview Schedule* as the diagnostic instrument—a 1-year incidence rate of 1.7 per 1000 habitants was found for the "psychotic affective syndrome" group (34). This looks like a high incidence rate, close to the 2.0 per 1000 habitants per year rate of schizophrenia, but it is important to remark that the "psychotic affective syndrome" group is not a diagnosis equivalent to schizoaffective disorder, because 59% of the patients included in that group only experienced psychotic symptoms while they were having a mood episode.

Most of the studies that have examined the prevalence rates of schizoaffective disorder were conducted in clinical settings. Therefore, we can only estimate prevalence rates. The clinical setting bias has also created a really inconsistent picture. Taken together, we can only say that the prevalence ratio of schizophrenia to schizoaffective disorder seems to be 2 to 1. If this was really the case, it would mean that the schizoaffective disorder diagnosis represented a clinically significant population (35). More studies, especially population surveys, are needed to clarify the prevalence issue.

Considering demographic factors, some general conclusions can be made. Firstly, that there appear to be more females than males in the schizoaffective group, Berner and Lenz (36) estimated that the male to female ratio ranged from 0.3:1 to 1:1 depending on the diagnostic tool used in each study. Secondly, the age of onset, as in the outcome studies, seems to locate the schizoaffective disorder in between schizophrenia and mood disorders. For example, in a study conducted by Marneros et al. (37), the median ages of onset were the following: 24 years for schizophrenia, 29 years for schizoaffective disorder, and 35 years for mood disorders. Once again, we have to remark that these results can be greatly influenced by the diagnostic criteria employed, especially when we compare RDC criteria vs. DSM criteria (36). It also seems that gender has an effect on the age of onset, with women tending to have an older age of onset.

Schizoaffective patients have an increased risk of death when compared with general population. Several factors contribute to this pre-occupying fact. The excess of mortality has been related to infections, cardiovascular diseases, neoplasms, and specially suicide (38). The suicide risk of schizoaffective patients, a substantial and enduring one, resembles the suicide risk for patients with mood disorders (39).

The presence of precipitating events, one of the defining characteristics of Kasanin's "acute schizoaffective psychoses" (4), has been replicated in several studies. Even more, it seems that schizoaffective patients are the ones who have a higher rate of precipitating factors, such as stressors or life events, when compared with schizophrenia or affective patients (34).

THE TREATMENT OF SCHIZOAFFECTIVE DISORDER

Although many controversies about schizoaffective disorder are currently unresolved, what is quite clear from the studies conducted on this topic is that patients who meet modern diagnostic criteria for the disorder suffer from substantial morbidity and mortality. Because of this suffering, clear treatment criteria are needed, but once again, the realization and interpretation of the studies conducted to establish these criteria are difficulted by those controversies mentioned before (40). Not many relevant articles are found when a search through the literature is done. And in the few articles found, the low number of patients included and the use of different diagnostic manuals and inclusion of different subgroups of patients affect the external validity. It is important to keep these considerations in mind when trying to review the available data in order to create treatment protocols for schizoaffective patients.

General Considerations

When confronting a case that seems a schizoaffective disorder, the clinician should consider the following points before choosing any treatment option.

Current Clinical Features

As it has been mentioned before, the schizoaffective disorder diagnosis is a cross-sectional one. An exhaustive assessment of current symptoms (type, duration, and temporal relationship between mood and psychotic symptoms) is needed to be sure that this new episode is actually a schizoaffective episode. It is important to be sure about the diagnosis, not only because of the treatment implications but also because of the different prognosis implications of the different endogenous psychosis. It has been remarked that in clinical practice many psychiatrists tend to be too flexible when diagnosing schizoaffective disorder, changing diagnosis from schizophrenia and mood disorder into schizoaffective disorder just because in a new episode a single psychotic or affective symptom appears (41). It is important to distinguish pure depressive symptoms from negative symptoms and from medication side effects such as neuroleptic-induced dysphoria or akathisia–akinesia or anhedonia, as the treatment options are different for each of these conditions. Sometimes, the clinical picture is vague mainly because negative symptoms and side effects can promote the appearance of secondary depressive symptoms due to the impairment in psychosocial functioning that they create. Depressive-like symptoms may also represent a "prodromal" stage of a new psychotic descompensation. The same happens when trying to distinguish clear symptoms of mania such as elevated mood, increase in pleasurable activities or increase in goal-directed activities from general agitation symptoms, that can be found during any acute schizophrenic episode, such as irritability, psychomotor agitation, insomnia, pressured speech or grandiose delusions; or from the psychomotor agitation and insomnia produced by akathisia. Also of great importance is the evaluation of how the symptoms progress once the treatment has been initiated.

Previous Illness Course

An assessment of the clinical features that were present during previous episodes and in between those episodes (residual symptoms) is highly recommended (42). An earlier course more consistent with schizophrenia or with mood disorder will surely help to decide the treatment options for the current episode.

Substance Abuse

The abuse of different type of drugs, due to acute intoxications or to withdrawal periods, can modify the typical clinical course of schizophrenia or of a mood disorder. Screening for toxic agents should always be done before considering a definitive diagnosis and a long-term treatment plan (41).

Psychopharmacological Options

The schizoaffective disorder clinical picture, a mixture of psychotic and affective symptoms, determines the psychopharmacological options for its treatment; the main options are the following.

Lithium

Several investigations have given support to the widely used strategy of combining lithium plus an antipsychotic for the treatment of an episode of schizoaffective disorder bipolar type (42–44). In general, lithium seems to be a good treatment option, alone or in combination with antipsychotics, for treating patients that present psychotic symptoms with excitement, over activity and euphoria. But when the patients are extremely agitated, lithium alone may not be sufficient and the combination with an antipsychotic is necessary (45). Currently, the use of lithium for schizoaffective disorder unipolar type is not supported by any controlled study, this is why this use of lithium can only be speculated through small studies that have investigated the use of lithium for the treatment of depressive symptoms in schizophrenia (46).

Anticonvulsants

Most of the data for the use of carbamazepine and valproate comes from open trails. These studies suggest that carbamazepine and valproate may be a treatment option for schizoaffective disorder bipolar type (40). In two controlled studies, carbamazepine presented only modest benefits (47,48). Due to the lack of controlled studies showing a clear efficacy for carbamazepine and valproate, they can only be recommended as second choice in combination treatments; for example, when lithium plus an antipsychotic has not been enough to control the clinical picture (as in difficult cases where mixed affective symptoms are present), or if lithium cannot be used because of unbearable side effects or contraindications. Paradoxically, in recent years, a decline in the use of lithium and an increase in the use of valproate for schizoaffective disorders have been reported (49). Probably, this situation is related with a general trend in the use of valproate instead of lithium for mood disorders A trend that seems to be motivated, mainly in the United States, by the clinicians perception that valproate is as useful as lithium but at the same time safer and easier to prescribe. New anticonvulsants such as gabapentin, lamotrigine, topiramate, and tiagabine are currently being investigated as potential treatments for mood disorders (50), but no recommendation can be made for their use in schizoaffective disorder until controlled studies are conducted. At the present time, they seem to be used in refractory cases where combinations of conventional treatments have failed.

Antidepressants

No controlled study has demonstrated an advantage of antidepressants, in monotherapy or in combination with antipsychotics, over antipsychotics alone in the treatment of schizoaffective disorder unipolar type (42), and even one study suggested that adding an antidepressant to a patient with florid psychotic symptoms may worsen the psychotic picture (51). With this information at hand, antidepressants should be left for treating post-psychotic depression or depressive episodes without psychotic exacerbation—different clinical conditions that cannot be considered a schizoaffective disorder—where they have clearly proved their utility (52). Anyway, when adding antidepressants to antypsychotic medication, the clinician needs to remember that each of these treatments can influence the metabolism of the other. To prevent possible complications, the clinician should monitor plasma levels if possible, routinely screen for side effects and adverse reactions, avoid rapid dosage increases, be aware of the potential for increases in the half-lives of each pharmacological agent, and before starting any combination treatment consider pre-existing physical conditions which could be problematic. The few available data of new antidepressants (SSRI, venlafaxine, and mirtazapine) as treatment options for schizoaffective disorders are not sufficient in order to draw conclusions about them, further research is needed.

Conventional Antipsychotics

Antipsychotics have proved in several controlled trials to be an effective treatment option for schizoaffective patients, both bipolar and unipolar types (40,42). Their main disadvantages are: their side effects profile that—as it has been mentioned before—can sometimes be confounded with mood symptoms and their lack of a clear thymoleptic effect that makes that, in many cases, the addition of another medication is needed in order to treat persistent affective symptoms.

New Generation Antipsychotics

This new group of antipsychotics, with an improved pharmacological profile when compared with conventional antipsychotics, has created a great expectancy, as their improved profile could make them the first-line treatment for schizoaffective disorder. In general, the serotoninergic activity that these antipsychotics have, make them able to modulate the dopaminergic blockade at the nigroestriatal level (52) and, as a consequence of this modulation, they have a much more favorable side effect profile, without loosing antipsychotic efficacy. This translates less adverse effects such as akathisia, akinesia, and anhedonia that can directly or indirectly contribute to depressive symptomatology. New generation antipsychotics are also superior in the treatment of secondary negative symptoms and they may even have some direct antidepressant effect on their own (53). The treatment of acute mania is another clinical condition in which new generation antipsychotics have shown their efficacy, in monotherapy and also as an adjunctive treatment (54). Main new generation antipsychotics are considered here separately as treatment options for schizoaffective disorder.

Clozapine. The conclusion of several open (55–57) and one double-blind randomized (58) studies is that clozapine is an optimal treatment for schizoaffective disorder, especially the bipolar type, as it has efficacy in treating positive, negative, and affective—specially manic—symptoms without the risk of generating adverse effects that could create or mimic depressive symptoms. Even more, pooling data from these studies, it seems that schizoaffective patients show a greater response to clozapine when compared with pure schizophrenia patients (40). These findings have to be considered as preliminary, since only one of the studies was a double-blind randomized study [and the number of patients included in this study ($n = 11$) is too low]. Clozapine has also been reported to be an effective acute antimanic agent in several open-label prospective studies on bipolar disorder (59,60); and a maintenance option for patients with a treatment-refractory illness, as it was confirmed in a study that included bipolar and schizoaffective patients (61). Another point to remember when considering clozapine as a treatment option is that double-blind randomized studies have demonstrated that clozapine significantly reduces suicidal behavior in schizophrenia and schizoaffective patients (62). These data suggest that clozapine would be a first-line treatment option when a high risk of suicide is detected in these patients. The risk of agranulocytosis, and the regular blood tests that are required, is the main problem that clinicians face today in order to prescribe clozapine, and this is why in most of the guidelines and protocols that are elaborated by groups of experts, clozapine is considered as a second- or third-line treatment (63).

Risperidone. Several open trials have evaluated the efficacy of risperidone in the treatment of schizoaffective patients. In general, risperidone seems to be an effective treatment for both types of schizoaffective disorders (64,65). In two double-blind randomized studies risperidone was as effective as haloperidol, alone or combined with amytriptyline, in treating schizoaffective disorder unipolar type (66,67). At the same time, several double-blind randomized studies have established the efficacy of risperidone, alone (68,69) or as an adjunctive treatment (70,71) for acute mania. When adherence to treatment is low, the new risperidone-sustained release formula may be a good treatment option.

Olanzapine. In a large double-blind prospective international study, Olanzapine demonstrated its superiority over haloperidol in the management of both types of schizoaffective disorders (72). Olanzapine has also proved to be superior to conventional antipsychotics in trials that studied response of negative and depressive symptoms to treatment in schizophrenia. Several double-blind randomized studies have also established the efficacy of Olanzapine, alone (73,74) or as an adjunctive treatment (75) for acute mania.

Ziprasidone. This new generation antipsychotic has established its effectiveness for treating positive, negative, and depressive symptoms during acute episodes of schizophrenia and schizoaffective disorder (76). In another trial that only included schizoaffective patients, ziprasidone exerted a clear reduction in psychotic and mood symptoms, both manic and depressive, when compared with placebo (77). One double-blind randomized study has established the efficacy of ziprasidone in monotherapy (78) for acute mania.

Other New Generation Antipsychotics. Quetiapine and aripiprazole have established their efficacy for alleviating acute manic symptoms in bipolar disorder (54), additional studies are needed to demonstrate their efficacy for schizoaffective disorder.

Benzodiazepines

If the schizoaffective patient presents with agitation or high levels of anxiety, benzodiazepines can be considered as an adjunctive treatment because of their efficacy, safety, and tolerability. Benzodiazepines allow a rapid sedative effect, and when they are used, the initial dosage of antipsychotic drugs is reduced and the titration can be done in a slower and safer way. Oral or intramuscular (preferably lorazepam or midazolam because of their complete and rapid absorption, with onset of their therapeutic effect at 15–30 min) high-potency benzodiazepines can be used for controlling agitation (79). Lorazepam and clonazepam have proved to be effective as adjunctive treatments for acute mania (80).

Psychopharmacological Combination Treatments

After presenting the several psychopharmacological treatment options for schizoaffective disorder, we now make some proposals about combination of different strategies in clinical practice. As we said before, the clinical practitioner has to consider, before prescribing any medication, the current clinical features and the previous illness course. With these two variables in the equation, the following treating scenarios may appear.

First Illness Episode

In this situation, there is no previous course to guide the treatment decision, so the clinical features are the only tool to guide the treatment choice. The first step is to use a new generation antipsychotic because of their, previously described, antipsychotic and thymoleptic properties. All new generation antipsychotics except clozapine (because of the agranulocytosis side effect) can be used. Two things have to be remembered when prescribing a new generation antipsychotic to an antipsychotic "naïve" patient. First, low doses of antipsychotics are the best treatment option. In PET studies, these low doses are able to produce a D2 receptor occupancy higher than 60%, the threshold for antipsychotic effects, but lower than 80%, the threshold for acute extrapyramidal side effects (81); in clinical studies, low doses produced good remission rates (82)—with a reduced incidence of side effects and secondary negative symptoms, which may promote compliance (82). Because of these data, a 2003 *Expert Consensus Guideline* recommends the following doses (mg/day) for the acute treatment of a first episode psychosis: aripiprazole (10–20), olanzapine (10–20), quetiapine (300–600), risperidone (2.5–5), and ziprasidone (100–160) (63). Second, when possible treatment should be started with a really low dose (100 mg chlorpromazine equivalents per day), this dose should be slowly increased monitoring the level of response and possible side effects in order to find the lowest effective dose (83). Once an adequate dose has been found, the clinician should wait 3 to 4 weeks before assessing the clinical situation. If after this period of time all symptoms have remitted, maintenance treatment with the antipsychotic is indicated and benzodiazepines, if used, should be tapered down. If psychotic symptoms persist and adherence is not an issue, the antipsychotic should be increased to its recommended higher dose and the patient monitored for another 3 to 6 weeks, if after this period of time psychotic symptoms are still present switching to another new generation antipsychotic is the recommended option, and after two trials with different antipsychotics, clozapine should be considered (63). If psychotic symptoms remit, but affective symptoms remain active, the clinician has to consider adding new treatments. If depressed mood is present, antidepressants should be the option, specially the newer ones because of their lower side effect profile. Interactions with the current antipsychotic treatment must be considered. If manic symptoms are the problem, a mood stabilizer should be added. Lithium, valproate, and carbamazepine are the options. Valproate seems to be the best choice because of its rapid symptom response with less adverse effects when a loading dose is used (30 mg/kg/day on days 1 and 2, then 20 mg/kg/day on days 3–10), and because it has proved to be an effective adjunct to antipsychotics (84). Lithium has a delayed onset of action of at least 5 to 7 days and full effect is not expected until 2 to 3 weeks of treatment (85), and although carbamazepine has a shorter delayed of onset and it seems more effective for treating psychotic mania when compared with lithium (86), its many interactions with antipsychotics make carbamazepine a second-line option.

Schizoaffective Episode in a Typically Schizophrenic Course

If the patient was not taking any treatment or was been treated with conventional antipsychotics, starting or switching treatment to a new generation antipsychotic should be the first treatment option. If a new generation antipsychotics has already been used, switching to another one is the correct treatment option, considering Clozapine if no effectiveness appears after the second new generation antipsychotic has been used at adequate doses during the proper time. The acute treatment dosing recommendations for this situation are higher than the ones made for first episodes: aripiprazole (15–30 mg/day), clozapine (400–600 mg/day), olanzapine (15–25 mg/day), quetiapine (500–800 mg/day), risperidone (4.0–6.5 mg/day), and ziprasidone (140–180 mg/day) (63). The general rules for using adjunctive treatments are the same as the ones indicated for first episodes.

Schizoaffective Episode in a Typically Unipolar Mood Disorder Course

For a unipolar-type schizoaffective episode, the rational choice is combining a new antidepressant with a new generation antipsychotic [as these drugs may have an anxiolytic and anti-irritability effect and their 5HTt antagonism may augment the antidepressant efficacy (87)]. If the schizoaffective episode is a bipolar-type one, stopping a current treatment with an antidepressant and starting a new generation antipsychotic should be the first treatment option. If this treatment alone or with a benzodiazepine is not enough, a mood stabilizer should be added.

Schizoaffective Episode in a Typically Bipolar Mood Disorder Course

A mood stabilizer should be the basic treatment for this clinical scenario. A new generation antipsychotic should be added, and if affective symptoms persist antidepressants and other mood stabilizers should be considered.

These clinical scenarios have been presented in a simplified way trying to clarify the treatment options. But in clinical daily practice, things might be much more complicated, patients might be already taking several treatments when the episode starts, or because some patients present with treatment-resistant symptoms that demand really complicated pharmacological regimes with different agents used at their higher doses. In these situations, clinicians need to cautiously monitor symptoms and side effects, always considering possible interactions between different treatment options, available plasma levels (lithium, valproate, carbamazepine, and clozapine), and renal and liver function.

As there are no controlled studies on maintenance treatment for schizoaffective disorder, no clear recommendations can be made on this subject (40). The most rational approach is to use general maintenance rules: once the symptoms have totally remitted, treatments should be reduced one by one to a minimal maintenance effective dose for preventing relapse and lower the side effects (88).

Non-Psychopharmacological Treatments

Other treatment options that should be considered for schizoaffective patients are the following.

Electroconvulsive Therapy

The presence of affective clinical features has always been considered as a predictor of positive response to electroconvulsive therapy in psychotic patients. In view with this clinical impression, there is only one study that has investigated the response of schizoaffective patients to electroconvulsive therapy. Ries et al. (89) found that nine patients who were medication-resistant manifested a strong relief of their symptoms with electroconvulsive therapy. These results suggest that treatment-refractory patients with marked psychotic and affective symptoms, especially if confusion is present, should be considered candidates for electroconvulsive therapy.

Assertive Community Treatment

The primary goals of Programs of Assertive Community Treatment are (90) to treat persistent symptoms, to prevent new acute episodes, to enhance quality of life, to improve social and vocational functioning, and to help families providing care. All these services are provided in an "out of office" and in a highly individualized way. The target population for this intervention is:

- Patients with persistent and severe mental illness (schizophrenia, bipolar disorder, and schizoaffective disorder mainly).
- Severe mental illnesses that create significant functional impairments.
- Patients who present one or more of the following problems: high use of psychiatric in-patient or emergency services, persistent severe symptoms, substance abuse, inability to meet basic survival needs, or criminal involvement. With these severe problems, these patients cannot be successfully treated in traditional office-based services.

Although there are no controlled studies that examine the efficacy of this type of treatment in schizoaffective patients, it is obvious that some of the schizoaffective patients do have these problems and are candidates for assertive community treatment programs.

Cognitive Therapy

No controlled studies have been conducted to measure the efficacy of this psychotherapeutic approach with schizoaffective patients alone, but cognitive therapy has proved to be a useful tool for treating affective—both depressive and manic—and psychotic persistent symptoms (91,92). These symptoms can be targeted with this therapy when detected in a schizoaffective patient.

Relapse Prevention

Schizoaffective patients have been included with schizophrenia patients in controlled studies where programs for relapse prevention (these programs usually consist in: psychoeducation for patients and family, active monitoring for prodromal symptoms, crisis clinical interventions, and coping skills training) have shown to be effective in detecting and preventing relapse (93).

Family Therapy

This therapy has proved to be an effective therapy for families of patients with severe mental disorders such as schizophrenia and bipolar illness, this is why models of this therapy, as the ones developed by Hogarty (94) or McFarlane (95), can be recommended for families of schizoaffective patients.

CONCLUSIONS

Despite the fact that schizoaffective and atypical psychoses are unsatisfactory diagnostic categories with low predictive validity and little longitudinal stability, the case is that we cannot afford to eliminate the diagnosis because many patients in our clinic do not fulfill diagnostic criteria for schizophrenia or mood disorder. As Marneros and Tsuang (96) mention, the heterogeneity of this disorder is not only a result of the different definitions and different samples, but a phenomenon per se. This is expected since we are dealing with a manic and a depressive type, with a productive and a non-productive type, with monomorphous and polymorphous types, and so on.

This intermediate psychotic area or "cases in between" may reflect the dimensional expression of psychiatric symptoms reflecting brain dysfunctions changing over time. The placing of cases on a continuum helps the offset the problem that, once a diagnostic scheme is in place it allows changes in diagnosis as the brain disease, manifested by psychiatric symptoms, affects different functions in the affected brain.

REFERENCES

1. Tsuang MT, Marneros A. Schizoaffective psychosis: questions and directions. In: Marneros A, Tsuang MT, eds. Schizoaffective Psychoses. Berlin: Springer-Verlag, 1986.
2. Kraepelin E. Dementia Praecox and Paraphrenia, Together with Manic Depressive Insanity [translated from original texts by the Classics of Psychiatry and Behavioral Sciences Library]. Delran, NJ: Gryphon Editions, 1993.
3. Bleuler E. Dementia Praecox or the Group of the Schizophrenias. New York: International University Press, 1950.
4. Kasanin J. The acute schizoaffective psychoses. Am J Psychiatry 1933; 113:97–126.
5. Brockington IF, Leff JP. Schizo-affective psychosis: definitions and incidence. Psychol Med 1979; 9:91–99.
6. Levitt JJ, Tsuang MT. The heterogeneity of schizoaffective disorder: implications for treatment. Am J Psychiatry 1988; 145:926–936.
7. Marneros A, Rohde A, Desiter A, Risse A. Features of schizoaffective disorders: the "cases-in-between." In: Marneros A, Tsuang MT, eds. Schizoaffective Psychoses. Berlin: Springer-Verlag, 1986.
8. Spitzer RL, Endicott J, Robinds E. Research Diagnostic Criteria. New York: New York State Psychiatric Institute, 1975.
9. Schneider K. Clinical Psychopathology [translated by M. W. Hamilton]. New York: Grune and Stratton, 1959.
10. Diagnostic and Statistical Manual of Mental Disorders. 3rd ed, rev. Washington, DC: American Psychiatric Press, 1987.
11. Diagnostic and Statistical Manual of Mental Disorders. 4th ed. Washington, DC: American Psychiatric Press, 1994.

12. Diagnostic and Statistical Manual of Mental Disorders. 4th ed, rev. Washington, DC: American Psychiatric Press, 2002.
13. Peralta V, Cuesta MJ. The nosology of psychotic disorders: a comparison among competing classification systems. Schizophr Bull 2003; 29(3):413–425.
14. Pope HG Jr, Lipinsky JF. Diagnosis of schizophrenia and manic-depressive illness: a reassessment of the specificity of "schizophrenic" symptoms in the light of current research. Arch Gen Psychiatry 1978; 39:157–162.
15. Carpenter WT, Strauss JS, Muleh S. Are there pathognomonic symptoms in schizophrenia? An empiric investigation of Schneider's first-rank symptoms. Arch Gen Psychiatry 1973; 28(6):847–852.
16. Angst J. Today's perspective on Kraepelin's nosology of endogenous psychoses. Eur Arch Psychiatry Clin Neurosci 1993; 243:164–170.
17. Andreasen NC, Flaum M, Arndt S. Positive and negative symptoms: assessment and validity. In: Marneros A, Andreasen NC, Tsuang MT, eds. Negative Versus Positive Schizophrenia. New York: Springer, 1991:28–51.
18. Ricca V, Galassi F, La Malfa G. Assessment of basic symptoms in schizophrenia, schizoaffective and bipolar disorders. Psychopathology 1997; 30:53–58.
19. Brockington IF, Meltzer HY. The nosology of schizoaffective psychosis. Psychiatr Dev 1983; 4:317–338.
20. Lapensée MA. A review of schizoaffective disorder: I. Current concepts. Can J Psychiatry 1992; 37:335–346.
21. Fowler RC. Remitting schizophrenia as a variant of affective disorder. Schizophr Bull 1978; 4:68–77.
22. Gershon ES, Delisi LE, Hamovit J. A controlled family study of chronic psychoses schizophrenia and schizoaffective disorder. Arch Gen Psychiatry 1988; 45:328–336.
23. Tsuang MT. Morbidity risk of schizophrenia and affective disorders among first-degree relatives of patients with schizoaffective disorder. Br J Psychiatry 1991; 158:165–170.
24. Bertelsen A, Gottesman II. Schizoaffective psychosis: genetic clues to classification. Am J Med Genet 1995; 60:7–11.
25. Cardno AG, Rijsdijk FV, Sham PA, Murray RM, McGuffin P. A twin study of genetic relationship between psychotic symptoms. Am J Psychiatry 2002; 159:539–545.
26. Kendler KS, Karkowski-Shuman L, O'Neill FA, Straub RE, MacLean CHJ, Walsh D. Resemblance of psychotic symptoms and syndromes in affected sibling pairs from the Irish study of high-density schizophrenia families: Evidence for Possible Etiologic Heterogeneity. Am J Psychiatry 1997; 154:191–198.
27. Samson JA, Simpson JC, Tsuang MT. Outcome of schizoaffective disorders. Schizophr Bull 1988; 14:543–554.
28. Kendler KS, McGuire M, Gurneberg AM, Walsh D. Examining the validity of DSM-III-R schizoaffective disorder and its putative subtypes in the Roscommon family study. Am J Psychiatry 1995; 152:755–764.
29. Marneros A, Rohde A, Deister A. Frequency and phenomenology of persisting alterations in affective, schizoaffective and schizophrenia disorders: a comparison. Psychopathology 1998; 31:23–28.
30. Harrow M, Grossman LS, Herbener ES. Ten-year outcome: patients with schizoaffective disorders, schizophrenia, affective disorders and mood-incongruent psychotic symptoms. Br J Psychiatry 2000; 177:421–426.
31. Evans JD, Heaton RK, Paulsen JS, McAdams LA, Heaton SC, Jeste DV. Schizoaffective disorder: a form of schizophrenia or affective disorder? J Clin Psychiatry 1999; 60: 874–882.
32. Coryell W, Keller M, Lavori P, Endicott J. Affective syndromes, psychotic features, and prognosis I. Depression. Arch Gen Psychiatry 1990; 47:651–657.
33. Coryell W, Keller M, Lavori P, Endicott J. Affective syndromes, psychotic features, and prognosis II. Mania. Arch Gen Psychiatry 1990; 47:658–662.

34. Tien AY, Eaton WW. Psychopathologic precursors and sociodemographic risk factors for the schizophrenia syndrome. Arch Gen Psychiatry 1992; 49:37–46.
35. Tsuang MT, Simpson JC, Fleming JA. Schizoaffective disorder. In: Gelder MG, López-Ibor JJ Jr, Andreasen NC, eds. New Oxford Textbook of Psychiatry. New York: Oxford University Press, 2000:400–412.
36. Berner P, Lenz G. Definitions of schizoaffective psychosis: mutual concordance and relationship to schizophrenia and affective disorders. In: Marneros A, Tsuang MT, eds. Schizoaffective Psychosis. New York: Springer, 1986:31–49.
37. Marneros A, Deister A, Rohde A. Psychopathological and social status of patients with affective, schizophrenic and schizoaffective disorders alter long-term course. Acta Psychiatr Scand 1990; 82:352–358.
38. Tsuang MT, Simpson JC, Fleming JA. Epidemiology of suicide. Int Rev Psychiatry 1992; 4:117–129.
39. Angst J, Stassen HH, Gross G. Suicide in affective and schizoaffective disorders. In: Marneros A, Tsuang MT, eds. Affective and Schizoaffective Disorders. New York: Springer, 1990:168–185.
40. McElroy SL, Keck PE, Strakowski SM. An overview of the treatment of schizoaffective disorder. J Clin Psychiatry 1999; 60(suppl 5):16–21.
41. Escamilla MA. Diagnosis and treatment of mood disorders that co-occur with schizophrenia. Psychiatr Serv 2001; 52:911–919.
42. Levinson DF, Umapathy C, Musthaq M. Treatment of schizoaffective disorder and schizophrenia with mood symptoms. Am J Psychiatry 1999; 156:1138–1148.
43. Biederman J, Lerner Y, Belmaker RH. Combination of lithium carbonate and haloperidol in schizoaffective disorder. Arch Gen Psychiatry 1979; 36:327–333.
44. Siris SG. The treatment of schizoaffective disorder. In: Dunner DL, ed. Current Psychiatry Therapy II. Philadelphia: W. B. Saunders, 1996:196–201.
45. Braden W, Fink EB, Qualls CB, Ho CK, Samuels WO. Lithium and chlorpromazine in psychotic inpatients. Psychiatry Res 1982; 7:69–81.
46. Lerner Y, Mintzer Y, Schestatzky M. Lithium combined with haloperidol in schizophrenic patients. Br J Psychiatry 1988; 153:359–362.
47. Okuma T, Yamashita I, Takahashi R, Itoh H, Kurihara M, Otsuki S, Watanabe S, Sarai K, Hazama H, Inanaga K. A double-blind study of adjunctive carbamazepine versus placebo on excited states of schizophrenic and schizoaffective disorders. Acta Psychiatr Scand 1989; 80:250–259.
48. Placidi GF, Lenzi A, Lazzerini F, Cassano GB, Akiskal HS. The comparative efficacy and safety of carbamazepine versus lithium: a randomized, double-blind 3-year trial in 83 patients. J Clin Psychiatry 1986; 47:490–494.
49. Fenn HH, Robinson D, Luby V, Dangel C, Buxton E, Beatty M, Kraemer H, Yesavage JA. Trends in pharmacotherapy of schizoaffective and bipolar affective disorder: a 5-year naturalistic study. Am J Psychiatry 1996; 153:711–713.
50. McElroy SL, Keck PE Jr. Pharmacological agents for the treatment of acute bipolar mania. Biol Psychiatry 2000; 48:539–557.
51. Kramer MS, Vogel WH, DiJohnson C, Dewey DA, Sheves P, Cavicchia S, Litle P, Schmidt R, Kimes I. Antidepressants in "depressed" schizophrenic inpatients: a controlled trial. Arch Gen Psychiatry 1989; 46:922–928.
52. Kapur S, Remington G. Serotonin–dopamine interaction and its relevance to schizophrenia. Am J Psychiatry 1996; 153:466–476.
53. Siris SG, Bench C. Depression and schizophrenia. In: Hirsch SR, Weinberger DR, eds. Schizophrenia. 2nd ed. Oxford: Blackwell Science Ltd, 2003:142–167.
54. Keck PE Jr, Manji HK. Current and emerging treatment for acute mania and long-term prophilaxis for bipolar disorder. In: Davis KL, Charney D, Coyle JT, Nemeroff CH, eds. Neuropsychopharmacology: The Fifth Generation of Progress. Philadelphia: Lippincott Williams & Wilkins, 2002:1109–1118.

55. Naber D, Hippius H. The European experience with the use of clozapine. Hosp Comm Psychiatry 1990; 41:886–890.
56. Mc Elroy Sl, Dessain EC, Pope HG Jr, Cole JO, Keck PE Jr, Frankenberg FR, Aizley HG, O'Brien S. Clozapine in the treatment of psychotic mood disorders, schizoaffective disorder, and schizophrenia. J Clin Psychiatry 1991; 52:411–414.
57. Banov MD, Zarate CA, Tohen M, Scialabba D, Wines JD, Kolbrener M, Kim J, Cole JO. Clozapine therapy in refractory affective disorders: polarity predicts response in long-term follow-up. J Clin Psychiatry 1994; 55:295–300.
58. Malhotra AK, Litman RE, Su TP. Clozapine response in schizoaffective disorder. New Research Program and Abstracts of the 146th Annual Meeting of the American Psychiatric Association, San Francisco, CA, May 24,1993.
59. Calabrese JR, Kimmel SE, Woyshville MJ, Rapport DJ, Faust CJ, Thompson PA, Meltzer HY. Clozapine for treatment-refractory mania. Am J Psychiatry 1996; 153: 759–762.
60. Barbini B, Scherillo P, Benedetti F, Crespi G, Colombo C, Smeraldi E. Response to clozapine in acute mania is more rapid than that of chlorpromazine. Int Clin Psychopharmacol 1997; 12:109–112.
61. Suppes T, Webb A, Paul B, Carmody T, Kraemer H, Rush AJ. Clinical outcome in a randomized one-year trial of clozapine versus treatment as usual for patients with treatment-resistant illness and a history of mania. Am J Psychiatry 1999; 156:1164–1169.
62. Meltzer HY, Alphs L, Green AI, Altamura AC, Anand R, Bertoldi A, Bourgeois M, Chouinard G, Islam MZ, Kane J, Krishnan P, Lindenmayer JP, Potkin S. Clozapine treatment for suicidality in schizophrenia. Arch Gen Psychiatry 2003; 60:82–91.
63. Kane JM, Leucht S, Carpenter D, Docherty JP. The Expert Consensus Guidelines Series: optimizing pharmacologic treatment of psychotic disorders. J Clin Psychiatry 2003; 64(suppl 12):4–100.
64. Keck PE Jr, Wilson DR, Strakowski SM, McElroy SL, Kizer DL, Balistreri TM, Holtman HM, Depreist M. Clinical predictors of acute risperidone response in schizophrenia, schizoaffective disorders and psychotic mood disorders. J Clin Psychiatry 1995; 56:466–470.
65. Masand PS, Xiaohong W, Gupta S, Schwartz TL, Subhdeep V, Hameed A. Comparison of risperidone and olanzapine in bipolar and schizoaffective disorders. J Clin Psychiatry 2002; 4:70–73.
66. Ceskova E, Svetska J. Double-blind comparison of risperidone and haloperidol in schizophrenic and schizoaffective psychosis. Pharmacopsychiatry 1993; 26:121–124.
67. Müller-Siecheneder F, Müller MJ, Hillert A, Szegedi A, Wetzel H, Benkert O. Risperidone versus haloperidol and amitriptyline in the treatment of patients with a combined psychotic and depressive syndrome. J Clin Psychopharmacol 1998; 18:111–120.
68. Segal J, Berk M, Brook S. Risperidone compared with both lithium and haloperidol in mania: a double-blind randomized controlled trial. Clin Neuropharmacol 1998; 21:176–180.
69. Hirschfeld R, Keck P, Karcher K, Kramer M, Grossman F. Rapid antimanic effect of risperidone monotherapy: a 3-week multicenter, double-blind, placebo controlled trial. Bipolar Disord 2003; 5:53; abstract P84.
70. Sachs GS, Grossman F, Ghaemi SN, Okamoto A, Bowden CL. Combination of a mood stabilizer with risperidone or haloperidol for treatment of acute mania: a double-blind, placebo-controlled comparison of efficacy and safety. Am J Psychiatry 2002; 159:1146–1154.
71. Yatham LN, Grossman F, Augustyns F, Vieta E, Ravindran A. Mood stabilisers plus risperidone or placebo in the treatment of acute mania. cInternational, double-blind, randomised controlled trial. Br J Psychiatry 2003; 182:141–147.
72. Tran PV, Tollefson GD, Sanger TM, Lu Y, Berg PH, Beasley Cm Jr. Olanzapine versus haloperidol in the treatment of schizoaffective disorder. Acute and long-term therapy. Br J Psychiatry 1999; 174:15–22.

73. Berk M, Ichim L, Brook S. Olanzapine compared to lithium in mania: a double-blind randomized controlled trial. Int Clin Psychopharmacol 1997; 12:109–112.
74. Tohen M, Sanger TM, Mc Elroy SL, Tollefson GD, Chengappa KN, Daniel DG, Petty F, Centorrino F, Wang R, Grundy SL, Greaney MG, Jacobs TG, David SR, Toma V. Olanzapine versus placebo in the treatment of acute mania. Am J Psychiatry 1999; 156:702–709.
75. Tohen M, Chengappa KN, Suppes T. Efficacy of olanzapine in combination with valproate or lithium in the treatment of mania in patients partially nonresponsive to valproate or lithium monotherapy. Arch Gen Psychiatry 2002; 59:62–69.
76. Daniel DG, Zimbroff DL, Potkin SG, Reeves KR, Harrigan EP, Lakshminarayanan M. The Ziprasidone Study Group. Ziprasidone 80 mg/day and 160 mg/day in the acute exacerbation of schizophrenia and schizoaffective disorder: a 6-week placebo-controlled trial. Neuropsychopharmacology 1999; 20:491–505.
77. Keck PE Jr, Reeves KR, Harrigan EP, the Ziprasidone Study Group. Ziprasidone in the short-term treatment of patients with schizoaffective disorder: results from two double-blind, placebo-controlled, multicenter studies. J Clin Psychopharmacol 2001; 21:27–35.
78. Keck PE Jr, Versiani M, Potkin S, West SA, Giller E, Ice K, the Ziprasidone Study Group. Ziprasidone in the treatment of acute bipolar mania: a three-week, placebo-controlled, double-blind, randomized trial. Am J Psychiatry 2003; 160:741–748.
79. Allen MH. Managing the agitated psychotic patient: a reappraisal of the evidence. J Clin Psychiatry 2000; 61(suppl 14):11–20.
80. Sachs GS. Bipolar mood disorder: practical strategies for acute and maintenance phase treatment. J Clin Psychopharmacol 1996; 16(2):32S–47S.
81. Kapur S, Zypursky RB, Remington G. Clinical and theoretical implications of 5-ht2 and D2 receptor occupancy of clozapine, risperidone, and olanzapine in schizophrenia. Am J Psychiatry 1999; 156:286–293.
82. Kopala LC, Kimberley PG, Honer WG. Extrapiramidal signs and clinical symptoms in first-episode schizophrenia: response to low-dose risperidone. J Clin Psychopharmacol 1997; 17:308–312.
83. Aitchinson KJ, Meehan K, Murray RM. Prescribing for a first episode of schizophrenia-like psychosis. In: First Episode on Psychosis. London: Martin Dunitz, 1999:43–66.
84. Mc Elroy SL, Keck PE, Stanton SP, Tugrul KC, Bennett JA, Strakowski SM. A randomized comparison of divalproex oral loading versus haloperidol in the initial treatment of acute psychotic mania. J Clin Psychiatry 1996; 57(4):142–146.
85. Aitchinson KJ, Meehan K, Murray RM. Prescribing for a first episode of affective psychosis. In: First Episode on Psychosis. London: Martin Dunitz, 1999:67–82.
86. Bazire S. C4.5 drug interactions. In: Psychotropic Drug Directory 2003/04. Salisbury: Fivepin Publishing Limited, 2003:271–370.
87. Thase ME. What role do atypical antipsychotics drugs have in treatment-resistant depression? J Clin Psychol 2002; 63(2):95–103.
88. Baldessarini RJ, Cohen BM, Teicher MH. Significance of neuroleptic dose and plasma level in the pharmacological treatment of psychosis. Arch Gen Psychiatry 1988; 45:79–90.
89. Ries RK, Wilson L, Bokan JA, Chiles JA. ECT in medication resistant schizoaffective disorder. Comprehensive Psychiatry 1981; 22:167–173.
90. Allness DJ, Knoedler WH. The PACT Model of Community-Based Treatment for Persons with Severe and Persistent Mental Illnesses: a Manual for PACT Start-Up. Arlington: NAMI, 1998.
91. Chadwick P, Birchwood M, Trower P. Cognitive Therapy for Delusions, Voices and Paranoia. Chichester: Wiley, 1996.
92. Lam DH, Jones SH, Hayward P, Bright JA. Cognitive Therapy for Bipolar Disorder. Chichester: Wiley, 1999.
93. Herz MI, Lamberti S, Mintz J, Scott R, O'Dell SP, McCartan L, Nix G. A program for relapse prevention in schizophrenia. Arch Gen Psychiatry 2000; 57:277–283.

94. Hogarty GE. Personal Therapy for Schizophrenia and Related Disorders. New York: The Guilford Press, 2002.
95. McFarlane WR. Multifamiliy Groups in the Treatment of Severe Psychiatric Disorders. New York: The Guilford Press, 2002.
96. Marneros A, Tsuang MT. Schizoaffective psychosis: present level and future perspectives. In: Marneros A, Tsuang MT, eds. Schizoaffective Psychoses. Berlin: Springer-Verlag, 1986.

16
Treatment of Bipolar Disorder in Children and Adolescents

Karen Dineen Wagner
Division of Child and Adolescent Psychiatry, Department of Psychiatry and Behavioral Sciences, University of Texas Medical Branch, Galveston, Texas, U.S.A.

INTRODUCTION

Bipolar disorder in children and adolescents is a serious illness that significantly disrupts a child's emotional, social, and academic development. It is important to identify effective treatments for this childhood disorder. To date, there are very little controlled data available about pharmacotherapy or psychotherapy for the treatment of pediatric bipolar disorder. This chapter provides an up-to-date status of the treatment of bipolar disorder in children and adolescents.

PHARMACOTHERAPY

Lithium

There is one small double-blind placebo-controlled trial for adolescents with bipolar disorder and substance dependence (1). Twenty-five outpatients were randomized to lithium or placebo for a 6-week trial. Measures used to assess outcome included the Schedule for Affective Disorders and Schizophrenia for School-Aged Children, Children's Global Assessment Scale (C-GAS) (2) and the Diagnostic and Statistical Manual of Mental Disorders (3rd edition) Revised (3) criteria for substance dependence. Significantly, more of the lithium treated patients showed improvement in global functioning than for the placebo group. The mean serum level for lithium responders was 0.9 meq/L. Adverse effects more common in the lithium group than the placebo group were polydipsia and polyuria.

There is a substantial amount of uncontrolled information regarding the use of lithium for bipolar disorder. In case series and case reports, clinical responses have ranged from 50% to 100% (4). In the largest open trial to date (5), 100 adolescents with an acute manic episode were treated with lithium for 4 weeks. The mean dose of lithium at the end of week 4 was 1.355 mg/day with a mean lithium serum level of 0.93 meq/L. Sixty-three percent of the adolescents had a positive response defined as $\geq$33% reduction in the Young Mania Rating Scale (YMRS) (6) from baseline and a rating of much improved or very much improved on the clinical global impression-improvement (CGI-I) (7) items. Remission of mania, defined as an YMRS score ≤6, was achieved by 26 of the adolescents. The most common side effects were weight gain, polydipsia, polyuria, headache, tremor, gastrointestinal pain, nausea, vomiting, anorexia, and diarrhea.

Common side effects of lithium include polydipsia, polyuria, nausea, vomiting, headache, weight gain, diarrhea, tremor, and acne. Less common but more serious side effects include renal function abnormalities, such as proteinuria, nephrogenic diabetes insipidus, neurotoxicity, hypothyroidism, cardiac conduction abnormalities, and leukocytosis (8).

Divalproex Sodium

There is one multi-site open study of divalproex treatment for children and adolescents aged 7 to 19 years with a diagnosis of bipolar disorder I or II, manic or mixed episode (9). Forty patients received divalproex treatment over a 2- to 8-week period. Divalproex was initiated at dosage of 15 mg/kg/day and titrated to achieve a serum blood level of 45–125 μg/mL. Twenty-two subjects (61%) showed ≥50% improvement in the Mania Rating Scale during the open-label period. Of the 23 subjects who discontinued the study, 6 (15%) discontinued for ineffectiveness, 6 (15%) for intolerance, 6 (15%) for non-compliance, and 6 (15%) for other reasons. The most common adverse events were headache, nausea, vomiting, diarrhea, and somnolence. In other case reports, case series and single-site open studies, response rates to divalproex treatment pediatric bipolar disorder have ranged from 66% to 83% (4).

To assess the long-term effectiveness and safety of divalproex in children aged 4 to 18 years with bipolar disorder, a retrospective chart review was conducted (10). Fifteen outpatients received divalproex (mean dose 966 per day; mean serum level 79.4 μg/mL) for a mean duration of 1.4 years. Eight (53%) patients had a moderate to marked improvement on the CGI-I Scale. Six (40%) discontinued divalproex, mostly due to weight gain.

Common side effects of divalproex sodium are nausea, vomiting, sedation, and weight gain. Less common but more serious side effects include pancreatitis, hepatic failure, thrombocytopenia, behavioral changes, and alopecia (11). There have been reports of an association of divalproex with polycystic ovarian syndrome in women with epilepsy who were treated in youth with divalproex (12,13). However, this association has not been found for women treated with divalproex for bipolar disorder (14).

Carbamazepine

In an active comparator study, 42 children and adolescents aged 8 to 18 years with bipolar I or II disorder, mixed or manic episode, were randomized to carbamazepine, lithium, or divalproex for 6- to 8-week treatment (15). Mean serum carbamazepine level was 7.1 μg/L, mean serum lithium level was 0.9 meq/L, and mean divalproex serum level was 82.8 μg/L. Response was defined as ≥50% reduction in the YMRS from baseline and a score of much or very much improved on the CGI-Bipolar Disorder Scale. The response rates for carbamazepine, lithium, and divalproex were 38%, 38%, and 53%, respectively. There were no statistically significant differences among these response rates. Nausea was the most common adverse effect in all treatment groups. Other side effects included sedation in the carbamazepine and divalproex groups; rash and dizziness in the carbamazepine group; and increased appetite, polyuria, and diarrhea in the lithium group. These side effects were assessed to be mild to moderate and well tolerated by most subjects.

Common side effects of carbamazepine are nausea, vomiting, dizziness, sedation, and rash (4). More serious side effects include hepatoxicity, aplastic anemia, agranulocytosis, and multiple drug interactions (16).

Oxcarbazepine

The effectiveness of adjunctive treatment with oxcarbazepine has been examined in a retrospective chart review of 44 patients, ages 6 to 18 years, with bipolar disorder, depression, or anxiety disorder. Eight-six percent of patients had clinical improvement defined as much or very much improved on the CGI. Side effects included sedation and dizziness (17).

Common side effects of oxcarbazepine include headache, dizziness, somnolence, fatigue, nausea, and vomiting. Hyponatremia, which is reversible with oxcarbazepine discontinuation, may occur (11).

Risperidone

In an open-label 8-week study, 30 outpatients aged 6 to 17 years with bipolar disorder I or II, manic or mixed episode were treated with risperidone (18). Risperidone was initiated at a dose of 0.25 mg/day for children up to 12 years of age to a maximum dose of 2 mg/day. For children over 12 years, risperidone was initiated at a dose of 0.5 mg/day to a maximum of 4 mg/day. The mean endpoint dose of risperidone was 1.3 mg/day. Nine subjects dropped from the study, two were lost to follow-up, and seven were discontinued because they could not be stabilized on risperidone monotherapy. There was a significant reduction in YMRS scores over the trial.

The effectiveness of risperidone and olanzapine were assessed in 12 pre-schoolers with bipolar disorder in an open-label 8-week study (19). Risperidone was initiated at 0.25 mg/day and increased to a maximum dose of 2 mg/day. Olanzapine was initiated at 1.25 mg/day and increased to a maximum dose of 10 mg/day. Eight children received risperidone and four children received olanzapine. By week 8, there was a significant improvement in scores on the YMRS. No difference was found in effectiveness between the two atypical neuroleptics. The most common adverse effects were headache, insomnia, and stomachache.

In a retrospective chart review of 28 outpatient children and adolescents aged 4 to 17 with bipolar disorder who were treated with risperidone for an average of 6 months, 82% showed clinical improvement in mania and aggression and 69% showed improvement in psychosis (20).

Common side effects of risperidone include sedation and weight gain. Less common side effects include hepatoxicity, orthostasis, hyperprolactinemia, constipation, dizziness, and tachycardia, and extrapyramidal symptoms at high doses (11).

Olanzapine

In an open-label 8-week trial, 23 children and adolescents ranging in age from 5 to 14 years with a diagnosis of bipolar disorder I or II, mixed or manic, received olanzapine treatment (21). The mean dose of olanzapine at endpoint was 9.6 mg/day. Based upon a response of $\geq$30% reduction in the YMRS and the CGI-S mania score $\leq$3, 61% of the subjects had a positive response to treatment. The most frequently reported adversc events were increased appetite, somnolence, abdominal pain, and weight gain.

Common side effects of olanzapine include sedation and weight gain. Less common side effects include orthostasis, constipation, tachycardia, gastrointestinal side effects, diabetes, hyperlipidemia, increased appetite, and hepatic transaminase elevation (11).

Quetiapine

Quetiapine has been studied as adjunctive treatment to divalproex in a double-blind placebo-controlled 6-week study (22). In this study, 30 adolescents with bipolar I disorder, mixed or manic episode, aged 12 to 18 years who were hospitalized received divalproex 20 mg/kg/day. The subjects were concurrently randomized to adjunctive quetiapine, which was titrated to 450 mg/day or to placebo. Response was defined as a $\geq$50% reduction in the YMRS score from baseline to endpoint. There was a significantly greater response in the divalproex–quetiapine-treated group (87%) than the divalproex–placebo group.

Side effects of quetiapine include somonolence, tachycardia, orthostasis, dizziness, constipation, weight gain, dyspepsia, dry mouth, and cataracts (11).

Topiramate

The efficacy of topiramate in adolescents with acute mania was assessed in a randomized double-blind placebo-controlled multi-center trial (23). Fifty-six patients participated in this study, which was designed as a 200-patient study. However, the study was terminated after randomizing 56 patients because the adult mania trials with topiramate failed to show efficacy. Adolescents were randomized to topiramate and titrated to 400 mg/day (mean daily dose of topiramate 278 mg/day at endpoint) or to placebo. There was no statistically significant difference between the topiramate group and placebo group in the change in YMRS score from baseline to endpoint. Mean CGI-I scores were significantly better at endpoint for topiramate-treated patients than for the placebo group. The most common adverse events in the topiramate-treated group were anorexia, nausea, diarrhea, paresthesia, and somnolence.

In a retrospective chart review of 26 youths with bipolar disorder ranging in age from 5 to 21 years who received adjunctive topiramate over a 1- to 30-month period, 73 of these patients showed improvement in mania defined as $\geq$50% reduction in the YMRS score (24). Adverse effects included cognitive disturbance and weight gain.

Common side effects of topiramate include weight loss, sedation, headache, gastrointestinal side effects, paresthesias, muscle aches, impaired concentration, and nervousness. Potential side effects of more concern include hepatotoxicity, renal stones, and glaucoma (11).

Gabapentin

There are no data available specific to the use of gabapentin for pediatric bipolar disorder. However, in a retrospective study of 18 adolescents ranging in age from 3 to 18 years, which included 16 adolescents with bipolar features or schizoaffective disorder who failed prior mood stabilizer treatment, 16 of these patients had cessation of cycling and, of these, 6 reported improved mood when treated with gabapentin in doses ranging from 900 to 2400 mg/day (25).

Side effects of gabapentin include somnolence, fatigue, headache, weight gain, nausea, ataxia, dizziness, and nystagmus (11).

Lamotrigine

Lamotrigine as an adjunctive therapy in the treatment of 22 adolescents with refractory bipolar depression was assessed in a 6-week open study (26). Response was defined as a $\geq$50% reduction in the Hamilton Depression Rating Scale (27) score at endpoint as compared with baseline. Sixteen (72%) of these adolescents had a positive response to a combination of lamotrigine (50–100 mg/day) and divalproex during the treatment period. Approximately 10% of subjects developed a rash.

Side effects of lamotrigine include nausea, vomiting, ataxia, and constipation. The incidence of serious rash including Stevens–Johnson syndrome is increased with the use of high doses of lamotrigine in combination with divalproex (11).

Clozapine

Ten hospitalized adolescents aged 12 to 17 years with a severe acute mania or mixed episodes who had failed prior trials of mood stabilizers and antipsychotics received clozapine either as monotherapy or in combination with a mood stabilizer in 15- to 28-day open trial (28). Clozapine doses range from 75 to 300 mg/day. Significant improvement in mood symptoms based upon scores on the YMRS, Brief Psychiatric Rating Scale, C-GAS, and CGI-Severity of Illness scores were found. Side effects included hyperphagia, weight gain, sedation, and enuresis.

Common side effects of clozapine include sedation, dizziness, increased salivation, constipation, tachycardia, increased appetite, and weight gain. Potentially serious side effects include agranulocytosis and petit mal seizures (11).

Combination Pharmacotherapy

There is increased interest in evaluating whether combination pharmacotherapy is more effective than monotherapy or whether monotherapy can be maintained for a sustained period of time for a child with bipolar disorder. Kowatch et al. (29) conducted a continuation study from their acute treatment comparison of a single mood stabilizer (lithium, divalproex, or carbamazepine). Thirty-five children and adolescents who had participated in the acute-phase treatment continued in a 6-week open extension study. For those patients who were treatment non-responders at the end of the acute phase, alternative treatment options included switching mood stabilizers or augmenting with another mood stabilizer, a stimulant, an antidepressant, or an atypical antipsychotic. It was found that during the extension phase, 20 (58%) required combination pharmacotherapy with one or two mood stabilizers and either a stimulant, an atypical antipsychotic or an antidepressant. Moreover, the response rate (80%) to combination treatment with two mood stabilizers was high for these patients who had not responded to monotherapy with a mood stabilizer.

The effectiveness of combination lithium and divalproex sodium was assessed in an open-label study with 96 children and adolescents, ages 5 to 17 years, with bipolar I or II disorder (30). Significant improvement on all outcome measures including the YMR-S, Children's Depression Rating Scale-Revised, and CGAS was found by week 8 and at the end of the study. The mean study duration was 11.3 weeks. Forty-two (47%) patients met remission criteria, which was defined as four contiguous weekly ratings of YMRS ≤12.5, CDRS-R ≤40, and CGAS ≥51, clinical stability, and no evidence of mood cycling. At study end, the mean daily dose of divalproex was 862.5 mg/day with a mean blood level of 79.8 μg/L. The mean dose of lithium at study end was 923.3 mg/day with a lithium level of 0.9 meq/L. Fifteen (16.7%) patients were withdrawn from the study due to medication intolerance. Adverse effects included ataxis/neurological side effects, elevated thyrotropin level, proteinuria, enuresis, emesis, and dysphoria, which was thought attributable to lithium. Medication discontinuations thought attributable to divalproex were increased transaminases and worsening manic symptoms with increased divalproex dose. The most common side effects occurring in at least 20% of the subjects included emesis, enuresis, stomach pain, tremor, increased thirst, headache, nausea, sedation, increased appetite, and diarrhea.

The use of adjunctive antipsychotic medication and its optimal duration for bipolar psychosis was assessed in an open study with lithium and adjunctive antipsychotic medication (31). Twenty-eight adolescents with bipolar I disorder, manic or mixed episode with psychotic features received open treatment with lithium and adjunctive antipsychotic medication. If psychotic symptoms resolved, the antipsychotic medication dose was gradually decreased and discontinued after 4 weeks of therapeutic lithium levels (0.6–1.2 meq/L). Sixty-four percent of the patients showed clinical improvement after 4 weeks on combination treatment. Only 14 of the 28 adolescents were clinically stable enough to have their antipsychotic medication discontinued. Of those 14, 6 (42%) had a clinically significant exacerbation of symptoms on lithium monotherapy, which required resumption of their adjunctive antipsychotic medication.

As noted previously, adjunctive quetiapine to divalproex treatment resulted in a higher response rate (87%) compared to the response rate for the divalproex and placebo group (53%) for adolescents with bipolar I or II disorder (22).

Treatment Duration

The optimal duration of pharmacotherapy for children and adolescents with bipolar disorder has not been established. However, in an 18-month naturalistic prospective follow-up of 37 adolescents with bipolar I disorder, manic episode, who had been stabilized with lithium during inpatient hospitalization (32), 13 of these patients discontinued lithium therapy shortly after discharge. The relapse rate was 92% in the treatment-non-compliant patients compared to 37% in the treatment-compliant patients. Therefore, it is recommended that mood stabilizer treatment continue for a minimum of 18 months following symptom remission of a manic or hypomanic episode in children.

ELECTROCONVULSIVE THERAPY

A literature review of 20 youths under the age of 18 years of age with mania who had received electroconvulsive therapy reported a response rate of 80% (33). In a 3.5-year follow-up of 10 adolescents treated with ECT of whom five had bipolar disorder, manic or mixed with psychotic features, no cognitive impairment was found at long-term follow-up compared to a psychiatric comparison group (34). In a 2- to 9-year follow-up of five adolescents with mania who received ECT, there were no differences in school achievement compared with a psychiatric control group (35).

PSYCHOEDUCATION

Multi-family psychoeducation group (MFPG) program for childhood mood disorders has been developed by Fristad et al. (36). This is a six-session, manual-driven MFPG therapy program for families of children or adolescents with a mood disorder. The sessions include both family meetings and separate meetings with the parent and child. There is training in communication, cognitive–behavioral interventions, and social problem-solving strategies. In a study designed to assess the impact of adjunctive MFPG on mood-disordered children aged 8 to 11 years and their families (37), 35 children and 47 parents were randomly assigned to receive either MFPG plus treatment as usual or a 6-month wait list condition plus treatment as usual. At 6-month follow-up, the MFPG plus treatment families reported increased parental knowledge about childhood mood symptoms, increased positive family interactions as reported by parents, increased perceptions of parental support as reported by children, and increased utilization of appropriate services by families.

Focused family therapy (FFT) is a psychosocial treatment for families with a bipolar member. The components of FFT include education about coping with the illness and training in communication and problem-solving skills. FFT was originally developed for families with an adult member who had bipolar disorder and is currently being modified for use with families who have bipolar adolescents (38).

SUMMARY

At this time, there are insufficient controlled data to empirically guide treatment decisions for bipolar disorder in children and adolescents. The most studied medications in this age group are lithium and divalproex. Atypical antipsychotics, used either as monotherapy or as an adjunctive treatment, have shown some effectiveness for treatment of manic and hypomanic episodes. Children with bipolar disorder often need combination treatments with mood stabilizers and/or atypical antipsychotics.

There are a number of areas that require further investigation in order to advance treatment for pediatric bipolar disorder. There is a glaring need for large-scale double-blind placebo-controlled trials of mood stabilizers in this age group. Similarly, comparative trials of these mood stabilizers are warranted. It is important to determine whether initial monotherapy or combination therapy results in greater efficacy. The role of adjunctive psychoeducation to psychopharmacotherapy versus pharmacotherapy alone requires further investigation. Maintenance studies of mood stabilizers would assist in establishing optimal treatment duration for youths with bipolar disorder.

REFERENCES

1. Geller B, Cooper TB, Sun K, Zimerman B, Frazier J, Williams M, Heath J. Double-blind and placebo-controlled study of lithium for adolescent bipolar disorders with secondary substance dependency. J Am Acad Child Adolesc Psychiatry 1998; 37(2):171–178.
2. Shaffer D, Gould MS, Brasic J, Ambrosini P, Fisher P, Bird H, Aluwahlia S. A children's global assessment scale (CGAS). Arch Gen Psychiatry 1983; 40:1228–1231.
3. American Psychiatric Association. Diagnostic and Statistical Manual of Mental Disorders. 3rd ed—revised. Washington, DC: APA, 1987.

4. Wagner KD. Management of bipolar disorder in children and adolescents. Psychopharmacol Bull 2002; 36(4):151–159.
5. Kafantaris V, Coletti DJ, Dicker R, Padula G, Kane JM. Lithium treatment of acute mania in adolescents: a large open trial. J Am Acad Child Adolesc Psychiatry 2003; 42(9):1038–1045.
6. Young RC, Biggs JT, Ziegler VE, Meyer DA. A rating scale for mania: reliability, validity and sensitivity. Br J Psychiatry 1978; 133:429–435.
7. Guy W. Clinical Global Impressions. ECDEU Assessment Manual for Psychopharmacology. Rockville, MD: Rev. National Institute of Mental Health, 1976.
8. Wagner KD. Treatment of childhood and adolescent disorders. In: Schatzberg AF, Nemeroff CB, eds. The American Psychiatric Publishing Textbook of Psychopharmacology. 3rd ed. Washington, DC: American Psychiatric Publishing, 2004:949–1007.
9. Wagner KD, Weller E, Carlson G, Sachs G, Biederman J, Frazier JA, Wozniak P, Tracy K, Weller RA, Bowden C. An open-label trial of divalproex in children and adolescents with bipolar disorder. J Am Acad Child Adolesc Psychiatry 2002; 41(10):1224–1230.
10. Henry CA, Zamvil LS, Lam C, Rosenquist KJ, Ghaemi SN. Long-term outcome with divalproex in children and adolescents with bipolar disorder. J Child Adolesc Psychopharmacol 2003; 13:523–529.
11. Wolf WV, Wagner KD. Bipolar disorder in children and adolescents. CNS Spectr 2003; 8(12):954–959.
12. Isojarvi JI, LaatikainenTJ, Pakarinen AJ, Juntunen KT, Myllyla VV. Polycystic ovaries and hyperandrogenism in women taking valproate for epilepsy. N Engl J Med 1993; 329(19):1383–1388.
13. Isojarvi JI, LaatikainenTJ, Knif M, Pakarinen AJ, Juntunen KTS, Myllyla VV. Obesity and endocrine disorders in women taking valproate for epilepsy. Ann Neurol 1996; 39(5):579–584.
14. Rasgon NL, Altshuler LL, Gudeman D, Burt VK, Tanavoli S, Hendrick V, Korenman S. Medication status and polycystic ovary syndrome in women with bipolar disorder: a preliminary report. J Clin Psychiatry 2000; 61(3):173–178.
15. Kowatch RA, Suppes T, Carmody TJ, Bucci JP, Hume JH, Kromelis M, Emslie GJ, Weinberg WA, Rush AJ. Effect size of lithium, divalproex sodium, and carbamazepine in children and adolescents with bipolar disorder. J Am Acad Child Adolesc Psychiatry 2000; 39(6):713–720.
16. Davanzo PA, McCracken JT. Mood stabilizers in the treatment of juvenile bipolar disorder. Advances and controversies. Child Adolesc Psychiatr Clin North Am 2000; 9(1):159–182.
17. Reimherr JP, Rosen SJ, Leahy LF. Oxcarbazepine treatment in child and adolescent mood and anxiety disorders. Annual U.S. Psychiatric Congress, Las Vegas, NV, October 28–31, 2002.
18. Biederman J. Open-label study of risperidone in children with bipolar disorder. 16th Annual Meeting of the European College of Neuropsychopharmacology, Prague, Czech Republic, September 20–24, 2003.
19. Biederman J, Mick E, Faraone S, Johnson M, Murphy H. Open trial of atypical neuroleptics in preschoolers with bipolar disorder. 50th Annual Meeting of the American Academy of Child & Adolescent Psychiatry. Miami Beach, FL, October 14–19, 2003.
20. Frazier JA, Meyer MC, Biederman J, Wozniak J, Wilens TE, Spencer TJ, Kim GS, Shapiro S. Risperidone treatment for juvenile bipolar disorder: a retrospective chart review. J Am Acad Child Adolesc Psychiatry 1999; 38(8):960–965.
21. Frazier JA, Biederman J, Tohen M, Feldman PD, Jacobs TG, Toma V, Rater MA, Tarazi RA, Kim GS, Garfield SB, Sohma M, Gonzalez-Heydrich J, Risser RC, Nowlin ZM. A prospective open-label treatment trial of olanzapine monotherapy in children and adolescents with bipolar disorder. J Child Adolesc Psychopharmacol 2001; 11(3): 239–250.

22. Delbello MP, Schwiers ML, Rosenberg HL Strakowski SM. A double-blind, randomized, placebo-controlled study of quetiapine as adjunctive treatment for adolescent mania. J Am Acad Child Adolesc Psychiatry 2002; 41(10):1216–1223.
23. Del Bello MP, Kushner S, Wang D, Olson W, Capece JA, Fazzio L, Rosenthal N. Topiramate treatment for acute mania in children and adolescents with bipolar I disorder. 42nd Annual Meeting of the American College of Neuropsychopharmacology, San Juan, Puerto Rico, December 7–11, 2003.
24. Delbello M, Kowatch RA, Warner J, Rappaport K, Daniels J, Foster K, Nelson D, Strakowski S. Topiramate use for pediatric bipolar disorder: a retrospective chart review. Annual Meeting of the Institute of Psychiatric Service, Orlando, FL, October 2001.
25. Ryback RS, Brodasky L, Munasifi F. Gabapentin in bipolar disorder. J Neuropsychiatry Clin Neurosci 1997; 9(2):301.
26. Kusumakar V, Yatham LN. An open study of lamotrigine in refractory bipolar depression. Psychiatry Res 1997; 72:145–148.
27. Hamilton M. A rating scale for depression. J Neurol Neurosurg Psychiatry 1960; 23: 56–62.
28. Masi G, Mucci M, Millepiede S. Clozapine in adolescent inpatients with acute mania. J Child Adolesc Psychopharmacol 2002; 12(2):93–99.
29. Kowatch RA, Sethuraman G, Hume JH, Kromelis M, Weinberg WA. Combination pharmacotherapy in children and adolescents with bipolar disorder. Biol Psychiatry 2003; 53(11):978–984.
30. Findling RL, McNamara NK, Gracious BL, Stansbrey RJ, Calabrese JR. Combination lithium and divalproex sodium in pediatric bipolarity. J Am Acad Child Adolesc Psychiatry 2003; 42:895–901.
31. Kafantaris V, Coletti DJ, Dicker R, Padula G, Kane JM. Adjunctive antipsychotic treatment of adolescents with bipolar psychosis. J Am Acad Child Adolesc Psychiatry 2001; 40(12):1448–1456.
32. Strober M, Morrell W, Lampert C, Burroughs J. Relapse following discontinuation of lithium maintenance therapy in adolescents with bipolar I illness: a naturalistic study. Am J Psychiatry 1990; 147:457–461.
33. Rey JM, Walter G. Half a century of ECT use in young people. Am J Psychiatry 1997; 154(5):595–602.
34. Cohen D, Taieb O, Flament M, Benoit N, Chevert S, Corcos M, Fossati P, Jeammet P, Allilaire JF, Basquin M. Absence of cognitive impairment at long-term follow-up in adolescents treated with ECT for severe mood disorder. Am J Psychiatry 2000; 157:460–462.
35. Taieb O, Flament MF, Chevret S, Jeammet P, Allilaire JF, Mazet P, Cohen D. Clinical relevance of electroconvulsive therapy (ECT) in adolescents with severe mood disorder: evidence from a follow-up study. Eur Psychiatry 2002; 17:206–212.
36. Fristad MA, Gavazzi SM, Soldano KW. Multi-family psychoeducation groups for childhood mood disorders: a program description and preliminary efficacy data. Contemp Fam Ther 1998; 20:385–402.
37. Fristad MA, Goldberg-Arnold JS, Gavazzi SM. Multi-family psychoeducation groups in the treatment of children with mood disorders. J Marit Fam Ther 2003; 29:491–504.
38. Taylor DO, Miklowitz DJ, George EL, Axelson D, Birmaher B, Brent D. Modifying focused family therapy for adolescents with bipolar disorder. 5th International Conference on Bipolar Disorder, Pittsburgh, PA, June 12–14, 2003.

17

Treatment of Bipolar Disorder in Late Life

Mark Rapoport, Ayal Schaffer, and Kenneth I. Shulman
Department of Psychiatry, Sunnybrook & Women's College Health Sciences Centre, University of Toronto, Toronto, Canada

INTRODUCTION

There are three broad groups of older bipolar patients. The first group is comprised of patients whose illness began early in life and persisted into old age. The second group is made up of individuals with earlier onset of depression and then a long latency before mania becomes manifest. Finally is the important group of late onset mania (secondary mania) (1). Studies of elderly inpatient bipolars reveal a high prevalence of comorbidity, particularly neurological disorders. This has served to cloud issues of diagnosis and nosology (2) and hence management. The Diagnostic and Statistical Manual of Mental Disorders (DSM-IV) (3) describes "a mood disorder due to a general medical condition" (293.83) but how can we be sure that "the disturbance is the direct physiologic consequence of a general medical condition?" The concept of secondary mania implies that cerebral organic factors are primarily responsible for the emerging manic syndrome (4). Similarly, neurologists tend to use the term "disinhibition syndromes" to describe a condition that is virtually identical to that of secondary mania. Because of the high prevalence of neurologic comorbidity, this scenario is very common in old age (5), and diagnostic clarity is still wanting in this murky area.

The clinical features of mania found in older adults do not appear to differ in a qualitative way from mixed age individuals except for the higher prevalence of cognitive impairment (6). While similar symptoms emerge in an older cohort compared to a mixed age population, the older patients tend towards symptoms of lesser severity and intensity.

Bipolar disorder by its very nature is a fluctuating illness, and its management requires balancing a variety of elements. Not only must treatment address the emergence of manic or depressive symptoms, but also take into account factors such as cognitive deficits, medical comorbidity, and suicide risk.

The mainstay of treatment for bipolar disorder has been the use of mood-stabilizing medications, and in particular, lithium. The definition of a mood stabilizer itself remains in question. Traditionally, medications that were efficacious in the treatment of mania were considered mood stabilizers, yet this may no longer be sufficient. Bauer and Mitchner (7) have proposed a "two-by-two" definition that requires efficacy in the treatment of acute mania, the treatment of acute depression, prevention of mania, and prevention of depression. While lithium is currently the only treatment with evidence in each of these domains, we are in the midst of a dramatic rise in the available treatments for the acute and maintenance phases of bipolar disorder. Treatment options beyond lithium now include several anticonvulsant medications, atypical antipsychotics, as well as short-term psychotherapeutic modalities.

As a lifelong illness, particular attention must be paid to issues of treatment safety and tolerability in patients with bipolar disorder. Furthermore, there has been a positive trend among studies towards use of more clinically relevant outcome measures such as remission, quality of life measures, and most importantly, suicide. This chapter outlines the current state of knowledge in the treatment of bipolar disorder in the elderly, and whenever possible will explore issues beyond efficacy in acute treatment.

MOOD STABILIZERS

There are no randomized controlled trials to inform the treatment of mania in late life. There has been a marked shift over the last decade away from the use of lithium towards the anticonvulsants, and a recent epidemiological study of elderly patients in Ontario confirmed this trend among older patients with no previous history of dementia or convulsive disorders (8). A steady decline in new lithium users was mirrored by a steady increase in the use of valproic acid users between 1993 and 2000, and in 1997, the number of new valproic acid users surpassed new lithium users (8).

Lithium (9,10), valproic acid (11,12), lamotrigine (13,14), olanzapine (15,16), and quetiapine (17,18) have each been approved by various regulatory agencies for the treatment of bipolar disorder in adults, and there has been some data as well for risperidone (19). However, the pivotal studies either excluded elderly patients, or elderly patients were not analyzed as a sub-sample.

Lithium

Evidence for Lithium

Although there have been no randomized trials of lithium for the treatment of depression or mania in the context of bipolar disorder in the elderly (20), uncontrolled naturalistic and retrospective data suggest that lithium has efficacy in the elderly that is comparable to younger populations (21–24). Similarly, there are no randomized studies of lithium for prophylaxis in elderly patients with bipolar disorder. However, in a two-year placebo-controlled study of elderly patients with unipolar major depressive disorder who had achieved remission with antidepressant monotherapy, the addition of lithium substantially delayed relapse (25).

Lithium Dosing Considerations and Toxicity

Age-related decline in creatinine clearance and glomerular filtration rate, as well as a reduction in volume of distribution can substantially delay the clearance of lithium (26), and increase its half-life (27). Lithium toxicity and significant adverse effects have been reported in the elderly with serum levels in the "normal" range for younger adults (28), as pharmacodynamic sensitivity seems to be increased in old age (20). In a recent cross-sectional study, lithium toxicity was seen in 8.1% of older patients treated with lithium (29), and older patients with medical illness represent a particular population in which lithium is poorly tolerated (30). Dosing of lithium in the elderly should likely be reduced to at least half that in younger patients (31), because of pharmacokinetic and pharmacodynamic changes with age. Lithium is generally started at a dose of 150 mg/day, with gradual upward titration to 300 mg/day (32). There has been disagreement in the literature as to the appropriate serum lithium levels for older adults: clinical guidelines generally recommend levels of 0.5 mmol/L (27), and while lithium may be better tolerated at this level, a recent paper suggested that higher levels may be needed for remission of symptoms (33). Lithium levels greater than 0.8 mmol/L are likely to produce significant side effects or toxicity (20).

Adverse Effects

Although adverse effects of lithium are similar in the elderly compared to younger patients, the central nervous system effects can be more prominent, and these include tremor, cognitive deficits (20), and cerebellar abnormalities (34). Other adverse effects including weight gain, nausea, polyuria, hyperglycemia, and cardiac conduction abnormalities can also be particularly problematic (32). Treatment-emergent hypothyroidism may be of particular concern in the elderly. In a cross-sectional community study, 32% of older patients treated with lithium were on thyroxine treatment or had laboratory evidence of hypothyroidism (29).

Monitoring

Before starting lithium, baseline investigations should include renal function tests, electrolytes, thyroid function, blood glucose, and possibly an electrocardiogram. Although these tests, in addition to lithium levels, should be monitored regularly, a recent survey of older adults in Cambridge, U.K. mental health system, identified wide variability in the frequency of monitoring (29). Lithium levels should be monitored with particular care when patients become ill or dehydrated. There are many concurrent medications that can potentially interact with lithium. In particular, angiotensin converting enzyme (ACE) inhibitors, calcium channel blockers, thiazide and loop diuretics, and non-steroidal anti-inflammatory drugs, can increase lithium levels, leading to toxicity (2,35).

Anticonvulsants

Valproate and Carbamazepine: Evidence

Randomized controlled trials of anticonvulsants have been conducted for the treatment of aggression in patients with dementia, and while carbamazepine was effective in a small six-week study (36), valproate showed no benefit over placebo in that population (37). Notwithstanding the lack of effect of valproate in dementia, the medication appears to be well tolerated in patients with dementia (37–39). Nonetheless, thus far there have been only retrospective studies and case series of valproate (20,40–42), and two case reports of carbamazepine for the treatment of bipolar disorder in old age (43,44). A recent report also points to the potential utility of intravenous sodium valproate for acute mania in older adults (45). The largest retrospective study of valproate restricted to elderly patients with bipolar disorder hospitalized for acute mania was conducted by Chen et al. (33). Patients, age 55 and over, treated with lithium ($n = 30$) were compared to valproate-treated patients ($n = 29$). Patients treated with lithium were more likely to be rated as improved compared to those treated with valproate (67% vs. 38%). However, there were no differences between the groups when sub-analyses were conducted of patients with supposedly "therapeutic" levels (≥0.8 mmol/L of lithium or 65–90 μg/mL of valproate) or patients with mixed mania. As discussed above, the definition of "therapeutic" levels of lithium in the older patient is controversial.

With suicide rates being higher with advancing age, and particularly with the presence of a psychiatric illness (46), the impact of mood-stabilizer treatment on suicide risk is particularly important. A recent study in a younger population identified a 2.7 times higher risk of death by suicide among patients treated with divalproex compared with lithium, and a 1.7 times higher risk of non-fatal attempts resulting in hospitalization (47). This requires further exploration in the elderly population. With such little evidence for the efficacy of valproate in older adults with bipolar disorder, the rapid shift in prescription patterns away from lithium is of some concern (8).

Valproate and Carbamazepine: Dosing and Adverse Effects

Valproic acid in the form of divalproex has been clinically seen to be well tolerated at mean doses ranging between 1000 and 1500 mg/day (2). Typical starting doses are 125–250 mg twice daily, with gradual upward titration. The value of serum monitoring in the elderly is unclear, but in one study of younger adults, levels above 350 μmol/L were associated with a greater likelihood of antimanic effect (48), and one retrospective case series in the elderly showed that increased serum levels are associated with greater efficacy (49).

The main side effects of valproate are sedation and gastrointestinal disturbance, which can be mitigated by use of a lower dose (20). Other side effects include tremor and weight gain, muscle weakness, thrombocytopenia, rash, elevated ammonia level, and SIADH, with hepatotoxicity and pancreatitis in rare cases (32). Lab evaluation with liver enzymes, CBC, and ECG is needed prior to starting valproate and these should be monitored over time (40).

Carbamazepine in the elderly is generally started at a dose of 100 mg twice per day, gradually titrating upward to 400–800 mg/day (50). The most common side effects of carbamazepine are sedation, dizziness, nausea, and rash. However, serious side effects include ataxia, nystagmus, leukopenia, agranulocytosis, anticholinergic side effects, Stevens–Johnson's syndrome, and hyponatremia pose particular concern in the elderly (32,40). Lab evaluation is similar to that with valproate.

An understanding of drug interactions with the anticonvulsants is important in the elderly as they are often on numerous medications. As there is no data on these interactions specifically in the elderly, readers are referred to Chapter 19 of this volume for a discussion of these.

Other Anticonvulsants

Little data are currently available regarding the use of gabapentin and lamotrigine in the treatment of bipolar disorder in the elderly. In non-geriatric patients with bipolar disorder, the only controlled trial of gabapentin monotherapy was negative (51), and it is now recommended only as adjunctive treatment. While one case series (52) and one case report (53) found gabapentin to be well tolerated and helpful in geriatric mania, another case series for bipolar depression was negative (54). Gabapentin, which is not metabolized or bound to protein, has a favorable adverse effect profile in the elderly with epilepsy (55). The most common side effects are somnolence, dizziness, ataxia, and fatigue, with less common gastrointestinal side effects and myalgia (32). Typical starting doses for older patients would be 25 mg twice daily.

There is good evidence for the use of lamotrigine monotherapy for the acute and prophylactic treatment of non-geriatric bipolar depression, although predictably data are limited in the elderly (13,14). Lamotrigine was added with good effect to divalproex in a case study of the treatment of a rapid-cycling elderly bipolar patient (56), and was shown to be effective in an open-label study of treatment-refractory bipolar disorder that included elderly patients (57). In a study, which pooled 13 clinical trials of lamotrigine in elderly patients with epilepsy, lamotrigine was well tolerated, with adverse effects less common than in carbamazepine (49% vs. 72%), particularly with lower rates of somnolence and rash (58). Common side effects of lamotrigine in the adult clinical trials include headaches and rash. Side effects of insomnia, memory impairment, and somnolence may be particularly salient for the elderly (32). Typical dosing for adults is: 25 mg for the first week, then 50 mg for two weeks, then increase by 50–100 mg every two weeks to a target dose of 200 mg. The target dose may need to be lower in the elderly, but data are lacking. If lamotrigine is used in combination with valproic acid, the dose is cut in half, whereas if it is used with carbamazepine, the dosage is doubled. The risk of Stevens–Johnson's Syndrome with lamotrigine is low [approximately 1:5000 (59)], but may be higher in combination with valproate (32). While there are preliminary data for topiramate and oxcarbazepine in the treatment of bipolar disorder (60,61), experience with these in the elderly is limited to patients with epilepsy (55) and a case report of adjunctive topiramate for bipolar disorder (62). While oxcarbazepine is generally well tolerated in older adults with epilepsy, hyponatremia is a concern (55,63). Cognitive side effects of topiramate may be particularly problematic for older adults (55,64). More information is needed regarding the efficacy of these newer anticonvulsants for older adults with bipolar disorder before they are recommended for clinical use.

ANTIPSYCHOTICS

In some acutely manic older patients, lithium and the anticonvulsant medications discussed above are insufficient in providing rapid relief of agitation, psychosis, and aggression. As such, use of antipsychotic medications can be critical. The risk of tardive dyskinesia with typical antipsychotics is increased in patients with bipolar disorder (65), and up to five- to sixfold in older patients (66). As such, adjuvant typical antipsychotic treatment is potentially problematic in the elderly. Furthermore, the elderly may be particularly vulnerable to extrapyramidal symptoms, anticholinergic side effects, and orthostatic hypotension, which are common with typical antipsychotic use (67). Recent research suggests the utility of atypical antipsychotics as mood stabilizers for adults with acute mania (68). However, elderly patients were either excluded or not analyzed separately (some of the studies included patients up to the age of 70) in the large-scale trials of risperidone, olanzapine, and quetiapine for the treatment of mania.

While there are no controlled trials of atypical antipsychotics for mania in late life, case reports and small case series suggest some benefit to clozapine (69), olanzapine (70), risperidone (71), and quetiapine (72). In a recent double-blind controlled trial of olanzapine and risperidone in elderly patients with schizophrenia, both these medications were well tolerated, and there were no differences in clinical outcomes between the groups (73). The median doses used were 2 mg/day of risperidone and 10 mg/day of olanzapine, and extrapyramidal symptoms were reduced over the course of the trial. There is growing evidence that the atypical antipsychotics may be effective in the long-term management of bipolar disorder in younger adults (15,74). Given the absence of controlled literature on atypical antipsychotics in older bipolar patients, readers seeking information about side effects, drug interactions, and monitoring should turn to Chapter 20 of this volume.

ANTIDEPRESSANTS

As per clinical guidelines in younger patients with bipolar disorder (75), the depressed phase of bipolar disorder is generally managed in old age by the use of mood stabilizers. However, in many patients with bipolar disorder, major depressive episodes can be chronic and refractory to mood-stabilizing medication. As such, antidepressants are often used. The risk of antidepressant-induced mania, as seen in younger patients with bipolar disorder, must be balanced with the risk of refractory depression. To date, only one published retrospective study has examined antidepressant use among older adults with bipolar disorder, finding "likely" antidepressant-induced mania in 19.3% of older patients admitted for mania (76). However, this study-examined patients admitted prior to 1990, and as such, the risk of mania with SSRIs and other newer antidepressants was not examined.

Newer antidepressants, including the SSRIs, have become increasingly used over the last 10 years in older adults, while prescriptions for tricyclic and other older antidepressants are declining (77). In the elderly, significantly lower doses of antidepressants are generally used, particularly when initiating a treatment trial, but the medication should be gradually titrated upwards to clinical effect, if tolerated (78). Detailed information about side effects, drug interactions, and monitoring of antidepressants is presented in Chapter 22 of this volume.

ELECTROCONVULSIVE THERAPY

For severe episodes of mania or major depression, particularly with psychosis or active suicidal ideation, or for patients who cannot tolerate pharmacotherapy, electroconvulsive therapy (ECT) should be considered as an option. Although the use of ECT in the elderly with bipolar disorder has been described (79), its use has not systematically been examined. Nonetheless, ECT appears to be beneficial and well tolerated in older patients with major depressive disorder, with a recent large open trial reporting remission rate of 71.3% in patients age 65 and over, with a rapid rate of response (80).

PSYCHOSOCIAL TREATMENTS

As the manic and depressed phases of bipolar disorder wreak havoc on the interpersonal lives and psychosocial functioning of older patients, non-pharmacological therapy is particularly important. Medications, as described above, have potent adverse effects, and compliance is enhanced by a therapeutic alliance with a psychiatrist and multidisciplinary treatment team (75). While cognitive behavioral therapy (CBT), psychoeducation, family therapy, and interpersonal therapy (IPT) have been seen as important for adults (81,82), data are predictably lacking in older patients with bipolar disorder. Nonetheless, lithium with adjuvant CBT was found to reduce patient's scores on depression ratings in the acute treatment and continuation phases of major depression in older patients (83), and while further research is clearly needed in older patients with bipolar disorder, the use of CBT should be considered.

CONCLUSION

Relatively limited evidence for the use of pharmacotherapy and psychotherapy for older bipolar adults reveals a major deficit in our current level of knowledge. Clinical trials that include older subjects as well as pharmacoepidemiological data should inform our management of bipolar disorders in later life. In particular, as we understand the relationship between cerebrovascular disease in bipolar disorder in late life, other medical interventions may be essential to consider as part of management. Indeed, the need for a close relationship of medical, psychiatric, and psychosocial care in older patients with bipolar disorder is a paradigm for all psychiatric disorders in old age.

REFERENCES

1. Tohen M, Shulman KI, Satlin A. First-episode mania in late life. Am J Psychiatry 1994; 151(1):130–132.
2. Shulman KI, Herrmann N. Manic syndromes in old age. In: Jacoby R, Oppenheimer C, eds. Psychiatry in the Elderly. Oxford, UK: Oxford University Press, 2002:683–695.
3. American Psychiatric Association. Diagnostic and Statistical Manual of Mental Disorders. Washington, DC: APA, 1994.
4. Krauthammer C, Klerman GL. Secondary mania: manic syndromes associated with antecedent physical illness or drugs. Arch Gen Psychiatry 1978; 35(11):1333–1339.
5. Shulman KI, Tohen M, Satlin A, Mallya G, Kalunian D. Mania compared with unipolar depression in old age. Am J Psychiatry 1992; 149(3):341–345.
6. Broadhead J, Jacoby R. Mania in old age: a first prospective study. Int J Geriatr Psychiatry 1990; 5:215.
7. Bauer MS, Mitchner L. What is a "mood stabilizer?" An evidence-based response. Am J Psychiatry 2004; 161(1):3–18.
8. Shulman KI, Rochon P, Sykora K, Anderson G, Mamdani M, Bronskill S, Tran CT. Changing prescription patterns for lithium and valproic acid in old age: shifting practice without evidence. BMJ 2003; 326(7396):960–961.
9. Goodwin FK, Murphy DL, Bunney WE Jr. Lithium-carbonate treatment in depression and mania. A longitudinal double-blind study. Arch Gen Psychiatry 1969; 21(4):486–496.
10. Stokes PE, Shamoian CA, Stoll PM, Patton MJ. Efficacy of lithium as acute treatment of manic-depressive illness. Lancet 1971; 1(7713):1319–1325.
11. Bowden CL, Brugger AM, Swann AC, Calabrese JR, Janicak PG, Petty F, Dilsaver SC, Davis JM, Rush AJ, Small JG, et al. Efficacy of divalproex vs lithium and placebo in the treatment of mania. The Depakote Mania Study Group. JAMA 1994; 271(12):918–924.
12. Bowden CL, Calabrese JR, McElroy SL, Gyulai L, Wassef A, Petty F, Pope HG Jr, Chou JC, Keck PE Jr, Rhodes LJ, Swann AC, Hirschfeld RM, Wozniak PJ. A randomized, placebo-controlled 12-month trial of divalproex and lithium in treatment of outpatients with bipolar I disorder. Divalproex Maintenance Study Group. Arch Gen Psychiatry 2000; 57(5):481–489.
13. Calabrese JR, Bowden CL, Sachs G, Yatham LN, Behnke K, Mehtonen OP, Montgomery P, Ascher J, Paska W, Earl N, DeVeaugh-Geiss J. A placebo-controlled 18-month trial of lamotrigine and lithium maintenance treatment in recently depressed patients with bipolar I disorder. J Clin Psychiatry 2003; 64(9):1013–1024.

14. Calabrese JR, Bowden CL, Sachs GS, Ascher JA, Monaghan E, Rudd GD. A double-blind placebo-controlled study of lamotrigine monotherapy in outpatients with bipolar I depression. Lamictal 602 Study Group. J Clin Psychiatry 1999; 60(2):79–88.
15. Tohen M, Ketter TA, Zarate CA, Suppes T, Frye M, Altshuler L, Zajecka J, Schuh LM, Risser RC, Brown E, Baker RW. Olanzapine versus divalproex sodium for the treatment of acute mania and maintenance of remission: a 47-week study. Am J Psychiatry 2003; 160(7):1263–1271.
16. Tohen M, Jacobs TG, Grundy SL, McElroy SL, Banov MC, Janicak PG, Sanger T, Risser R, Zhang F, Toma V, Francis J, Tollefson GD, Breier A. Efficacy of olanzapine in acute bipolar mania: a double-blind, placebo-controlled study. The Olanzipine HGGW Study Group. Arch Gen Psychiatry 2000; 57(9):841–849.
17. Jones M. Quetiapine monotherapy for acute mania associated with bipolar disorder [abstr]. American Psychiatric Association Annual Meeting, San Francisco, CA, 2003.
18. Sachs G, Mullen J, Devine N, et al. Quetiapine versus placebo as adjunct to mood stabilizer for the treatment of acute bipolar mania [abstr]. 3rd European Stanley Foundation Conference on Bipolar Disorder, Freiburg, Germany, 2002.
19. Yatham LN, Binder C, Riccardelli R, Leblanc J, Connolly M, Kusumakar V. Risperidone in acute and continuation treatment of mania. Int Clin Psychopharmacol 2003; 18(4):227–235.
20. Shulman KI, Herrmann N. The nature and management of mania in old age. Psychiatr Clin N Am 1999; 22(3):649–665.
21. van der Velde C. Effectiveness of lithium carbonate in the treatment of manic-depressive illness. Am J Psychiatry 1970; 127:345–351.
22. Schaffer C, Garvey M. Use of lithium in acutely manic elderly patients. Clin Gerontol 1984; 3:58–60.
23. Shulman K, Post F. Bipolar affective disorder in old age. Br J Psychiatry 1980; 136: 26–32.
24. Himmelhoch JM, Neil JF, May SJ, Fuchs CZ, Licata SM. Age, dementia, dyskinesias, and lithium response. Am J Psychiatry 1980; 137(8):941–945.
25. Wilkinson D, Holmes C, Woolford J, Stammers S, North J. Prophylactic therapy with lithium in elderly patients with unipolar major depression. Int J Geriatr Psychiatry 2002; 17(7):619–622.
26. Hardy BG, Shulman KI, Mackenzie SE, Kutcher SP, Silverberg JD. Pharmacokinetics of lithium in the elderly. J Clin Psychopharmacol 1987; 7(3):153–158.
27. Shulman KI, Mackenzie S, Hardy B. The clinical use of lithium carbonate in old age: a review. Prog Neuropsychopharmacol Biol Psychiatry 1987; 11(2–3):159–164.
28. Murray N, Hopwood S, Balfour DJ, Ogston S, Hewick DS. The influence of age on lithium efficacy and side-effects in out-patients. Psychol Med 1983; 13(1):53–60.
29. Head L, Dening T. Lithium in the over-65s: who is taking it and who is monitoring it? A survey of older adults on lithium in the Cambridge Mental Health Services catchment area. Int J Geriatr Psychiatry 1998; 13(3):164–171.
30. Stoudemire A, Hill CD, Lewison BJ, Marquardt M, Dalton S. Lithium intolerance in a medical-psychiatric population. Gen Hosp Psychiatry 1998; 20(2):85–90.
31. Foster JR. Use of lithium in elderly psychiatric patients: a review of the literature. Lithium 1992; 3:77–93.
32. Jacobson SA, Pies RW, Greenblatt DJ. Mood stabilizers. In: Jacobson SA, Pies RW, Greenblatt DJ, eds. Handbook of Geriatric Psychopharmacology. Washington, DC: American Psychiatric Publishing, 2002:187–248.
33. Chen ST, Altshuler LL, Melnyk KA, Erhart SM, Miller E, Mintz J. Efficacy of lithium vs. valproate in the treatment of mania in the elderly: a retrospective study. J Clin Psychiatry 1999; 60(3):181–186.
34. Manto M, Godaux E, Jacquy J, Hildebrand JG. Analysis of cerebellar dysmetria associated with lithium intoxication. Neurol Res 1996; 18(5):416–424.

35. Juurlink D, Mamdani M, Kopp A, Rochon P, Shulman K, Redelmeier D. Drug-induced lithium toxicity in the elderly: a population-based study. J Am Geriatr Soc 2004; 52:1–5.
36. Tariot PN, Erb R, Podgorski CA, Cox C, Patel S, Jakimovich L, Irvine C. Efficacy and tolerability of carbamazepine for agitation and aggression in dementia. Am J Psychiatry 1998; 155(1):54–61.
37. Sival RC, Haffmans PM, Jansen PA, Duursma SA, Eikelenboom P. Sodium valproate in the treatment of aggressive behavior in patients with dementia—a randomized placebo controlled clinical trial. Int J Geriatr Psychiatry 2002; 17(6):579–585.
38. Herrmann N. Valproic acid treatment of agitation in dementia. Can J Psychiatry 1998; 43(1):69–72.
39. Porsteinsson AP, Tariot PN, Erb R, Gaile S. An open trial of valproate for agitation in geriatric neuropsychiatric disorders. Am J Geriatr Psychiatry 1997; 5(4):344–351.
40. Sajatovic M. Treatment of bipolar disorder in older adults. Int J Geriatr Psychiatry 2002; 17(9):865–873.
41. Mordecai DJ, Sheikh JI, Glick ID. Divalproex for the treatment of geriatric bipolar disorder. Int J Geriatr Psychiatry 1999; 14(6):494–496.
42. Noaghiul S, Narayan M, Nelson JC. Divalproex treatment of mania in elderly patients. Am J Geriatr Psychiatry 1998; 6(3):257–262.
43. Schneier HA, Kahn D. Selective response to carbamazepine in a case of organic mood disorder. J Clin Psychiatry 1990; 51(11):485.
44. Kellner MB, Neher F. A first episode of mania after age 80. Can J Psychiatry 1991; 36(8):607–608.
45. Regenold WT, Prasad M. Uses of intravenous valproate in geriatric psychiatry. Am J Geriatr Psychiatry 2001; 9(3):306–308.
46. Conwell Y. Management of suicidal behavior in the elderly. Psychiatr Clin N Am 1997; 20(3):667–683.
47. Goodwin FK, Fireman B, Simon GE, Hunkeler EM, Lee J, Revicki D. Suicide risk in bipolar disorder during treatment with lithium and divalproex. JAMA 2003; 290(11): 1467–1473.
48. Bowden CL, Janicak PG, Orsulak P, Swann AC, Davis JM, Calabrese JR, Goodnick P, Small JG, Rush AJ, Kimmel SE, Risch SC, Morris DD. Relation of serum valproate concentration to response in mania. Am J Psychiatry 1996; 153(6):765–770.
49. Niedermier JA, Nasrallah HA. Clinical correlates of response to valproate in geriatric inpatients. Ann Clin Psychiatry 1998; 10(4):165–168.
50. McDonald WM. Epidemiology, etiology, and treatment of geriatric mania. J Clin Psychiatry 2000; 61(suppl 13):3–11.
51. Frye MA, Ketter TA, Kimbrell TA, Dunn RT, Speer AM, Osuch EA, Luckenbaugh DA, Cora-Ocatelli G, Leverich GS, Post RM. A placebo-controlled study of lamotrigine and gabapentin monotherapy in refractory mood disorders. J Clin Psychopharmacol 2000; 20(6):607–614.
52. Sethi MA, Mehta R, Devanand DP. Gabapentin in geriatric mania. J Geriatr Psychiatry Neurol 2003; 16(2):117–120.
53. Sheldon LJ, Ancill RJ, Holliday SG. Gabapentin in geriatric psychiatry patients. Can J Psychiatry 1998; 43(4):422–423.
54. Robillard M, Conn D. Gabapentin use in geriatric patients with depression and bipolar illness. Can J Psychiatry 2001; 46(8):764.
55. Willmore LJ. Choice and use of newer anticonvulsant drugs in older patients. Drugs Aging 2000; 17(6):441–452.
56. Kusumakar V, Yatham LN. Lamotrigine treatment of rapid cycling bipolar disorder. Am J Psychiatry 1997; 154(8):1171–1172.
57. Calabrese JR, Bowden CL, McElroy SL, Cookson J, Andersen J, Keck PE Jr, Rhodes L, Bolden-Watson C, Zhou J, Ascher JA. Spectrum of activity of lamotrigine in treatment-refractory bipolar disorder. Am J Psychiatry 1999; 156(7):1019–1023.

58. Giorgi L, Gomcz G, O'Neill F, Hammer AE, Risner M. The tolerability of lamotrigine in elderly patients with epilepsy. Drugs Aging 2001; 18(8):621–630.
59. Messenheimer J. The incidence of AED-related Stevens-Johnson Syndrome in the German Registry of Serious Cutaneous Reactions [abstr]. American Academy of Neurology 2002.
60. Ghaemi SN, Berv DA, Klugman J, Rosenquist KJ, Hsu DJ. Oxcarbazepine treatment of bipolar disorder. J Clin Psychiatry 2003; 64(8):943–945.
61. Chengappa KN, Gershon S, Levine J. The evolving role of topiramate among other mood stabilizers in the management of bipolar disorder. Bipolar Disord 2001; 3(5): 215–232.
62. Madhusoodanan S, Bogunovic O, Brenner R, Gupta S. Use of topiramate as an adjunctive medication in an elderly patient with treatment-resistant bipolar disorder. Am J Geriatr Psychiatry 2002; 10(6):759.
63. Kutluay E, McCague K, D'Souza J, Beydoun A. Safety and tolerability of oxcarbazepine in elderly patients with epilepsy. Epilepsy Behav 2003; 4(2):175–180.
64. Aldenkamp AP, De Krom M, Reijs R. Newer antiepileptic drugs and cognitive issues. Epilepsia 2003; 44(suppl 4):21–29.
65. Kane JM. Tardive dyskinesia in affective disorders. J Clin Psychiatry 1999; 60(suppl 5): 43–47; discussion 48–49.
66. Jeste DV. Tardive dyskinesia in older patients. J Clin Psychiatry 2000; 61(suppl 4):27–32.
67. Naranjo CA, Herrmann N, Mittmann N, Bremner KE. Recent advances in geriatric psychopharmacology. Drugs Aging 1995; 7(3):184–202.
68. Yatham LN. Efficacy of atypical antipsychotics in mood disorders. J Clin Psychopharmacol 2003; 23(3 suppl 1):S9–S14.
69. Shulman RW, Singh A, Shulman KI. Treatment of elderly institutionalized bipolar patients with clozapine. Psychopharmacol Bull 1997; 33(1):113–118.
70. Street J, Tollefson G, Tohen M, Sanger TM, Clark WS, Gannon KS, Wei H. Olanzapine for psychotic conditions in the elderly. Psychiatr Ann 2000; 30(3):191–196.
71. Madhusoodanan S, Brecher M, Brenner R, Kasckow J, Kunik M, Negron AE, Pomara N. Risperidone in the treatment of elderly patients with psychotic disorders. Am J Geriatr Psychiatry 1999; 7(2):132–138.
72. Madhusoodanan S, Brenner R, Alcantra A. Clinical experience with quetiapine in elderly patients with psychotic disorders. J Geriatr Psychiatry Neurol 2000; 13(1):28–32.
73. Jeste DV, Barak Y, Madhusoodanan S, Grossman F, Gharabawi G. International multisite double-blind trial of the atypical antipsychotics risperidone and olanzapine in 175 elderly patients with chronic schizophrenia. Am J Geriatr Psychiatry 2003; 11(6): 638–647.
74. Vieta E, Goikolea JM, Corbella B, Benabarre A, Reinares M, Martinez G, Fernandez A, Colom F, Martinez-Aran A, Torrent C. Risperidone safety and efficacy in the treatment of bipolar and schizoaffective disorders: results from a 6-month, multicenter, open study. J Clin Psychiatry 2001; 62(10):818–825.
75. American Psychiatric Association. Practice guideline for the treatment of patients with bipolar disorder (revision). Am J Psychiatry 2002; 159(4):1–50.
76. Young RC, Jain H, Kiosses DN, Meyers BS. Antidepressant-associated mania in late life. Int J Geriatr Psychiatry 2003; 18(5):421–424.
77. Mamdani MM, Parikh SV, Austin PC, Upshur RE. Use of antidepressants among elderly subjects: trends and contributing factors. Am J Psychiatry 2000; 157(3):360–367.
78. Alexopoulos GS, Katz IR, Reynolds CF, Carpenter D, Docherty JP. Pharmacotherapy of depressive disorders in older patients. Postgraduate Medicine, 2001:1–86.
79. Mukherjee S, Sackeim HA, Schnur DB. Electroconvulsive therapy of acute manic episodes: a review of 50 years' experience. Am J Psychiatry 1994; 151(2):169–176.
80. Kellner C. The efficacy of ECT in major depression: findings from phase 1 of the C.O.R.E. ECT Study. Int Psychogeriatr 2003; 15(suppl 2):151.

81. Zaretsky AE, Segal ZV, Gemar M. Cognitive therapy for bipolar depression: a pilot study. Can J Psychiatry 1999; 44(5):491–494.
82. Rothbaum BO, Astin MC. Integration of pharmacotherapy and psychotherapy for bipolar disorder. J Clin Psychiatry 2000; 61(suppl 9):68–75.
83. Wilson KC, Scott M, Abou-Saleh M, Burns R, Copeland JR. Long-term effects of cognitive-behavioural therapy and lithium therapy on depression in the elderly. Br J Psychiatry 1995; 167(5):653–658.

18
Lithium in Bipolar Disorder

Paul Grof
Bipolar Research Unit, University of Ottawa, Royal Ottawa Hospital, Ottawa, Ontario, Canada

INTRODUCTION

Lithium can produce dramatic benefits for patients with bipolar disorders. It is the treatment of choice for individuals suffering from the classical, episodically recurring type of bipolar disorder, particularly for their long-term stabilization. Lithium is also suitable for a therapeutic trial in some other types of bipolar illnesses. Presenting a balanced, evidence-based perspective on this fascinating salt, however, poses a challenge, given the major controversies that have been raging about the use of lithium in the literature. Over the past four decades, investigators and clinicians have made a variety of observations under different experimental designs, and their interpretations and conclusions reflect their varied experience. In the late 1960s and 1970s, lithium was used in patients with bipolar disorders diagnosed primarily according to the Kraepelinian tradition, after a careful exclusion of all other psychiatric diagnoses, comorbidities, and the pre-emption of those with mood-incongruent psychotic symptoms. The outcome of lithium clinical trials from that time period was very satisfactory and the findings replicable. Bipolar illness suddenly became treatable with medication, lithium being the first effective agent; the management of bipolar disorder changed from episodic to long term; and biological concepts in psychiatry received a major boost of confidence, reflected in a huge expansion of research activities.

However, as it commonly happens, the success of lithium has also sown the seeds of its gradual fall from grace. Clinicians full of new hope experimented with lithium in all varieties of mood disorders and the concept of bipolar disorders expanded accordingly. Between 1967 and 2003, epidemiological studies noted a 10-fold increase in the prevalence of diagnosed bipolar disorders.

The more recent use of lithium in the 1990s in the expanded bipolar population resulted in a much lower treatment success and in new phenomena, such as a rebound after discontinuation, a seeming loss of efficacy after the re-introduction of lithium, and increased frequency of side effects. In parallel with the euphoria about newly discovered treatment alternatives, the use of lithium gradually faded and disappeared from some of the post-graduate curricula. As a result, a physician in North America may now complete residency in psychiatry without ever having treated a single patient with lithium, a substance that used to be labeled as the most effective medication in psychiatry. The resulting lack of competence in the use of lithium only compounds the discrepancies seen in clinical practice.

Dealing with these complex issues would require more allotted space. This chapter will be limited to the use of lithium primarily as a treatment of choice for the classical type of bipolar disorder. As a secondary application, the benefits of lithium will be explored in the context of other bipolar conditions, where it is best applied in time-limited trials with clearly defined objectives. The text will be focusing on what transpires during lithium treatment administered to patients properly selected and adequately monitored during lithium treatment.

The literature on the psychiatric use of lithium has mushroomed dramatically over the past 40 years and exceeds 24,000 publications. Only representative examples from the voluminous material can be included here, not comprehensive listings; all references in this text should be read as prefaced by "for instance, e.g." Knowledge gathered from randomized, controlled clinical trials, as well as from large series of replicated observations, has been included, as evidence-based medicine must integrate all relevant material (1).

HISTORICAL BACKGROUND

In the 19th century, lithium was used in medicine for several indications and, in Denmark, Lange administered it to depressed patients but had no successor in this approach. In 1949, the first report on the successful use in a small group of manic patients was published by an Australian John Cade (2). In Denmark, Schou et al. (3) were able to confirm Cade's observation in a double-blind, placebo-controlled study, the first of its kind in psychopharmacology. The publication of lithium's mood stabilizing effect, demonstrated in a long-term open study, had to wait another 13 years (4). Regulatory agencies waited much longer: they accepted the recurrence-preventing effect only after a series of double-blind studies fully demonstrated it, starting with Baastrup et al. (5). It was in particular Schou's pioneering, systematic research, which, after heated debates, convinced the psychiatric community to accept lithium as an effective treatment for the prophylaxis of recurrent mood disorders (6).

The triumphs of lithium treatment in the management of many manic-depressive disorders brought a great deal of optimism into psychiatry. Lithium has since then remained the standard prophylactic and antimanic treatment for bipolar disorders. During the past four decades, its strong impact stimulated a new wave of interest in mood disorders, triggered a vigorous search for alternative treatments, and accelerated reformulation of psychiatric diagnoses and classification.

The introduction of lithium into psychiatric practice has had a major impact on modern psychiatry (7). Lithium provided support for the view that bipolar illness has important biological roots and strengthened the need for careful diagnosis and for attention to the clinical course of illness. Lithium inaugurated the psychopharmacological revolution and energized the links between bedside and bench research. The successful treatment outcome generated useful pharmacoeconomic data, and the striking benefits from lithium treatment played an important impetus for patient advocacy and self-help groups. In developed countries, one to two persons per thousand have been treated with lithium and the marked reduction in suffering, as well as in healthcare costs, has been well documented (8).

The widespread use of lithium around the world has added a number of new observations. To wit, it became clear that lithium works prophylactically best in classical, fully remitting, and episodically recurring bipolar disorders and in unipolar disorders that mimic them. It also offers a score of other benefits in psychiatry and medicine and can reduce mortality and suicidal behavior. As with other psychotropics over time, many possible side effects have been observed as well, some common, others idiosyncratic. Recently, the increased acceptance of lithium's antisuicidal effect and neuroprotective properties have re-ignited interest in its clinical use, particularly in long-term treatment.

CLINICAL EFFECTS AND INDICATIONS

The initial controversy as to whether lithium is an effective mood stabilizer energized investigators to intensely explore and resolve the issue. When lithium finally achieved wide acceptance, it was welcomed as a treatment that had the best-demonstrated efficacy among then-available psychiatric treatments.

Lithium was initially thought to be a drug specific for manic-depressive illness. However, the initially narrow range of lithium's wingspread in affective disorders quickly broadened, adding to its well-demonstrated antimanic and prophylactic benefits potent antiaggressive effects (9,10), antipsychotic potential, (11–13) antisuicidal and mortality-reducing ability (14–16), and antidepressant effects (17–19). All of them have application in the treatment of bipolar disorder.

Mood Stabilizing, "Prophylactic" Effect

This benefit of long-term lithium treatment has been well documented in a large series of pivotal studies, open and then controlled, and performed in the late 1960s and early 1970s (20,21) (Table 1).

These trials included mostly patients diagnosed as bipolar according to the Kraepelinian tradition. All other diagnoses had to be excluded first, meaning that patients with comorbidities and mood-incongruent psychotic symptoms were eliminated and the remaining patients had a mostly episodic, remitting course of illness.

In this series of studies, the recurrences of abnormal moods were significantly reduced in about three-quarters of patients, either prevented fully or rendered fewer in frequency. Particularly convincing drug–placebo difference, unparalleled in psychiatry, emerged from a double-blind discontinuation study by Baastrup et al. (5). When patients suffering from recurrent bipolar and unipolar disorders were initially stabilized on lithium and then randomly assigned to lithium or placebo, it was the placebo-assigned patients who suffered recurrence.

Table 1 Efficacy of Long-Term Lithium Treatment

Diagnosis	Medication	Number of patients	Percentage of patients with recurrences during the first year of study
Bipolar	Lithium	186	20
	Placebo	187	73

Data combined from the first nine double-blind controlled trials.

Several features characterized these early clinical trials and differentiated them from later lithium investigations: the expected number of both manias and depressions was significantly reduced; toxicity was observed only with elevated lithium levels; after lithium was discontinued, in remission no rebound was observed (22,23); subsequent recurrences developed gradually and the benefit was reproducible by re-instituting lithium.

In contrast with the findings from the first two decades of lithium use, the literature on lithium from the past 20 years paints a different, rather pessimistic picture. In brief, the outcome in the recent lithium studies suggests that lithium does not help either much anymore (24) or not at all (25), and that initial benefits may not be enduring (26). Furthermore, Suppes et al. (27) reported that discontinuation of lithium is often followed promptly by an intense rebound, suggesting an increase in the intensity of illness. Thus, the earlier perception of lithium as an effective, highly valued, stabilizing treatment for bipolar disorders has changed mostly to that of a questionably useful substance of fleeting benefit.

This unexpected shift for the worse appears to have reflected several factors such as a dramatic broadening of the bipolar diagnostic category; unwillingness to recognize that naturalistic studies test effectiveness rather than efficacy (28); and accumulation of treatment-resistant mood disorders in academic research centers (29). Deshauer et al. (30) have shown that the early and recent studies of lithium's efficacy are not directly comparable because of methodological differences, and that recent studies favored other drugs by using pre-randomization open phases.

Lithium prophylaxis remains the treatment of choice for recurrent, typical episodic mood disorders. The most important characteristic of the conditions responsive to lithium prophylaxis is episodic course, i.e., the episodes of mania and depression alternating with periods of complete remission. During such remissions, the patients not only return to pre-morbid functioning in their employment and in their family, but also free of any affective as well as non-affective symptoms. The typical psychopathological presentation of a mood disorder also helps predicting lithium response: intense sadness or euphoria, changing of vital functions such as appetite, sleep, and sexual functioning, and mood-congruent alterations of thinking. A family history of episodic mood disorders further increases the probability of successful prophylaxis (31).

If the patient is correctly selected according to the earlier-mentioned criteria, the response is relatively predictable in most patients, regardless of the preceding severity of illness or its duration. An excellent, sustained response of a typical, frequently recurring episodic bipolar disorder to lithium prophylaxis is one of the most gratifying experiences a treating psychiatrist may have.

In recent years, there has been much confusion in the literature about the continuing efficacy of long-term lithium treatment in DSM-IV-diagnosed bipolar disorders (32). Studies have shown that lithium remains highly effective for the typical, classical bipolar disorder for which it was originally proven as beneficial (33). The efficacy of lithium given to psychiatric patients loosely diagnosed with a bipolar spectrum disorders has not been established, but seems low. For example, a recent study of DSM-IV-diagnosed bipolar disorders suggests that about one-third of patients may actually benefit from long-term lithium (34). In heterogeneous bipolar populations, the efficacy of lithium may be difficult or impossible to demonstrate in clinical trials (25).

Antimanic Effect

Lithium is now considered a standard treatment for acute manic phase of bipolar disorder. Its value in this indication was earlier well established against both placebo and typical neuroleptics (35) and, more recently, has been extensively evaluated against atypical neuroleptics and antiepileptics. In parallel with the lingering discussions about lithium's stabilizing efficacy, recent findings about its antimanic effect have been less uniform, some questioning and others confirming (36) lithium's superiority over placebo. Though clinically there seems to be an association between the antimanic and prophylactic effect of lithium, the issue of whether the benefit unfolds in the same patients has not been systematically investigated. Clinically, lithium also seems to exert a non-specific, over-activity reducing action, reaching beyond the range of bipolar manias.

In clinical practice, lithium treatment should be considered as one of the alternatives in the treatment of acute mania or hypomania. The response in typical manias often takes 10 to 14 days. Mania, however, is an acute event requiring a prompt intervention; it is, therefore, usually preferable to start the treatment with a combination of a neuroleptic and an antiepileptic. An adequate dosage of the combination can bring the acute symptoms of mania under quicker control, and it is then easier to initiate the long-term treatment with lithium. This is particularly important in manic patients who have not been taking fluids and eating properly and could react abnormally to the initiation of intensive lithium treatment, even with a shutdown of the kidney function.

Antidepressant Effect of Lithium

The antidepressant effect of lithium was first reported by Vojtechovsky (37) and later confirmed by Mendels (17) and others. Its efficacy for bipolar depression has been proven, but the findings have not been generally accepted. It is important to keep this possibility in mind particularly in depressed bipolar and "pseudo-unipolar" patients ("pseudo-unipolar" patients have clinical characteristics of bipolar illness but have not as yet experienced the manic polarity). Not only both these types of patients respond poorly to antidepressants, but also often the treatment with antidepressants worsens both the acute and long-term presentation of the illness (38).

Antisuicidal Effect and the Reduction of Mortality

There is now a growing body of data supporting the conclusions that long-term lithium administration significantly reduces suicidal behavior of bipolar patients and diminishes their high mortality to a level indistinguishable from that of the general population (14,15). The antisuicidal effect has also been supported by findings from a comparative, long-term study of lithium and carbamazepine, in which only lithium-treated patients remained completely free of suicide (39). These findings from individual studies were further strengthened by large meta-analyses (16). It is interesting that the antisuicidal effect may be present over and above the stabilizing lithium treatment (40), even in non-responders to lithium's mood stabilizing action.

Other Effects of Lithium Relevant for Bipolar Disorder

Lithium's antipsychotic and antiaggressive properties can be utilized particularly in patients with atypical presentations of bipolar illness.

Antipsychotic effect. Both acute and long-term antipsychotic effects of lithium have been described best by Garver and colleagues (11,41) in schizophrenias and schizophreniform psychoses and demonstrated by many others (42,43) in schizoaffective psychoses. In Garver et al. studies, a striking clearing of psychotic manifestations, even of mood-incongruent ones, was seen during treatment with lithium alone. Excellent responses to acute treatment with lithium alone were described in nearly one-third of such patients. Lithium responders fared well, without any introduction of neuroleptics during hospitalization, and could be discharged essentially symptom-free. Maintained treatment with lithium alone could also avert further episodes in many patients. Of those patients who had to be re-admitted, about half showed again a concordant response to acute lithium treatment.

Although this antipsychotic effect of lithium bears some superficial resemblance to the stabilizing benefit in classical bipolars, there are marked differences. First, patients benefiting from the antipsychotic effect experience in long-term treatment a reduction of manias but no reduction in their depressive episodes (44). Second, the antimanic effect of lithium is on re-admission reproducible only in about half of the patients (41), whereas in the other half, neuroleptics are needed. Third, lithium toxicity may develop even with therapeutic lithium levels. Finally, after discontinuation, patients frequently experience early, magnified recurrences (44,45).

Cycloid psychoses meet the DSM-IV diagnostic criteria for bipolar disorder and have been described to respond well to lithium maintenance (46).

Antiaggressive effect. In a series of studies spearheaded in particular by Sheard (9,10), the antiaggressive effect of lithium has been widely documented. Several different populations were studied, ranging from a variety of psychiatric populations and mentally retarded subjects to penitentiary prisoners. Sheards, as well as others who systematically investigated the antiaggressive effect of lithium, argued persuasively that the subjects who benefited did not suffer from bipolar illness: the lithium effect was distinctly different.

*Children of a lithium-responsive bipolar parent*s who are suffering from episodic emotional problems (such as intermittent insomnia, anxiety, panic, phobias, conduct disorder, etc.) may respond best to lithium, regardless of psychopathology and intensity of problems (47).

Roots of Controversies About Lithium's Clinical Use in Bipolar Disorders

In recent years, we have lived with a paradox. On the one hand, lithium is considered the golden standard for the treatment of bipolar illness and utilized as such in the clinical trials of new, promising compounds. On the other hand, it is also viewed and described in the literature as the medication associated with a low efficacy in bipolar disorders and a high-potential toxicity. Thus, the prevailing practice has recently been to use lithium mainly in combinations with newer drugs, in order to make it work. To comprehend this contradiction, it is important to appreciate the issues involved.

Prior to the discovery of the stabilizing effect of lithium in the early 1970s, the course of bipolar disorders was considered completely capricious (48) and not responsive to any medication. After the introduction of lithium into clinical practice, numerous bipolar patients with long histories became fully stabilized. Regardless of the severity of their illness, the patients who responded often became completely well, returned back to their profession and family, and were completely free of any further symptoms of mental illness. Even patients who had been hospitalized many times, or had psychotic episodes, or were dysfunctional for long periods of time responded well, as long as they had the right, episodic type of illness.

Those excellent outcomes contrasted strikingly with the usual effects of antidepressants and neuroleptics and resulted in several, written or implicit, assumptions: that lithium is a specific treatment for bipolar disorder, i.e., it is a good practice to treat any kind of bipolar disorder with lithium; that lithium has only one type of action and therefore could not work for other conditions; that benefit from lithium demonstrates underlying bipolarity; that the absence of frequent recurrences during lithium treatment always demonstrates benefit from lithium. Over time, all these assumptions turned out either incorrect or simplistic, requiring an important qualification. However, the impact of these assumptions on the use of lithium treatment of bipolar disorders and the interpretation of outcomes lingers on.

Over the years, these assumptions markedly influenced the shift in psychiatric thinking and experimentation. They led to re-diagnosing of a number of psychiatric patients as bipolars (49,50), to findings of a much lower efficacy of lithium both in naturalistic studies and double-blind trials, and to a presumption of a loss of lithium efficacy over time and rebound effect on discontinuation.

While full prophylactic effect is probably available only in episodic mood disorders, lithium has a variety of demonstrated benefits: prophylactic, antimanic, antidepressant augmenting, antisuicidal, antiaggressive. Recurrent mood disorders have an extremely variable course, and a reliable prediction of the course is possible only statistically for a larger group of higher risk patients. The phenomena observed when lithium is used in atypical bipolar and cycloid and other psychotic patients, such as poor reproducibility of prophylactic effect and rebound after discontinuation, cannot be automatically generalized to other types of illness.

There has been much evidence over the past 35 years that there is not one but several bipolar disorders (51–54). The heterogeneity grew further with DSM-IV and the bipolar spectrum disorders. Then, the practical problem is that clinicians now very often treat with lithium—and include into clinical trials—types of bipolar disorder, for whom lithium has never been proven effective.

Some controversies about lithium treatment of bipolar disorders are due to misunderstandings about the natural course of bipolar illness. In order to evaluate the effect of long-term treatment on an individual bipolar patient, it is important to have a reasonably realistic idea as to what would happen without long-term treatment. Unfortunately, in these days, very few clinicians actually see an untreated course of bipolar illness and, therefore, underestimate both the capriciousness and the inter-individual variability of the natural course.

There are unfortunate consequences of wrong assumptions. For example, when a clinician treats a lithium-unresponsive bipolar patient and erroneously attributes 2 years free of recurrences to the benefit of lithium instead of natural illness course, later recurrences can be incorrectly interpreted as a loss of lithium's efficacy. However, investigators, who have worked with demonstrably lithium-responsive patients, have not found any loss of efficacy later during the course of illness (33,55).

ADVERSE EFFECTS OF LITHIUM TREATMENT

Lithium has a potential to induce a score of adverse effects. In the literature, lithium treatment has often been associated with many side effects and toxicity, because it

Table 2 Frequency of Common Side Effects in Patients Responding to Long-Term Lithium Treatment

Side effects	Percentage of patients
Increased thirst	28
Nocturia	26
Weight gain	16
Hypothyroidism	15
Polyuria	12
Gastrointestinal distress	8
Hand tremor	5
Goiter	3

Two hundred and five patients treated for more than 1 year, research program.

may exert many well-documented impacts on the biology of the human body. Therefore, it can, depending on the circumstances, lead to a number of adversities: neurological, cardiovascular, endocrine, nephrological, gastrointestinal, metabolic, and dermatological.

Yet, when used properly in long-term treatment of the classical type of bipolar disorder, most patients tolerate it quite well (Table 2) and, in addition, the unwanted effects of lithium can be avoided or minimized by proper dosing of the drug and conscientious monitoring.

For practice, we need to differentiate between several types of side effects: (1) those likely to occur during the first few weeks of acute treatment, (2) side effects common during long-term administration, (3) less common side effects during long-term administration, and (4) toxicity indicators that can crop up during the administration of lithium, which is inappropriate either in the dosage or for the type of the patient's disorder.

Initial Phase

During the first few weeks of acute lithium administration, side effects are more common. In particular, patients often report increased thirst, more frequent urination, and fine tremor. Mild gastrointestinal side effects, such as nausea, anorexia, and diarrhea, are not infrequent; they can be significantly reduced by slow-release lithium preparations.

Common Side Effects During Long-Term Administration

At least one-third of the patients may experience increased thirst and fluid intake, and a smaller percentage may exhibit increased urinary frequency, nocturia, polyuria, slight trembling of hand, and significant weight gain. These symptoms need medical attention only if they persist or become bothersome.

Increased thirst and fluid intake and accompanying polyuria result both from the direct effect of lithium of the thirst center and from reduced renal concentrating ability. Much investigative work has gone into evaluating the effects of lithium, as a light metal, on the kidney function (56). There is no convincing evidence that lithium administration reduces glomerular filtration rate, as long as the patient has a normal kidney function to start with. The reduction of tubular function, and of urine concentrating ability, is common and appears to be dose related, but its clinical significance is not clear, unless the resulting polyuria is excessive.

Cognitive side effects may also be more common, but they are usually difficult to differentiate from sub-clinical depressive complaints or worries. Complaints of mild cognitive impairment, such as less efficient memory, are common on lithium but not supported by neuropsychological findings. The relationship to treatment is usually unconvincing, and an explanation through sub-clinical depressive symptoms is often more plausible. Lithium often causes benign T-wave changes, benign leukocytosis, and platelet count elevation.

In general, if the type of bipolar disorder is correctly selected for long-term treatment and the dosage is properly adjusted for the individual patient, most patients tolerate long-term lithium treatment without much subjectively noticeable adversity (Table 2). The reports in the literature offer much longer lists and higher percentages but, unfortunately, do not differentiate between side effects in patients who have been correctly chosen, monitored, and are receiving an appropriately low dosage of lithium and those who receive lithium on inadequate indication and in higher dosage. These patients often receive lithium in combination with other drugs, and the decision that one actually causes the side effect is often arbitrary.

There is a striking difference in the emergence and intensity of side effects between lithium responders and non-responders, not only in the subjective report of patients but also in objective findings. To wit, the average 24-hour urine volume of non-responders was markedly larger than that of lithium responders, despite comparable plasma lithium levels (57). It is, therefore, important to differentiate between the tolerable side effects of correctly indicated and carried out lithium prophylaxis and the variety of side effects that may develop during loosely indicated or incorrectly performed lithium trials. Most side effects of long-term lithium treatment are dosage dependent—increasing with higher dosage and plasma level—and will, therefore, increase if the patient is treated with lithium aggressively.

Less Common Side Effects During Lithium Treatment

Skin problems associated with lithium may include acne, rash, hair loss, and psoriasis. Causal relationship to psoriasis remains somewhat unclear, mainly because psoriasis is so common in the general population. Sporadically, hyperparathyroidism with elevated plasma calcium has been observed. Infrequently, the effects of lithium on cardiac function have been noted and may lead to arrhythmia, sinus node function impairment, ventricular irritability, and conduction disturbances. These changes are usually reversible when lithium is discontinued.

Lithium Toxicity

At high lithium levels, dysphoria, lethargy, intellectual inability, reduced spontaneity, and seizures may develop. The most serious adversity that can develop during lithium treatment is lithium toxicity (58). In essence, toxicity develops when either the patients continue receiving a dosage higher than the patients' lithium clearance can manage or if their ability to excrete lithium becomes reduced, for example, by dehydration or by drug interactions. The diagnosis is primarily a clinical task, but because clinical symptoms vary individually, the serial serum lithium levels in the toxic range are usually critical for the correct diagnosis. In a patient treated with lithium, neurological symptoms such as severe tremor or confusion and gastrointestinal symptoms such as vomiting and diarrhea must cause concern. Neurological symptoms may also resemble a stroke or other localized manifestations.

Fortunately, clinical experience has shown that lithium intoxication can usually be avoided by careful screening and monitoring, as well as by patient education. It is important to ensure that the dosage of lithium is carefully monitored and tailored to the patient's lithium excretory capacity and that the patient is educated well about the principles of lithium treatment. In our program, we have not seen a single case of lithium intoxication among our lithium-treated bipolar patients during the past 25 years.

The treatment of choice for lithium intoxication is hemodialysis (59).

Balancing Benefits and Side Effects

Overall, mood disorders carry with them a significant morbidity and mortality. A clinician considering lithium treatment for an individual patient must balance possible adverse effects against the likelihood of minimized recurrences and suicidal acts. Alternative approaches, with their risks and benefits, must also be taken into consideration. The degree of side effects of correctly performed lithium maintenance treatment compares favorably with other medications used in the treatment of mood disorders.

Physician's training and experience with lithium treatment and with regular monitoring also play a role in the manifestation and impact of side effects. Finally, corrective strategies are available for most common lithium side effects and are described in detail in the literature (60).

SPECIAL SITUATIONS

During the treatment of bipolar patients, there are special situations that require special considerations and may pose an increase risk of adverse effects, e.g., pregnancy, travel, or the use of lithium in combination with medications that markedly influence lithium's excretion.

Lithium Interactions

Lithium has a potential to interact with a number of drugs, such as amphetamines, ACE inhibitors, calcium channel blockers, fluoxetine, haloperidol, metronidazole, and xanthines. For practice, the important interactions to keep in mind are lithium's interaction with diuretics, such as furosemide and hydrochlorothiazide, and interaction with non-steroidal anti-inflammatory drugs, such as indocin and phenylbutazolidin. Anti-inflammatories reduce and diuretics delay the renal excretion of lithium, thereby increasing the risk of toxicity. Co-administration of lithium with these medications requires close and monitoring, more frequent serum lithium levels, and often a reduction of lithium dosage.

Lithium in Pregnancy

Animal studies and clinical registries of lithium's teratogenic potential had initially suggested that lithium should be avoided during the first trimester of the pregnancy, because of an increased risk of cardiac malformations. From these early observations, it was concluded that a pregnant woman should receive lithium during the first trimester of pregnancy only if there is no other way of controlling malignant bipolar illness. All involved should be carefully consulted and included in such decision.

Recently, more systematic studies have, however, indicated less teratogenicity than initially alleged, and perhaps even clinically insignificant (61). In any case, lithium in pregnancy is less risky than several other commonly used medications for bipolar disorders, such as valproate or carbamazepine.

Lithium and Travel

Patients on lithium may be in an increased danger when traveling in high-altitude and high-temperature areas because of dehydration and loss of sodium by excessive sweating. Lithium dosage may have to be reduced and salt intake increased.

MANAGEMENT OF LITHIUM TREATMENT

Screening for Treatment

The extent of adequate screening for lithium treatment depends primarily on the medical condition of the patient and the psychiatric intent: does the bipolar patient require acute or long-term treatment? If, for example, a patient is young and healthy, with negative medical history and normal physical examination, then normal serum creatinine, TSH, and routine urine may be considered adequate for a short-term antimanic treatment. On the other hand, for long-term, stabilizing lithium treatment, a comprehensive evaluation is highly advisable. It should include a complete medical history and a full set of laboratory investigations, both focusing in particular on areas that could be potentially influenced by lithium, as outlined in what follows.

Such a caution is necessary because lithium can potentially influence many systems, as outlined earlier. However, equally important, a comprehensive screening should be performed for medico-legal reasons. When interpreting any abnormal laboratory finding that may emerge during lithium treatment, it is very helpful to have baseline values taken at screening.

Comprehensive screening for lithium therapy includes: (A) Evaluating, by comprehensive psychiatric assessment, if the patient suffers from a lithium responsive condition or, alternatively, if lithium is indicated as a treatment trial for a pre-determined period of time.

(B) Evaluating safety: (a) Assessing medical history with regard to cardiovascular, neurological, endocrine, gastrointestinal kidney, and skin disorders. Of particular concern are heart disorders associated with conduction disorders and arrhythmia, hypertension, Parkinson's illness, hypothyroidism, gastrointestinal disorders associated with diarrhea, kidney disorders, and psoriasis. (b) Performing laboratory tests of the above systems. Comprehensive laboratory assessment should include EKG with blood pressure and pulse, TSH, plasma calcium, body weight and height, serum creatinine and BUN, complete blood count, creatinine clearance, 24 urine collections, and urine creatinine.

Planning and Educating

It is advisable to include both the patients and their partners into the planning of long-term lithium treatment. The disruptions induced by bipolar disorder are very demanding on families and human partnerships. Recovery can be equally stressful as becoming ill because it may require major adjustments, e.g., the couple must renegotiate their roles, obligations, or lifestyle. Because of dynamic shifts in the relationship, some couples require supportive psychotherapy in dealing with such adaptations.

Providing a patient with sufficient information about the illness and treatment alternatives is extremely important for the success of long-term treatment, for compliance with medication and for safety of lithium treatment. There is a variety of patient guides readily available. The instruction book by Schou (62) on lithium treatment has been accepted particularly well by patients and their families.

Monitoring

During each visit, the clinician should assess any changes in the patient's mental and physical state, check on the dosage of lithium and of all other medications, discuss medication compliance, and review recent serum lithium levels.

Clinical and laboratory monitoring of long-term lithium-treated patients should persevere systematically as long as lithium treatment continues. This surveillance remains the responsibility of the prescribing clinician or clinic. To avoid lithium intoxication, clinicians should counteract conditions under which the renal lithium clearance changes, for example, dehydration and a low sodium intake, and also treatment with diuretics, antihypertensive drugs, and non-steroid anti-inflammatory drugs.

Serum lithium levels can guide the dosage, and the optimum amount of lithium maintains the concentration above the efficacy threshold and below the level giving troublesome side effects. The effective concentration for long-term treatment appears wider than initially recommended and ranges between 0.4 and 0.9 mEq/L of standardized 12-hour serum lithium. Both the dosage and the serum level need to be chosen according to the age, sex, dosage regimen, and the clinical condition and response of the individual. Usually, serial serum lithium determinations are employed to determine the patient's lithium concentration; however, they leave the clinician at the mercy of the patient's compliance. Therefore, helpful predictive procedures of the lithium dosage have been developed for achieving specific serum lithium concentrations more easily.

Combination of Lithium with Psychotherapy and Other Modalities

Supportive psychotherapy that ensures good therapeutic relationship is always helpful during lithium treatment. Most bipolar patients can resolve their remaining individual and marital issues on their own, once they have been stabilized. Some patients, however, need to receive systematic individual or marital psychotherapy in addition to lithium treatment, particularly if the illness led to a dysfunctional marriage or family.

Lithium, Combinations, and Alternatives

The accomplishments of prophylactic lithium in mood disorders has stimulated extensive search for other alternatives, in particular for lithium non-responsive and atypical mood disorders. The options that we as clinicians have acquired for stabilizing treatment of bipolar disorders have increased exponentially in recent years, to a dozen of

Table 3 Characteristics of Responders to Long-Term Lithium Treatment

Clinical course: episodic, fully remitting, predominance of depressions
Family history: bipolar disorders, with episodic course
Comorbidity: as common as in the general population
Presentation: classical, as described in earlier textbooks (e.g., depressions with sadness, manias with euphoria, absence of mood-incongruent psychotic symptoms)

Source: From Ref. 31.

promising substances. These medications include in particular carbamazepine, valproic acid, lamotrigine, clozapine, risperidone, olanzapine, quetiapine, newer atypical antipsychotics, and other substances described in more detail in other chapters.

Although current practice relies heavily on drug combinations, many bipolar patients can be successfully stabilized if the initial monotherapy is carefully selected according to the patient's clinical characteristics. There is a growing body of evidence indicating that unequivocal responders to long-term monotherapy such as lithium, lamotrigine, or atypical neuroleptics, each have a very different clinical profile including clinical presentation, course of illness, comorbidity, and, in particular, family history.

Responders to lithium stabilization present with depressive and manic episodes of the classical type, without mood-incongruent symptoms, clearly sad depressions, and often euphoric manias. In their family history, they tend to have bipolar disorders with an episodic course. They, themselves, have an episodic full-remitting course and, if the course has been extensive, one can usually see a predominance of depressions over manias. Finally, in these patients, comorbid conditions such as, e.g., alcoholism and drug addiction are as common as in the general population (Table 3).

Furthermore, there is a growing body of literature that in bipolar patients good responses to lithium, antiepileptics, and atypical neuroleptics are relatively selective and often mutually exclusive. The patients who respond well to a particular long-term monotherapy have often failed on other monotherapies and treatment strategies. For example, excellent lithium responders failed on long-term carbamazepine and vice versa (63). Post et al. (64) made a similar observation: most patients with a good acute response to carbamazepine had a clear history of non-response to lithium. Bowden et al. (36) found that previous lithium responders did well on lithium but not on divalproex. Similarly, Swann et al. (65) noted that responders to valproate had evidence of prior non-response to lithium. Tohen et al. (66) observed that olanzapine succeeded in patients failed previously on lithium and divalproex. Despite some methodological limitations of these observations, together they provide a credible picture of a degree of selectivity among these medications.

PUTATIVE MECHANISMS OF ACTION

Lithium exerts a large number of well-established biological effects on a multitude of organs, especially the brain. Early work explored possible deficiency or excess states of neurotransmitters, whereas more recently, attention shifted more to regulatory systems in the brain. The main yield of earlier research was evidence of lithium's ability to stabilize or enhance serotonergic activity (67,68). Moving beyond direct neurotransmitter effects, explorations revealed lithium having a multitude of actions at the post-synaptic level, particularly on G-proteins and second messenger systems, especially on phosphatidylinositol, protein kinase C, and intracellular calcium.

For some time, the most widely accepted mechanism of action of lithium was its inhibitory effect on phosphoinositol system, particularly on the synthesis of inositol, resulting in depletion of inositol with profound effects on neuronal signal transduction pathways. Recently, it has become increasingly appreciated that lithium also influences the regulation of gene expression and produces a marked increase in the expression of selected neuroprotective proteins, as well as enhances neuroplasticity and cell resilience (69,70).

Despite three decades of extensive investigations, it remains unclear which neurobiological mechanisms are actually responsible for the beneficial effects of lithium. In particular, it remains unresolved which of the many well-documented neurobiological effects are specific to the patients exhibiting an excellent response to lithium prophylaxis. In the meantime, a hunt for convincing mechanisms of lithium's action continues. Hopefully, once we understand how lithium actually achieves mood stabilization in bipolar patients, we will be able to develop new treatment strategies and improve dramatically the management of bipolar disorders.

SUMMARY

To sum up, lithium can be utilized in a variety of indications in psychiatry and medicine, but its unique value is in long-term treatment of the classical type of bipolar illness, with recurrent episodic, fully remitting course. In this particular indication, no effective substitute has been found to date. The antisuicidal and mortality reducing effects of lithium are also of particular value. Although it can potentially induce a large number of side effects, if lithium is administered to correctly selected bipolar patients in a properly tailored dosage, it is generally well tolerated, with the exception of idiosyncratic reactions. There are several misconceptions about lithium treatment that prevail in the literature, and these misconceptions result mostly from the lack of appreciation of the variety of lithium actions, of the heterogeneity of bipolar disorders, and of the capricious natural course. Further advances in the understanding of lithium treatment are limited by the lack commercial interest, despite its unique value.

Despite several plausible and promising hypotheses, the mechanism of stabilizing action of lithium in bipolar disorders remains undetected.

REFERENCES

1. Jenicek M. Clinical Case Reporting in Evidence-Based Medicine. 2nd ed. New York, NY: Oxford University Press, 2001.
2. Cade J. Lithium salts in the treatment of psychotic excitement. Med J Aust 1949; 36: 349–352.
3. Schou M, Juel-Nielsen N, Stromgren E, Voldby H. The treatment of manic psychoses by the administration of lithium salts. J Neurol Neurosurg Psychiatr 1954; 17:250–260.
4. Baastrup PC, Schou M. Lithium as a prophylactic agent: its effect against recurrent depressions and manic-depressive psychosis. Arch Gen Psychiatry 1967; 16:162–172.
5. Baastrup PC, Poulsen JC, Schou M. Prophylactic lithium: double blind discontinuation in manic-depressive and recurrent-depressive disorders. Lancet 1970; 2:326.
6. Johnson FN. The History of Lithium Therapy. London: The MacMillan Press Ltd, 1984.
7. Goodwin FK, Ghaemi SN. The impact of the discovery of lithium on psychiatric thought and practice in the USA and Europe. Aust N Z J Psychiatry 1999; 33:S54–S64.

8. Reifman A, Wyatt RJ. Lithium: a brake in the rising cost of mental illness. Arch Gen Psychiatry 1980; 37:385–388.
9. Sheard MH. The effect of lithium and other ions on aggressive behavior. Mod Probl Pharmacopsychiatry 1978; 13:53–68.
10. Sheard MH. Clinical pharmacology of aggressive behavior. Clin Neuropharmacol 1984; 7:173–183.
11. Garver DL, Hirschowitz J, Fleishman R, Djuric PE. Lithium response and psychoses: a double-blind, placebo-controlled study. Psychiatr Res 1984; 12:57–68.
12. Garver DL, Kelly K, Fried KA, Magnusson M, Hirschowitz J. Drug response patterns as a basis of nosology for the mood-incongruent psychoses (the schizophrenias). Psychol Med 1988; 18:873–885.
13. Lenz G, Lovrek A, Thau K, Topitz A, Denk A, Simhandl C, et al. Lithium prophylaxis of schizoaffective disorders (in German). Wien Med Wochenschr 1987; 137:5.
14. Muller-Oerlinghausen B, Ahrens B, Grof E, Grof P, Lenz G, Schou M, et al. The effect of long-term lithium treatment on the mortality of patients with manic-depressive and schizoaffective illness. Acta Psychiatr Scand 1992; 86:218–222.
15. Coppen A, Bailey J, Houston B, Silcocks P. Lithium and mortality: a 15-year follow-up. Clin Neuropharmacol 1992; 15:448A–449A.
16. Tondo L, Jamison KR, Baldessarini RJ. Effect of lithium maintenance on suicidal behavior in major mood disorders. Ann N Y Acad Sci 1997; 836:339–351.
17. Mendels J. Lithium in the treatment of depression. Am J Psychiatry 1976; 133:373–378.
18. de Montigny C. Lithium addition in refractory depression. In: Nolen WA, Zohar J, Roose SP, Amsterdam JD, eds. Refractory Depression: Current Strategies and Future Directions. Chichester: John Wiley and Sons, 1994:47–57.
19. Price LH, Charney DS, Heninger GR. Variability of response to lithium augmentation in refractory depression. Am J Psychiatry 1986; 143:1387–1392.
20. Schou M. Trends in lithium treatment and research during the last decade. Pharmacopsychiatria 1982; 15:128–130.
21. Schou M. Perspectives on lithium treatment of bipolar disorder: action, efficacy, effect on suicidal behavior. Bipolar Disord 1999; 1:5–10.
22. Schou M, Thomsen K, Baastrup PC. Studies on the course of recurrent endogenous affective disorders. Int Pharmacopsychiatr 1970; 5:100–106.
23. Grof P, Cakuls P, Dostal T. Lithium drop-outs: a followup study of the patients who discontinued prophylactic lithium. Int J Pharmacopsychiatr 1971; 5:162–169.
24. Prien RF, Gelenberg AJ. Alternatives to lithium for the preventative treatment of bipolar disorder. Am J Psychiatry 1989; 146(7):840–848.
25. Bowden CL, Calabrese JR, McElroy SL, et al. A randomized, placebo-controlled, 12-month trial of divalproex and lithium in treatment of out-patients with bipolar I disorder. Arch Gen Psychiatry 2000; 57:481–489.
26. Post RM, Leverich GS, Altshuler L, Mikalauskas K. Lithium-discontinuation-induced refractoriness: preliminary observations. Am J Psychiatry 1992; 149(12):1727–1729.
27. Suppes T, Baldessarini RJ, Faedda GL, Tohen M. Risk of recurrence following discontinuation of lithium treatment in bipolar disorder. Arch Gen Psychiatry 1991; 48: 1082–1088.
28. Guscott R, Taylor L. Lithium prophylaxis in recurrent affective illness. Efficacy, effectiveness and efficiency [see comments] [review]. Br J Psychiatry 1994; 164:741–746.
29. Grof P. Has the effectiveness of lithium changed? Impact of the variety of lithium's effects. Neuropsychopharmacology 1998; 19:183–188.
30. Deshauer D, Fergusson D, Duffy A, Albuquerque J, Grof P. Lithium monotherapy in bipolar illness: factors influencing differences in outcome reports. Bipolar Disorders. In press.
31. Grof P, Duffy A, Cavazzoni P, Grof E, Garnham J, MacDougall M, et al. Is response to prophylactic lithium a familial trait? J Clin Psychiatry 2002; 63:942–947.

32. Baldessarini RJ, Tondo L. Does lithium treatment still work? Evidence of stable responses over three decades. Arch Gen Psychiatry 2000; 57:187–190.
33. Berghoefer A, Mueller-Oerlinghausen B. No loss of efficacy after discontinuation and reinstitution of long-term lithium treatment. Biol Psychiatry 1997; 42:78S.
34. Garnham JS, Munro A, Teehan A, Slaney A, Duffy A, MacDougall M, et al. Naturalistic study of outcome of mood stabilizing treatment in bipolar disorder. Eur Neuropsychopharmacol 2003; 13(suppl 4):S201.
35. Goodwin FK, Jamison KR. Manic-Depressive Illness. Oxford: Oxford University Press, 1990.
36. Bowden CL, Brugger AM, Swann AC, Calabrese JR, Janicak PG, Petty F, et al. Efficacy of divalproex vs lithium and placebo in the treatment of mania. The Depakote Mania Study Group. JAMA 1994; 271(12):918–924.
37. Vojtechovsky M. Zkusenosti s lecbou solemi lithia. Problemy Psychiatrie v Praxi a ve Vyzkumu. Prague: Czechoslovak Medical Press, 1957:216–224.
38. Ghaemi SN, Ko J, Goodwin FK. "Cade's disease" and beyond: misdiagnosis, antidepressant use, and a proposed definition for bipolar spectrum disorder. Can J Psychiatry 2002; 47(2):125–134.
39. Greil W, Ludwig-Mayerhofer W, Erazo N, Schöchlin C, Schmidt S, Engel RR, et al. Lithium versus carbamazepine in the maintenance treatment of bipolar disorders—a randomized study. J Affect Disord 1997; 43:151–161.
40. Ahrens B, Grof P, Moller HJ, Muller-Oerlinghausen B, Wolf TH. Extended survival of patients on long-term lithium treatment. Can J Psychiatry 1995; 40:241–246.
41. Garver DL, Hutchinson LJ. Psychosis, lithium-induced antipsychotic response, and seasonality. Psychiatr Res 1988; 26:279–286.
42. Angst J, Weis P, Grof P, Baastrup PC, Schou M. Lithium prophylaxis in recurrent affective disorders. Br J Psychiatry 1970; 116:604–614.
43. Lenz G, Wolf R, Simhandl C, Topicz A, Berner P. Long-term prognosis and recurrence prophylaxis of schizoaffective psychoses (in German). In: Marneros A, ed. Schizoaffektive Psychosen (Tropon Symposium). Vol. IV. Berlin: Springer, 1989:55–66.
44. Grof P. Lithium discontinuation in typical and atypical affective disorders. Collegium Internationale Neuropsychopharmacologicum Meeting, Washington 1994, Abstracts, 237.
45. Lenz G, Lovrek A, Thau K, Topitz A, Denk A, Simhandl C, et al. Lithium-withdrawal study in schizoaffective patients. In: Birch NJ, ed. Lithium: Inorganic Pharmacology and Psychiatric Use. Oxford: IRL Press Ltd, 1988.
46. Perris P, Smigan L. The use of lithium in the long term morbidity suppressing treatment of cycloid and schizoaffective psychoses. In: Pichot P, Berner P, Wolf R, Thau K, eds. Psychiatry: the State of the Art. New York: Plenum, 1985:375–380.
47. Duffy A, Deshauer D, Alda M, Grof P. Exploratory study of stabilizing treatment among the affected offspring of well characterized bipolar parents: observations supporting selective effectiveness. Bipolar Disord 2004. Submitted.
48. Lader MH. Prophylactic lithium? Lancet 1968; II:103.
49. Baldessarini RJ. Frequency of diagnosis of schizophrenia versus affective disorders from 1944 to 1968. Am J Psychiatry 1970; 127:759–763.
50. Stoll AL, Tohen M, Baldessarini RJ, Goodwin DC, Stein S, Katz S, et al. Shifts in diagnostic frequencies of schizophrenia and major affective disorders at six North American psychiatric hospitals, 1972–1988. Am J Psychiatry 1993; 150:1668–1673.
51. Angst J. The course of affective disorders. II. Typology of bipolar manic-depressive illness. Archiv Psychiatr Nervenkrankheiten 1978; 226:65–73.
52. Bellivier F, et al. Age at onset in bipolar I affective disorder: further evidence for three subgroups. Am J Psychiatry 2003; 160(5):999–1001.
53. Schurhoff F, Bellivier F, Jouvent R, Mouren-Simeoni M, Bouvard M, Allilaire J, et al. Early and late onset bipolar disorders: two different forms of manic-depressive illness? J Affect Disord 2000; 58:215–221.

54. Alda M. The phenotypic spectra of bipolar disorder. Eur Neuropsychopharmacol 2004; 14:S94–S99.
55. Tondo L, Baldessarini RJ, Floris G, Rudas N. Effectiveness of restarting lithium treatment after its discontinuation in bipolar I and bipolar II disorders. Am J Psychiatry 1997; 154:548–550.
56. Schou M. Lithium treatment and kidney function. Ugeskr Laeger 1990; 152:2343–2345.
57. Grof P, Grof E, Hux M. Side effects of responders and nonresponders to longterm stabilization. Proceedings, 33rd Annual Meeting of the CPA, 1983:96.
58. Schou M, Amdisen A, Baastrup PC. Clinical and serum level monitoring in lithium therapy and lithium intoxication. In: Cooper TB, Gershon ES, Kline N, eds. Lithium: Controversies and Unresolved Issues. Amsterdam: Excerpta Medica, 1979.
59. Amdisen A, Schou M. Lithium. Side Eff Drug Annu 1979; 3:22–25.
60. Grof P, O'Sullivan K. Somatic side effects of long-term lithium treatment. In: Stancer, et al., eds. Guidelines for the Use of Psychotropic Drugs. New York: Spectrum, 1984: 105–118.
61. Schou M. Treating recurrent affective disorders during and after pregnancy: what can be taken safely? Drug Saf 1998; 18:143–152.
62. Schou M. Lithium Treatment of Mood Disorders, a Practical Guide. 6th ed. Karger, 2004.
63. Grof P. Lithium update: selected issues. In: Ayd F, Taylor JT, Taylor BT, eds. Affective Disorders Reassessed. Baltimore: Ayd Medical Publications, 1983.
64. Post RM, Denicoff KD, Frye MA, Everich GS. Re-evaluating carbamazepine prophylaxis in bipolar disorder. Br J Psychiatry 1997; 170:202–204.
65. Swann AC, Bowden CL, Calabrese JR, Dilsaver SC, Morris DD. Mania: differential effects of previous depressive and manic episodes on response to treatment. Acta Psychiatr Scand 2000; 101:444–451.
66. Tohen M, Chengappa KNR, Suppes T, Zarate CA, Calabrese JR, Bowden CL, et al. Efficacy of olanzapine in combination with valproate or lithium in the treatment of mania in patients partially nonresponsive to valproate or lithium monotherapy. Arch Gen Psychiatry 2002; 59:62–69.
67. Muller-Oerlinghausen B. Lithium long-term treatment: does it act via serotonin? Pharmacopsychiatria 1985; 18:214–217.
68. Goodwin G. Mechanism of action of lithium. Curr Opin Psychiatry 1988; 1:72–75.
69. Manji HK, Moore GJ, Rajkowska G, Chen G. Neuroplasticity and cellular resilience in mood disorders. Mol Psychiatry 2000; 5:578–593.
70. Manji HK, Young LT. Structural plasticity and neuronal resilience: are these targets for mood stabilizers and antidepressants in the treatment of bipolar disorder? Bipolar Disord 2002; 4(2):77–79.

19
The Use of Anticonvulsants in the Treatment of Bipolar Disorder

Paolo Brambilla
Department of Pathology and Experimental and Clinical Medicine, Section of Psychiatry, University of Udine School of Medicine, Udine, Italy

Jair C. Soares
Division of Mood and Anxiety Disorders, Department of Psychiatry, University of Texas Health Science Center at San Antonio, San Antonio, Texas, U.S.A.

ABSTRACT

The available literature on the use of anticonvulsants in the treatment of bipolar patients is summarized here, and perspectives and directions for future research and therapeutic development in this area are discussed. Carbamazepine and valproate have been shown to be effective in the acute antimanic treatment of bipolar disorder, and are the first-choice treatments for lithium-refractory patients. Valproate has been approved by the FDA in the United States as an antimanic agent. While the efficacy of these drugs in the acute treatment of the illness has been satisfactorily documented, double-blind randomized studies are still necessary to evaluate the long-term effectiveness of both anticonvulsants, although there are some controlled data to support their efficacy for maintenance, mostly for valproate. Newer anticonvulsants, such as gabapentin, lamotrigine, and topiramate have been investigated in the past few years as possible alternatives for bipolar individuals. Controlled double-blind studies failed to support the antimanic effects of gabapentin. On the contrary, whereas the antimanic efficacy of lamotrigine needs to be confirmed in double-blind studies, this agent has been shown to be effective in the pharmacological management of the depressive phase of the illness, as well as a maintenance treatment, recently resulting on FDA approval for the maintenance treatment of bipolar disorder in the Unite States. Topiramate, due to induced weight loss, may represent a potential alternative for treatment-resistant bipolar patients with obesity or drug-induced weight gain. However, its antimanic action is still unconfirmed as there is no controlled evidence to support its efficacy.

INTRODUCTION

In 1949, the Australian psychiatrist John Cade (1) suggested that lithium had therapeutic effects in the treatment of bipolar patients. Lithium is still the gold standard in the treatment of bipolar disorder, with an overall response rate for typical mania between 60% and 90% (2–4). On the contrary, the response rates are lower for patients with atypical features, such as psychotic symptoms, mixed state, rapid cycling illness, comorbid substance abuse, and personality disorders (5–7). Therefore, considering the high percentage of poor or non-responders, as well as patients who are intolerant to lithium's side effects, in recent years there has been a growing interest on new pharmacological alternatives for the treatment of bipolar disorder.

Anticonvulsant medications have been examined since the early 1970s as potential mood stabilizers for bipolar disorder. These drugs are the first alternatives as acute antimanic and long-term agents for the treatment of bipolar patients refractory to lithium (8). In particular, carbamazepine and valproate have been investigated as potential mood stabilizers since the 1970s and are first-line alternatives to lithium. Most recently, newer anticonvulsants such as lamotrigine, gabapentin, topiramate, and tiagabine have been examined in preliminary studies as possible options in the treatment of this disorder (9). Other possible treatment choices for refractory patients also include antipsychotics and calcium antagonists (10). In particular, the efficacy of several atypical antipsychotics has been demonstrated in controlled studies and their use for the management of acute mania, either as monotherapy or part of combination treatment, has become increasingly popular.

Here we summarized the available literature on the use of anticonvulsants in the treatment of bipolar patients and discussed the perspectives and directions for future research and therapeutic development in this area.

FIRST-GENERATION ANTICONVULSANTS

Carbamazepine

Psychopharmacology

Carbamazepine, chemically related to the antidepressant imipramine, is a neutral and lipophilic compound (11). After 2 to 3 weeks of treatment, the plasma levels may drop 20–30%, because carbamazepine auto-induces its own metabolism through the induction of the cytochrome P450 hepatic system (isoform CYP 3A3/4) (12) (Table 1). Its most important metabolite, the 10,11-epoxide-carbamazepine, also has anticonvulsant properties, and is excreted in the urine, as well as carbamazepine. The most common dose-related side effects are neurological symptoms such as diplopia, blurred vision, fatigue, nausea, and ataxia. Less frequent side effects are skin rashes, leukopenia, thrombocytopenia, hyponatremia, and liver enzyme

Table 1 Pharmacokinetics

	Carbamazepine	Valproate	Gabapentin	Lamotrigine	Topiramate
Absorption (hr)	6–24	2–8	2–3	1–3	1–4
Bioavailability (%)	58–87	68–100	35–60	98	> 80
Protein binding (%)	70–80	90	0	55	15
Half-life (hr)	18–55	10–16	6–7	15–70	18–23

Table 2 Mechanisms of Action

	Carbamazepine	Valproate	Gabapentin	Lamotrigine	Topiramate
GABA	Enhanced	Enhanced	Enhanced	Uncertain	Enhanced
Glutamate	Inconsistent	Inconsistent	Inconsistent	Decrease	Effective
Blockade Na^+ voltage-dependent channels	Effective	Effective	Uncertain	Effective	Effective
Modulate Ca^{2+} channels	Inconsistent	Not effective	Effective	Effective	Effective

Abbreviation: GABA, gamma-aminobutyric acid.

elevations. Idiosyncratic side effects are agranulocytosis, aplastic anemia, hepatic failure, exfoliative dermatitis, and pancreatitis.

Carbamazepine is the most effective agent for inhibiting the kindling phenomenon in animal models in the limbic system and temporal lobe regions, which may explain its efficacy in treating epilepsy and psychiatric disorders (13). It diminishes gamma-aminobutyric acid (GABA) and dopamine turnover, blocks norepinephrine uptake and voltage-dependent sodium channels, and has a vasopressin-agonist-like activity (14,15) (Table 2). Carbamazepine also interferes with post-synaptic signal-tranduction mechanisms, and has been shown to inhibit G-proteins, the cGMP/cAMP second-messenger systems, and calcium (Ca^{2+}) calmodulin protein kinase activity (16,17).

In acutely ill patients, the dosage may be increased by 200 mg/day up to 800–1000 mg/day, according to treatment response and side effects. The maintenance doses may range from 200 to 1600 mg/day. Suggested therapeutic serum levels ranged from 4 to 12 μg/mL, similarly to the ones utilized for epileptic patients, although no available studies have found a clear correlation between serum level and clinical response in affective patients.

Efficacy

Acute Trials in Mania. Uncontrolled prospective studies [response rates: 46% (18); 70% (19); 86% (20); 83% (21); 32% (22); 66% (23); 63% (24)] and retrospective studies [response rates: 40% (25); 64% (26); 89.5% (27); 57% (28)] suggested antimanic effects of carbamazepine in resistant bipolar patients.

Subsequently, randomized double-blind studies (21,29–41) and randomized open studies (42–44) showed antimanic response of carbamazepine in bipolar patients (Table 3). Carbamazepine was administered in conjunction with neuroleptics or other drugs and as monotherapy. In comparison to lithium, carbamazepine was found to have inferior (35) or similar response in manic and mixed bipolar patients (34,38,39). Also, the efficacy of carbamazepine monotherapy was not superior to placebo in three small studies (29,31,36), whereas in a recent large, multicenter study, carbamazepine monotherapy was significantly superior to placebo in treating manic or mixed bipolar patients (41). Similar efficacy in the treatment of mania was also found when carbamazepine was compared to chlorpromazine (37), haloperidol (21,40,43), and valproate (30,44). Interestingly, carbamazepine has also been found to be comparable to lithium in the treatment of children and adolescents with bipolar disorder (45).

Table 3 Controlled Studies with Carbamazepine in Mania

Study	Design	Duration	Treatment	Subjects	Responders
Okuma et al. (37)	r, db	3 weeks	CBZ vs. CPZ	60 ICD-IX BP and monopolar manic pts, 36 years (16–70)	17 CBZ (53%), 12 CPZ (43%)
Ballenger and Post (29)	db, placebo	6 weeks	CBZ/placebo/CBZ	Nine RDC BP pts, 33 years (24–53)	Five CBZ (56%), three placebo (60%)
Grossi et al. (32)	r, db	3 weeks	CBZ vs. CPZ	37 DSM-III BP pts, 45 ± 15 years	10 CBZ (56%), 10 CPZ (68%)
Klein et al. (33)	r, db	5 weeks	CBZ+HAL vs. HAL + placebo	43 RDC pts: 22 BP, 11 SA, 10 SKZ, 34 years (20–70)	BPRS improvement in CBZ + HAL group (18%) superior than placebo + HAL group (11%)
Muller and Stoll (21)	r, db	2 weeks	oxCBZ vs. HAL	20 manic pts, age not reported	50% BRMAS improvement in both groups
Sethi and Tiwari (42)	r	4 weeks	CBZ vs. CPZ	10 DSM-III BP pts, 36 ± 6 years	Five CBZ (100%), five CBZ (100%)
Emrich et al. (30)	r, db, off-on-off	Variable duration	Placebo/oxCBZ or VPA/placebo	12 ICD-IX pts: 5 BP, 7 SA, 29 years (17–53)	Four oxCBZ (57%), three VPA pts (60%)
Goncalves and Stoll (31)	r, db, placebo	3 weeks	CBZ vs. placebo	12 ICD-IX pts: 7 BP, 5 SA, 43 years (22–65)	Four CBZ (67%), three placebo (50%)
Stoll et al. (43)	r	3 weeks	CBZ vs. HAL	58 ICD-IX pts: 34 manic, 24 SA, 40 ± 13.4 years	12 manic CBZ (75%), seven SA CBZ (54%), 12 manic HAL (67%), seven SA HAL (64%)
Lenzi et al. (34)	r, db	3 weeks	CPZ + CBZ vs. Li + CBZ	30 DSM-III pts: 22 BP, 3 SA, five other diagnoses, 39 ± 14 years	50% CGI and some BPRS factors improvement in both groups
Lerer et al. (35)	r, db	4 weeks	CBZ vs. Li	34 DSM-III BP pts, 40 years (23–65)	Four CBZ (27%), 11 Li (58%)

Moller et al. (36)	r, db	3 weeks	CBZ + HAL vs. placebo + HAL	20 ICD-IX pts: 12 manic, eight schizomanic, 33 ± 13 years	50% BRMAS improvement in both groups
Okuma et al. (38)	r, db	4 weeks	CBZ vs. Li	101 DSM-III BP pts, 36 years (19–70)	30 CBZ (62%), 30 Li (60%)
Small et al. (39)	r, db	8 weeks	CBZ vs. Li	48 DSM III-R BP pts, 39 years (22–73)	Eight CBZ (33%), eight Li (33%)
Small et al. (40)	r, db	8 weeks	Li + CBZ vs. Li + HAL	33 DSM-III-R BP pts, 37 years (19–62)	50% MRS improvement in both groups
Kowatch et al. (45)	r	6 weeks	CBZ vs. VPA vs. Li	42 DSM-IV BP pts, 11 ± 3 years	Five CBZ (38%), eight VPA (53%), five Li (36%)
Vasudev et al. (44)	r	4 weeks	CBZ vs. VPA	30 DSM-III-R BP pts	Eight CBZ (53%), 11 VPA (73%)
Weisler et al. (41)	r, db	3 weeks	CBZ vs. placebo	204 DSM-III-R BP pts, 38 ± 11 years	42 CBZ (42%), 23 placebo (22%)

Abbreviations: r, randomized; db, double blind; pts, patients; BP, bipolar; SA, schizoaffective; SKZ, schizophrenic; CBZ, carbamazepine; VPA, valproate; HAL, haloperidol; oxCBZ, ox-carbamazepine; Li, lithium; CPZ, chloropromazine; CGI, Clinical Global Impression; BRMAS, Bech–Rafaelsen Mania Scale; BPRS, Brief Psychiatric Rating Scale; MRS, Mania Rating Scale.

Acute Trials in Depression. Uncontrolled prospective [response rates: 39% (46); 40% (47); 53% (48); rates not reported (49); 92% (50); 38% (51)], and retrospective studies [response rate: 44% (52); 44% (53); 74% (27)] suggested the efficacy of carbamazepine as monotherapy or as adjunctive treatment for bipolar depression.

Placebo-controlled studies reported the efficacy of carbamazepine in treating bipolar depression as an add-on to antidepressants or as a monotherapy (29,54). It was also found to have comparable efficacy to trimipramine (55) or lithium augmentation (56) (Table 4). A small, randomized study found imipramine superior to carbamazepine in depressed affective patients (42).

Prophylaxis Trials. Several uncontrolled prospective [response rates: 75% (57); 33% (58); 68% (22); 86% (59); 46% (60); 57% (61); 83% (62); 63% (63)], and retrospective studies suggested carbamazepine's prophylactic effect in bipolar patients [response rates: not reported (64); 24% (65); 67% (66); 21% (67)]. Carbamazepine was used in combination with lithium, or as adjunctive therapy to other medications. Most of the patients were lithium-resistant or intolerant; rapid cycling patients also responded. Three retrospective studies have shown similar antimanic and antidepressant prophylactic effects with carbamazepine compared to lithium [response rates: 67% vs. 56% (66); 21% vs. 15% (66)]. Three open studies found comparable long-term efficacy of carbamazepine and lithium in bipolar patients (68–70) (Table 5), whereas Greil and collaborators (78–80) found a significantly higher overall prophylactic response of lithium compared to carbamazepine in bipolar disorder type I, particularly when taking into consideration inter-episodic morbidity, drop-out, and re-hospitalization (81).

Randomized, double-blind, controlled studies have shown prophylactic effects of carbamazepine similar to lithium (72–75) and superior to placebo (71) (Table 5). However, better antimanic efficacy of lithium compared to carbamazepine has also been reported (25,76,77).

Valproate

Psychopharmacology

Valproic acid is a simple branched-chain carboxylic acid. It does not induce its own metabolism, is mostly glucuronidated, and less than 20% is oxidatively metabolized (β, ω, and ω1 oxidation) (82) (Table 1). Common dose-related side effects are gastrointestinal distress, tremors, sedation, weight gain, increased appetite, hair loss, and hepatic transaminase elevations. The use of the enteric-coated divalproex sodium instead of valproic acid or sodium valproate reduces the gastrointestinal complaints, possibly improving patients' compliance. Other potential side effects may possibly include polycystic ovaries or hyperandrogenism (83), and rarely irreversible hepatic failure, pancreatitis, and thrombocytopenia.

Valproate may increase the GABA brain concentration through the enhancement of GABA synthesis and the inhibition of GABA catabolism. It has also been reported that valproate increases glutamate–aspartate transporter, decrease glutamate transporter-1, GABA transporter-1 and -3, affecting glutamate removal and increasing GABA concentrations (84). These effects could eventually modulate a proposed GABAergic abnormality in manic-depressive illness (85). Valproate also inhibits the phenomenon of kindling, enhances serotonin (5-HT) neurotransmission, and blocks voltage-dependent sodium (Na^+) channels (86,87) (Table 2). It has also been shown that valproate inhibits specific steps in second-messenger signal transduction pathways (cGMP, protein kinase C, phosphatidylinositol systems, and

Table 4 Controlled Trials with Carbamazepine in Depression

Study	Design	Duration	Treatment	Subjects	Responders
Ballenger and Post (29)	db, placebo	6 weeks	Placebo/CBZ/placebo	13 RDC pts: seven BP, four UP, two SA, 45 years (27–63)	Five CBZ (38%), one placebo (20%)
Neumann et al. (55)	r	4 weeks	CBZ vs. TRI	12 BP or UP pts, 48 years (29–63)	50% HDRS and SPES improvement in both groups
Sethi and Tiwari (42)	r	4 weeks	CBZ vs. IMI	11 DSM-III BP or UP pts, 42±6 years	Three CPZ (60%), four IMI (80%)
Post et al. (54)	r, db, placebo	8 weeks	Placebo/CBZ/placebo	35 DSM-III pts: 24 BP, 11 UP, 41±13 years	20 CBZ (57%;): 15 BP (62%), five UP (45%), nine placebo (45%)
Rybakowski et al. (56)	r	4 weeks	CBZ vs. Li	59 DSM-IV pts: 18 BP, 41 UP, 49±12 years	16 CBZ (57%), 21 Li (68%)

Abbreviations: r, randomized; db, double blind; CBZ, carbamazepine; pts, patients; BP, bipolar; UP, unipolar; SA, schizoaffective; IMI, imipramine; TRI, trimipramine; Li, lithium; HDRS, Hamilton Depression Rating Scale; SPES, Structured Psychopathological Rating Scale.

Table 5 Controlled Trials with Carbamazepine in Prophilaxys

Study	Design	Duration	Treatment	Subjects	Responders
Double-blind trials					
Okuma et al. (71)	r, db, placebo	1 year	CBZ vs. placebo	22 ICD-IX BP pts, 43 years (21–64)	Six CBZ (50%), two placebo (20%)
Placidi et al. (72)	r, db	3 years	CBZ vs. Li	83 DSM-III pts: 54 BP or UP, 29 SA, 41 ± 12 years	2/3 of the patients in each group
Watkins et al. (73)	r, db	1.5 years	CBZ vs. Li	52 DSM-III BP or UP pts, 20–60 years	16 CBZ (62%), 15 Li (58%)
Elphick et al. (25)	r, db, c.o.	9 months	CBZ vs. Li, trial interrupted for severe CBZ side effects	20 manic-depressive pts, 17–70 years	Three CBZ (21%), eight Li (62%)
Lusznat et al. (74)	r, db	1 year	CBZ vs. Li	54 DSM-III pts: 52 BP, two SA	Nine CBZ (33%), five Li (19%)
Coxhead et al. (75)	r, db	1 year	CBZ vs. Li	31 DSM-III BP pts, 48 ± 12 years (23–66)	Seven CBZ (47%), seven Li (44%)
Denicoff et al. (76)	First year: r, db; second year: c.o., db; third year: db, frst and second year Li or CBZ monotherapy, third year Li + CBZ	52 DSM-III-R BP pts, 41 ± 11 years (19–75)	11 (24% of 46) in CBZ group, 14 (28% of 50) in Li group, six (52% of 31) in Li + CBZ group		
Hartong et al. (77)	r, db	2 years	CBZ vs. Li	94 DSM-III-R BP pts, 42 ± 14 years	29 CBZ (58%), 32 Li (73%)

Open trials					
Cabrera et al. (69)	Open	1.2 years	oxCBZ vs. Li	14 ICD-X pts: eight BP, two SA, 40 years (21–61)	Four oxCBZ (50%), three Li (50%)
Bellaire et al. (68)	Open	2 years	CBZ vs. Li	139 pts: 85 BP, 37 UP, 17 SA, 44± 13 years	34 CBZ (49%), 42 Li (61%)
Simhandl et al. (70)	r	2 years	CBZ vs. Li	84 DSM-III-R pts: 52 BP, 32 UP, 42± 13 years	15 CBZ (50%), 12 Li (43%)
Greil et al. (78–80); Kleindienst and Greil 2002 (81)	r	2.5 years	CBZ vs. Li	171 DSM-IV BP pts, 40 years	20 CBZ (24%), 34 Li (40%), 50% higher risk of failure with CBZ than Li in BP-I, but not in BP-II or BP-NOS

Abbreviations: r, randomized; db, double blind; c.o., cross-over; CBZ, carbamazepine; oxCBZ, ox-carbamazepine; pts, patients; BP, bipolar; UP, unipolar; SA, schizoaffective; Li, lithium; RCBP, rapid cycling bipolar; BP-NOS, bipolar not otherwise specified.

arachidonic acid) (88,89) and increases the expression of endoplasmic reticulum stress proteins (90,91). Interestingly, chronic valproate treatment may have neurotrophic/neuroprotective effects by increasing the expression of the neuroprotective protein bcl-2, by inhibiting the glycogen synthase kinase 3β (GSK-3β), which may play a role in neuronal death, and by stimulating MAP kinases activity, which may be involved in neurotrophic events (92).

Serum concentrations within 50–100 μg/mL are suggested for a better therapeutic response with valproate and to minimize the adverse effects. Starting generally with 250 mg orally twice a day, the dosage may be quickly titrated up till reaching therapeutic serum levels in 7 to 10 days.

Efficacy

Acute Trials in Mania. Efficacy of valproate alone or as adjunctive therapy in the treatment of resistant manic or mixed bipolar patients has been suggested in prospective [response rates: not reported (93); 64% (94); 41% (95); 86% (96); 62% (97); 80% (98); 89% (99)] and retrospective [response rates: 83% (100); 44% (101); not reported (102); 76% (103)] studies. Valproate was also suggested to be effective in the treatment of bipolar subjects with rapid cycling disorder (99,101,103), with comorbid substance dependence (93), and in the treatment of adolescent (97,104) and elderly patients (104).

Controlled studies have examined the acute antimanic efficacy of valproate monotherapy (Table 6). Superior effects to placebo were reported (106,108,110), although two small off–on–off studies showed comparable effects (30,105). Similar efficacy was found vs. lithium (108,107), carbamazepine (30,44), or olanzapine (111). Loading strategies with valproate have been investigated as potentially useful to speed the onset of response and potentially decrease the length of hospitalization (109,113,114). Interestingly, valproate has been found to be comparable to lithium in the treatment of mixed or manic episodes in children and adolescents with bipolar disorder (45) and superior to placebo in diminishing anger/hostility in women with borderline personality disorder and comorbid bipolar II disorder (115).

Acute Trials in Depression. Antidepressant effects of valproate monotherapy have been suggested in mood-stabilizer-naïve bipolar II patients [$N = 19$; response rates = 63% (116)] and in unipolar patients [$N = 33$; response rates: 58% (117)]. A randomized, double-blind study did not find significant differences between valproate plus lithium and paroxetine plus valproate or lithium in depressed bipolar patients (112) (Table 6).

Prophylactic Trials. Uncontrolled prospective [response rates: 75% (105); 71% (118); 25% (119); not available (30); 27% (95); 79% (120); not available (121); 72% (122)] and retrospective [response rates: 65% (100); 91% (123); 34% (124); 77% (125); 75% (126)] studies suggested prophylactic effects of valproate in bipolar patients when administered alone or as adjunctive treatment. Most of the patients in these studies were resistant to lithium and/or carbamazepine. Long-term valproate efficacy was also suggested in rapid cycling (118,120) and cyclothymic patients (120).

A large 1-year randomized, double-blind study found no differences among lithium, valproate, or placebo in the prophylaxis of bipolar disorder type I (127). Nonetheless, the dropout rates with valproate were significantly lower than with lithium or placebo in this study (termination rates: 62% vs. 75% vs. 76%, respectively). One small, randomized study found significantly fewer relapses with

Table 6 Short-Term Controlled Trials with Valproate

Study	Design	Duration	Treatment	Subjects	Responders
Prospective studies in mania					
Brennan et al. (105)	off-on-off	2 weeks	Placebo/VPA/ placebo	Eight acute manic pts	Six VPA (75%), five placebo (83%)
Emrich et al. (30)	r, db, off–on–off	Variable	Placebo/oxCBZ or VPA/placebo	12 ICD-IX pts: five BP, seven SA, 29 years (17–53)	Three VPA (60%), four oxCBZ (57%)
Pope et al. (106)	r, db, placebo	3 weeks	VPA vs. placebo	36 DSM-III-R BP pts, 37 ± 13 years (18–62)	Nine VPA (53%), two placebo (11%)
Freeman et al. (107)	r, db	3 weeks	VPA vs. Li	27 DSM-III-R BP pts	Nine VPA (64%), 12 Li (92%)
Bowden et al. (108)	r, db, placebo	3 weeks	VPA vs. Li vs. placebo	179 RDC BP pts, 40 ± 11 years	33 VPA (48%), 18 Li (50%), 18 placebo (24%)
McElroy et al. (109)	r	7 days	VPA vs. HAL	36 DSM-III-R BP pts, 36 ± 13 years	10 VPA (48%), five Hal (33%)
Muller-Oerlinghausen et al. (110)	r, db	3 weeks	VPA + NL vs. placebo + NL	136 ICD-X pts: 64 BP, 45 SA, 27 other diagnoses of mania, 38 ± 12 years	70% VPA + NL, 46% placebo + NL
Vasudev et al. (44)	r	4 weeks	VPA vs CBZ	30 DSM-III-R BP pts	11 VPA (73%), Eight CBZ (53%)
Zajecka et al. (111)	r, db	3 weeks	VPA vs. OLA	120 DSM-IV BP pts, 38.5 ± 12 years	Similar improvement of MRS, HAM-D, and BPRS
Prospective study in depression					
Young et al. (112)	r, db	6 weeks	VPA + Li vs. PRX + VPA or +Li	27 DSM-IV BP pts, 40 ± 12 years	11 VPA + Li (69%), 10 PRX + VPA or PRX + Li, (91%)

Abbreviations: r, randomized; db, double blind; VPA, valproate; CBZ, carbamazepine; oxCBZ, ox-carbamazepine; Li, lithium; HAL, haloperidol; NL, neuroleptic; OLA, olanzapine; PRX, paroxetine; pts, patients; BP, bipolar; SA, schizoaffective; MRS, Mania Rating Scale; HAM-D, Hamilton Rating Scale For Depression; BPRS, Brief Psychiatric Rating Scale.

Table 7 Controlled Trials with Valproate in Prophylaxis

Study	Design	Duration	Treatment	Subjects	Responders
Prospective					
Solomon et al. (128)	r	1 year	Li + placebo vs. Li + VPA	12 DSM-III-R BP pts, 40 years (30–65)	Zero VPA + Li relapsed, five Li + placebo relapsed
Bowden et al. (127)	r, db	1 year	VPA vs. Li vs. placebo	372 DSM-III-R BP pts, 39 ± 8 years	No efficacy differences among the three groups
Retrospecitve					
Ghaemi and Goodwin (129)		94 weeks	VPA vs. Li	30 DSM-III-R BP pts	Nine VPA (53%), seven Li (54%)

Abbreviations: r, randomized; db, double blind; VPA, valproate; Li, lithium; pts, patients; BP, bipolar.

valproate plus lithium compared to placebo plus lithium (128), whereas a retrospective study reported similar efficacy with valproate or lithium (129) (Table 7).

Comments: The antimanic effects of carbamazepine and valproate in the treatment of bipolar disorder have been extensively evaluated in the last three decades in several randomized, double-blind controlled studies, which mostly reported efficacy comparable with lithium. A meta-analysis study including only randomized double-blind controlled studies did not find any significant differences between lithium, valproate, and carbamazepine in treating acute mania in manic-depressive illness (130). Carbamazepine was the first anticonvulsant for which a mood-stabilizing effect was demonstrated, and has been, for that reason, more extensively studied than valproate in affective patients to this date. Nonetheless, valproate, based on its demonstrated antimanic effects and favorable pharmacokinetic and side-effect profile, may be preferable to carbamazepine as an alternative for lithium non-responders. Also, there are more controlled maintenance data for valproate compared to carbamazepine, where evidence for efficacy in the maintenance treatment comes mostly from relatively small studies. Valproate has been approved by the FDA for treatment of mania in bipolar disorder.

The acute efficacy of carbamazepine and valproate in treating bipolar depression has been suggested in small studies, but to this date, no parallel, randomized, double-blind, placebo-controlled studies are available. Nonetheless, available uncontrolled and controlled data suggest that these agents may have potential antidepressant effects when added to antidepressant drugs. However, large double-blind controlled studies are needed to evaluate their role as monotherapy. Bipolar depression is a challenging clinical condition, for which available treatments are often unsatisfactory. In the management of depressed bipolar subjects, for patients already on full doses of mood-stabilizing agents, antidepressants, whenever needed, should be considered. For this purpose, tricyclic antidepressants should be avoided, as they may result in higher rates of switch to mania. A possible alternative is the addition of an anticonvulsant to the primary mood stabilizer, which may result in appropriate therapeutic response, without the need of adding an antidepressant drug, as those carry the risk of inducing a switch into mania. The specific role of newer anticonvulsant medications in the management of bipolar depression should be further investigated in controlled studies, as these agents may offer a very important alternative to the use of antidepressant drugs in the pharmacological management of this phase of the illness.

Conversely, the long-term effectiveness of carbamazepine and valproate has not been conclusively demonstrated yet and needs to be confirmed. Specifically, a large long-term double-blind, placebo-controlled study evaluating the efficacy of carbamazepine in bipolar disorder is still not available. The prophylactic efficacy of valproate in bipolar patients is also not conclusively demonstrated, as the only double-blind, parallel group, placebo-controlled study found no significant differences between valproate, lithium, and placebo in the long-term treatment of bipolar patients (127). However, the valproate group had better secondary outcomes than the placebo group, with longer duration of prophylaxis and less premature discontinuation from the study for any major affective episode. So, the prophylactic efficacy of carbamazepine and valproate in the long-term treatment of bipolar patients, while suggested by smaller studies, is still not conclusively demonstrated in large double-blind, placebo-controlled studies.

SECOND-GENERATION ANTICONVULSANTS

Gabapentin

Psychopharmacology

Gabapentin is structurally related to the neurotransmitter gamma-aminobutyric acid (GABA) (Table 1). It is excreted by the kidney. The most common side effects are sedation, dizziness, ataxia, diplopia, fatigue, nystagmus, headache, gastrointestinal upset, and amnesia. Rarely reported side effects are renal impairment, thyroiditis, ejaculatory failure, and anorgasmia.

Gabapentin may enhance GABAergic transmission by increasing GABA synthesis, probably through the activation of glutamic acid decarboxilase (131), GABA release, GABA turnover, and by reducing GABA degradation (131,132). It may also limit the firing of neuronal sodium channels and bind to the alfa2δ sub-unit of brain voltage-dependent Ca^{2+} channels, which may lead to decreased glutamate and aspartate release and to reduced activation of AMPA receptors (133–135) (Table 2).

Efficacy

Open prospective [response rates: 71% (136); 76% (137); 71% (138); 60% (139); 67% (140); 78% (141); 48% (142); 64% (143); not available (144)] and retrospective [response rates: 30% (145); 92% (146)] studies suggested acute antimanic effects of gabapentin in bipolar disorder, mostly as add-on therapy. On the contrary, Vieta et al. (147) did not find evidence of significant effects of gabapentin administration on manic symptoms. Also, in double-blind, controlled studies, gabapentin, administered as monotherapy or as an add-on therapy, had similar (148) or less (149) antimanic effects compared to placebo in treatment-resistant bipolar patients (Table 8).

Gabapentin was suggested to be effective in bipolar depression (140,147,150) and as adjunctive maintenance treatment in resistant bipolar patients (141,143, 144,150) in naturalistic uncontrolled studies.

Table 8 Controlled Trials of Gabapentin

Study	Design	Duration (weeks)	Treatment	Subjects	Responders
Pande et al. (149)	r, db, placebo	10	GBP + VPA and/or Li vs. placebo + VPA and/or Li	117 DSM-IV BP I pts, 39 ± 10 years (17–73)	Significant greater decrease in YMRS for "placebo group"
Obrocea et al. (148)	r, db, placebo	6	LMT vs. GBP vs. placebo, two subsequent c.o.	45 DSM-IV pts: 35 BP, 10 UP, 39 ± 10.5 years (20–67)	11 GBP (28%), 20 LMT (51%), eight placebo (21%)

Abbreviations: r, randomized; db, double blind; LMT, lamotrigine; GBP, gabapentin; VPA, valproate; Li, lithium; pts, patients; BP, bipolar; YMRS, Young Mania Rating Scale.

Overall, the available controlled evidence with gabapentin in bipolar disorder is disappointing and there is no support for its efficacy in the treatment of this disorder.

Lamotrigine

Psychopharmacology

Lamotrigine is a phenyltriazine derivative; it is glucoronidated by the liver to inactive glucuronide conjugates and it is excreted in the urine (151) (Table 1). The most frequent side effects are dizziness, headache, nausea, tremor, somnolence, asthenia, insomnia, and skin rash, which is a main cause for withdrawing the treatment. Severe skin rashes, including Stevens–Johnson syndrome and toxic epidermal necrolysis occur in about one of 300 adults and one of 100 children, and seem to be increased by concurrent valproate use (152).

Lamotrigine decreases both glutamate and aspartate release, probably mediated by the blockade of voltage-sensitive Ca^{2+} and Na^{+} channels and by nitric oxide mechanisms (153–155). Also, it has been suggested that lamotrigine enhances GABA release and downregulates 5-HT1A receptor-mediated adenylyl cyclase response in rat cortex (156,157) (Table 2).

Efficacy

Acute Trials. Antimanic effects of lamotrigine as adjunctive treatment has been suggested by prospective open studies in refractory bipolar patients [response rates: 43% (158); 62% (159); 71% (160); 67% (161); 50% (162)]. Acute mood-stabilizing effects of lamotrigine have also been found in bipolar patients with rapid cycling (160,163–165) and in those with cocaine dependence (166). Controlled studies also evaluated the mood-stabilizing effects of lamotrigine in bipolar disorder. No significant differences were found in the treatment of acute manic patients among lamotrigine monotherapy, lithium, or olanzapine in a small double-blind study (167), suggesting similar efficacy of lamotrigine to lithium or olanzapine in the treatment of mania. However, one placebo-controlled, double-blind study produced negative findings (168). Another double-blind, placebo-controlled, crossover study found lamotrigine monotherapy to be significantly superior than gabapentin or placebo in the treatment of refractory bipolar or unipolar patients (148) (Table 9).

Lamotrigine was also suggested to be effective in treatment-refractory depressed bipolar patients [response rates: 73% (175); 56% (162)]. A multicenter, randomized, double-blind, placebo-controlled study showed greater acute antidepressant efficacy in depressed bipolar I patients with lamotrigine compared to placebo [response rates: 51% vs. 37% (169)]. Moreover, preliminary findings from a large, randomized, double-blind study in depressed unipolar patients showed significantly higher antidepressant effects of lamotrigine compared to placebo (170) (Table 9). Bryant-Comstock et al. (176) also reported that lamotrigine was more effective than placebo in improving quality of life in depressed bipolar patients.

Prophylactic Trials. Long-term mood-stabilizing effects of lamotrigine in bipolar disorder have also been reported [response rates: 60% (165); not available (177); 65% (178); 69% (179)]. Long-term efficacy of lamotrigine monotherapy for bipolar disorder has been reported in controlled double-blind studies to be greater than placebo and comparable to lithium, with particular efficacy for those with depression (173,174) or rapid cycling (171,172) (Table 9).

The available controlled data with lamotrigine document its efficacy in the treatment of the depressive phase and in the maintenance phase of the treatment; these data resulted on its approval in 2003 for the maintenance treatment of bipolar disorder.

Topiramate

Psychopharmacology

Topiramate is a sulfamate-substituted derivative of the monosaccharide d-fructose; it does not affect liver enzymes and it is excreted unchanged in the urine (180) (Table 1). Most common side effects are paresthesias, somnolence, fatigue, dizziness, ataxia, anxiety, and cognitive and gastrointestinal disturbances. Weight loss occurs in about 20% of patients, and rarely kidney stones are reported (181).

Topiramate reduces the seizure threshold and the after-charge duration in the amygdala-kindled rat (182), blocking the spread of seizures. It may increase cerebral GABA concentrations in humans (183) and enhance GABAergic transmission by binding to allosteric $GABA_A$ receptors, probably through a non-benzodiazepine mechanism, and through effects on second-messenger systems (183–185). Also, topiramate may inhibit brain glutamate release by antagonizing AMPA/kainate type of glutamate receptors, possibly interacting with intracellular intermediaries, and may reduce Na^+ and l-type Ca^{2+} channel neuronal activities (186–188) (Table 2). It is also suggested to be an inhibitor of the enzyme carbonic anhydrase (189).

Efficacy

Acute antimanic effects of topiramate as adjunctive treatment in refractory bipolar patients have been reported in several open studies (190–198) (Table 10). However, recent unpublished double-blind controlled trials in the manic phase, presented in scientific meetings, have not demonstrated efficacy. Interestingly, patients treated with this medication also experience weight loss. Topiramate was also effective in patients resistant to gabapentin and/or lamotrigine (190,203) and in rapid cycling patients (190,191,203,204). Antidepressant (199,200) and long-term effects (198,201,202)

Table 9 Controlled Trials of Lamotrigine

Study	Design	Duration	Treatment	Subjects	Responders
Mania					
Anand et al. (168)	r, db, placebo	8 weeks	LMT ± Li vs. placebo	16 BP pts	Five LMT (62%), four placebo (50%)
Berk (167)	db, r	4 weeks	LMT vs. Li vs. OLA	45 DSM-IV manic pts, 20–59 years	Significant improvement in MRS for all groups
Obrocea et al. (148)	r, db, placebo	6 weeks	LMT vs. GBP vs. placebo, Two subsequent c.o.	45 DSM-IV pts: 35 BP, 10 UP, 39 ± 10.5 years (20–67)	11 GBP (28%), 20 LMT (51%), eight placebo (21%)
Depression					
Calabrese et al. (169)	r, db, placebo	7 weeks	LMT vs. placebo	195 DSM IV BP pts, 42 years (19–75)	66 LMT (51%): 34 LMT 200 mg and 32 LMT 50 mg, 24 placebo (37%)
Laurenza et al. (170)	r, db, placebo	8 weeks	LMT vs. DMI vs. placebo	437 DSM-IV UP pts	Statistically difference for both LMT and DMI vs. placebo on HDRS
Long term					
Calabrese et al. (171)	r, db, placebo	6 months	LMT vs. placebo	180 DSM-IV RCBP pts, 38 years (18–64)	37 LMT (41%), 23 placebo (26%)
Walden et al. (172)	Open, pro	52 weeks	LMT vs. Li	14 DSM-IV RCBP pts, 40.5 years (22–55)	Six LMT (86%), three Li (43%)
Bowden et al. (173)	r, db, placebo	76 weeks	LMT vs. Li vs. placebo	175 DSM-IV BP pts, 41 years	31 LMT (53%), 28 Li (61%), 21 placebo (30%)
Calabrese et al. (174)	r, db, placebo	76 weeks	LMT vs. Li vs. placebo	463 DSM-IV BP pts, 43 years	Intervention free at 1 year; Depression: LMT (57%), Li (46%), placebo (45%); Mania: LMT (77%), Li (86%), placebo (72%)

Abbreviations: r, randomized; db, double blind; pro, prospective; LMT, lamotrigine; GBP, gabapentin; OLA, olanzapine; Li, lithium; DMI, desmethylimipramine; pts, patients; BP, bipolar; RCBP, rapid cycling bipolar; UP, unipolar; MRS, Mania Rating Scale; HDRS, Hamilton Depression Rating Scale; QLDS, Quality of Life in Depression Scale.

Table 10 Trials of Topiramate

Study	Duration	Treatment	Subjects	Responders
Prospective				
Chengappa et al. (190)	5 weeks	TPM adjunctive treatment	20 DSM-IV pts: 18 BP, two SA, 43 ± 14 years (21–67)	12 (60%)
van Kammen et al. (193)	4 weeks	TPM monotherapy	11 BP pts, 42 years	Five (46%)
Kusumakar et al. (191)	16 weeks	TPM ± Li or VPA	19 RCBP pts	Eight (42%)
McElroy et al. (192)	Acute: 10 weeks; Maintenance: 42 weeks	TPM adjunctive treatment	54 DSM-IV BP pts, two SA	22 acute (41%), 12 long term (22%)
Calabrese et al. (194)	4 weeks	TPM monotherapy	10 DSM-IV BP pts, 43 years (22–64)	Three (30%)
Grunze et al. (195)	3 weeks	TPM adjunctive treatment on/off/on design	11 DSM-IV BP pts, 39 ± 10 years (24–64)	Eight (73%)
Bozikas et al. (196)	4 weeks	TPM adjunctive treatment	14 DSM-IV BP pts, 41 years (24–69)	Eight (73%)
Guille and Sachs (197)	22.4 weeks	TPM adjunctive treatment	14 DSM-IV BP pts, 37 years (16–51)	Eight (73%)
McIntyre et al. (199)	r, 8 weeks	TPM vs. buproprion, as adjunctive treatment	36 DSM-IV BP pts, 41 years (29–55)	10 LMT (56%), 11 buproprion (59%)
Vieta et al. (200)	24 weeks	TPM adjunctive treatment	33 DSM-IV BP and one SA pts, 42 ± 16 years	16 (47%)
Vieta et al. (198)	12 weeks	TPM adjunctive treatment	19 DSM-IV BP type II pts, 43 years (22–60)	10 (53%)
Vieta et al. (201)	48 weeks	TPM plus risperidone	58 DSM-IV BP pts, 41 ± 11 years	36 (62%)
Vieta et al. (202)	48 weeks	TPM plus olanzapine	24 DSM-IV BP and four SA pts, 43 ± 12 years	13 (50%)
Retrospective				
Marcotte (203)	16 weeks	TPM adjunctive treatment	58 DSM-IV pts: 44 RCBP, nine SA, five other diagnosis, 45 ± 16 years (10–90)	35 (60%): 23 RCBP (52%), seven SA (78%), five other (100%)

Abbreviations: r, randomized; TPM, topiramate; VPA, valproate; Li, lithium; pts, patients; BP, bipolar; SA, schizoaffective; RCBP, rapid cycling bipolar.

of topiramate in bipolar patients have also been suggested, but large double-blind, placebo-controlled studies are needed for confirmation of these effects.

Therefore, despite its interesting side-effects profile, as far as causing weight loss, which is often desirable among bipolar patients, there is no controlled evidence to support the efficacy of topiramate in the treatment of any phase of the illness.

Others

Tiagabine has been suggested as a potential adjunctive drug in the treatment of refractory bipolar patients in clinical case series (205–207), but not in two other small open trials (208,209). Up to this point, no controlled studies have examined its potential use in the treatment of bipolar disorder. Mishory et al. (210), in a randomized, double-blind, placebo-controlled study, found more substantial improvement in manic symptoms in refractory bipolar patients treated with a combination of phenytoin and haloperidol. In two uncontrolled open studies, only one-third of the resistant bipolar patients responded to primidone (211,212). Five of 15 manic patients showed marked improvement under treatment with zonisamide, an anticonvulsant developed in Japan, administered concurrently with other psychotropic drugs (213).

Comments: Acute antimanic effects of gabapentin in bipolar disorder were suggested in open trials, but controlled double-blind studies failed to confirm that. Therefore, this agent does not seem to have a clear role in the pharmacological management of mania. In regard to lamotrigine, the suggestions of antimanic efficacy come from naturalistic studies, but need to be documented in large double-blind controlled ones. There is evidence from both open and controlled studies suggesting therapeutic effects of lamotrigine in the treatment of bipolar depression, in the management of rapid cycling patients, as well as the maintenance phase of the treatment. This new evidence resulted on its recent approval by the FDA for the maintenance treatment of bipolar disorder in the United States. Thus, available findings suggest that this is a promising new agent that may have important role in the treatment of refractory cases of the disorder and possibly in the management of bipolar depression. A limitation in its use is the potential for induction of skin rashes (in about 10% of the cases), which can rarely be severe, such as Stevens–Johnson syndrome and toxic epidermal necrolysis. The occurrence of skin reactions may be increased by the combination of lamotrigine with valproate. No controlled data are available for topiramate in the treatment of bipolar patients, even though open studies suggested acute antimanic actions and effects in treatment-resistant bipolar patients. Due to the resulting weight loss (214), which seems to be already noticeable after only a few weeks of its therapeutic use, topiramate may be a promising new medication (215,216), as an adjunctive to first-line treatments in resistant patients, especially in those with obesity or drug-induced weight gain (198,201). However, as a monotherapy treatment for mania, its potential is limited considering that recently conducted large double-blind trials failed to document its efficacy. Nonetheless, if proven effective for the treatment of any phase of the disorder, it could have a unique role in the management of bipolar patients, where weight gain is a very common and often debilitating side effect for virtually every other available mood-stabilizing agent. Double-blind controlled studies are eagerly waited to further examine the efficacy of topiramate in bipolar disorder.

CONCLUSIONS

The available literature shows that there is good support for the efficacy of first-generation anticonvulsant agents in the treatment of bipolar patients. Valproate has become, in most places, the first choice for lithium-resistant patients, as it is easier to use, better tolerated as far as side effects, and generally safer than carbamazepine (217). Valproate or carbamazepine may be added to lithium or used as monotherapy. For refractory bipolar patients, there are also other useful anticonvulsants of second generation, like gabapentin, lamotrigine, and topiramate as possible alternatives. However, since the efficacy of these newer agents as monotherapy in the management of bipolar disorder is still under investigation, they should preferably be added to lithium or to first-generation anticonvulsants. Whereas gapapentin does not seem to have antimanic efficacy, there is robust evidence to support lamotrigine as an effective antidepressive and maintenance treatment for bipolar disorder. Topiramate could be an attractive alternative for patients who experience medication-related weight gain, a side effect that often contributes to patient's non-compliance, what makes it a particularly promising new agent; nonetheless, its efficacy has not been demonstrated in controlled studies for any phase of the illness. Last, future-controlled studies will also need to evaluate the potential prophylactic efficacy of these agents.

Thus, anticonvulsants of first and second generation have a very important role in the management of lithium-refractory bipolar and schizoaffective patients. These agents could initially be administered concurrently with lithium, to attempt to augment lithium's efficacy, and subsequently could be used alone, if patients respond to it. However, in clinical practice, monotherapy in the management of bipolar patients may not be commonly found, as a substantial proportion of these patients eventually needs a combination of pharmacological agents (218). When combination treatment is utilized, the serum levels of carbamazepine, valproate, or lithium should be carefully monitored, in order to reach the suggested therapeutic levels and avoid toxicity that would result from high medication doses.

Future research that will examine the mechanisms involved in therapeutic response in bipolar disorder will be very important. The elucidation of the mechanisms of action of anticonvulsant medications in bipolar patients is likely to contribute substantially to improve the understanding of the pathophysiology of this disorder and to guide future efforts in drug development in this field.

REFERENCES

1. Cade JFJ. Lithium salts in the treatment of psychotic excitement. Med J Aust 1949; 14:349–352.
2. Himmelhoch JM, Mulla D, Neil JF, Detre TP, Kupfer DJ. Incidence and significance of mixed affective states in a bipolar population. Arch Gen Psychiatry 1976; 33:1062–1066.
3. Maj M. The effect of lithium in bipolar disorder: a review of recent research evidence. Bipolar Disord 2003; 5:180–188.
4. Soares JC, Gershon S. The lithium ion: a foundation for psychopharmacological specificity. Neuropsychopharmacology 1998; 19:167–182.
5. Abou-Saleh MT, Coppen A. Who responds to prophylactic lithium? J Affect Disord 1986; 10:115–125.

6. Gaviria M, Flaherty J, Val E. A comparison of bipolar patients with and without a borderline personality disorder. Psychiatr J Univ Ott 1982; 7:190–195.
7. Prien RF, Potter WZ. NIMH workshop report on treatment of bipolar disorder. Psychopharmacol Bull 1990; 26:409–427.
8. Brambilla P, Barale F, Soares JC. Perspectives on the use of anticonvulsants in the treatment of bipolar disorder. Int J Neuropsychopharmacol 2001; 4:421–446.
9. Brambilla P, Soares JC. The pharmacological treatment of acute mania. In: Dunner DL, Rosenbaum J, eds. Psychiatric Clinics of North America: Annual of Drug Therapy. Vol. 8. Philadelphia, PA: W.B. Saunders Company, 2001:155–180.
10. Brambilla P, Barale F, Soares JC. Atypical antipsychotics and mood stabilization in bipolar disorder. Psychopharmacology (Berl) 2003; 166:315–332.
11. Birkhimer LJ, Curtis JL, Jann MW. Use of carbamazepine in psychiatric disorders. Clin Pharm 1985; 4:425–434.
12. Kerr BM, Thummel KE, Wurden CJ, Klein SM, Kroetz DL, Gonzalez FJ, Levy RH. Human liver carbamazepine metabolism. Role of CYP3A4 and CYP2C8 in 10,11-epoxide formation. Biochem Pharmacol 1994; 47:1969–1979.
13. Post RM, Uhde TW, Putnam FW, Ballenger JC, Berrettini WH. Kindling and carbamazepine in affective illness. J Nerv Ment Dis 1982; 170:717–731.
14. Post RM, Rubinow DR, Uhde TW. Biochemical mechanisms of action of carbamazepine in affective illness and epilepsy. Psychopharmacol Bull 1984; 20:585–589.
15. Purdy RE, Julien RM, Fairhurst AS, Terry MD. Effect of carbamazepine on the in vitro uptake and release of norepinephrine in adrenergic nerves of rabbit aorta and in whole brain synaptosomes. Epilepsia 1977; 18:251–257.
16. Avissar S, Schreiber G, Aulakh CS, Wozniak KM, Murphy DL. Carbamazepine and electroconvulsive shock attenuate beta-adrenoceptor and muscarinic cholinoceptor coupling to G proteins in rat cortex. Eur J Pharmacol 1990; 189:99–103.
17. Manji HK, Moore GJ, Chen G. Clinical and preclinical evidence for the neurotrophic effects of mood stabilizers: implications for the pathophysiology and treatment of manic-depressive illness. Biol Psychiatry 2000; 48:740–754.
18. Elphick M. An open clinical trial of carbamazepine in treatment-resistant bipolar and schizo-affective psychotics. Br J Psychiatry 1985; 147:198–200.
19. Folks DG, King LD, Dowdy SB, Petrie WM, Jack RA, Koomen JC, Swenson BR, Edwards P. Carbamazepine treatment of selected affectively disordered inpatients. Am J Psychiatry 1982; 139:115–117.
20. Kramlinger KG, Post RM. Adding lithium carbonate to carbamazepine: antimanic efficacy in treatment-resistant mania. Acta Psychiatr Scand 1989; 79:378–385.
21. Muller AA, Stoll K. Carbamazepine and oxcarbamazepine in the treatment of manic syndromes—studies in Germany. In: Emrich HM, Okuma T, Muller AA, eds. Anticonvulsants in Affective Disorders. Amsterdam: Excerpta Medica, 1984:139–147.
22. Okuma T, Kishimoto A, Inoue K, Matsumoto H, Ogura A. Anti-manic and prophylactic effects of carbamazepine (Tegretol) on manic depressive psychosis. A preliminary report. Folia Psychiatr Neurol Jpn 1973; 27:283–297.
23. Okuma T, Yamashita I, Takahashi R, Itoh H, Kurihara M, Otsuki S, Watanabe S, Sarai K, Hazama H, Inanaga K. Clinical efficacy of carbamazepine in affective, schizoaffective, and schizophrenic disorders. Pharmacopsychiatry 1989; 22:47–53.
24. Post RM, Uhde TW, Roy-Byrne PP, Joffe RT. Correlates of antimanic response to carbamazepine. Psychiatry Res 1987; 21:71–83.
25. Elphick M, Lyons F, Cowen PJ. Low tolerability of carbamazepine in psychiatric patients may restrict its clinical usefulness. J Psychopharmacol 1988; 2:1–4.
26. Jann MW, Saklad SR, Ereshefsky L. Carbamazepine for patients with affective target symptoms [letter]. Drug Intell Clin Pharm 1984; 18:81.
27. Centorrino F, Albert MJ, Berry JM, Kelleher JP, Fellman V, Line G, Koukopoulos AE, Kidwell JE, Fogarty KV, Baldessarini RJ. Oxcarbazepine: clinical experience with hospitalized psychiatric patients. Bipolar Disord 2003; 5:370–374.

28. Ghaemi SN, Berv DA, Klugman J, Rosenquist KJ, Hsu DJ. Oxcarbazepine treatment of bipolar disorder. J Clin Psychiatry 2003; 64:943–945.
29. Ballenger JC, Post RM. Carbamazepine in manic-depressive illness: a new treatment. Am J Psychiatry 1980; 137:782–790.
30. Emrich HM, Dose M, von Zerssen D. The use of sodium valproate, carbamazepine and oxcarbazepine in patients with affective disorders. J Affect Disord 1985; 8:243–250.
31. Goncalves N, Stoll KD. Carbamazepine in manic syndromes. A controlled double-blind study. Nervenarzt 1985; 56:43–47.
32. Grossi E, Sacchetti E, Vita A, Conte G, Faravelli C, Hautman G, Zerbi D, Mesina AM, Drago F, Motta A. Carbamazepine vs chloropromazine in mania: a double blind trial. In: Emrich HM, Okuma T, Muller AA, eds. Anticonvulsants in Affective Disorders. Amsterdam: Excerpta Medica, 1984:177–187.
33. Klein E, Bental E, Lerer B, Belmaker RH. Carbamazepine and haloperidol v placebo and haloperidol in excited psychoses. A controlled study. Arch Gen Psychiatry 1984; 41: 165–170.
34. Lenzi A, Lazzerini F, Grossi E, Massimetti G, Placidi GF. Use of carbamazepine in acute psychosis: a controlled study. J Int Med Res 1986; 14:78–84.
35. Lerer B, Moore N, Meyendorff E, Cho SR, Gershon S. Carbamazepine versus lithium in mania: a double-blind study. J Clin Psychiatry 1987; 48:89–93.
36. Moller HJ, Kissling W, Riehl T, Bauml J, Binz U, Wendt G. Double blind evaluation of the antimanic properties of carbamazepine as a comedication to haloperidol. Prog Neuropsychopharmacol Biol Psychiatry 1989; 13:127–136.
37. Okuma T, Inanaga K, Otsuki S, Sarai K, Takahashi R, Hazama H, Mori A, Watanabe M. Comparison of the antimanic efficacy of carbamazepine and chlorpromazine: a double-blind controlled study. Psychopharmacology 1979; 66:211–217.
38. Okuma T, Yamashita I, Takahashi R, Itoh H, Otsuki S, Watanabe S, Sarai K, Hazama H, Inanaga K. Comparison of the antimanic efficacy of carbamazepine and lithium carbonate by double-blind controlled study. Pharmacopsychiatry 1990; 23:143–150.
39. Small JG, Klapper MH, Milstein V, Kellams JJ, Miller MJ, Marhenke JD, Small IF. Carbamazepine compared with lithium in the treatment of mania. Arch Gen Psychiatry 1991; 48:915–921.
40. Small JG, Klapper MH, Marhenke JD, Milstein V, Woodham GC, Kellams JJ. Lithium combined with carbamazepine or haloperidol in the treatment of mania. Psychopharmacol Bull 1995; 31:265–272.
41. Weisler RH, Kalali AH, Ketter TA. A multicenter, randomized, double-blind, placebo-controlled trial of extended-release carbamazepine capsules as monotherapy for bipolar disorder patients with manic or mixed episodes. J Clin Psychiatry 2004; 65:478–484.
42. Sethi BB, Tiwari SC. Carbamazepine in affective disorders. In: Emrich HM, Okuma T, Muller AA, eds. Anticonvulsants in Affective Disorders. Amsterdam: Excerpta Medica, 1984:167–176.
43. Stoll KD, Bisson HE, Fischer E, et al. Carbamazepine versus haloperidol in manic syndromes—first report of a multicentric study in Germany. In: Shagas C, Josiassen RC, Bridger WH, et al., eds. Biological Psychiatry 1985. Amsterdam: Elsevier, 1986:332–334.
44. Vasudev K, Goswami U, Kohli K. Carbamazepine and valproate monotherapy: feasibility, relative safety and efficacy, and therapeutic drug monitoring in manic disorder. Psychopharmacology (Berl) 2000; 150:15–23.
45. Kowatch RA, Suppes T, Carmody TJ, Bucci JP, Hume JH, Kromelis M, Emslie GJ, Weinberg WA, Rush AJ. Effect size of lithium, divalproex sodium, and carbamazepine in children and adolescents with bipolar disorder. J Am Acad Child Adolesc Psychiatry 2000; 39:713–720.
46. Dilsaver SC, Swann SC, Chen YW, Shoaib A, Joe B, Krajewski KJ, Gruber N, Tsai Y. Treatment of bipolar depression with carbamazepine: results of an open study. Biol Psychiatry 1996; 40:935–937.

47. Ketter TA, Post RM, Parekh PI, Worthington K. Addition of monoamine oxidase inhibitors to carbamazepine: preliminary evidence of safety and antidepressant efficacy in treatment-resistant depression. J Clin Psychiatry 1995; 56:471–475.
48. Kramlinger KG, Post RM. The addition of lithium to carbamazepine. Antidepressant efficacy in treatment-resistant depression. Arch Gen Psychiatry 1989; 46:794–800.
49. Post RM, Uhde TW, Ballenger JC, Chatterji DC, Greene RF, Bunney WE Jr. Carbamazepine and its 10,11-epoxide metabolite in plasma and CSF. Relationship to antidepressant response. Arch Gen Psychiatry 1983; 40:673–676.
50. Prasad AJ. Efficacy of carbamazepine as an antidepressant in chronic resistant depressives. J Indian Med Assoc 1985; 83:235–237.
51. Roy-Byrne P, Uhde TW, Post RM, Joffe RT. Relationship of response to sleep deprivation and carbamazepine in depressed patients. Acta Psychiatr Scand 1984; 69:379–382.
52. Cullen M, Mitchell P, Brodaty H, Boyce P, Parker G, Hickie I, Wilhelm K. Carbamazepine for treatment-resistant melancholia. J Clin Psychiatry 1991; 52:472–476.
53. Nassir Ghaemi S, Ko JY, Katzow JJ. Oxcarbazepine treatment of refractory bipolar disorder: a retrospective chart review. Bipolar Disord 2002; 4:70–74.
54. Post RM, Uhde TW, Roy-Byrne PP, Joffe RT. Antidepressant effects of carbamazepine. Am J Psychiatry 1986; 143:29–34.
55. Neumann J, Seidel K, Wunderlich H-P. Comparative studies of the effect of carbamazepine and trimipramine in depression. In: Emrich HM, Okumna T, Muller AA, eds. Anticonvulsants in Affective Disorders. Amsterdam: Excerpta Medica, 1984:160–166.
56. Rybakowski JK, Suwalska A, Chlopocka-Wozniak M. Potentiation of antidepressants with lithium or carbamazepine in treatment-resistant depression. Neuropsychobiology 1999; 40:134–139.
57. Kishimoto A, Ogura C, Hazama H, Inoue K. Long-term prophylactic effects of carbamazepine in affective disorder. Br J Psychiatry 1983; 143:327–331.
58. Nolen WA. Carbamazepine, a possible adjunct or alternative to lithium in bipolar disorder. Acta Psychiatr Scand 1983; 67:218–225.
59. Post RM, Uhde TW, Ballenger JC, Squillace KM. Prophylactic efficacy of carbamazepine in manic-depressive illness. Am J Psychiatry 1983; 140:1602–1604.
60. Post RM, Leverich GS, Rosoff AS, Altshuler LL. Carbamazepine prophylaxis in refractory affective disorders: a focus on long-term follow-up. J Clin Psychopharmacol 1990; 10:318–327.
61. Shukla S, Cook BL, Miller MG. Lithium-carbamazepine versus lithium-neuroleptic prophylaxis in bipolar illness. J Affect Disord 1985; 9:219–222.
62. Stuppaeck C, Barnas C, Miller C, Schwitzer J, Fleischhacker WW. Carbamazepine in the prophylaxis of mood disorders. J Clin Psychopharmacol 1990; 10:39–42.
63. Svestka J, Nahunek K, Ceskova E, Korbicka J. Carbamazepine prophylaxis of affective psychoses (intraindividual comparison with lithium carbonate). Activ Nerv Suppl (Praha) 1985; 27:261–262.
64. Di Costanzo E, Schifano F. Lithium alone or in combination with carbamazepine for the treatment of rapid-cycling bipolar affective disorder. Acta Psychiatr Scand 1991; 83:456–459.
65. Fawcett J, Kravitz HM. The long-term management of bipolar disorders with lithium, carbamazepine, and antidepressants. J Clin Psychiatry 1985; 46:58–60.
66. Kishimoto A. The treatment of affective disorder with carbamazepine: prophylactic synergism of lithium and carbamazepine combination. Prog Neuropsychopharmacol Biol Psychiatry 1992; 16:483–493.
67. Okuma T. Effects of carbamazepine and lithium on affective disorders. Neuropsychobiology 1993; 27:138–145.
68. Bellaire W, Demisch K, Stoll K-D. Carbamazepine vs lithium. Einsatz in der prophylaxe rezidivierender affektiver und schizoaffectiver psychosen. Munch Med Wochenschr 1990; 132:82–86.

69. Cabrera JF, Muhlbauer HD, Schley J, Stoll KD, Muller-Oerlinghausen B. Long-term randomized clinical trial on oxcarbamazepine vs lithium in bipolar and schizoaffective disorders: preliminary reports. Pharmacopsychiatry 1986; 19:282–283.
70. Simhandl C, Denk E, Thau K. The comparative efficacy of carbamazepine low and high serum level and lithium carbonate in the prophylaxis of affective disorders. J Affect Disord 1993; 28:221–231.
71. Okuma T, Inanaga K, Otsuki S, Sarai K, Takahashi R, Hazama H, Mori A, Watanabe S. A preliminary double-blind study on the efficacy of carbamazepine in prophylaxis of manic-depressive illness. Psychopharmacology 1981; 73:95–96.
72. Placidi GF, Lenzi A, Lazzerini F, Cassano GB, Akiskal HS. The comparative efficacy and safety of carbamazepine versus lithium: a randomized, double-blind 3-year trial in 83 patients. J Clin Psychiatry 1986; 47:490–494.
73. Watkins SE, Callender K, Thomas DR, Tidmarsh SF, Shaw DM. The effect of carbamazepine and lithium on remission from affective illness. Br J Psychiatry 1987; 150:180–182.
74. Lusznat RM, Murphy DP, Nunn CM. Carbamazepine vs lithium in the treatment and prophylaxis of mania. Br J Psychiatry 1988; 153:198–204.
75. Coxhead N, Silverstone T, Cookson J. Carbamazepine versus lithium in the prophylaxis of bipolar affective disorder. Acta Psychiatr Scand 1992; 85:114–118.
76. Denicoff KD, Smith-Jackson EE, Disney ER, Ali SO, Leverich GS, Post RM. Comparative prophylactic efficacy of lithium, carbamazepine, and the combination in bipolar disorder. J Clin Psychiatry 1997; 58:470–478.
77. Hartong EG, Moleman P, Hoogduin CA, Broekman TG, Nolen WA. Prophylactic efficacy of lithium versus carbamazepine in treatment-naive bipolar patients. J Clin Psychiatry 2003; 64:144–151.
78. Greil W, Kleindienst N, Erazo N, Muller-Oerlinghausen B. Differential response to lithium and carbamazepine in the prophylaxis of bipolar disorder. J Clin Psychopharmacol 1998; 18:455–460.
79. Greil W, Kleindienst N. Lithium versus carbamazepine in the maintenance treatment of bipolar II disorder and bipolar disorder not otherwise specified. Int Clin Psychopharmacol 1999; 14:283–285.
80. Greil W, Kleindienst N. The comparative prophylactic efficacy of lithium and carbamazepine in patients with bipolar I disorder. Int Clin Psychopharmacol 1999; 14:277–281.
81. Kleindienst N, Greil W. Inter-episodic morbidity and drop-out under carbamazepine and lithium in the maintenance treatment of bipolar disorder. Psychol Med 2002; 32:493–501.
82. Zaccara G, Messori A, Moroni F. Clinical pharmacokinetics of valproic acid—1988. Clin Pharmacokinet 1988; 15:367–389.
83. Soares JC. Valproate treatment and the risk of hyperandrogenism and polycystic ovaries. Bipolar Disord 2000; 2:37–41.
84. Ueda Y, Willmore LJ. Molecular regulation of glutamate and GABA transporter proteins by valproic acid in rat hippocampus during epileptogenesis. Exp Brain Res 2000; 133:334–339.
85. Brambilla P, Perez J, Barale F, Schettini G, Soares JC. GABAergic dysfunction in mood disorders. Mol Psychiatry 2003; 8:721–737, 715.
86. McElroy SL, Keck PE Jr, Pope HG Jr, Hudson JI. Valproate in psychiatric disorders: literature review and clinical guidelines. J Clin Psychiatry 1989; 50(suppl):23–29.
87. Shiah IS, Yatham LN, Lam RW, Zis AP. Effects of divalproex sodium on 5-HT1A receptor function in healthy human males: hypothermic, hormonal, and behavioral responses to ipsapirone. Neuropsychopharmacology 1997; 17:382–390.
88. Hahn CG, Friedman E. Abnormalities in protein kinase C signaling and the pathophysiology of bipolar disorder. Bipolar Disord 1999; 2:81–86.
89. Chang MC, Contreras MA, Rosenberger TA, Rintala JJ, Bell JM, Rapoport SI. Chronic valproate treatment decreases the in vivo turnover of arachidonic acid in brain

phospholipids: a possible common effect of mood stabilizers. J Neurochem 2001; 77: 796–803.
90. Chen B, Wang JF, Young LT. Chronic valproate treatment increases expression of endoplasmic reticulum stress proteins in the rat cerebral cortex and hippocampus. Biol Psychiatry 2000; 48:658–664.
91. Bown CD, Wang JF, Young LT. Increased expression of endoplasmic reticulum stress proteins following chronic valproate treatment of rat C6 glioma cells. Neuropharmacology 2000; 39:2162–2169.
92. Sassi RB, Soares JC. Emerging therapeutic targets in bipolar mood disorder. Expert Opin Ther Targets 2001; 5:587–599.
93. Brady KT, Sonne SC, Anton R, Ballenger JC. Valproate in the treatment of acute bipolar affective episodes complicated by substance abuse: a pilot study. J Clin Psychiatry 1995; 56:118–121.
94. Brown R. U.S. experience with valproate in manic depressive illness: a multicenter trial. J Clin Psychiatry 1989; 50(suppl):13–16.
95. Guscott R. Clinical experience with valproic acid in 22 patients with refractory bipolar mood disorder [letter]. Can J Psychiatry 1992; 37:590.
96. McFarland BH, Miller MR, Straumfjord AA. Valproate use in the older manic patient. J Clin Psychiatry 1990; 51:479–481.
97. Papatheodorou G, Kutcher SP, Katic M, Szalai JP. The efficacy and safety of divalproex sodium in the treatment of acute mania in adolescents and young adults: an open clinical trial. J Clin Psychopharmacol 1995; 15:110–116.
98. Prasad AJ. The role of sodium valproate as an anti-manic agent. Pharmatherapeutica 1984; 4:6–8.
99. Sharma V, Persad E, Mazmanian D, Karunaratne K. Treatment of rapid cycling bipolar disorder with combination therapy of valproate and lithium. Can J Psychiatry 1993; 38:137–139.
100. Fogelson DL, Jacobson S, Sternbach H. A retrospective study of valproate in private psychiatric practice. Ann Clin Psychiatry 1991; 3:315–320.
101. McElroy SL, Keck PE Jr, Pope HG Jr. Sodium valproate: its use in primary psychiatric disorders. J Clin Psychopharmacol 1987; 7:16–24.
102. Stoll AL, Banov M, Kolbrener M, Mayer PV, Tohen M, Strakowski SM, Castillo J, Suppes T, Cohen BM. Neurologic factors predict a favorable valproate response in bipolar and schizoaffective disorders. J Clin Psychopharmacol 1994; 14:311–313.
103. Tohen M, Castillo J, Pope HG Jr, Herbstein J. Concomitant use of valproate and carbamazepine in bipolar and schizoaffective disorders. J Clin Psychopharmacol 1994; 14:67–70.
104. Papatheodorou G, Kutcher SP. Divalproex sodium treatment in late adolescent and young adult acute mania. Psychopharmacol Bull 1993; 29:213–219.
105. Brennan MJW, Sandyk E, Borsook D. Use of sodium valproate in the management of affective disorders: basic and clinical aspects. In: Emrich HM, Okumna T, Muller AA, eds. Anticonvulsants in Affective Disorders. Vol. 56–65. Amsterdam: Excerpta Medica, 1984.
106. Pope HG Jr, McElroy SL, Keck PE Jr, Hudson JI. Valproate in the treatment of acute mania. A placebo-controlled study. Arch Gen Psychiatry 1991; 48:62–68.
107. Freeman TW, Clothier JL, Pazzaglia P, Lesem MD, Swann AC. A double-blind comparison of valproate and lithium in the treatment of acute mania. Am J Psychiatry 1992; 149:108–111.
108. Bowden CL, Brugger AM, Swann AC, Calabrese JR, Janicak PG, Petty F, Dilsaver SC, Davis JM, Rush AJ, Small JG, et al. Efficacy of divalproex vs lithium and placebo in the treatment of mania. The Depakote Mania Study Group. JAMA 1994; 271:918–924.
109. McElroy SL, Keck PE, Stanton SP, Tugrul KC, Bennett JA, Strakowski SM. A randomized comparison of divalproex oral loading versus haloperidol in the initial treatment of acute psychotic mania. J Clin Psychiatry 1996; 57:142–146.

110. Muller-Oerlinghausen B, Retzow A, Henn FA, Giedke H, Walden J. Valproate as an adjunct to neuroleptic medication for the treatment of acute episodes of mania: a prospective, randomized, double-blind, placebo-controlled, multicenter study. European Valproate Mania Study Group. J Clin Psychopharmacol 2000; 20:195–203.
111. Zajecka JM, Weisler R, Sachs G, Swann AC, Wozniak P, Sommerville KW. A comparison of the efficacy, safety, and tolerability of divalproex sodium and olanzapine in the treatment of bipolar disorder. J Clin Psychiatry 2002; 63:1148–1155.
112. Young LT, Joffe RT, Robb JC, MacQueen GM, Marriott M, Patelis-Siotis I. Double-blind comparison of addition of a second mood stabilizer versus an antidepressant to an initial mood stabilizer for treatment of patients with bipolar depression. Am J Psychiatry 2000; 157:124–126.
113. Keck PE Jr, McElroy SL, Tugrul KC, Bennett JA. Valproate oral loading in the treatment of acute mania. J Clin Psychiatry 1993; 54:305–308.
114. Grunze H, Erfurth A, Amann B, Giupponi G, Kammerer C, Walden J. Intravenous valproate loading in acutely manic and depressed bipolar I patients. J Clin Psychopharmacol 1999; 19:303–309.
115. Frankenburg FR, Zanarini MC. Divalproex sodium treatment of women with borderline personality disorder and bipolar II disorder: a double-blind placebo-controlled pilot study. J Clin Psychiatry 2002; 63:442–446.
116. Winsberg ME, DeGolia SG, Strong CM, Ketter TA. Divalproex therapy in medication-naive and mood-stabilizer-naive bipolar II depression. J Affect Disord 2001; 67: 207–212.
117. Davis LL, Kabel D, Patel D, Choate AD, Foslien-Nash C, Gurguis GN, Kramer GL, Petty F. Valproate as an antidepressant in major depressive disorder. Psychopharmacol Bull 1996; 32:647–652.
118. Calabrese JR, Woyshville MJ, Kimmel SE, Rapport DJ. Predictors of valproate response in bipolar rapid cycling. J Clin Psychopharmacol 1993; 13:280–283.
119. Denicoff KD, Smith-Jackson EE, Bryan AL, Ali SO, Post RM. Valproate prophylaxis in a prospective clinical trial of refractory bipolar disorder. Am J Psychiatry 1997; 154:1456–1458.
120. Jacobsen FM. Low-dose valproate: a new treatment for cyclothymia, mild rapid cycling disorders, and premenstrual syndrome. J Clin Psychiatry 1993; 54:229–234.
121. Puzynski S, Klosiewicz L. Valproic acid amide in the treatment of affective and schizoaffective disorders. J Affect Disord 1984; 6:115–121.
122. Semademi GW. Etude clinique de l'effect normothymique du dipropylacetamide. Acta Psychiatrica Belgica 1976; 76:458–466.
123. Hayes SG. Long-term use of valproate in primary psychiatric disorders. J Clin Psychiatry 1989; 50(suppl):35–39.
124. Lambert PA. Acute and prophylactic therapies of patients with affective disorders using valpromide (dipropylacetamide). In: Emrich HM, Okumna T, Muller AA, eds. Anticonvulsants in Affective Disorders. Amsterdam: Excerpta Medica, 1984.
125. Niedermier JA, Nasrallah HA. Clinical correlates of response to valproate in geriatric inpatients. Ann Clin Psychiatry 1998; 10:165–168.
126. Schaff MR, Fawcett J, Zajecka JM. Divalproex sodium in the treatment of refractory affective disorders. J Clin Psychiatry 1993; 54:380–384.
127. Bowden CL, Calabrese JR, McElroy SL, Gyulai L, Wassef A, Petty F, Pope HG Jr, Chou JC, Keck PE Jr, Rhodes LJ, Swann AC, Hirschfeld RM, Wozniak PJ. A randomized, placebo-controlled 12-month trial of divalproex and lithium in treatment of outpatients with bipolar I disorder. Divalproex Maintenance Study Group. Arch Gen Psychiatry 2000; 57:481–489.
128. Solomon DA, Ryan CE, Keitner GI, Miller IW, Shea MT, Kazim A, Keller MB. A pilot study of lithium carbonate plus divalproex sodium for the continuation and maintenance treatment of patients with bipolar I disorder. J Clin Psychiatry 1997; 58:95–99.

129. Ghaemi SN, Goodwin FK. Long-term naturalistic treatment of depressive symptoms in bipolar illness with divalproex vs. lithium in the setting of minimal antidepressant use. J Affect Disord 2001; 65:281–287.
130. Emilien G, Maloteaux JM, Seghers A, Charles G. Lithium therapy in the treatment of manic-depressive illness. Present status and future perspectives. A critical review. Arch Int Pharmacodyn Ther 1995; 330:251–278.
131. Czuczwar SJ. GABA-ergic system and antiepileptic drugs. Neurol Neurochir Pol 2000; 33:13–20.
132. Taylor CP. Emerging perspectives on the mechanism of action of gabapentin. Neurology 1994; 44:S10–S16; discussion S31–S32.
133. Dooley DJ, Mieske CA, Borosky SA. Inhibition of K(+)-evoked glutamate release from rat neocortical and hippocampal slices by gabapentin. Neurosci Lett 2000; 280:107–110.
134. Fink K, Meder W, Dooley DJ, Gothert M. Inhibition of neuronal Ca(2+) influx by gabapentin and subsequent reduction of neurotransmitter release from rat neocortical slices. Br J Pharmacol 2000; 130:900–906.
135. Gee NS, Brown JP, Dissanayake VU, Offord J, Thurlow R, Woodruff GN. The novel anticonvulsant drug, gabapentin (Neurontin), binds to the alpha2delta subunit of a calcium channel. J Biol Chem 1996; 271:5768–5776.
136. Altshuler LL, Keck PEJ, McElroy SL, Suppes T, Brown ES, Denicoff K, Frye M, Gitlin M, Hwang S, Goodman R, Leverich G, Nolen W, Kupka R, Post R. Gabapentin in the acute treatment of refractory bipolar disorder. Bipolar Disord 1999; 1:61–65.
137. Cabras PL, Hardoy MJ, Hardoy MC, Carta MG. Clinical experience with gabapentin in patients with bipolar or schizoaffective disorder: results of an open-label study. J Clin Psychiatry 1999; 60:245–248.
138. Erfurth A, Kammerer C, Grunze H, Normann C, Walden J. An open label study of gabapentin in the treatment of acute mania. J Psychiatr Res 1998; 32:261–264.
139. Hardoy MJ, Hardoy MC, Carta MG, et al. Gabapentin in the treatment of bipolar disorders. Bipolar Disord 1999; 1:34.
140. Knoll J, Stegman K, Suppes T. Clinical experience using gabapentin adjunctively in patients with a history of mania or hypomania. J Affect Disord 1998; 49:229–233.
141. McElroy SL, Soutullo CA, Keck PE Jr, Kmetz GF. A pilot trial of adjunctive gabapentin in the treatment of bipolar disorder. Ann Clin Psychiatry 1997; 9:99–103.
142. Perugi G, Toni C, Ruffolo G, Sartini S, Simonini E, Akiskal H. Clinical experience using adjunctive gabapentin in treatment-resistant bipolar mixed states. Pharmacopsychiatry 1999; 32:136–141.
143. Schaffer CB, Schaffer LC. Gabapentin in the treatment of bipolar disorder [letter]. Am J Psychiatry 1997; 154:291–292.
144. Sokolski KN, Green C, Maris DE, DeMet EM. Gabapentin as an adjunct to standard mood stabilizers in outpatients with mixed bipolar symptomatology. Ann Clin Psychiatry 1999; 11:217–222.
145. Ghaemi SN, Katzow JJ, Desai SP, Goodwin FK. Gabapentin treatment of mood disorders: a preliminary study. J Clin Psychiatry 1998; 59:426–429.
146. Ryback RS, Brodsky L, Munasifi F. Gabapentin in bipolar disorder [letter]. J Neuropsychiatry Clin Neurosci 1997; 9:301.
147. Vieta E, Martinez-Aran A, Nieto E, Colom F, Reinares M, Benabarre A, Gasto C. Adjunctive gabapentin treatment of bipolar disorder. Eur Psychiatry 2000; 15:433–437.
148. Obrocea GV, Dunn RM, Frye MA, Ketter TA, Luckenbaugh DA, Leverich GS, Speer AM, Osuch EA, Jajodia K, Post RM. Clinical predictors of response to lamotrigine and gabapentin monotherapy in refractory affective disorders. Biol Psychiatry 2002; 51: 253–260.
149. Pande AC, Crockatt JC, Janney CA, Werth JL, Tsaroucha G. Gabapentin in bipolar disorder: a placebo-controlled trial of adjunctive therapy. Bipolar Disord 2000; 2: 249–255.

150. Young LT, Robb JC, Hasey GM, MacQueen GM, Patelis Siotis I, Marriott M, Joffe RT. Gabapentin as an adjunctive treatment in bipolar disorder. J Affect Disord 1999; 55: 73–77.
151. Cohen AF, Land GS, Breimer DD, Yuen WC, Winton C, Peck AW. Lamotrigine, a new anticonvulsant: pharmacokinetics in normal humans. Clin Pharmacol Ther 1987; 42:535–541.
152. Guberman AH, Besag FM, Brodie MJ, Dooley JM, Duchowny MS, Pellock JM, Richens A, Stern RS, Trevathan E. Lamotrigine-associated rash: risk/benefit considerations in adults and children. Epilepsia 1999; 40:985–991.
153. Afanas'ev I, Kudrin V, Rayevsky KS, Varga V, Saransaari P, Oja SS. Lamotrigine and carbamazepine affect differently the release of D-[3H]aspartate from mouse cerebral cortex slices: involvement of NO. Neurochem Res 1999; 24:1153–1159.
154. Leach MJ, Marden CM, Miller AA. Pharmacological studies on lamotrigine, a novel potential antiepileptic drug: II. Neurochemical studies on the mechanism of action. Epilepsia 1986; 27:490–497.
155. Xie X, Hagan RM. Cellular and molecular actions of lamotrigine: possible mechanisms of efficacy in bipolar disorder. Neuropsychobiology 1998; 38:119–130.
156. Cunningham MO, Jones RS. The anticonvulsant, lamotrigine decreases spontaneous glutamate release but increases spontaneous GABA release in the rat entorhinal cortex in vitro. Neuropharmacology 2000; 39:2139–2146.
157. Vinod KY, Subhash MN. Lamotrigine induced selective changes in 5-HT(1A) receptor mediated response in rat brain. Neurochem Int 2002; 40:315–319.
158. Fogelson DL, Sternbach H. Lamotrigine treatment of refractory bipolar disorder. J Clin Psychiatry 1997; 58:271–273.
159. Hoopes S. Lamotrigine in the treatment of bipolar depression and affective disorders: clinical experience in 218 patients [abstr]. Bipolar Disord 1999; 1:35.
160. Kusumakar V, Yatham LN. Lamotrigine treatment of rapid cycling bipolar disorder. Am J Psychiatry 1997; 154:1171–1172.
161. Lafer B, Tamada RS, Issler CK, Amaral JAMS, Moreno RA. Lamotrigine in treatment-refractory bipolar disorder. A Brazilian experience [abstr]. Bipolar Disord 1999; 1:39.
162. Sporn J, Sachs G. The anticonvulsant lamotrigine in treatment-resistant manic-depressive illness. J Clin Psychopharmacol 1997; 17:185–189.
163. Bowden CL, Calabrese JR, McElroy SL, Rhodes LJ, Keck PE Jr, Cookson J, Anderson J, Bolden-Watson C, Ascher J, Monaghan E, Zhou J. The efficacy of lamotrigine in rapid cycling and non-rapid cycling patients with bipolar disorder. Biol Psychiatry 1999; 45:953–958.
164. Calabrese JR, Fatemi SH, Woyshville MJ. Antidepressant effects of lamotrigine in rapid cycling bipolar disorder. Am J Psychiatry 1996; 153:1236.
165. Calabrese JR, Bowden CL, McElroy SL, Cookson J, Andersen J, Keck PE Jr, Rhodes L, Bolden-Watson C, Zhou J, Ascher JA. Spectrum of activity of lamotrigine in treatment-refractory bipolar disorder. Am J Psychiatry 1999; 156:1019–1023.
166. Brown ES, Nejtek VA, Perantie DC, Orsulak PJ, Bobadilla L. Lamotrigine in patients with bipolar disorder and cocaine dependence. J Clin Psychiatry 2003; 64:197–201.
167. Berk M. Lamotrigine and the treatment of mania in bipolar disorder. Eur Neuropsychopharmacol 1999; 9:119–123.
168. Anand A, Oren DA, Berman RM, et al. Lamotrigine treatment of lithium failure outpatient mania. A double blind placebo controlled trial. Bipolar Disord 1999; 1:23.
169. Calabrese JR, Bowden CL, Sachs GS, Ascher JA, Monaghan E, Rudd GD. A double-blind placebo-controlled study of lamotrigine monotherapy in outpatients with bipolar I depression. Lamictal 602 Study Group. J Clin Psychiatry 1999; 60:79–88.
170. Laurenza A, Asnis G, Beaman M, Hudson J, Khan A, Londborg P, Monaghan E, Rudd D. A double blind, placebo controlled study supporting the efficacy of lamotrigine (lamictal) in unipolar depression [abstr]. Bipolar Disord 1999; 1:39–40.

171. Calabrese JR, Suppes T, Bowden CL, Sachs GS, Swann AC, McElroy SL, Kusumakar V, Ascher JA, Earl NL, Greene PL, Monaghan ET. A double-blind, placebo-controlled, prophylaxis study of lamotrigine in rapid-cycling bipolar disorder. Lamictal 614 Study Group [in process citation]. J Clin Psychiatry 2000; 61:841–850.
172. Walden J, Schaerer L, Schloesser S, Grunze H. An open longitudinal study of patients with bipolar rapid cycling treated with lithium or lamotrigine for mood stabilization. Bipolar Disord 2000; 2:336–339.
173. Bowden CL, Calabrese JR, Sachs G, Yatham LN, Asghar SA, Hompland M, Montgomery P, Earl N, Smoot TM, DeVeaugh-Geiss J. A placebo-controlled 18-month trial of lamotrigine and lithium maintenance treatment in recently manic or hypomanic patients with bipolar I disorder. Arch Gen Psychiatry 2003; 60:392–400.
174. Calabrese JR, Bowden CL, Sachs G, Yatham LN, Behnke K, Mehtonen OP, Montgomery P, Ascher J, Paska W, Earl N, DeVeaugh-Geiss J. A placebo-controlled 18-month trial of lamotrigine and lithium maintenance treatment in recently depressed patients with bipolar I disorder. J Clin Psychiatry 2003; 64:1013–1024.
175. Kusumakar V, Yatham LN. An open study of lamotrigine in refractory bipolar depression. Psychiatry Res 1997; 72:145–148.
176. Bryant-Comstock L, Chang CN, Phillips S. Quality of life improvement in bipolar depressed patients treated with lamotrigine [abstr]. Bipolar Disord 1999; 1:25–26.
177. Fatemi SH, Rapport DJ, Calabrese JR, Thuras P. Lamotrigine in rapid-cycling bipolar disorder. J Clin Psychiatry 1997; 58:522–527.
178. Suppes T, Brown ES, McElroy SL, Keck PE Jr, Nolen W, Kupka R, Frye M, Denicoff KD, Altshuler L, Leverich GS, Post RM. Lamotrigine for the treatment of bipolar disorder: a clinical case series. J Affect Disord 1999; 53:95–98.
179. McElroy SL, Zarate CA, Cookson J, Suppes T, Huffman RF, Greene P, Ascher J. A 52-week, open-label continuation study of lamotrigine in the treatment of bipolar depression. J Clin Psychiatry 2004; 65:204–210.
180. Doose DR, Walker SA, Gisclon LG, Nayak RK. Single-dose pharmacokinetics and effect of food on the bioavailability of topiramate, a novel antiepileptic drug. J Clin Pharmacol 1996; 36:884–891.
181. Rosenfeld WE. Topiramate: a review of preclinical, pharmacokinetic, and clinical data. Clin Ther 1997; 19:1294–1308; discussion 1523–1524.
182. Wauquier A, Zhou S. Topiramate: a potent anticonvulsant in the amygdala-kindled rat. Epilepsy Res 1996; 24:73–77.
183. Kuzniecky R, Hetherington H, Ho S, Pan J, Martin R, Gilliam F, Hugg J, Faught E. Topiramate increases cerebral GABA in healthy humans. Neurology 1998; 51:627–629.
184. Gordey M, DeLorey TM, Olsen RW. Differential sensitivity of recombinant GABA(A) receptors expressed in *Xenopus oocytes* to modulation by topiramate. Epilepsia 2000; 41: S25–S19.
185. White HS, Brown SD, Woodhead JH, Skeen GA, Wolf HH. Topiramate modulates GABA-evoked currents in murine cortical neurons by a nonbenzodiazepine mechanism. Epilepsia 2000; 41:S17–S20.
186. Gibbs JW III, Sombati S, DeLorenzo RJ, Coulter DA. Cellular actions of topiramate: blockade of kainate-evoked inward currents in cultured hippocampal neurons. Epilepsia 2000; 41:S10–S16.
187. Hanaya R, Sasa M, Ujihara H, Ishihara K, Serikawa T, Iida K, Akimitsu T, Arita K, Kurisu K. Suppression by topiramate of epileptiform burst discharges in hippocampal CA3 neurons of spontaneously epileptic rat in vitro. Brain Res 1998; 789:274–282.
188. Zhang X, Velumian AA, Jones OT, Carlen PL. Modulation of high-voltage-activated calcium channels in dentate granule cells by topiramate. Epilepsia 2000; 41:S52–S60.
189. Dodgson SJ, Shank RP, Maryanoff BE. Topiramate as an inhibitor of carbonic anhydrase isoenzymes. Epilepsia 2000; 41:S35–S39.

190. Chengappa KNR, Rathore D, Levine J, Atzert R, Solai L, Parepally H, Levin H, Moffa N, Delaney J, Brar JS. Topiramate as add-on treatment for patients with bipolar mania. Bipolar Disord 1999; 1:42–53.
191. Kusumakar V, Yatham LN, O'Donovan C, Kutcher SP. Topiramate augmentation in women with refractory rapid cycling bipolar disorder and significant weight gain from previous treatment. Bipolar Disord 1999; 1:38–39.
192. McElroy SL, Suppes T, Keck PE, Frye MA, Denicoff KD, Altshuler LL, Brown ES, Nolen WA, Kupka RW, Rochussen J, Leverich GS, Post RM. Open-label adjunctive topiramate in the treatment of bipolar disorders. Biol Psychiatry 2000; 47:1025–1033.
193. van Kammen DP, Calabrese JR, Shelton MD, et al. Topiramate in severe treatment refractory mania. Bipolar Disord 1999; 1:56.
194. Calabrese JR, Keck PE Jr, McElroy SL, Shelton MD. A pilot study of topiramate as monotherapy in the treatment of acute mania. J Clin Psychopharmacol 2001; 21: 340–342.
195. Grunze HC, Normann C, Langosch J, Schaefer M, Amann B, Sterr A, Schloesser S, Kleindienst N, Walden J. Antimanic efficacy of topiramate in 11 patients in an open trial with an on–off–on design. J Clin Psychiatry 2001; 62:464–468.
196. Bozikas VP, Petrikis P, Kourtis A, Youlis P, Karavatos A. Treatment of acute mania with topiramate in hospitalized patients. Prog Neuropsychopharmacol Biol Psychiatry 2002; 26:1203–1206.
197. Guille C, Sachs G. Clinical outcome of adjunctive topiramate treatment in a sample of refractory bipolar patients with comorbid conditions. Prog Neuropsychopharmacol Biol Psychiatry 2002; 26:1035–1039.
198. Vieta E, Sanchez-Moreno J, Goikolea JM, Torrent C, Benabarre A, Colom F, Martinez-Aran A, Reinares M, Comes M, Corbella B. Adjunctive topiramate in bipolar II disorder. World J Biol Psychiatry 2003; 4:172–176.
199. McIntyre RS, Mancini DA, McCann S, Srinivasan J, Sagman D, Kennedy SH. Topiramate versus bupropion SR when added to mood stabilizer therapy for the depressive phase of bipolar disorder: a preliminary single-blind study. Bipolar Disord 2002; 4: 207–213.
200. Vieta E, Torrent C, Garcia-Ribas G, Gilabert A, Garcia-Pares G, Rodriguez A, Cadevall J, Garcia-Castrillon J, Lusilla P, Arrufat F. Use of topiramate in treatment-resistant bipolar spectrum disorders. J Clin Psychopharmacol 2002; 22:431–435.
201. Vieta E, Goikolea JM, Olivares JM, Gonzalez-Pinto A, Rodriguez A, Colom F, Comes M, Torrent C, Sanchez-Moreno J. 1-year follow-up of patients treated with risperidone and topiramate for a manic episode. J Clin Psychiatry 2003; 64:834–839.
202. Vieta E, Sanchez-Moreno J, Goikolea JM, Colom F, Martinez-Aran A, Benabarre A, Corbella B, Torrent C, Comes M, Reinares M, Brugue E. Effects on weight and outcome of long-term olanzapine-topiramate combination treatment in bipolar disorder. J Clin Psychopharmacol 2004; 24:374–378.
203. Marcotte D. Use of topiramate, a new anti-epileptic as a mood stabilizer. J Affect Disord 1998; 50:245–251.
204. Gordon A, Price LH. Mood stabilization and weight loss with topiramate. Am J Psychiatry 1999; 156:968–969.
205. Kaufman KR. Adjunctive tiagabine treatment of psychiatric disorders: three cases. Ann Clin Psychiatry 1998; 10:181–184.
206. Schaffer LC, Schaffer CB. Tiagabine and the treatment of refractory bipolar disorder [letter]. Am J Psychiatry 1999; 156:2014–2015.
207. Schaffer LC, Schaffer CB, Howe J. An open case series on the utility of tiagabine as an augmentation in refractory bipolar outpatients. J Affect Disord 2002; 71:259–263.
208. Grunze H, Erfurth A, Marcuse A, Amann B, Normann C, Walden J. Tiagabine appears not to be efficacious in the treatment of acute mania. J Clin Psychiatry 1999; 60: 759–762.

209. Suppes T, Chisholm KA, Dhavale D, Frye MA, Altshuler LL, McElroy SL, Keck PE, Nolen WA, Kupka R, Denicoff KD, Leverich GS, Rush AJ, Post RM. Tiagabine in treatment refractory bipolar disorder: a clinical case series. Bipolar Disord 2002; 4:283–289.
210. Mishory A, Yaroslavsky Y, Bersudsky Y, Belmaker RH. Phenytoin as an antimanic anticonvulsant: a controlled study. Am J Psychiatry 2000; 157:463–465.
211. Hayes SG. Barbiturate anticonvulsants in refractory affective disorders. Ann Clin Psychiatry 1993; 5:35–44.
212. Schaffer LC, Schaffer CB, Caretto J. The use of primidone in the treatment of refractory bipolar disorder. Ann Clin Psychiatry 1999; 11:61–66.
213. Kanba S, Yagi G, Kamijima K, Suzuki T, Tajima O, Otaki J, Arata E, Koshikawa H, Nibuya M, Kinoshita N, et al. The first open study of zonisamide, a novel anticonvulsant, shows efficacy in mania. Prog Neuropsychopharmacol Biol Psychiatry 1994; 18:707–715.
214. Bray GA, Hollander P, Klein S, Kushner R, Levy B, Fitchet M, Perry BH. A 6-month randomized, placebo-controlled, dose-ranging trial of topiramate for weight loss in obesity. Obes Res 2003; 11:722–733.
215. Gupta S, Masand PS, Frank B, Turner KL, Keller P. Topiramate in bipolar and schizoaffective disorder: mood stabilizing properties in treatment refractory patients [abstr]. Int J Neuropsychopharmacol 2000; 3(S1):334.
216. Carpenter LL, Leon Z, Yasmin S, Price LH. Do obese depressed patients respond to topiramate? A retrospective chart review. J Affect Disord 2002; 69:251–255.
217. Richens A, Davidson DL, Cartlidge NE, Easter DJ. A multicentre comparative trial of sodium valproate and carbamazepine in adult onset epilepsy. Adult EPITEG Collaborative Group. J Neurol Neurosurg Psychiatry 1994; 57:682–687.
218. Levine J, Chengappa R, Brar JS, et al. Psychotropic drug prescription patterns among patients with bipolar I disorder. Bipolar Disord 2000; 2:120–130.

20
Atypical Antipsychotics in Bipolar Disorder

Siegfried Kasper
Department of General Psychiatry, Medical University of Vienna, Wien, Austria

INTRODUCTION

In Europe, the first so-called atypical antipsychotic, clozapine, was studied as early as the years 1961 and 1962 at the universities of Bern/Switzerland as well as Vienna/Austria in chronic schizophrenia (1), and the first beneficial effects of clozapine (double-blind study in comparison to levomepromazin) in mania and acute schizophrenia were published by Angst et al. (2) in 1971. Thereafter, clozapine was mainly used in acute schizophrenia, and it was not until the mid-1990s that atypical antipsychotics were studied systematically for treatment of bipolar disorder (3). There were a few early case reports about risperidone in the beginning 1990s, which even suggested that risperidone causes manic switches in specifically vulnerable patients (4), a finding which was opposed soon thereafter by observations obtained in larger sample sizes (5).

The rationale to use atypical antipsychotics in affective disorders stems from the pharmacodynamic profile of these compounds, which is mainly focused on antidopaminergic and 5-HT2 blocking properties. Although this mechanism is the major mechanism of action, and for ease of understanding also called DSA (dopamine serotonin antagonism), there are a number of other pharmacodynamic properties also involved in the mechanism of action of atypical antipsychotics. The different pharmacodynamic properties of these compounds and their respective side-effect profiles are outlined in Table 1.

The term atypical antipsychotic was first introduced in the 1970s when it became evident from animal as well as patient studies that clozapine did not exhibit the extrapyramidal symptomatology seen with, for instance, haloperidol. Later, with the introduction of the newer atypical antipsychotics such as olanzapine, quetiapine, risperidone, sertindole, ziprasidone, and zotepine, it emerged that these compounds, in comparison with typical neuroleptics, do not only have a reduced or even non-existing extrapyramidal symptom profile but are, additionally to their antipsychotic properties, also effective for negative, affective, and cognitive symptoms in schizophrenia (6).

Table 1 Pharmacodynamics and Side Effects of Atypical Antipsychotics

	Receptor binding						Side effects			
Drug name	D1	D2	5-HT2A	α-1	Ach	Hist	EPS	Prolactin	Weight gain	Sedation
Haloperidol	–	+++	+	+	–	–	+++	+++	+	+
Amisulpride	(+)	+++	–	–	–	–	+(+)	+++	+	+
Aripiprazole	N/A	++	++	+	–	(+)	+(–)	–	+	+
Clozapine	++	+(+)	+++	++	+++	++	–	–	+++	+++
Olanzapine	+	++	+++	+(+)	++	++	+	+	+++	++
Quetiapine	+	+	+++	++	–	++	–	–	+(+)	++
Risperidone	+	++	+++	+	–	(+)	+(+)	++	+(+)	+
Ziprasidone	+	++	+++	+(+)	–	(+)	+	+	+	+

+++, Very high/severe; ++, moderate; +, weak/mild; –,none.
Abbreviations: Ach, acetylcholine; Hist, histamine; N/A, not available.

TREATMENT OF MANIA

Lithium and divalproex have been considered the first-line treatment for acute mania in a number of treatment recommendations (7–10). However, in clinical practice, specifically in Europe, it was apparent that typical neuroleptics like haloperidol or zuclopenthixol are used to a larger extent, specifically as these compounds can also be administered intravenously or in a depot formulation (11,12). Owing to the depressiogenic effect of typical neuroleptics and the availability of atypical antipsychotics, which overcome these problems, there was a rapid change in clinical practice towards the usage of the newer compounds. In non-compliant manic patients, the intravenously applicable haloperidol and the depot formulation of zuclopenthixol have, however, still a role for antimanic treatment.

Monotherapy with Antipsychotics

The available studies of controlled monotherapy trials for atypical antipsychotics are presented in Table 2.

In the development program of *olanzapine*, researchers reported two similarly designed studies of a 3- versus 4-week duration (13,14). In both studies, there was a highly significant difference between olanzapine and placebo. A 50% reduction in the Young Mania Rating Scale (YMRS) was apparent in 49% for olanzapin and 24% for placebo-treated patients in the first study. In the second study, the response and remission rates with olanzapine were 65% and 61%, respectively, compared with 42% and 36% with placebo. The mean dosage used in these studies was 15 mg. The statistically significant difference between placebo and olanzapine emerged after only 1 week of treatment and continued during the 3- and 4-week trial. The sub-classification of patients according to their clinical presentation as rapid versus non-rapid cycling, pure mania versus mixed states, and psychotic versus non-psychotic mania, revealed no differences in their antimanic response to olanzapine.

Risperidone was also investigated in two large multicenter trials (19,20). Both trials, one carried out in the United States (19) and the other in India (20), revealed a statistically highly significant difference between risperidone and placebo. The onset of improvement in the YMRS score occurred as early as day 3 of the study period. The dosage used in both studies was between 1 and 6 mg/day.

Quetiapine in a dose range of up to 800 mg/day was investigated in two large identically designed three-arm studies with placebo control and active comparator (either lithium or haloperidol) (21,22). In both studies, the efficacy of quetiapine was similar to the active comparator in all efficacy measurements, and a statistically highly significant difference to placebo was found. The analysis of the pooled data (24) from these two 12-week monotherapy studies of quetiapine revealed that from day 4 onwards there was a statistically significant reduction in manic symptoms as measured by the YMRS. The effect was substantiated by day 24 and further increased by day 84. There was also no hint that patients in the study population on active treatment exhibited depressive symptoms or suffered a depressive relapse during that treatment period.

Ziprasidone used in a high initial dosage of 160 mg/day (achieved within 2 days) showed a significant reduction in manic symptoms 2 days after treatment initiation (17). This reduction was maintained throughout the study period, and mania ratings from baseline to endpoint exhibited a 54% improvement of the symptomatology. This finding has been replicated in a 21-day randomized, double-blind, placebo-controlled trial (18).

Table 2 Summary of Double-Blind, Randomized, Placebo-Controlled Monotherapy Trials of Atypical Antipsychotics in Bipolar Mania

					Outcome measurements from baseline to end of study vs. placebo					
Agent	Study	*n*	Dose range	Duration (weeks)	Primary efficacy variable	Result	*p*-Value	Secondary efficacy variables	Result	*p*-Value
Olanzapine	Tohen et al., 1999 (13)	139	5–20 mg/day	3	YMRS (D 21)	>	0.02	CGI-BP mania	>	0.02
								PANSS total	>	0.02
								PANSS positive	>	0.04
								HAMD	=	0.87
Olanzapine	Tohen et al., 2000 (14)	115	5–20 mg/day	4	YMRS (D 28)	>	< 0.001	CGI-BP mania	>	< 0.001
								PANSS total	>	< 0.001
								PANSS positive	>	< 0.001
								HAMD	=	0.09
Aripiprazole	Keck et al., 2003 (15)	262	30–15 mg/day	3	YMRS (D 21)	>	0.002	CGI-BP	>	0.001
								CGI-BP mania	>	0.001
								CGI-BP depression	>	0.03
Aripiprazole	Carson et al., 2004 (16)	272	30 mg	3	YMRS (D 21)	>	0.01	CGI-BP	>	0.01
								PANSS hostility	>	0.01
Ziprasidone	Keck et al., 2003 (17)	210	40–80 mg twice daily	3	MRS (D 21)	>	< 0.005	CGI-BP	>	< 0.001
								improvement	>	< 0.001
								PANSS positive	>	< 0.005
								GAF		
Ziprasidone	Segal et al., 2003 (18)	139	40–80 mg twice daily	3	MRS (D 21)	>	0.01	CGI-BP	>	0.001

Risperidone	Hirschfeld et al., 2003 (19)	279	1–6 mg/day	3	YMRS (D 21)	>	< 0.001	CGI-BP severity	>	< 0.001
								PANSS activation	>	< 0.001
								GAS	>	< 0.001
Risperidone	Khanna et al., 2003 (20)	290	1–6 mg/day	3	YMRS (D 21)	>	< 0.001	*	*	*
Quetiapine	Brecher and Huizar, 2003 (21)	302	Up to 800 mg/day	12	YMRS (D 21)	>	< 0.001	CGI-BP improvement	>	< 0.001
								PANSS total	>	< 0.001
								PANSS activation	>	< 0.001
								MADRS	>	0.002
Quetiapine	Paulsson and Huizar, 2003 (22)	302	Up to 800 mg/day	12	YMRS (D 21)	>	< 0.001	CGI-BP improvement	>	0.003
								PANSS total	>	< 0.001
								PANSS activation	>	0.001
								MADRS	>	0.008

Note: > indicates that atypical was significantly better than placebo; = indicates that atypical was not different from placebo.

*Data not provided.

Abbreviations: CGI-BP, Clinician Global Impressions Severity of Bipolar Disorder Scale; GAF, Global-Assessment-of-Functioning Scale; GAS, Global Assessment Scale Score; HAMD, Hamilton Rating Scale for Depression; MADRS, Montgomery–Asberg Depression Rating Scale; MRS, Mania Rating Scale; PANSS, Positive and Negative Syndrome Scale; YMRS, Young Mania Rating Scale.

Source: Ref. 23.

Aripiprazole in a dosage of 30 mg/day was able to alleviate symptoms of acute manic or mixed episodes of bipolar disorder compared with placebo (15). The early onset on day 4, which was observed with other atypical antipsychotics, was also apparent. Aripiprazole also demonstrated its efficacy and safety in the treatment of acute mania or mixed episodes in another large multicenter, double-blind study of 272 patients (16). A pooled analysis of three 3-week, double-blind, multicenter placebo-controlled studies revealed that there is no difference in efficacy of aripiprazole if manic patients were classified either as manic or as suffering from mixed episodes, rapid-cycling bipolar disorder, each with or without psychotic symptoms (25).

Combination Studies

In clinical practice, large proportions of patients with mania receive combination (e.g., from the beginning of pharmacotherapy) or adjunctive treatment (e.g., at a later time point) when they are considered unresponsive to monotherapy or have exhausted first-line monotherapy treatment options (Table 3). There are only a few controlled trials comparing one particular combination regimen with another, but there is growing clinical evidence of the effectiveness of combination therapy in patients with mania who are unresponsive to one or more medications. Controlled combination studies have been conducted for olanzapine, risperidone, and quetiapine.

The combination of *olanzapine* with lithium or divalproex has been shown to be more effective than lithium and valproic acid monotherapy alone for treatment of bipolar mania (30). In this study, the combination with olanzapine co-therapy was initiated when patients were unresponsive to more than 2 weeks of lithium or divalproex therapy. This regimen exhibited a significantly higher improvement in total YMRS scores from baseline to end of study compared with lithium or divalproex monotherapy plus placebo. The response rate for olanzapine co-therapy was also significantly higher with rates of 67.7% versus 44.7% with monotherapy ($p < 0.001$). There were also higher improvements in the Hamilton rating scale for depression (HAMD-21) for olanzapine co-therapy compared with monotherapy.

Two independent trials were performed to establish the efficacy of *risperidone* in combination with mood stabilizers for treatment of acute mania (26,27). It emerged that the combination of risperidone plus lithium or divalproex was significantly more efficacious compared with lithium or divalproex plus placebo and as efficacious as haloperidol plus lithium or divalproex for treating manic symptoms in patients with manic or mixed episodes (26). In a second study, in which risperidone was used in combination with lithium, divalproex, or carbamazepine, there was no statistically significant difference at the primary endpoint, which was defined as a change from baseline in YMRS score at study end compared with placebo plus mood stabilizer. However, in a post hoc analysis excluding carbamazepine-treated patients, there was a statistically significant difference. Additionally, 61% of patients in the risperidone co-therapy group were "much," "more," or "very much" improved, compared with 31% of patients in the placebo group. At the end of the study, significantly greater improvement in the hostility and thought disturbance subscales of the Brief Psychiatric Rating Scale (BPRS) was apparent in the risperidone co-therapy group compared with the placebo-treated group ($p < 0.05$).

The combination therapy of *quetiapine* with lithium or divalproex revealed a statistically higher effect when quetiapine was added (compared to lithium). The

Table 3 Summary of Placebo-Controlled, Randomized, Double-Blind Adjunctive Therapy Trials of Atypical Antipsychotics in Bipolar Mania

Study	Study drugs (*n*)	Dose range	Duration (weeks)	Outcome measures: Primary efficacy variable	Result	Secondary efficacy variables	Result
Tohen et al., 2002 (16)	Li + OLZ (76) DVP + OLZ (153) Li + placebo (41) DVP + placebo (73)	5–20 mg/day (OLZ) 50–125 μg/mL (DVP) 0.6–1.2 mEq/L (Li)	3	YMRS	OLZ + Li/DVP > Li/DVP	Remission, time to remission, clinical response HAMD, PANSS (total, positive, negative, cognitive), CGI-BP (overall, mania)	OLZ + Li/DVP > Li/DVP
Sachs et al., 2002 (26)	Placebo + Li/DVP (51) RISP + Li/DVP (52) HAL + Li/DVP (53)	0.6–1.4 mEq/L (Li) 50–120 μg/mL (DVP) 4–6 mg/day (RISP) 4–12 mg/day (HAL)	3	YMRS	RISP + Li/DVP > Li/DVP; HAL + Li/DVP > Li/DVP; RISP + Li/DVP = HAL + Li/DVP	CGI severity	RISP + Li/DVP > Li/DVP; HAL + Li/DVP > Li/DVP; RISP + Li/DVP = HAL + Li/DVP
Yatham et al., 2003 (27)	Placebo + Li/DVP/CBZ (75) RISP + Li/DVP/CBZ (75)	1–6 mg/day (RISP)	3	YMRS	RISP + Li/DVP/CBZ not statistically superior to Li/DVP/CBZ	CGI-BP, BPRS, HAMD	RISP + Li/DVP/CBZ > Li/DVP/CBZ
Mullen et al.,	Placebo + Li/DVP	0.7–1.0 mEq/L (Li)	3	YMRS	QTP + Li/DVP > Li/DVP	Remission, response CGI-	QTP + Li/DVP

(*Continued*)

Table 3 Summary of Placebo-Controlled, Randomized, Double-Blind Adjunctive Therapy Trials of Atypical Antipsychotics in Bipolar Mania (*Continued*)

				Outcome measures			
Study	Study drugs (*n*)	Dose range	Duration (weeks)	Primary efficacy variable	Result	Secondary efficacy variables	Result
2003 (28)	(100) QTP + Li/DVP (91)	50–100 µg/mL(DVP) Up to 800 mg/day (QTP)				BP (severity of illness, global improvement), PANSS (aggression risk subscale)	> Li/DVP
						PANSS (total, positive and negative subscale scores)	QTP + Li/DVP = Li/DVP
Mullen and Paulsson, 2003 (29) (pooled analysis)	Placebo + Li/ DVP (205) QTP + Li/DVP (197)	0.7–1.0 mEq/L (Li) 50–100 µg/L (DVP) Up to 800 mg/day (QTP)	3	YMRS	QTP + Li/DVP > Li/DVP	Remission, response CGI-BP, response GAS	QTP + Li/DVP > Li/DVP

Remission, YMRS score ≤12; Response, ≥ reduction in total YMRS score.
Abbreviations: BPRS, Brief Psychiatric Rating Scale; CGI-BP, Clinician Global Impressions Severity of Bipolar Disorder Scale; CBZ, carbamazepine; DVP, divalproex; GAS, Global Assessment Scale Score; HAL, haloperidol; HAMD, Hamilton Rating Scale for Depression; Li, lithium; OLZ, olanzapine; PANSS, Positive and Negative Syndrome Scale; QTP, quetiapine; RISP, risperidone; YMRS, Young Mania Rating Scale.
Source: Ref. 23.

effect was apparent in the total score of the YMRS as well as in response calculations. Interestingly, there was also a statistically significant improvement in the PANSS supplemental aggression scores compared with placebo. A pooled analysis of combination studies of quetiapine-treated patients showed significantly greater reduction in mean YMRS scores compared with patients receiving placebo plus lithium or divalproex (29). Furthermore, the pooled analyses revealed that these differences were apparent as early as in the first week of treatment.

Tolerability

Bases of the pharmacodynamic properties and the resulting tolerability profiles of these compounds are summarized in Table 1. Although the magnitude of antimanic effects across placebo-controlled mania studies is remarkably similar among atypical antipsychotics, there is evidence from controlled mania studies as well as from the use of atypical antipsychotics in schizophrenia that there are differences with respect to safety and tolerability profiles (6,31–34).

Clozapine and olanzapine have as the most prominent side effects somnolence, dry mouth, increased appetite, and weight gain (35,36). Increased appetite and weight gain can be problematic in some patients because of the increased risk of diabetes and also other components of the metabolic syndrome (31,34,37,38).

Dose-dependent extrapyramidal side effects (39) as well as increased prolactin levels, moderate weight gain, headache, and dizziness can be a problem with risperidone administration (40,41).

Treatment with quetiapine can be associated with somnolence and postural hypotension. Quetiapine has a placebo level incidence of EPS and prolactin elevation (42,43). Furthermore, long-term data revealed minimal weight gain (44).

Ziprasidone treatment can be associated with sedation and prolongation of the QTC interval (17), and aripiprazole treatment has been associated with akathisia, insomnia, and gastrointestinal disturbances (15). Both medications—ziprasidone and aripiprazole—have not been associated with increases in weight gain or an increase in serum prolactin levels.

Guidelines for Treatment of Mania Including Atypical Antipsychotics

There are a number of published guidelines from Europe (6,10,26,45), the United States (7), and international and worldwide (32) guidelines. These guidelines are driven by the trend towards evidence-based medicine. The probably most useful guidelines are those that do not directly recommend specific treatments but offer a framework of principles that practitioners can use together with their clinical judgment to formulate an appropriate treatment plan (10).

Guidelines are usually not followed by colleagues in hospital settings, as has been shown by Lim et al. (46) in North America and by Letmaier et al. (47) in Europe. For instance, these reports revealed that only one-third of bipolar I (manic or depressed) patients with psychotic features were discharged on medications recommended by expert guidelines as the preferred treatment, and in nonpsychotic manic patients, these figures dropped to one out of six. There are several barriers, which keep clinicians away from using guidelines and these problems range from lack of awareness to frustration with confusing or cumbersome guidelines.

The practice guidelines released by the American Psychiatric Association (7), British Association for Psychopharmacology (45), and the World Federation of

Societies of Biological Psychiatry (WFSBP) (32) are evidence-based. The American Psychiatric Association guidelines recommend lithium or valproate with an antipsychotic agent as first-line therapy for severe manic episodes, and for less severe manic episodes, monotherapy with lithium, valproate, or atypical antipsychotics is recommended. Short-term administration of benzodiazepines is also recommended to control agitation in manic episodes. The guidelines specifically outline that atypical antipsychotics are preferred over typical neuroleptics because of their favorable side-effect profile.

The guidelines of the British Association for Psychopharmacology (45) recommend for initial treatment of an acute manic episode an antipsychotic or valproate, followed by a combination of lithium or valproate with an antipsychotic if symptoms are inadequately controlled. For less severe manic episodes, lithium or carbamazepine is recommended. Atypical antipsychotics are also recommended to control psychoses during a manic or mixed episode.

The Texas Medication Algorithm Project (TMAP) has its goals in symptomatic remission, full return of psychosocial functioning, and prevention of relapse and recurrences (48). In this program, the first choice between lithium, divalproex, or olanzapine is for patients presenting with euphoric mania/hypomania or psychotic mania. For mixed or dysphoric mania, divalproex or olanzapine is recommended.

TREATMENT OF BIPOLAR DEPRESSION

Introduction

Bipolar depression as a specific treatment indication was overlooked for a long time, and in the study protocols of bipolar disorder, mania received more attention (49). Only now is bipolar depression emerging as an area of interest, because it is apparent that in the long term, bipolar patients suffer mostly from the depressive component (50,51). Epidemiological studies reveal that bipolar depression is generally under-diagnosed or misdiagnosed as unipolar depression (52,53). New treatment modalities, including not only lamotrigine, but also atypical antipsychotics, have ameliorated treatment for this indication (54).

Lithium and lamotrigine were classified as first-line treatments for the management of bipolar depression as published by a recent international consensus group (54). In this publication, category I evidence for a compound was given if the agent exhibited evidence from randomized, placebo-controlled trial(s) in the treatment of acute bipolar depression (or breakthrough mania) and in the long-term treatment for both poles of illness in recently depressed and recently manic patients. Agents meeting category II evidence had to have randomized placebo-controlled trial(s) in the acute phase for which the patient is being treated or randomized, placebo-controlled trial(s) in the long-term treatment from one pole of illness that suggest(s) no mood destabilization. Finally, agents meeting category III evidence had to have randomized controlled trial(s) in any phase of bipolar disorder treatment. Using this approach, it emerged that lithium and lamotrigine are meeting the criteria for category I evidence for treatment of bipolar depression and olanzapine, or that the combination of olanzapine and fluoxetine meets category II evidence.

The results of lamotrigine and lithium trials are reviewed elsewhere, as the focus of this chapter is on the usage of atypical antipsychotics.

Olanzapine and the combination of olanzapine and fluoxetine met the criteria for category II, with acute and limited long-term study data available. The evidence from a randomized, placebo-controlled 8-week trial (55) revealed that olanzapine and the olanzapine–fluoxetine combination were effective treatments for bipolar I depression. Interestingly, the combination of olanzapine–fluoxetine was superior to olanzapine alone, and both groups were significantly different from placebo. In this study, over 700 patients were studied who suffered from bipolar I depression and had a score of at least 20 on the MADRS. Not only absolute numbers from MADRS differed significantly between the three treatment arms, there were also statistically significant higher rates of response and remission. There are open-label data existing for the effectiveness of olanzapine and the olanzapine–fluoxetine combination as maintenance treatments for bipolar I depression (55).

Quetiapine exerted therapeutic efficacy against anxiety and depressive symptoms in the long-term treatment of patients with schizophrenia (56). It was, therefore, logical to also assess its therapeutic properties in patients meeting DSM-IV criteria for bipolar depression over an 8-week, double-blind treatment phase, comparing it to placebo (quetiapine was given in a fixed dose of either 300 or 600 mg in 542 patients) (57). Patients in both dosage groups had a statistically significantly greater improvement in mean MADRS scores vs. placebo at every assessment, starting with the first evaluation and sustained through end point. There were also statistically significantly more patients considered responders (more than 50% decrease from baseline MADRS score) from week 2 through the end of the study. There was no difference in treatment-emergent mania between the quetiapine and placebo groups, and the most common adverse events were dry mouth, sedation, somnolence, dizziness, and constipation. These data encourage to further study the role of antipsychotics in affective disorders also with the focus on depressive symptomatology.

Because atypical antipsychotics also have a potent antidepressant mechanism of action, it is likely that other atypical antipsychotics such as aripiprazole, risperidone, ziprasidone, and zotepine also exert antidepressant properties. So far, these substances have not been studied systematically for the indication of bipolar depression.

Long-Term Perspective

Bipolar disorder is considered a life-long illness, and recommendations include that patients who respond to their first-line treatment should continue that treatment for the long term. However, in order to base these recommendations on study evidence, it is important to note that placebo-controlled evidence is only available for the efficacy and safety of lithium for 2 years (58), lamotrigine for 18 months (59,60), olanzapine in recently manic patients for 1 year (61), and aripiprazole in recently manic patients for 26 weeks (62).

Olanzapine has also been studied in a double-blind fashion compared with lithium (63), indicating a lower frequency of relapse into mania and a similar frequency for relapse into depression within 1 year. The 47-week comparison between olanzapine and divalproex revealed no difference in maintenance treatment (64). The addition of olanzapine to lithium or divalproex resulted in a significantly lower time to relapse compared with lithium or divalproex alone over an 18-month observation period (65). The aripiprazole maintenance trial [26 weeks] of patients with a recent episode of mania indicated a statistically significant superior efficacy compared with placebo (62).

No double-blind long-term studies are as yet available for other atypical antipsychotics. However, open-label evidence from these compounds indicates that atypical antipsychotics are a valuable choice. For quetiapine, ziprasidone, and zotepine, there is a need for further long-term studies to establish their role for prophylaxis as monotherapy or combination treatment with mood stabilizers like lithium, divalproex, or lamotrigine.

REFERENCES

1. Klimke A, Klieser E. Clozapin—Geschichtliche Entwicklung und aktuelle Fragen. In: Naber D, Müller-Spahn F, eds. Clozapin. Pharmakologie und Klinik eines Atypischen Neuroleptikums. Eine kritische Bestandsaufnahme. Stuttgart, New York: Schattauer, 1992:3–10.
2. Angst J, Jaenicke U, Padrutt A, Scharfetter C. Ergebnisse eines Doppelblindversuches von HF 1854 [8-Chlor-11-(4-methyl-1-piperazinyl]-5H-dibenzo(b,e)[1,4]diazepin) im Vergleich zu Levomepromazin. Pharmakopsychiatrie 1971; 4:192–200.
3. Keck PE, McElroy SL, Strakowski SM. Anticonvulsants and antipsychotics in the treatment of bipolar disorder. J Clin Psychiatry 1998; 59(suppl 6):74–81.
4. Dwight MM, Keck PEJ, Stanton SP, Strokowski SM, McElroy SL. Anti-depressant activity and mania associated with risperidone treatment of schizoaffective disorder. Lancet 1994; 344:554–555.
5. Stoll AL. Risperidone and the risk of switch into mania. In: Ayd FJ, ed. The Art of Rational Risperidone Therapy. Baltimore, MD: Ayd Medical Communications, 1997: 121–127.
6. Kasper S, Tauscher, J, Aschauer H, Danzinger R, Friedl EJ, Friedrich M, Haring C, Kalousek M, Kapfhammer HP, König P, Lehofer M, Platz T, Schubert H, Simhandl C, Stuppäck C, Tauscher-Wisniewski S, Windhager E, Wolf W. Bipolare Störungen. Medikamentöse Therapie. Konsensus-Statement State of the Art 2003. CliniCum psy Sonderausgabe. November 2003.
7. American Psychiatric Association. Practice guidelines for the treatment of patients with bipolar disorder (revision). Am J Psychiatry 2002; 159[4 suppl]:1–50.
8. Bauer MS, Callahan AM, Jampala C, Petty F, Sajatovic M, Schaefer V, Wittlin B, Powell BJ. Clinical practice guidelines for bipolar disorder from the Department of Veterans Affairs. J Clin Psychiatry 1999; 60:9–21.
9. Frye MA, Altshuler LL. Selection of initial treatment for bipolar disorder, manic phase. In: Rush AJ, ed. Clinical Decision Trees in the Pharmacotherapy of Mood Disorders. Vol. 25. Basel: Karger, 1994:88–113.
10. Kasper S, Zohar J, Stein DJ, eds. Decision Making in Psychopharmacology. London: Martin Dunitz, 2002.
11. Chou JC, Zito JM, Vitrai J, Craig TJ, Allingham BH, Czobor P. Neuroleptics in acute mania: a pharmacoepidemiologic study. Ann Pharmacother 1996; 30:1396–1398.
12. Tohen M, Zhang F, Taylor CC, Burns P, Zarate C, Sanger T, Tollefson G. A meta-analysis of the use of typical antipsychotic agents in bipolar disorder. J Aff Disord 2001; 65:85–93.
13. Tohen M, Sanger TM, McElroy SL, Tollefson GD, Chengappa KN, Daniel DG, Petty F, Centorrino F, Wang R, Grundy SL, Greaney MG, Jacobs TG, David SR, Toma V. Olanzapine versus placebo in the treatment of acute mania. Olanzapine HGEH Study Group. Am J Psychiatry 1999; 156:702–709.
14. Tohen M, Jacobs TG, Grundy SL, McElroy SL, Banov MC, Janicak PG, Sanger T, Risser R, Zhang F, Toma V, Francis J, Tollefson GD, Breier A. Efficacy of olanzapine in acute bipolar mania: a double-blind, placebo-controlled study. The Olanzapine HGGW Study Group. Arch Gen Psychiatry 2000; 57:841–849.
15. Keck PE, Marcus R, Tourkodimitris S, Ali M, Liebeskind A, Saha A, Ingenito G. on behalf of the Aripiprazole Study Group. A placebo-controlled, double-blind study of the

efficacy and safety of aripiprazole in patients with acute bipolar mania. Am J Psychiatry 2003; 160:1651–1658.
16. Carson W, Sachs G, Sanchez R, Marcus R, Kujawa M, Archibald D, Iwamoto T. Aripiprazole vs. placebo for the treatment of acute mania in patients with bipolar disorder. Int J Neuropsychopharmacol 2004; 7(suppl 1):S332.
17. Keck PE, Versiani M, Potkin S, West SA, Giller E, Ice K. Ziprasidone in the treatment of acute bipolar mania: a three-week, placebo-controlled, double-blind, randomized trial. Am J Psychiatry 2003; 160:741–748.
18. Segal S, Riesenberg RA, Ice K, English P. Ziprasidone in mania: a 21-day randomized, double-blind, placebo controlled trial. Eur Neuropsychopharmacol 2003; 13(suppl 4): S345–S346.
19. Hirschfeld R, Keck P, Karcher K, Kramer M, Grossman F. Rapid antimanic effect of risperidone monotherapy: a 3-week multicenter, double-blind, placebo-controlled trial. Bipolar Disord 2003a; 5(suppl 1):53.
20. Khanna S, Vieta E, Lyons B, Grossman F, Kramer M. Risperidone monotherapy in acute bipolar mania. Bipolar Disord 2003; 5(suppl 1):60.
21. Brecher M, Huizar K. Quetiapine vs placebo for acute mania associated with bipolar disorder (STAMP 1). Bipolar Disord 2003; 5(suppl 1):35.
22. Paulsson B, Huizar K. Quetiapine monotherapy vs placebo for acute bipolar mania (STAMP 2). Bipolar Disord 2003; 5(suppl 1):74.
23. Kasper S, Attarbaschi T. Treatment options for bipolar mania. Clinical approaches. Bipolar Disord 2004; 3:24–32.
24. Jones M, Huizar K. Quetiapine monotherapy for acute mania associated with bipolar disorder (STAMP 1 and STAMP 2). Bipolar Disord 2003; 5(suppl 1):57.
25. Marcus R, McQuade R, Sanchez R, Carson W, Kostic D, Abou-Gharbia N, Jody D, Iwamoto T, Hardy S. Efficacy of aripiprazole in sub-populations of bipolar disorder patients with acute mania: a pooled analysis. Int J Neuropsychopharmacol 2004; 7(suppl 1):S160–S161.
26. Sachs GS, Grossman F, Ghaemi SN, Okamoto A, Bowden CL. Combination of a mood stabilizer with risperidone or haloperidol for treatment of acute mania: a double-blind, placebo-controlled comparison of efficacy and safety. Am J Psychiatry 2002; 159: 1146–1154.
27. Yatham LN, Grossman F, Augustyns I, Vieta E, Ravindran A. Mood stabilisers plus risperidone or placebo in the treatment of acute mania. International, double-blind, randomised controlled trial.. Br J Psychiatry 2003; 182:141–147.
28. Mullen J, Devine N, Sweitzer D. Quetiapine adjunctive therapy for acute mania associated with bipolar disorder (SIAM). Bipolar Disord 2003; 5(suppl 1):70.
29. Mullen J, Paulsson B. Quetiapine in combination with mood stabilizer for the treatment of acute mania associated with bipolar disorder. Bipolar Disord 2003; 5(suppl 1):70.
30. Tohen M, Chengappa KN, Suppes T, Zarate CA Jr, Calabrese JR, Bowden CL, Sachs GS, Kupfer DJ, Baker RW, Risser RC, Keeter EL, Feldman PD, Tollefson GD, Breier A. Efficacy of olanzapine in combination with valproate or lithium in the treatment of mania in patients partially nonresponsive to valproate or lithium monotherapy. Arch Gen Psychiatry 2002; 59:62–69.
31. Allison DB, Mentore JL, Heo M, Chandler LP, Cappelleri JC, Infante MC, Weiden PJ. Antipsychotic-induced weight gain: a comprehensive research synthesis. Am J Psychiatry 1999; 156:1686–1696.
32. Grunze H, Kasper S, Goodwin G, Bowden C, Baldwin D, Licht R, Vieta E, Möller HJ, on behalf of the WFSBP Task Force on Treatment Guidelines for Bipolar Disorders (Akiskal H, Allain H, Ayuso-Gutierrez J, Bech P, Benkert O, Berk M, Bitter I, Bourgeois M, Burrrows G, Calabrese J, Cassano G, Cetkovich-Bakmas M, Cookson J, da Costa D, George M, Goodwin F, Heinze G, Higuchi T, Hirschfeld R, Hoeschl C, Holsboer-Trachsler E, Jamison K, Katona C, Keller M, Kulhara P, Kupfer D, Lecrubier Y, Leonard B, Lingjaerde O, Lublin H, Maj M, Mendlewicz J, Mitchell P, Montgomery S,

Nemeroff C, Nolen W, Nutt D, Paykel E, Philipp M, Post R, Puzynski S, Rihmer Z, Rybakowski J, Vestergaard P, Walden J, Whybrow P, Yamada K). World Federation of Societies of Biological Psychiatry (WFSBP) guidelines for biological treatment of bipolar disorders, part II: treatment of mania. World J Biol Psychiatry 2003; 4:5–13.

33. Bobes J, Rejas J, Garcia-Garcia M, Rico-Villademoros F, Garcia-Portilla MP, Fernandez I, Hernandez G, on behalf of the EIRE Study Group. Weight gain in patients with schizophrenia treated with risperidone, olanzapine, quetiapine or haloperidol: results of the EIRE study. Schizophr Res 2003; 62:77–88.
34. Sernyak MJ, Leslie DL, Alarcon RD, Losonczy MF, Rosenheck R. Association of diabetes mellitus with use of atypical neuroleptics in the treatment of schizophrenia. Am J Psychiatry 2002; 159:561–566.
35. McElroy SL, Frye MA, Suppes T, Dhavale D, Keck PE, Leverich GS, Altshuler L, Denicoff KD, Nolen WA, Kupka R, Grunze H, Walden J, Post RM. Correlates of overweight and obesity in 644 patients with bipolar disorder. J Clin Psychiatry 2002; 63: 207–213.
36. Gianfrancesco F, White R, Wang RH, Nasrallah HA. Antipsychotic-induced type 2 diabetes: evidence from a large health plan database. J Clin Psychopharmacol 2003; 23:328–335.
37. Elmslie JL, Silverstone JT, Mann JI, Williams SM, Romans SE. Prevalence of overweight and obesity in bipolar patients. J Clin Psychiatry 2000; 61:179–184.
38. Wirshing DA, Boyd JA, Meng LR, Ballon JS, Marder SR, Wirshing WC. The effects of novel antipsychotics on glucose and lipid levels. J Clin Psychiatry 2002; 63:856–865.
39. Owens DG. Extrapyramidal side effects and tolerability of risperidone: a review. J Clin Psychiatry 1994; 55(suppl):29–35.
40. Conley RR, Mahmoud R. A randomized double-blind study of risperidone and olanzapine in the treatment of schizophrenia or schizoaffective disorder. Am J Psychiatry 2001; 158:765–774.
41. Kleinberg DL, Davis JM, de Coster R, Van Baelen B, Brecher M. Prolactin levels and adverse events in patients treated with risperidone. J Clin Psychopharmacol 1999; 19:57–61.
42. Arvanitis LA, Miller BG. Multiple fixed doses of "Seroquel" (quetiapine) in patients with acute exacerbation of schizophrenia: a comparison with haloperidol and placebo. The Seroquel Trial 13 Study Group.. Biol Psychiatry 1997; 42:233–246.
43. Hamner MB, Arvanitis LA, Miller BG, Link CG, Hong WW. Plasma prolactin in schizophrenia subjects treated with Seroquel (ICI 204,636). Psychopharmacol Bull 1996; 32:107–110.
44. Brecher M, Rak I, Melvin K, Jones A. The long-term effect of quetiapine (Seroquel™) monotherapy on weight in patients with schizophrenia. Int J Psychiatry Clin Pract 2000; 4:287–291.
45. Goodwin GM, for the consensus group of the British Association for Psychopharmacology. Evidence-based guidelines for treating bipolar disorder: recommendations from the British Association for Psychopharmacology. J Psychopharmacol 2003; 17:149–173.
46. Lim PZ, Tunis SL, Edell WS, Jensik SE, Tohen M. Medication prescribing patterns for patients with bipolar I disorder in hospital settings: adherence to published practice guidelines. Bipolar Disord 2001; 3:165–173.
47. Letmaier M, Schreinzer D, Thierry N, Wolf R, Kasper S. Medikamentöse Behandlung akuter Manien. Eine retrospektive Datenanalyse stationärer Patienten von 1997 bis 1999. Nervenarzt 2004, 75:249–257.
48. Suppes T, Dennehy EB, Swann AC. Report of the Texas Consensus Conference Panel on Medication Treatment of Bipolar Disorder 2000. J Clin Psychiatry 2002; 63:288–299.
49. Goodwin F, Jamison K. Manic-Depressive Illness. New York: Oxford University Press, 1990.
50. Judd L, Akiskal H, Schettler P. The long-term natural history of the weekly symptomatic status of bipolar I disorder. Arch Gen Psychiatry 2002; 56:530–537.

51. Judd LL, Schettler PJ, Akiskal HS, Maser J, Coryell W, Solomon D, Endicott J, Keller M. Long-term symptomatic status of bipolar I vs. bipolar II disorders. Int J Neuropsychopharmacol 2003; 6:127–137.
52. Kessler RC, Rubinow DR, Holmes C, Abelson JM, Zhao S. The epidemiology of DSM-III-R bipolar I disorder in a general population survey. Psychol Med 1997; 27:1079–1089.
53. Hirschfeld RM, Calabrese JR, Weissman MM, Reed M, Davies MA, Frye MA, Keck PE, Lewis L, McElroy SL, McNulty JP, Wagner KD. Screening for bipolar disorder in the community. J Clin Psychiatry 2003; 64:53–59.
54. Calabrese JR, Kasper S, Johnson G, Tajima O, Vieta E, Yatham LN, Young AH. International consensus group on bipolar I depression treatment guidelines [ACADEMIC HIGHLIGHTS]. J Clin Psychiatry 2004; 65:569–579.
55. Tohen MF, Vieta E, Calabrese J, Ketter TA, Sachs G, Bowden C, Mitchell PB, Centorrino F, Risser R, Baker RW, Evans AR, Beymer K, Dube S, Tollefson GD, Breier A. Efficacy of olanzapine and olanzapine/fluoxetine combination in the treatment of bipolar I depression. Arch Gen Psychiatry 2003; 60:1079–1088.
56. Kasper S. Quetiapine is effective against anxiety and depressive symptoms in long-term treatment of patients with schizophrenia. Depress Anxiety 2004; 20:44–47.
57. Calabrese JR, Macfadden W, McCoy R, Minkwitz M, Wilson E, Mullen J. Double-blind, placebo-controlled study of quetiapine in bipolar depression. Int J Neuropsychopharmacol 2004; 7(suppl 1):S330–S331.
58. Prien RF, Caffey EM, Klett CH. Prophylactic efficacy of lithium carbonate in manic-depressive illness. Arch Gen Psychiatry 1973; 28:337–341.
59. Calabrese JR, Bowden C, Sachs G, Yatham LN, Behnke K, Mehtonen OP, Montgomery P, Ascher J, Paska W, Earl N, DeVeaugh-Geiss J, on behalf of the Lamictal 605 Study Group. A placebo-controlled 18-month trial of lamotrigine or lithium in the maintenance treatment in recently depressed patients bipolar I disorder. J Clin Psychiatry 2003; 64:1013–1024.
60. Bowden C, Calabrese JR, Sachs G, Yatham LN, Asghar SA, Hompland M, Montgomery P, Earl N, Smoot TM, DeVeaugh-Geiss J, on behalf of the Lamictal 606 Study Group. A placebo-controlled 18-month trial of lamotrigine and lithium maintenance treatment in recently manic or hypomanic patients with bipolar 1 disorder. Arch Gen Psychiatry 2003; 60:392–400.
61. Tohen M, Bowden C, Calabrese J, Chou J, Jacobs T, Baker RW, Williamson D, Evans AR. Olanzapine's efficacy for relapse prevention in bipolar disorder: a randomized double-blind placebo-controlled 12-month clinical trial. Bipolar Disord 2003; 5(suppl 1):89.
62. McQuade R, Sanchez R, Marcus R, Carson W, Rollin L, Iwamoto T, Stock E. Aripiprazole for relapse prevention in bipolar disorder: a 26-week placebo-controlled study. Int J Neuropsychopharmacol 2004; 7(suppl 1):S161.
63. Tohen M, Marneros A, Bowden C, Greil W, Koukopoulos A, Belmaker H, Jacobs T, Baker R, Williamson D, Evans A, Dossenbach M, McGee D, Cassano G. Olanzapine versus lithium in relapse prevention in bipolar disorder: a randomized double-blind controlled 12-month clinical trial. Bipolar Disord 2003; 5(suppl 1):89.
64. Tohen M, Ketter TA, Zarate CA, Suppes T, Frye M, Altshuler L, Zajecka J, Schuh L, Risser R, Brown E, Baker R. Olanzapine versus divalproex sodium for the treatment of acute mania and maintenance of remission: a 47-week study. Am J Psychiatry 2003; 160:1263–1271.
65. Tohen M, Chengappa KNR, Suppes T, Baker RW, Zarate C, Bowden C, Sachs G, Kupfer D, Ghaemi S, Feldman P, Risser R, Evans AR, Calabrese J. Relapse prevention in bipolar I disorder: 18-month comparison of olanzapine plus mood stabilizer versus mood stabilizer alone. Br J Psychiatry 2004; 184:334–345.

21
Is There a Role for Typical Neuroleptics in Bipolar Disorder?

H. J. Möller and Heinz Grunze
Department of Psychiatry, Ludwig–Maximilians University, Munich, Germany

INTRODUCTION

With the emergence of the atypical antipsychotics and the subsequent broadening of the treatment portfolio for acute mania, recent treatment guidelines seem to neglect typical neuroleptics as a treatment option or even discourage their use. Nevertheless, there is still a widespread clinical use, as demonstrated by several observational studies (1–4), which may well exceed the time frame of acute antimanic treatment (5). For example, a Medline-based review using publications between 1980 and 1999 on the naturalistic use of typical antipsychotics in bipolar disorder by Tohen et al. (3) showed that on average 90.7% of manic inpatients and 65.3% of outpatients received typical antipsychotics. At least in an outpatient population, a lower degree of severity of mania may be expected, which makes the extensive use of typical antipsychotics somewhat surprising. The reasons behind the use of typical antipsychotics may be plentiful: it may just be sticking to tradition, as especially older clinicians are more familiar with their use or it may be due to the fact that psychosis, including hallucinations, is part of severe stages of mania (6) and may occur in up to 40% of patients (7). Many clinicians may also associate typical antipsychotics not only with stronger antipsychotic effects, but also see them as more powerful against other symptoms of acute mania (irritability, agitation, impulsiveness, and aggression) than other treatment modalities. However, all these potential advantages of typical antipsychotics are based on clinical experience. Thus, it is important to review the existing data to elucidate whether this impression is also backed up by controlled studies.

One of the main reasons why treatment guidelines usually recommend the use of atypical antipsychotics or mood stabilizers as first-line treatment is the tolerability issue. Acute extrapyramidal symptoms, prolactin elevations, and tardive dyskinesias, as well as emerging depression, have been associated with the use of typical antipsychotics, not only in schizophrenic patients. Thus, the second part of this chapter will also review the available tolerability data for bipolar patients when taking typical neuroleptics. Balancing the arguments for efficacy against tolerability issues may finally lead to a more balanced view about the use of typical neuroleptics in bipolar disorder and how they may fit into treatment algorithms.

USE OF TYPICAL NEUROLEPTICS IN ROUTINE CLINICAL SETTINGS

After the introduction of chlorpromazine, typical antipsychotics were the traditional first-line treatment of acute mania at least far into the 1990s. Although the antimanic efficacy of lithium is well documented, the usual time lapse until lithium shows antimanic efficacy made mood stabilizers only a second choice treatment, either overlapping or following antipsychotic use after mania had resolved. This scenario changed slightly with the introduction of valproate, especially in the United States, as a reasonably well-tolerated and fast-acting antimanic agent. However, due to regulatory issues and clinical scepticism concerning valproate monotherapy in severely manic patients, typical antipsychotics remained the first-line clinical routine treatment in most European countries. However, even in the United States, a pharmacoepidemiological census by Chou et al. (4) showed that 92% of inpatients were treated with typical antipsychotics alone or in combination with mood stabilizers. Another census by Keck et al. (8) demonstrated that even in the United States, 67.5% of outpatients received typical antipsychotics, mostly in combination with a mood stabilizer. For Germany, two recent epidemiological studies should be mentioned. Reetz-Kokott and Müller-Öerlinghausen (1) investigated the use of typical antipsychotics in a university hospital setting. They reported that 93.5% of acutely manic inpatients received typical neuroleptics, 44.4% in monotherapy, and 49.1% in combination treatment regimens. The census of the drug-safety working group in Bavaria (AMÜP-Bayern) revealed that in 1998, 81% of inpatients in Bavarian state hospitals received antipsychotics, almost exclusively typical neuroleptics (9). A retrospective analysis of treatment modalities in inpatients at the University Hospital of Vienna from 1997 to 1999 demonstrated that also in an Austrian university setting, the use of typical antipsychotics is rather the rule than the exception (2). During the first 2 weeks in hospital, almost every patient received antipsychotics and the majority (>80%) were still on antipsychotics at discharge. The most commonly used antipsychotics were chlorprothixene (46%), followed by haloperidol (32%) and prothipendyl (26%). Antipsychotics, as well as other agents, were mostly used in combination treatment regimens. More than 60% received at least five different medications at admission and still more than 10% at discharge.

In addition, in other studies, the use of typical neuroleptics appears not to be limited to the time period of acute manic symptomatology. The median time of use in the meta-analysis of Tohen et al. (3) was 2.5 months, ranging from 1 week to 6 months. Sernyak et al. (5) evaluated 40 patients 6 months after discharge from hospital and recovery from acute mania and found that 95% were still receiving typical neuroleptics. This high number may be exceptional and may reflect treatment resistance to previously administered mood stabilizers, as discussed by the authors. Nevertheless, it is obvious that—even in academic settings, where recent treatment recommendations and algorithms should be well known—typical neuroleptics are still a major cornerstone of the treatment of acute mania and beyond.

EVIDENCE FROM CONTROLLED STUDIES FOR THE EFFICACY OF TYPICAL NEUROLEPTICS IN ACUTE MANIA

With the general acceptance of the use of typical neuroleptics in acute manic patients and its long-standing clinical tradition, obviously no one felt any pressing need to examine this class of drugs in sophisticated scientific studies. In addition, at the time of the emergence of typical neuroleptics in acute mania, regulatory issues did not stipulate such high scientific demands as they do today. Thus, until recently, there was only one placebo-controlled randomized trial for a typical neuroleptic, in this case chlorpromazine, in acutely manic patients (10). Other controlled studies were head-to-head comparisons of typical neuroleptics versus the mood stabilizers lithium (11–16), valproate (17), and carbamazepine (18,19). Comparing typical neuroleptics with lithium, the overall impression of these studies was a higher efficacy of lithium by the end of the treatment, usually after 3 weeks. A pooled analysis by Janicak et al. (20) reported a responder rate for lithium of 89% compared to 54% responders on typical neuroleptics; this difference was significantly different. However, the effect of typical neuroleptics on psychomotor agitation during the initial treatment week appeared better. In the Northwick Park Study (16), which compared lithium and pimozide in a sample of hospitalized acute agitated manic and schizophrenic patients, the authors concluded that lithium appeared only to affect mood, whereas pimozide controlled both mood and psychotic agitation. This differential profile is also reflected in the usual clinical practice to combine lithium treatment of acute mania with typical neuroleptics during the initial treatment, despite the described risk of neurotoxicity with this combination (21). In the only study comparing haloperidol with valproate (17), both treatment modalities were found to be equally effective, with valproate also acting on psychotic symptoms to a similar degree as haloperidol. However, this study is clearly limited by the small sample size and short duration. Neither of the two studies that compared carbamazepine with typical neuroleptics (18,19) found a significant difference between these treatment modalities.

Just recently, haloperidol has been increasingly used as a comparator in controlled studies of atypical antipsychotics. In the study by Segal et al. (22), treatment with risperidone (6 mg/day), lithium (800–1200 mg/day), or haloperidol (10 mg/day) was compared under double-blind, randomized conditions in acute mania for 4 weeks. No difference in efficacy was observed between these three agents; however, any conclusions from this study are clearly limited by the small sample size of 15 patients per study arm, the absence of a placebo control, and the extensive use of lorazepam for the whole study period.

In a more recent, well-powered but not placebo-controlled study, olanzapine was compared to haloperidol (23). For the primary efficacy criterion (reduction of the mania rating scale after week 6), haloperidol (flexible dose 3–15 mg) outperformed olanzapine significantly. For several secondary measures, e.g., the percentage of responders and remitters after week 12, no difference was observed between these two treatments.

Just recently, two placebo-controlled studies have been published in which haloperidol served as a comparator to either risperidone (24) or quetiapine (25). In the risperidone study, a mean modal dose of haloperidol of 8 ± 3.6 mg/day was equal to a mean modal dose of risperidone of 4.2 ± 1.7 mg/day for all efficacy parameters. Both treatments were significantly superior to placebo from week 1 onwards and throughout the whole 3-week trial. In the 12-week, double-blind, placebo-controlled study comparing quetiapine (fixed dose 600 mg/day), haloperidol (fixed dose 5 mg/day), and placebo, again both quetiapine and haloperidol were significantly better than placebo from week 1 onwards for the whole 12-week study period. In direct comparison, there was no significant difference between quetiapine and haloperidol. In a recent, yet unpublished study, haloperidol was compared to aripiprazol in the absence of a placebo-controlled group (26,27). The result of this study showing superiority of aripiprazol is hard to interpret as a mixed outcome criterion (being a responder and remaining in the study until the endpoint at week 12) was used. As anticholinergic drugs were not allowed in the study, it is likely that several patients on haloperidol dropped out due to tolerability problems, despite improvement of mania.

In summary, especially the more recent studies proved that haloperidol, used in dosages between 5 and 15 mg, appears to be as equally efficacious as recommended dosages of different atypical antipsychotics. These studies appear not to justify the common clinical practice of using high doses of haloperidol, which may not improve efficacy but only lead to tolerability problems. It remains an area of uncertainty whether even lower dosages of haloperidol, e.g., 1–5 mg/day, which are usually well below the EPS threshold, may already be equally efficacious, reasonably tolerated, and in times of increasing economical pressure also a cost-effective treatment of acute mania. This view is reflected in the recent guideline of the British Association of Psychopharmacology (28) and also backed up by the experimental finding that low-dose haloperidol is sufficient to reach a >70% D_2 receptor occupancy (29).

MAINTENANCE TREATMENT WITH TYPICAL NEUROLEPTICS IN BIPOLAR DISORDER

According to naturalistic data, between 68% and 95% of bipolar patients continue to receive typical neuroleptics for lengthy periods after acute treatment (3). However, the published controlled evidence in favor of such treatment is sparse. Data from older, controlled studies of typical neuroleptics as a maintenance treatment are not compelling (30–35). Those trials performed under controlled conditions, for example, the study by Esparon et al. (31), could not prove the benefit of long-term treatment with a typical neuroleptic, in this case, flupenthixol. The most recent study published by Zarate and Tohen (36) compared combination treatment with a mood stabilizer (lithium or valproate) and perphenazine against a mood stabilizer with placebo after remission from acute mania for 6 months. The outcome was significantly in favor of the mood stabilizer-alone treatment, with significantly more days until discontinuation and no relapses into depression, compared with a 21% relapse rate with continuation of perphenazine. There were no significant differences concerning relapses into mania. However, despite the double-blind, controlled nature of this study, all conclusions are clearly limited by the small number of patients ($n = 37$).

In conclusion, with the absence of convincing controlled data and keeping the increased risk of tardive dyskinesia and the potential "depressiogenic effect," as observed in schizophrenic patients, in mind, long-term maintenance treatment with typical neuroleptics cannot be generally recommended. However, selected patients who are prone to severe mania and where compliance has been a problem in the past may still be suitable candidates for depot formulations of typical neuroleptics, especially in cases where the long-term formulation of risperidone might not be suitable.

TOLERABILITY AND SAFETY

The main argument for the use of atypical neuroleptics in both schizophrenia and acute mania is their edge with respect to tolerability and safety issues. Extrapyramidal symptoms and sexual side effects due to prolactin elevation are often disruptive in the doctor–patient relationship and also question future treatment compliance.

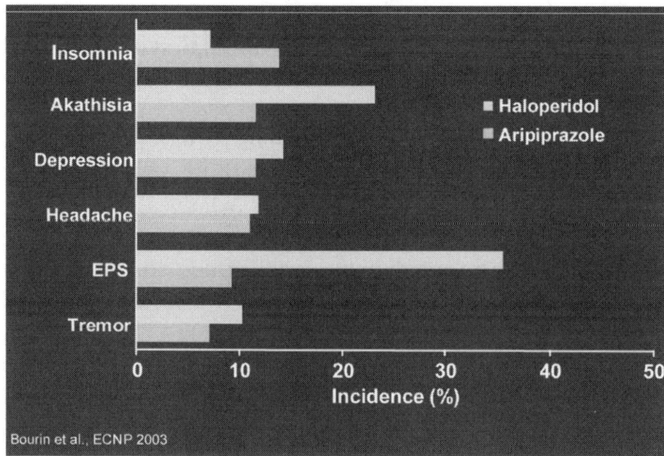

Figure 1 Spontaneously reported side effects > 10% in a double-blind, randomized 12-week study of aripiprazole vs. haloperidol in acute mania. Most obvious, EPS and akathisia occur more frequently with haloperidol when the concomitant use of anticholinergics is prohibited; otherwise, no striking difference can be seen comparing this typical and atypical neuroleptic medication. *Source*: Adapted from Ref. 27.

A dose-dependent prolactin elevation can be expected for all neuroleptics that mainly act on the dopaminergic system, including some atypicals such as risperidone and amisulpride when used in high dosages. In a recent controlled study comparing aripiprazole (mean dosage 21.6 mg/day) with haloperidol (mean dosage 11.1 mg/day) in acute mania (26,27), side effects observed in > 10% of patients, as depicted in Figure 1.

This study appears of special interest as it did not allow the use of adjunctive anticholinergics, which otherwise may mask the typical side effects of haloperidol. Thus, it clearly illustrates the problem of EPMS with typical neuroleptics, but otherwise the safety advantage appears just marginal for the modern atypical aripiprazole.

A more worrying aspect, however, is the risk of a malignant neuroleptic syndrome, which may occur in up to 1% of patients treated with typical neuroleptics, and the risk of tardive dyskinesia. Two reports in the mid-1970s described for the first time that affective disorder patients have an elevated risk compared with schizophrenics to develop tardive dyskinesias (37,38). Since then, several studies and retrospective reviews have been dedicated to the issue of tardive dyskinesia in mood-disorder patients. Prevalence rates of 26–64% have been described, depending on the duration of observation, neuroleptics, and dosages used, and instruments used to detect movement disorders (for an overview, see Ref. 39). In two studies, prevalence rates between mood disorder and schizophrenic patients were compared (40,41), both of which recorded a 1.3–1.8 times increased risk in mood-disorder patients. The underlying mechanism of this differential sensitivity to typical neuroleptics remains unclear; it has been speculated that it may have to do with the mode of usage. Whereas schizophrenic patients may rather have a pattern of low-dose, long-term, continuous use of typical neuroleptics, many bipolar patients exhibit a pattern of high-dose typical neuroleptics during acute episodes and discontinuation while in remission. In experimental animal settings, this mode of application appears to favor long-term side effects of typical neuroleptics. In conclusion, typical neuroleptics are associated with an increased risk of both acute extrapyramidal symptoms and long-term tardive dyskinesias. Issues like dosage and pattern of use may modulate this risk.

However, there are also arguments in favor of typical neuroleptics compared to many other treatment options, especially mood stabilizers like lithium and valproate, and many atypical antipsychotics. This includes the relative cardiac safety of haloperidol, which is of importance, especially in the initial treatment of mania where an ECG is usually not available. Furthermore, typical neuroleptics do not show a comparable degree of weight gain as some atypicals, for example, clozapine and olanzapine, and mood stabilizers such as lithium and valproate do. In addition, the risk of developing diabetes mellitus appears less compared with olanzapine and clozapine (42,43). However, also in the group of atypical antipsychotics, there are individual medications available, which are lacking these respective side effects.

CONCLUSIONS

Typical neuroleptics in monotherapy or in combination treatment have a long-standing tradition in the treatment of bipolar disorder, mainly in acute mania. By this, they are familiar to many clinicians and are still preferred to mood-stabilizer monotherapy or atypical antipsychotics, despite guideline recommendations. It would be over-simplified to assume that treating physicians are not aware of the arguments in favor of these other treatment options, as even in university hospital settings typical neuroleptics have a widespread use. Factors contributing to these treatment habits have been outlined in this chapter. They include the efficacy that has been proven more recently in a methodologically unambiguous way in acute manic patients, the possibility to control for acute side effects by administering anticholinergic drugs and flexible dosages below the EPS threshold, and finally the generally good cost-effectiveness relationship. For long-term maintenance treatment with typical neuroleptics, however, the scientific basis is not compelling. Maintenance with typical neuroleptics should rather be discouraged in the majority of bipolar patients and may only be an option for selected mania-prone or, as a depot, in otherwise non-compliant patients. Nevertheless, it does not appear justified to ban the use of typical neuroleptics in general, and future treatment guidelines should rather adopt a more differentiated view, as do the guidelines of the British Association of Psychopharmacology (28), for example.

REFERENCES

1. Reetz-Kokott U, Müller-Oerlinghausen B. Hat sich die medikamentose Behandlung der Manien im klinischen Alltag verändert? Retrospektive Analyse der Behandlungsmodalitäten und -ergebnisse in einer psychiatrischen Universitätsklinik. Nervenarzt 1996; 67:229–234.
2. Letmaier M, Schreinzer D, Thierry N, Wolf R, Kasper S. Medikamentöse Behandlung akuter Manie. Eine retrospektive Datenanalyse stationärer Patienten von 1997 bis 1999. Nervenarzt 2004; 75:249–257.
3. Tohen M, Zhang F, Taylor CC, Burns P, Zarate C, Sanger T, Tollefson G. A meta-analysis of the use of typical antipsychotic agents in bipolar disorder. J Affect Disord 2001; 65:85–93.

4. Chou JC, Zito JM, Vitrai J, Craig TJ, Allingham BH, Czobor P. Neuroleptics in acute mania: a pharmacoepidemiologic study. Ann Pharmacother 1996; 30:1396–1398.
5. Sernyak MJ, Griffin RA, Johnson RM, Pearsall HR, Wexler BE, Woods SW. Neuroleptic exposure following inpatient treatment of acute mania with lithium and neuroleptic. Am J Psychiatry 1994; 151:133–135.
6. Carlson GA, Goodwin FK. The stages of mania. A longitudinal analysis of the manic episode. Arch Gen Psychiatry 1973; 28:221–228.
7. Goodwin FK, Jamison KR. Manic-Depressive Illness. New York: Oxford University Press, 1990.
8. Keck PE, McElroy SL, Strakowski SM, Balistreri TM, Kizer DI, West SA. Factors associated with maintenance antipsychotic treatment of patients with bipolar disorder. J Clin Psychiatry 1996; 57:147–151.
9. Grunze H, Dobmeier M. Modul Therapie akuter Episoden. In: DGBS EV, ed. Deutsche Gesellschaft für Bipolare Störungen e.V. Weissbuch Bipolare Störungen in Deutschland. Hamburg: CP-Verlag, 2002:57–66.
10. Klein DF, Oak G. Importance of psychiatric diagnosis in prediction of clinical drug effects. Arch Gen Psychiatry 1967; 16:118–126.
11. Shopsin B, Gershon S, Thompson H, Collins P. Psychoactive drugs in mania. A controlled comparison of lithium carbonate, chlorpromazine, and haloperidol. Arch Gen Psychiatry 1975; 32:34–42.
12. Johnson G, Gershon S, Burdock EI, Floyd A, Hekimian L. Comparative effects of lithium and chlorpromazine in the treatment of acute manic states. Br J Psychiatry 1971; 119:267–276.
13. Spring G, Schweid D, Gray C, Steinberg J, Horwitz M. A double-blind comparison of lithium and chlorpromazine in the treatment of manic states. Am J Psychiatry 1970; 126: 1306–1310.
14. Platman SR. A comparison of lithium carbonate and chlorpromazine in mania. Am J Psychiatry 1970; 127:351–353.
15. Prien RF, Caffey EM, Klett CJ. Comparison of lithium carbonate and chlorpromazine in the treatment of mania. Report of the Veterans Administration and National Institute of Mental Health Collaborative Study Group. Arch Gen Psychiatry 1972; 26:146–153.
16. Johnstone EC, Crow TJ, Frith CD, Owens DG. The Northwick Park "functional" psychosis study: diagnosis and treatment response. Lancet 1988; 2:119–125.
17. McElroy SL, Keck PE, Stanton SP, Tugrul KC, Bennett JA, Strakowski SM. A randomized comparison of divalproex oral loading versus haloperidol in the initial treatment of acute psychotic mania. J Clin Psychiatry 1996; 57:142–146.
18. Okuma T, Inanaga K, Otsuki S, Sarai K, Takahashi R, Hazama H, Mori A, Watanabe M. Comparison of the antimanic efficacy of carbamazepine and chlorpromazine: a double-blind controlled study. Psychopharmacology 1979; 66:211–217.
19. Klein E, Bental E, Lerer B, Belmaker RH. Carbamazepine and haloperidol v placebo and haloperidol in excited psychoses. A controlled study. Arch Gen Psychiatry 1984; 41: 165–170.
20. Janicak PG, Newman R, Davis JM. Advances in the treatment of mania related disorders: a reappraisal. Psychiatry Ann 1992; 22:92–103.
21. Normann C, Brandt C, Berger M, Walden J. Delirium and persistent dyskinesia induced by a lithium-neuroleptic interaction. Pharmacopsychiatry 1998; 31:201–204.
22. Segal J, Berk M, Brook S. Risperidone compared with both lithium and haloperidol in mania: a double-blind randomized controlled trial. Clin Neuropharmacol 1998; 21: 176–180.
23. Tohen M, Goldberg JF, Gonzalez-Pinto Arrillaga AM, Azorin JM, Vieta E, Hardy-Bayle MC, Lawson WB, Emsley RA, Zhang F, Baker RW, Risser RC, Namjoshi MA, Evans AR, Breier A. A 12-week, double-blind comparison of olanzapine vs haloperidol in the treatment of acute mania. Arch Gen Psychiatry 2003; 60:1218–1226.

24. Smulevich AB, Khanna S, Eerdekens M, Karcher K, Kramer M, Grossman F. Acute and continuation risperidone monotherapy in bipolar mania: a 3-week placebo-controlled trial followed by a 9-week double-blind trial of risperidone and haloperidol. Eur Neuropsychopharmacol 2005; 15:75–84.
25. McIntyre RS, Brecher M, Paulsson B. Quetiapine as monotherapy for bipolar mania: A double blind randomized parallel group placebo controlled trial. Eur Neuropsychopharmacol.
26. Auby P, Marcus RN, Swannik R, McQuade RD, Iwamoto T, et al. Aripiprazole versus haloperidol for maintained treatment effect in acute mania. APA Annual Meeting Abstracts 2004; NR 467.
27. Bourin M, Auby P, Swanik E, Marcus R, McQuade R, et al. Aripiprazole vs. haloperidol for maintained treatment effect in acute mania. Eur Neuropsychopharmacol 2003; 13(suppl 4):333.
28. Goodwin GM. Evidence-based guidelines for treating bipolar disorder: recommendations from the British Association for Psychopharmacology. J Psychopharmacol 2003; 17:149–173.
29. Tauscher J, Kufferle B, Asenbaum S, Tauscher-Wisniewski S, Kasper S. Striatal dopamine-2 receptor occupancy as measured with [123I]iodobenzamide and SPECT predicted the occurrence of EPS in patients treated with atypical antipsychotics and haloperidol. Psychopharmacology (Berl) 2002; 162:42–49.
30. White E, Cheung P, Silverstone T. Depot antipsychotics in bipolar affective disorder. Int Clin Psychopharmacol 1993; 8:119–122.
31. Esparon J, Kolloori J, Naylor GJ, McHarg AM, Smith AH, Hopwood SE. Comparison of the prophylactic action of flupenthixol with placebo in lithium treated manic-depressive patients. Br J Psychiatry 1986; 148:723–725.
32. Naylor GJ, Scott CR. Depot injections for affective disorders. Br J Psychiatry 1980; 136:105.
33. Lowe MR, Batchelor DH. Depot neuroleptics and manic depressive psychosis. Int Clin Psychopharmacol 1986; 1(suppl 1):53–62.
34. Littlejohn R, Leslie F, Cookson J. Depot antipsychotics in the prophylaxis of bipolar affective disorder. Br J Psychiatry 1994; 165:827–829.
35. Ahlfors UG, Baastrup PC, Dencker SJ, Elgen K, Lingjaerde O, Pedersen V, Schou M, Aaskoven O. Flupenthixol decanoate in recurrent manic-depressive illness. A comparison with lithium. Acta Psychiatr Scand 1981; 64:226–237.
36. Zarate CA, Tohen M. Double-blind comparison of the continued use of antipsychotic treatment versus its discontinuation in remitted manic patients. Am J Psychiatry 2004; 161:169–171.
37. Davis KL, Berger PA, Hollister LE. Tardive dyskinesia and depressive illness. Psychopharmacol Commun 1976; 2:125–130.
38. Rosenbaum AH, Niven RG, Hanson NP, Swanson DW. Tardive dyskinesia: relationship with a primary affective disorder. Dis Nerv Syst 1977; 38:423–427.
39. Keck PE, McElroy SL, Strakowski SM, Soutullo CA. Antipsychotics in the treatment of mood disorders and risk of tardive dyskinesia. J Clin Psychiatry 2000; 61(suppl 4):33–38.
40. Kane JM, Smith JM. Tardive dyskinesia: prevalence and risk factors, 1959 to 1979. Arch Gen Psychiatry 1982; 39:473–481.
41. Yassa R, Nair V, Schwartz G. Tardive dyskinesia and the primary psychiatric diagnosis. Psychosomatics 1984; 25:135–138.
42. Cohen D. Atypical antipsychotics and new onset diabetes mellitus. An overview of the literature. Pharmacopsychiatry 2004; 37:1–11.
43. Fuller MA, Shermock KM, Secic M, Grogg AL. Comparative study of the development of diabetes mellitus in patients taking risperidone and olanzapine. Pharmacotherapy 2003; 23:1037–1043.

22
Antidepressants in Bipolar Disorder

Lori Pellegrino and Jack Gorman
Mount Sinai School of Medicine, New York, New York, U.S.A.

INTRODUCTION

Depression is a significant part of bipolar illness; bipolar patients spend much more time in a depressed state than in a manic state (49% compared with 12%) (1). As well, there is a high rate of suicide in bipolar patients (2). It is not unusual for a bipolar patient to be initially diagnosed with a major depressive episode, and even if a family history of affective disorder is obtained, these patients often receive a prescription for antidepressants (1,3). Clinician error also results in bipolar patients receiving antidepressants instead of mood stabilizers. In one naturalistic sample, 37% of patients were misdiagnosed as unipolar after already having had a hypomanic or manic episode (1).

Further making the treatment of bipolar depression difficult, there is a significant lack of research in this area. As of 2001, there were only seven blinded controlled trials of long-term antidepressant treatment (4). This chapter attempts to coordinate existing evidence and highlights new research that may be challenging clinical beliefs about antidepressant use in bipolar disorder.

CURRENT GUIDELINES ON ANTIDEPRESSANT USE IN BIPOLAR DISORDER

The 2002 APA Practice Guidelines for the treatment of bipolar depression recommend that antidepressants be initiated only after lithium, lamotrigine, or another mood stabilizer is initiated (5). For a depressive episode, which breaks through maintenance mood stabilizer therapy, the guidelines recommend first to maximize the maintenance therapy to high-normal levels. Should the depression persist, add-on medications such as lamotrigine, buproprion, or paroxetine should be tried. Alternatively, another SSRI or a monoamine oxidase inhibitor may be added. Tricyclic antidepressants are not recommended given their high rate of causing switch from depression to mania. If the depression does not remit, ECT is to be considered.

The APA guidelines do not comment on recommended length of antidepressant treatment. However, the expert consensus guidelines published in 1998 recommend a relatively rapid taper of the antidepressant medication after a 6- to

12-week trial. The argument against a continuation phase of the antidepressant is that of high switch rates to mania, hypomania, and rapid cycling (6).

EFFICACY IN BIPOLAR DISORDER VS. UNIPOLAR DISORDER

Given that there are data showing neurobiological differences between bipolar and unipolar patients (7), one poses the question: are antidepressants actually effective in bipolar patients? Three studies to date address this issue.

The first is a retrospective chart review of over 2000 inpatients who were admitted to a psychiatric unit between 1980 and 1992 (8). Unipolar and bipolar patients who were treated with antidepressants were compared. No difference in response rates was found between unipolar and bipolar patients as measured by depressive scales (depressive syndrome scale, GAS score) and days in the hospital. The sample was divided into subgroups of 4-year intervals and the same comparison was done, again yielding no significant differences in response to antidepressants between unipolar and bipolar patients. This latter calculation attempted to factor the change in standard antidepressant use over that 12-year period (during which a general switch from TCA/MAOI to SSRI usage occurred). Of note, the bipolar patients were mostly *not* on mood stabilizers. The bipolar patients did have lower apathy scores, and they also had higher mania rating scores—these differences were statistically significant. However, the mania score in bipolar I depressed patents was still smaller at discharge than at admission; the authors hypothesized that this elevated mania score was due to "unspecific" symptoms of depression such as psychomotor agitation.

The same research group then did a prospective naturalistic study comparing 50 bipolar and 50 unipolar depressed inpatients (matched for age, gender, duration of illness). Depressive, manic, and paranoid–hallucinatory symptoms were compared at discharge. Again, there were no differences between groups. However, the bipolar patients were more often on mood stabilizing therapy. An additional analysis compared unipolar and bipolar patients who were on both antidepressants and mood stabilizers, once more yielding no differences in symptom ratings. These two studies suggest that there is no difference in efficacy of antidepressants between unipolar and bipolar patients (9).

A recently published chart review comparing 41 bipolar and 37 unipolar depressed patients reported a 1.6 times lower response rate to antidepressants in the bipolar patients. No unipolar patients experienced manic switch or cycle acceleration, as compared with the bipolar patients (who switched at rates of 48.8% and 25.6% had cycle acceleration). A catch-all group of "miscellaneous" antidepressant agents were significantly less likely to be effective than the standard antidepressants; included in this former group were nefazodone, mirtazapine, D-amphetamine, isocarboxazide, and St. John's wort. As well, relapsing to depression after discontinuation of the antidepressant was 4.7 times as likely in the bipolar versus the unipolar group (10).

ANTIDEPRESSANT EFFICACY AS COMPARED WITH MOOD STABILIZER EFFICACY

What is now commonplace treatment of bipolar disorder, mood stabilizers as first-line treatment, is a relatively recent development. Throughout the 1970s and 1980s, a number of studies determined the current standard of care.

The first placebo-controlled, randomly assigned comparison of a TCA versus lithium was reported in 1973 (11). Bipolar patients stabilized much better on lithium monotherapy rather than imipramine monotherapy, and there was a significantly higher rate of imipramine-induced mania compared to placebo and lithium treatment. The same NIMH Group performed a large, double-blind, but uncontrolled, study comparing the use of lithium, imipramine, or a combination in the treatment of both unipolar and bipolar patients. In the bipolar group, the combination treatment and lithium as monotherapy were both superior to imipramine alone in preventing manic recurrences, and were equally effective as imipramine in preventing depressive recurrences. In this study, there was no advantage to using the combination treatment over lithium alone. As well, only 8% of the IMI patients were in remission by end of the two-year study, as compared with 33% of the other two groups (12).

Five years later, these results were reanalyzed using survival analysis with inquiry into the index episode (13). In patients with manic index episodes (i.e., were manic upon entry into the study), both lithium monotherapy and the combination treatment were superior to imipramine. In patients with depressive index episodes, the combination of lithium and imipramine was superior to the individual treatments. By doing a different statistical analysis, combination of antidepressant and mood stabilizer was shown to be superior to using lithium as sole treatment. A more recent study found that antidepressants and mood stabilizers were more effective, overall, if the mood state preceding the depression was euthymia (as opposed to mania or hypomania) (14).

Another early study looking at combination treatment vs. monotherapy with lithium was a randomized double-blind trial done in 1981 when 75 patients were treated with either lithium + imipramine or lithium + placebo. There was a slightly higher rate of relapse to depression in the lithium-only group; however, a higher rate of relapse to mania occurred in the combination treatment group (24% vs. 10.5%). These numbers were not statistically significant, but suggest that imipramine increases manic relapse, even when combined with lithium (15).

Other, more recent studies, found no differences in efficacy between treatment with a mood stabilizer alone or in combination with an antidepressant. In a small, double-blind, randomized but non-controlled trial, researchers found that adding paroxetine vs. a second mood stabilizer to lithium or valproate produced no difference in clinical outcome (16). The group hypothesized that because there were more dropouts in the double mood stabilizer group, the paroxetine may have had a slightly superior effect overall. It was proposed that the patients receiving two mood stabilizers dropped out of the study because they were experiencing more adverse side effects. There were no cases of mania in the group receiving paroxetine.

As well, in a small single-blind prospective trial, topiramate was compared with bupropion as adjunctive therapy to valproate or lithium. Both treatments were effective in lowering HAM-D scales. Patients were excluded if they were a serious suicide risk, excluding the most depressed patients (17). Another small study comparing lithium with a combination of lithium and amitryptiline showed no difference in efficacy (18).

In a large (119 patients) multicentered, double-blinded, randomized, placebo-controlled trial, it was the level of lithium that determined if antidepressants were efficacious. Nemeroff et al. (19) looked at paroxetine or imipramine in addition to lithium, and compared their efficacy at different lithium levels. At levels lower than 0.8 meq/L, both imipramine and paroxetine were equally superior to placebo.

However, when the lithium level was higher than 0.8 meq/L, neither antidepressant provided additional efficacy to lithium alone. These findings support the recommendation that optimizing the lithium level is a reasonable first step in treating bipolar depression.

In a much smaller sample, a difference in lithium level was not significant between patients who responded to mood stabilizers as compared with patients who needed antidepressants added to their mood stabilizer therapy (20). This group retrospectively looked at characteristics of patients who required different treatments for bipolar depression. Patients remitting on mood stabilizer therapy alone were more likely to be married, stabilized more quickly in the trial, had experienced a previous depressive episode more recently, and also presented with higher young mania rating scale scores. Patients on ongoing antidepressant therapy were excluded from this study. As well, patients who did not stabilize within 4 weeks of entering the study protocol were excluded from this study. Therefore, perhaps this study did not look at more seriously ill, treatment-refractory patients. There was no significant increased risk of mania in the antidepressant-treated patients.

Most, but not all, of the above studies show that antidepressants are only questionably helpful in the treatment of bipolar depression. Frenkle et al. (21) looked at length of depressive episodes to determine if they are shortened with antidepressant treatment. This was a retrospective chart review, and the median length of the major depressive episode was 66 days. There was no significant difference in length of the depressive episode between groups treated with antidepressant or mood stabilizer, although the antidepressant-treated group had a numerically longer median episode length. It was postulated that clinicians were attempting to find alternate treatments to depression (such as adding a second mood stabilizer) because of being hesitant to use an antidepressant, thus contributing to longer episode lengths. However, the start of the episode was determined as 14 days prior to first clinic visit, which skews the results towards a shorter duration of depression. Nor was there a significantly increased rate of switch in antidepressant-treated patients.

THE SWITCH TO MANIA

Clinicians are hesitant to use antidepressants in bipolar disorder because of concern that the patient will switch into mania or hypomania. Many factors in the literature make drawing definitive conclusions about particular switch rates difficult. Studies are done for different lengths of time, earlier studies did not separate unipolar from bipolar patients, and many studies are not placebo-controlled. It is also difficult to determine a "normal" switch rate for bipolar patients, further emphasizing the need for placebo-controlled studies.

The pattern of affective state sequence has been studied. The sequence of depression switching into mania is not the most frequent pattern of non-pharmacologically induced illness in bipolar disorder. In bipolar I patients, usually the patient's affective state flows from mania to depression to euthymia, not depression to mania (22).

A seminal review of the literature from 1920 to 1980 showed that switch rates on inpatient units rose from the pre-antidepressant era (1920–1959) to the "tricyclic era" (1959–1982), following introduction of antidepressants. For reasons that are not completely clear, Angst concluded that this increase in rate was not because of the use of antidepressant medication. However, though the numbers are too small to draw definitive conclusions, this study does suggest that antidepressants increase the rates of mania/hypomania (23). Wehr and Goodwin (24) conclude in an early review of the literature that antidepressants increase switch rate by 2 to 3 times.

This factor is supported by a number of studies. In Nemeroff et al.'s (19) study, 5% of patients switched on lithium monotherapy, versus 11% of patients who switched on imipramine at low serum lithium levels. Though Quitkin et al.'s 1981 (15) study did not have statistical significance, 24% of patients on imipramine became manic versus 10.5% of patients on placebo. Other studies report a higher rate of switch. In Ghaemi et al.'s (1) naturalistic study, 55% of patients on antidepressants experienced mania or hypomania.

The Stanley Foundation Bipolar Network has been doing a series of studies looking at antidepressant-induced mania. This group has proposed a definition of antidepressant-induced mania, a definition that has been picked up by subsequent studies. The criteria for antidepressant-induced mania are: (a) mania occurring within 8 weeks of antidepressant initiation, (b) antidepressant causing a change in the pattern of illness, or (c) antidepressant causing a change in severity of illness. In this retrospective study, the life charts of 51 treatment-refractory bipolar patients were evaluated. One-third (35%) of patients were rated as likely to have had an antidepressant-induced mania. Although 82% of patients on heterocyclics became manic, only 35% of these episodes were deemed antidepressant-induced by the above criteria. Of note, 72% of these patients were on no mood stabilizing agents, and 28% were on lithium. Altshuler et al. (25) thus noted, "One half of the total switch rate for patients taking tricyclics is attributable to the direct effects of TCA, while natural course accounts for the other half."

A double-blind, random, placebo-controlled trial by the same group published in 2001 looks at the switch rates in patients given antidepressants on top of mood stabilizer treatment, thus studying the current standard of care (26). Patients on mood stabilizer therapy were randomized to bupropion, venlafaxine, or sertraline treatment for a 10-week double-blind trial for depression, followed by a 1-year blinded continuation maintenance phase for responders (the non-responders were re-randomized). Of the 175 acute treatment trials, 25% switched into mania or hypomania, and in the continuation phase, 38.8% of the patients switched. We are currently awaiting the results of the unblinding of this trial (27).

Current research postulates a qualitative difference in antidepressant-associated mania. Stoll et al. (28) found, in a blind, retrospective study, that antidepressant-induced mania is generally that of a mixed state, with significant irritability, and it resolves quickly when the antidepressant is discontinued. The patients with antidepressant-induced mania had generally less severe psychopathology, required less nursing checks/interventions, and had less severe psychotic and bizarre symptoms. These researchers defined antidepressant-induced mania as having received at least 3 days of antidepressants within 2 weeks of admission for mania. The overall severity of the episode was less in patients manic from buproprion and MAOI as compared with those patients taking tricyclics or fluoxetine, but these differences were not statistically significant.

Risk Factors for Switching

Many studies comment on potential risk factors, which predict antidepressant-induced switching. The number of past manic episodes has been both associated with a higher risk of switching (29) and has not been associated (or negatively associated) with switch (25,30). Serretti and colleagues found that older age positively correlated with increased risk of switching (30), whereas other studies found that younger age either trended towards (25) or correlated with increased switch (31).

Index episode in illness has been studied as regards to whether it predicts antidepressant-induced switch. Serretti et al. (30) found depressive index episode in the illness to be a risk factor for switch. As well, a diagnosis of bipolar I (vs. bipolar II) was found to be more likely to switch. The presence of delusions was negatively correlated with switches (30).

Previous episode was also analyzed. In a naturalistic study, depressed patients who had previously been manic had a higher rate of switch when treated with either antidepressants or mood stabilizers (14). This study also showed that previously euthymic patients had a better response to either mood stabilizers or antidepressants.

In a naturalistic study done by Henry et al. (32), patients who switched to mania or hypomania on antidepressants were compared with those who did not switch. The study found that patients who were on lithium were significantly less likely to switch. There was no difference in switch rates between patients on other types of mood stabilizers and patients on no mood stabilizer therapy. As well, the number of previous episodes of mania was not a protective, or negative, indicator of the likelihood to switch. A hyperthymic temperament was associated with a greater risk of antidepressant-induced switching. This finding is consistent with an earlier review in which the same author hypothesized that bipolar patients who trend towards a hyperthymic temperament can predictably have manic rather than depressive episodes in general, despite antidepressant treatment (33).

A recent naturalistic chart review studying antidepressant-induced rapid cycling found that in women, antidepressant administration prior to first manic episode was significantly correlated with rapid cycling (this was not significant in men). There was no correlation between type of first episode (depressed/manic) and rapid cycling, negating the hypothesis that if a depressive episode heralded rapid cycling, the subsequent treatment with antidepressants would be a "red herring," falsely appearing to cause rapid cycling (34).

Arguments Against Antidepressant-Induced Switch

There is some remote and recent literature claiming that antidepressants do not, in spite of the above evidence, cause mania. In a chart review done in 1982 by Lewis and Winokur (35), antidepressants were associated with a non-significantly higher switch rate than mood stabilizers; however, the antidepressants did not induce mania more often than the spontaneous rate. The authors defined switching as within 6 months of treatment initiation, which may account for the lack of significant difference—6 months is a long interval (as compared to the 2-month interval as proposed by Altshuler) and may increase the amount of switching in the control group. As well, the number of patients in this study was small, and the treatment had been naturalistic. There is also an article of 10 case reports of patients on SSRIs who experienced a decrease in severity, duration, and/or frequency of their manic or hypomanic symptoms. Parker hypothesizes that the SSRIs had mood stabilizing properties in these patients (36). There are no prospective data to date confirming this hypothesis.

Switch Rates and Mood Stabilizers

A number of studies, including some quoted above, prove that mood stabilizers prevent antidepressant-induced manic switch. A naturalistic study examining depressive episodes done by Boerlin and colleagues compared patients on mood stabilizers with patients on mood stabilizers + antidepressants and found no significant difference in the switch rates between the groups. A retrospective chart review showed that being on TCA without a mood stabilizer significantly predicted switch to mania, and that mood stabilizers offered a statistically significant protective effect against manic switch (37).

CYCLE ACCELERATION

To date, no double-blind, randomized, placebo-controlled trials exist looking at the issue of whether antidepressant use in bipolar disorder causes cycle acceleration. A number of studies (most naturalistic) do look at this issue and imply this hypothesis is true. Wehr and Goodwin (38) wrote perhaps the first literature on rapid cycling induced by tricyclics in an article with five case reports of rapid cycling in bipolar women given tricyclics. The authors noted that co-administration of lithium did not prevent the rapid cycling.

A number of chart reviews have realized an association between antidepressant use and the development of rapid cycling (25,39,40). The time elapsed from onset of antidepressant use to development of rapid cycling ranged from 6 months (25) to 1 year (40). In one study, the rapid cycling course resolved in half of the patients when the tricyclics were discontinued but resumed again when tricyclics were reinstated (39). The incidence of antidepressant-induced rapid cycling ranged from 73% (39) to 26% (25) of those begun on antidepressants. Younger age predicted cycle acceleration in Altshuler et al.'s (25) study (though it only trended towards predicting antidepressant-induced mania). Female gender and bipolar II were overrepresented but not found to be statistically significant predictors of the development of rapid cycling (25). Koukopoulos et al. (40) argue that the prevalence of rapid cycling affective disorder has increased concurrently with the advent of antidepressant drugs.

The only prospective, but naturalistic, study focusing on cycle acceleration was performed by Ghaemi et al. in 2000 (1). Twenty-three percent of the 54 patients in this study experienced new or worsened cycle acceleration, and 55% became manic or hypomanic while treated with antidepressants. SSRIs were the most common antidepressant used in this study. The mean number of episodes increased from 3.9 to 9.8 (per annum) but episodes were sufficiently brief, and the absolute duration of illness dropped from 60% to 45% of a year. Thus, this study suggests a trend for spending less time ill when on antidepressants, albeit with a higher risk of becoming a rapid cycler. In this naturalistic study, there was an increased number of manic and depressive episodes in the antidepressant-treated patients, but this effect was not found to be statistically significant.

Some discussion also exists on whether cyclothymics switch to bipolar II disorder when treated with antidepressants (41). As part of his argument for the inclusion of cyclothymic disorder in the bipolar affective category, Akiskal and colleagues did a study following 46 cyclothymics and compared them with 50 bipolar I patients and 50 patients with personality disorders as controls. The study was naturalistic and lasted 2 to 3 years. Besides showing that cyclothymic patients and bipolar patients have similar family history patterns of specific affective illnesses, these two groups had similar rates of pharmacological (TCA) -induced hypomania. The rate of antidepressant-induced hypomania was statistically significant when compared with the switch rates of patients with personality disorders.

The Issue of Mixed State (Agitated Depression) and Temperament

Whether the type of depression predicts antidepressant-induced switch is also discussed in the literature, but to date only in case reports. Agitated depression, now also called mixed state, has been reported to have a higher incidence of switch rate (42). Koukopoulos' theory is quite interesting but is not yet supported by empirical studies: a hyperthymic (hypomanic) temperament, when superimposed with an endogenous or seasonal depression, produces an agitated depression. (Conversely, a person with a depressive temperament, who becomes manic, experiences a dysphoric mania.) The definition of mixed state varies. Bottlender et al. (43) defined mixed depressive factors as flight of ideas, racing thoughts, distractibility, aggression, irritability, logorrhea, increased social contact, and increased drive. Koukopoulous and Koukopoulos (42) propose the following to define agitated depression: a major depressive episode plus at least two of the following symptoms: motor agitation, psychic agitation or intense inner tension, or racing/crowded thoughts.

Though not done with a statistical analysis, in Koukopoulos et al.'s (40) retrospective study in 1983, temperament and course of rapid cycling were studied. Of the sample of 118 bipolar patients who were rapid cyclers, a patient with hyperthymic temperament was at risk of becoming a rapid cycler if given an antidepressant. Patients with cyclothymic temperaments were at less of a risk of developing rapid cycling if given antidepressants. One retrospective chart review of 158 bipolar I patients hospitalized for depression found that the presence of certain mixed depressive symptoms predicted antidepressant-induced switch. The antidepressants used in this study were TCAs (43).

TYPES OF ANTIDEPRESSANTS

This section explores the literature on each type of antidepressant, mostly with regards to the risk of causing manic switch and efficacy of the antidepressant for bipolar depression.

Tricyclic Antidepressants

We will be revisiting some of the literature mentioned above in our previous discussion of tricyclics. In one of the earlier retrospective chart reviews, switch rates were determined as: 22% of patients receiving ECT, 15% of patients receiving tricyclics, and 34% of patients who received no treatment at all on admission. This study concluded that there was no risk of switch with tricyclics. The general consensus throughout the ensuing 20 years of research on switch rates is that these data were skewed, not in the least because there was no randomized treatment, and no way to protect against selection bias (35).

Early studies compare the use of tricyclics as monotherapy in the treatment of bipolar depression (or as maintenance treatment). As discussed earlier, they often are studies of both bipolar and unipolar patients. A 2-year prospective, placebo-controlled, randomized trial comparing imipramine and lithium by Prien et al. in 1973 (11) showed that lithium was superior to imipramine and placebo in preventing affective episodes. Though statistical analysis was not done in this study, manic episodes occurred in 12% of patients on lithium, 33% of patients on placebo, and 67% of patients on imipramine. These early placebo-controlled trials are good indicators of rates of mania in untreated patients.

A study of bipolar patients comparing monotherapy with lithium or imipramine or the combination found that over the 2-year maintenance phase, lithium was the superior treatment in preventing depressive or manic episodes. Fifty-three percent of patients in the imipramine monotherapy group had a manic episode, vs. 28% and 26% of patients in the combination group and lithium monotherapy group, respectively (12). Another prospective, randomized study found no statistical difference between depressive and manic relapses in patients given lithium versus patients given lithium and imipramine (15). This same group did a placebo-controlled analysis using a lithium/imipramine combination compared with lithium and placebo. There was no difference in the incidence of depressive relapses. Female patients on the lithium/imipramine combination were at a significantly higher risk of becoming manic (44).

Just as the recent study by Nemeroff and colleagues showed that there was no additional efficacy to adding antidepressants to lithium at lower serum lithium levels, an earlier chart review showed that at lower serum lithium levels, there is a significantly higher incidence of tricyclic-induced switch to mania (45).

Monoamine Oxidase Inhibitors

The use of monoamine oxidase inhibitors remains a viable treatment alternative in psychiatric practice for those patients who are treatment-refractory and can follow the dietary restrictions. There are few studies looking at the efficacy and side effects of these medications in bipolar patients. One group performed studies on MAOI's ability to treat atypical, or anergic, depression in bipolar patients (motor retardation, fatigue, volitional inhibition, and reversed neurovegetative features). Both of these studies looked at antidepressants as monotherapy (again, limiting the results' application in current clinical practice). The first study done by this group was a small study looking at both bipolar and unipolar patients. Tranylcypromine was compared with placebo, and was shown to be efficacious in treating depression. No switches were observed in this 6-week trial (46). A second study, looking solely at bipolar patients with anergic bipolar depression, compared tranylcypromine with imipramine (no placebo). There was a significantly greater response in the patients treated with tranylcypromine, and there were equivalent switch rates (47).

The only placebo-controlled, randomized, double-blind study looking at a reversible MAOI (moclobemide) compared with imipramine in bipolar depressed patients also has limitations. In the total of 156 patients, there was no statistical difference in efficacy between the two medications. More patients on imipramine became manic than patients on moclobemide, but the difference was not statistically significant. The shortcoming of this study is that some, but not all, of these patients were on mood stabilizers. These differences were not worked into the statistical analysis, and obviously would give more credence and applicability to the utility of these findings in today's practice (48).

Despite the paucity of evidence of the utility and risks of MAOIs in the treatment of bipolar disorder, these medications remain a credible alternative to the first-line treatments of bipolar depression (5). The fact that these medications are still recommended, usually before the use of TCAs, in bipolar patients, should remind us that much of psychiatry's clinical practice in treating bipolar patients is still not based on evidence.

Selective Serotonin Reuptake Inhibitors

Again, a relatively small amount of evidence exists on SSRIs in bipolar depression, particularly concerning the use of SSRIs in addition to mood stabilizer therapy. Some case reports of either bipolar II depression or non-bipolar depression show that a dosage decrease of an SSRI resolves the treatment-emergent hypomania/mania (49,50). One case report of fluoxtine-induced mania at 10 mg/day showed that the mania resolved when the fluoxetine was decreased to 10 mg twice weekly (51).

A large meta-analysis of pooled data from pharmaceutical industry-sponsored studies looked at switch rates in both bipolar and unipolar patients (52). In the unipolar group, there were very low switch rates and no differences between SSRIs and TCAs. In the bipolar patient data, the rate of manic switch of patients on sertraline and paroxetine was no greater than placebo (3.7% vs. 4.2%), and was significantly lower than the switch rate on tricyclics (11.2%). This meta-analysis included no information on mood stabilizers, nor were there strict diagnostic criteria used for mania or hypomania.

A naturalistic study of 44 bipolar depressed patients attempted to look at risk factors for antidepressant-induced mania, and attempted to differentiate between patients on or off mood stabilizer therapy. One-quarter of the patients on SSRIs had switches to mania or hypomania, and no differences were found among types of SSRIs. There was a significantly lower incidence of mood switching on patients with lithium in comparison to patients receiving anticonvulsant mood stabilizer therapy or no mood stabilizer therapy (32).

A placebo-controlled, randomized study of unipolar vs. bipolar II patients looked at monotherapy of fluoxetine for various lengths of time (the longest interval being 1 year). Relapse rates to depression were similar across all groups. In the short-term treatment group, there was a 3.8% vs. 0.3% manic switch of bipolar vs. unipolar patients. In the long-term treatment group, there was a 3.6% vs. 0.8% manic switch. The conclusion of this study was that fluoxetine was safe and effective with a low rate of switch to mania; however, this study was limited to bipolar II patients (53).

Venlafaxine

In a class of its own, venlafaxine warrants its own discussion, and its own evidence. A number of case reports exist on venlafaxine-induced mania, and in a few cases, mania occurred on venlafaxine while it had not occurred while the patient was on an SSRI (54,55). One small non-placebo-controlled trial studied bipolar and unipolar patients being treated with venlafaxine. There was a significant reduction in depression in both groups and no switches to mania occurred over the 6-week trial (56). In an RCT comparing venlafaxine and paroxetine in bipolar I and II patients, no difference in efficacy was found, but a slightly higher switch rate was found in the venlafaxine group (57). Venlafaxine has the highest switch rate in the Stanley Network Foundation's double-blind, randomized, placebo-controlled trial comparing sertraline, buproprion, and venlafaxine (R. Post, personal communication, 2004).

Bupropion

Bupropion is considered by some, including the guidelines discussed above, to be the first-line antidepressant for bipolar depression. This recommendation is supported by a number of case reports and studies, but careful investigation of the literature shows that bupropion is itself not without risks in a bipolar population. One report of three cases showed successful use of bupropion in "difficult-to-treat" bipolar depressed patients—it did not cause mania in these three patients, and their depression was put into remission (58). It is also potentially helpful for bipolar II rapid cycling patients (59). However, there do exist some case reports of bupropion-related mania, specifically at high doses (>450 mg/day) (60).

A year-long prospective, naturalistic life-charting study looked at 69 patients who received 113 trials of antidepressants. Using the criteria for antidepressant-induced mania discussed above and defined by Altshuler and colleagues, the researchers found no difference in switch rates, nor cycle acceleration, in patients receiving SSRIs versus bupropion. This was a large trial, but was potentially subject to clinician bias as it was not blinded (61). Similarly, a small prospective trial consisting of the acute treatment of 11 depressed bipolar patients on baseline mood stabilizer therapy showed that 7 out of 11 patients responded to the bupropion within 6 weeks. However, 6 out of 11 of the patients overall (four of the non-responders) experienced hypomania or manic symptoms necessitating the discontinuation of the medication (62). The lack of stringency in both of these trials calls the results into question, but each of these trials do question bupropion's superiority to other antidepressants in the treatment of bipolar depression.

Some literature exists on the use of bupropion as maintenance treatment in bipolar disorder. It should be noted that "maintenance" treatment usually refers to studying patients for 1 year on a medication. One author published three case reports of bipolar patients maintained on bupropion for 1 year without affective episode: these patients relapsed to depression or mania within 8 weeks of bupropion discontinuation (63). As part of an open-label study of bupropion for the treatment of depression, 11 schizoaffective/bipolar patients were presented (64). These 11 patients were maintained on the medication for 1 year and had a significant decrease in affective episodes (some patients were taking concomitant treatment).

Though soon to be accompanied by more current data, the only double-blind trial to date comparing bupropion with tricyclic therapy was done by Sachs and colleagues. Bupropion and desipramine were randomly added to lithium or anticonvulsant treatment for an 8-week acute trial followed by a 1-year crossover trial. Similar efficacy was observed in both groups; however, there were more manic episodes in the TCA acute group (30% mania vs. 11%) and in the maintenance group (two TCA patients experienced manic episodes, vs. no bupropion patients) (65). This study, though rigorous by design, is limited by its small numbers.

Of note, we are currently awaiting the unmasking of the results of the Stanley Foundation Bipolar Network double-blind randomized placebo-controlled comparison of buproprion, sertraline, and venlafaxine. There was an acute phase of 10 weeks of medication, and apparent and possible responders were offered the opportunity for 1 year of continued treatment—the subsequent section in this chapter discuses new evidence recommending more lengthy treatment. In the acute phase, 12.6% of the patients became hypomanic, and 12.6% of the patients became manic. In the 1-year continuation phase, 17.9% of the patients became hypomanic and 20.9% of the patients became manic. However, 42% of these patients reported a history of rapid cycling, so this switch rate may not be more than expected (27).

Combination of Antidepressants

There have been no studies on the risk of using combined antidepressant treatments in causing a manic switch. However, to date at least two case reports exist. The first, by Gabbay et al. (66), is a report of a patient who switched to mania 3 days after paroxetine 20 mg was added to buproprion 400 mg po qd. It is postulated that cytochrome 2D6 interaction caused an increased level of the paroxetine. A second report was in a bipolar patient who became manic during a switch of antidepressants: buproprion was begun 4 days prior to the switch (200 mg/day) and fluoxetine was discontinued 2 days prior to the switch (67). This case of mania may have been caused by the combination of the buproprion and fluoxetine (because of fluoxetine's long $t_{1/2}$) or abrupt withdrawal of the fluoxetine (68).

Antidepressant Withdrawal

Less studied and understood is whether withdrawal of antidepressants causes a switch to mania. In a study of imipramine in bipolar II and unipolar depression, there was a 2.6% overall incidence of hypomania (no difference between the groups) (69). Sixty-six percent of these affective switches occurred upon withdrawal of the antidepressant. Other case reports discuss mania and hypomania upon tricyclic withdrawal—observed between 24 hours and 7 days of discontinuation (70,71). Cases have also been evaluated wherein the patients were on adequate mood stabilizer therapy, and cases have been observed upon discontinuation of SSRIs as well (67,72).

Henry (68) poses an interesting hypothesis about why withdrawal of antidepressants might cause mania. The author postulates that the discontinuation syndrome (often seen upon abrupt cessation of antidepressants) could cause or exacerbate mania. If such were true, then a slow taper of the antidepressant would be indicated even if hypomanic symptoms were beginning to manifest. One of the studies discussed above specifically ruled out discontinuation syndrome symptoms in the patients (72). Inquiring about symptoms such as dizziness, light-headedness, nausea, headache, and sensory disturbance can help differentiate between discontinuation syndrome and hypomania (73).

LENGTH OF ANTIDEPRESSANT TREATMENT

In the studies, which postulate that antidepressants worsen the course of bipolar disorder, it is often recommended that the antidepressants should be stopped as soon as the depression remits (24,41). Recent data call this common clinical practice into question.

Altshuler et al. (74) (Stanley Foundation) first did a retrospective study showing that termination of antidepressant treatment within 2 years of remission significantly increased the risk of depressive relapse. This group then tested the results of this study by following 84 bipolar patients who were responding successfully to antidepressant treatment (in addition to mood stabilizer therapy) for a major depressive episode. In the 1-year naturalistic study, the relapse rates to depression, as well as their switch rates, were compared based on whether they received antidepressant treatment for less than 6 months or longer than 6 months. The study was set up to exclude patients who would switch to mania within 2 months by admitting patients to the study only if they were at least 60 days into antidepressant treatment. The patients who received antidepressant treatment for less than 6 months had a significantly increased risk (four times greater) of relapse to depression within the next year. Additionally, the group with the shorter length of antidepressant treatment had a significantly higher rate of manic switch (75).

It was considered whether the discontinuation group (shorter treatment time) stopped their antidepressant treatment because they were switching into mania. However, Altshuler showed that between the two groups, the patients who became manic did not discontinue their antidepressants in concordance with the emergence of manic symptoms.

The earliest studies comparing tricyclics and mood stabilizers led researchers to believe the opposite to be true. In Prien et al.'s 1984 (12) study, the same percentage of patients on imipramine as on lithium had depressive episodes when treated for 1 year. Also, in Quitkin et al.'s (15) 1981 study, imipramine given for 1 year was ineffective in preventing long-term bipolar depression. However, these studies looked at groups on tricyclic monotherapy. As Altshuler's studies emphasize, one must always question the inferences suggested by scientific literature. These new data necessitate a rethinking of treatment guidelines and clinical practice, suggesting that if a patient is responding well after 2 months of antidepressant treatment, the antidepressant should be continued for at least 6 months.

CONCLUSION

As Moller and Grunze (76) argue in their paper, which questions "Have some guidelines gone too far in the restriction of antidepressants?," there still does not exist a mood stabilizer which is as effective as antidepressants for bipolar depression. The oldest literature shows that lithium is a relatively strong antidepressant; however, it is not adequate to prevent against bipolar depressions breaking through lithium maintenance treatment. Yet newer data, such as the study done by Nemeroff and colleagues, posits that using higher levels of lithium therapy makes antidepressants unnecessary. Evidence-based psychiatry has not compared the newer mood stabilizers, particularly lamotrigine, with antidepressants in bipolar depression (77).

This chapter leaves unsolved many questions about antidepressants in bipolar disorder. Current research is addressing some of these questions. The unblinded results of the comparison of sertraline, venlafaxine, and bupropion will be the most definitive data regarding manic switch and the newest antidepressants. Whether the difference in risk of switch between sertraline and bupropion will be statistically significant remains to be seen. It is not clear that SSRIs pose much more of a risk of manic switch than does bupropion. As well, the recent data on length of treatment suggest a change in treatment strategy as is currently practiced. Altshuler's evidence suggests that antidepressants must be tapered much more slowly than is done in clinical practice, so as not to precipitate a manic switch. Mania upon withdrawal of antidepressants is also poorly understood, as are the hypotheses about character type and risk of antidepressant-induced mania.

With the current level of evidence-based knowledge, antidepressants are still necessary in bipolar disorder. Though the risk of manic switch is lower with the newer antidepressants, and mania induced by antidepressants tends to be of lesser severity, patients with bipolar disorder must be educated about this potential outcome.

REFERENCES

1. Ghaemi SN, Boiman EE, Goodwin FK. Diagnosing Bipolar disorder and the effect of antidepressants: a naturalistic study. J Clin Psychiatry 2000; 61:804–808.
2. Simpson SG, Jamison KR. The risk of suicide in patients with bipolar disorders. J Clin Psychiatry 1999; 60(suppl 2):53–56.
3. Bowden CL. Strategies to reduce misdiagnosis of bipolar depression. Psychaitr Serv 2001; 52:51–55.
4. Ghaemi SN, Lenox MS, Baldessarini RJ. Effectiveness and safety of long-term antidepressant treatment in bipolar disorder. J Clin Psychiatry 2001; 62:565–569.
5. American Journal of Psychiatry Practice Guideline for the treatment of patients with bipolar disorder. Am J Psychiatry 2002; 159(4):1–50.
6. Frances AJ, Kahn D, Carpenter D, Docherty JP, Donovan SL. The expert consensus guidelines for treating depression in bipolar disorder. J Clin Psychiatry 1998; 59(suppl 4): 73–79.
7. Soares JC, Mann JJ. The anatomy of mood disorders—review of structural neuroimaging studies. Biol Psychiatry 1997; 41:86–106.
8. Moller HJ, Bottlender R, Grunze H, Strauss A, Wittmann J. Are antidepressants less effective in the acute treatment of bipolar I compared to unipolar depression? J Affect Disord 2001; 67:141–146.
9. Bottlender R, Rudolf D, Jager M, Strauss A, Moller HJ. Are bipolar I depressive patients less responsive to treatment with antidepressants than unipolar depressive patients? Results from a case control study. Eur Psychiatry 2002; 17:200–205.
10. Ghaemi SN, Rosenquist KJ, Ko JY, Baldassano CF, Kontos NJ, Baldessarini RJ. Antidepressant treatment in bipolar versus unipolar depression. Am J Psychiatry 2004; 161: 163–165.
11. Prien RF, KIett CJ, Caffey EM. Lithium carbonate and imipramine in prevention of affective episodes. Arch Gen Psychiatry 1973; 29:420–425.
12. Prien RF, Kupfer DJ, Mansky PA, Small JG, Tuason VB, Voss CB, Johnson WE. Drug therapy in the prevention of recurrences in unipolar and bipolar affective disorders. Arch Gen Psychiatry 1984; 41:1096–1104.
13. Shapiro DR, Quitkin FM, Fleiss JL. Response to maintenance therapy in bipolar illness: effect of index episode. Arch Gen Psychiatry 1989; 46:401–405.
14. MacQueen GM, Young LT, Marriott M, Robb J, Begin H, Joffe RT. Previous mood state predicts response and switch rates and patients with bipolar depression. Acta Psychiatr Scand 2002; 105:414–418.
15. Quitkin FM, Kane J, Rifkin A, Ramos-Lorenzi JR, Nayak DV. Prophylactic lithium carbonate with and without imipramine for bipolar I patients. Arch Gen Psychiatry 1981; 38:902–907.
16. Young LT, Joffe RT, Robb JC, MacQueen GM, Marriott M, Patelis-Siotis I. Double-blind comparison of addition of a second mood stabilizer versus an antidepressant to an initial mood stabilizer for treatment of patients with bipolar depression. Am J Psychiatry 2000; 157:124–126.
17. McIntyre RS, Mancini DA, McCann S, Srinivasan J, Sagman D, Kennedy SH. Topiramate versus bupropion SR when added to mood stabilizer therapy for the depressive phase of bipolar disorder: a preliminary single-blind study. Bipolar Disord 2002; 4: 207–213.
18. Johnstone EC, Owens DGC, Lambert MT, Crow TJ, Frith CD, Done DJ. Combination tricyclic antidepressant and lithium maintenance medication in unipolar and bipolar depressed patients. J Affect Disord 1990; 20:225–233.
19. Nemeroff CB, Evans DL, Gyulai L, Sachs GS, Gowden CL, Gergel IP, Oakes R, Pitts CD. Double-blind, placebo-controlled comparison of imipramine and paroxetine in the treatment of bipolar depression. Am J Psychiatry 2001; 158:906–912.

20. Fagiolini A, Frank E, Cherry CR, Houck PR, Novick DM, Buysse DJ, Kupfer DJ. Clinical indicators for the use of antidepressants in the treatment of bipolar I depression. Bipolar Disord 2002; 4:277–282.
21. Frenkle WG, Perlis RH, Deckersbach T, Grandin D, Gray SM, Sachs GS, Nierenberg AA. Bipolar depression: relationship between episode length and antidepressant treatment. Psychol Med 2002; 32:1417–1423.
22. Faedda GL, Baldessarini RJ, Tohen M, Strakowski SM, Waternaux C. Episode sequence in bipolar disorder and response to lithium treatment. Am J Psychiatry 1991; 148: 1237–1239.
23. Angst J. Switch from depression to mania—a record study over decades between 1920 and 1982. Psychopathology 1985; 18:140–154.
24. Wehr, TA, Goodwin FK. Can antidepressants cause mania and worsen the course of affective illness?. Am J Psychiatry 1987; 144:1403–1411.
25. Altshuler L, Post R, Leverich G, Mikalauskas K, Rosoff A, Ackerman L. Antidepressant-induced mania and cycle acceleration: a controversy revisited. Am J Psychiatry 1995; 152:1130–1138.
26. Post RM, Altshuler LL, Frye MA Suppes T, Rush AJ, Keck PE Jr, McElroy SL, Denicoff KD, Leverich GS, Kupka R, Nolen WA. Rate of switch in bipolar patients prospectively treated with second-generation antidepressants as augmentation to mood stabilizers. Bipolar Disord 2001; 3:259–265.
27. Post RM, Leverich GS, Altshuler LL, Frye MA, Suppes TM, Keck PE Jr, McElroy SL, Kupka R, Nolen WA, Grunze H, Walden J. An overview of recent findings of the Stanley Foundation Bipolar Network (part I). Bipolar Disord 2003; 5:310–319.
28. Stoll A, Mayer P, Kolbrener M, Goldstein E, Suplit B, Lucier J, Cohen B, Tohen M. Antidepressant-associated mania: a controlled comparison with spontaneous mania. Am J Psychiatry 1994; 141:1642–1645.
29. Boerlin, H, Gitlin M, Zoellner L, Hammen, C. Bipolar depression and antidepressant-induced mania: a naturalistic study. J Clin Psychiatry 1998; 59:374–379.
30. Serretti A, Artioli P, Zanardi R, Rossini D. Clinical features of antidepressant associated manic and hypomanic switches in bipolar disorder. Prog Neuropsychopharmacol Biol Psychiatry 2003; 27:751–757.
31. Nasrallah HA, Lyskowski J, Schroeder D. TCA-induced mania: differences between switchers and non-switchers. Biol Psychiatry 1982; 17(2):271–274.
32. Henry C, Sorbara F, Lacoste J, Gindre C, Leboyer M. Antidepressant-induced mania in bipolar patients: identification of risk factors. J Clin Psychiatry 2001; 62:255–294.
33. Henry C, Lacoste J, Bellivier F, Verdoux H, Bourgeois ML, Leboyer M. Temperament in bipolar illness: impact on prognosis. J Affect Disord 1999; 56:103–108.
34. Yildiz A, Sachs G. Do antidepressants induce rapid cycling? A gender-specific association. J Clin Psychiatry 2003; 64(7):814–818.
35. Lewis JL, Winokur G. The induction of mania: a natural history study with controls. Arch Gen Psychiatry 1982; 39:303–306.
36. Parker G. Do the newer antidepressants have mood stabilizing properties?. Aust N Z J Psychiatry 2002; 36:427–428.
37. Bottlender R, Rudolf D, Straus A, Moller HJ. Mood stabilizers reduce the risk of developing antidepressant-induced maniform states in acute treatment of bipolar I depressed patients. J Affect Disord 2001; 63:79–83.
38. Wehr TA, Goodwin FK. Rapid cycling in manic-depressive induced by tricyclic antidepressants. Arch Gen Psychiatry 1979; 36:555–559.
39. Wehr T, Sack D, Rosenthal N, Cowdry R. Rapid cycling affective disorder: contributing factors and treatment responses in 51 patients. Am J Psychiatry 1988; 145(2):179–184.
40. Koukopoulos A, Caliari B, Tundo A, Minnai G, Floris G, Regnialdi D, Tondo L. Rapid cyclers, temperament, and antidepressants. Compr Psychiatry 1983; 24:249–258.

41. Akiskal HS, Djenderedjian AH, Rosenthal RH, Khani MK. Cyclothymic disorder: validating criteria for inclusion in the bipolar affective group. Am J Psychiatry 1977; 134:1227–1233.
42. Koukopoulous A, Koukopoulos A. Agitated depression as a mixed state and the problem of melancholia. Psychiatr Clin N Am 1999; 22:547–564.
43. Bottlender R, Sato T, Kleindienst N, Straus A, Moller HJ. Mixed depressive features predict maniform switch during treatment of depression in bipolar I disorder. J Affect Disord 2004; 63:79–83.
44. Kane JM, Quitkin FM, Rifkin A, Ramos-Lorenzi JR, Saraf K, Howard A, Klein DF. Prophylactic lithium with and without imipramine for bipolar I patients: a double blind study. Psychopharmacol Bull 1981; 17(1):144–145.
45. Jann MW, Bitar AH, Rao A. Lithium prophylaxis of tricyclic-antidepressant-induced mania in bipolar patients. Am J Psychiatry 1982; 139(5):683–684.
46. Himmelhoch JM, Fuchs CZ, Symons BJ. A double-blind study of tranylcypromine treatment of major anergic depression. J Nerv Ment Dis 1982; 170(10):628–634.
47. Himmelhoch JM, Thase ME, Mallinger AG, Houck P. Tranylcypromine versus imipramine in anergic bipolar depression. Am J Psychiatry 1991; 148:910–916.
48. Silverstone T. Moclobemide vs. imipramine in bipolar depression: a multicentre double-blind clinical trial. Acta Psychiatr Scand 2001; 104:104–109.
49. Simpson SG, DePaulo R. Fluoxetine treatment of bipolar II depression. J Clin Psychopharmacol 1991; 11(1):322–332.
50. Rammasubbu R. Dose response relationship of SSRI treatment-emergent hypomania in depressive disorderes. Acta Psychiatr Scand 2001; 104:236–238.
51. Megna JL, Devitt PJ. Treatment of bipolar depression with twice-weekly fluoxetine: management of antidepressant-induced mania. Ann Pharmacother 2001; 35:45–47.
52. Peet M. Induction of mania with selective serotonin re-uptake inhibitors and tricyclic antidepressants. Br J Psychiatry 1994; 164:549–550.
53. Amsterdam JD, Garcia-Espana F, Fawcett J. Efficacy and safety of fluoxetine in treating bipolar II major depressive episode. J Clin Psychopharmacol 1998; 18(6):435–440.
54. Shulman RB, Scheftner WA, Nayudu S. Venlafaxine-associated mania. J Clin Psychopharmacol 2001; 21(2):239–241.
55. Stoner SC, Williams RJ, Worrel J, Ramlatchman L. Possible venlafaxine-induced mania. J Clin Psychopharmacol 1999; 19:184–185.
56. Amsterdam J. Efficacy and safety of venlafaxine in the treatment of bipolar II major depressive episode. J Clin Psychopharmacol 1998; 18(5):414–417.
57. Vieta E, Martinez-Aran A, Goikolea JM, Torrent C, Colom F, Benabarre A, Reinares M. A randomized trial comparing paroxetine and venlafaxine in the treatment of bipolar depressed patients taking mood stabilizers. J Clin Psychiatry 2002; 63:508–512.
58. Erfuth A, Michael N, Stadtland C, Arolt V. Bupropion as add-on strategy in difficult-to-treat bipolar depressive patients. Neuropsychobiology 2002; 45(suppl 1):33–36.
59. Haykal RF, Akiskal H. Bupropion as a promising approach to rapid cycling bipolar II patients. J Clin Psychiatry 1990; 51:450–455.
60. Goren JL, Levin GM. Mania with bupropion: a dose related phenomenon? Ann Pharmacother 2000; 34:619–621.
61. Joffe RT, MacQueen GM, Marriott M, Robb J, Begin J, Young LT. Induction of mania and cycle acceleration in bipolar disorder: effect of different classes of antidepressant. Acta Psychiatr Scand 2002; 105:427–430.
62. Fogelson DL, Bystritsky A, Pasnau R. Bupropion in the treatment of bipolar disorders: the same old story? J Clin Psychiatry 1992; 53:443–446.
63. Shopsin B. Bupropions prophylactic efficacy in bipolar affective illness. J Clin Psychiatry 1983; 44(5, sec 2):74–78.
64. Wright G, Galloway L, Kim J, Dalton M, Miller L, Stern W. Bupropion in the long-term treatment of cyclic mood disorders: mood stabilizing effects. J Clin Psychiatry 1985; 46:22–25.

65. Sachs GA, Lafer B, Stoll AL, Banov M, Thibault AB, Tohen M, Rosenbaum JF. A double-blind trial of bupropion versus desipramine for bipolar depression. J Clin Psychiatry 1994; 55:391–393.
66. Gabbay V, O'Dowd MA, Asnis GM. Combined antidepressant treatment: a risk factor for switching in bipolar patients. J Clin Psychiatry 2002; 63(4):367–368.
67. Zubieta JK, Demitrack MA. Possible bupropion precipitation of mania and a mixed affective state. J Clin Psychopharmacol 1991; 11(5):327–328.
68. Henry C. Response to combined antidepressant treatment: a risk factor for switching in bipolar patients. J Clin Psychiatry 2002; 63(4):368.
69. Kupfer DJ, Carpenter LL, Frank E. Possible role of antidepressants in precipitating mania and hypomania in recurrent depression. Am J Psychiatry 1988; 145:804–808.
70. Nelson JC, Schottenfeld RS, Conrad CD. Hypomania after desipramine withdrawal. Am J Psychaitry 1983; 140:624–625.
71. Mirin SM, Schatzberg AF, Creasey DE. Hypomania and mania after withdrawal of tricyclic antidepressants. Am J Psychiatry 1981; 138:87–89.
72. Goldstein TR, Frye MA, Denicoff KD, Smith-Jackson E, Leverich GS, Bryan AL, Ali OS, Post RM. Antidepressant discontinuation-related mania: critical prospective observation and theoretical implications in bipolar disorder. J Clin Psychiatry 1999; 60: 563–567.
73. Zajecka J, Tracy KA, Mitchell. Discontinuation symptoms after treatment with serotonin reuptake inhibitors: a literature review. J Clin Psychiatry 1997; 58:291–297.
74. Altshuler L, Kiriakos L, Calcagno J, Goodman R, Gitlin M, Frye M, Mintz J. The impact of antidepressant discontinuation versus antidepressant continuation on one-year risk for relapse of bipolar depression: a retrospective chart review. J Clin Psychiatry 2001; 62:512–616.
75. Altshuler L, Suppes T, Black D, Nolen WA, Keck PE, Frye MA, McElroy S, Kupka R, Grunze H, Walden J, Leverich G, Kenicoff K, Luckenbaugh D, Post R. Impact of antidepressant discontinuation after acute bipolar depression remission on rates of depressive relapse at 1-year follow-up. Am J Psychiatry 2003; 260:1252–1262.
76. Moller HJ, Grunze H. Have some guidelines for the treatment of acute bipolar depression gone too far in the restriction of antidepressants? Eur Arch Psychiatry Clin Neurosci 2000; 250:57–68.
77. Calabrese JR, Bowden CL, Sachs GS, Ascher JA, Monaghan E, Rudd GD. A double-blind placebo-controlled study of lamotrigine monotherapy in outpatients with bipolar I depression. J Clin Psychiatry 1999; 60:79–88.

23
Combination Therapy in Bipolar Disorder

Adrian J. Lloyd and Allan H. Young
School of Neurology, Neurobiology and Psychiatry, University of Newcastle upon Tyne, Royal Victoria Infirmary, Newcastle upon Tyne, U.K.

BACKGROUND

Monotherapy for bipolar disorder is well established as both acute and prophylactic treatment, the most familiar drugs used in these roles being lithium, sodium valproate, and carbamazepine (1–3). The choice of agent can be guided at least in part by the subtype of bipolar disorder, for instance, valproate possibly being more efficacious in rapid cycling illness than lithium (3–6). More recently, a literature is beginning to accumulate regarding the efficacy of other anticonvulsant drugs (1,4,7–14)—although gabapentin does not have evidence to support this action (15,16)—and also antipsychotic medication, particularly atypical antipsychotic drugs (17–20). Indeed, formal recognition of the value of such alternative agents in the treatment of bipolar disorder is now reaching the level at which, at least in the case of atypical antipsychotics, licenses are beginning to be granted to them specifically for this purpose.

The availability of an increasing number of medications with recognized mood-stabilizing capabilities opens an ever wider potential for their use in combination when a single agent has proved ineffective in either controlling acute illness or preventing illness relapse. A literature regarding combination treatment is gradually developing and informing practice (4,5,18,21–24), and an important trial of lithium and valproate as monotherapies and in combination is in progress (25), but, at present, empirical data remain scant (3,23,26).

A further aspect of bipolar illness often necessitating the use of more than one drug is a persistent depressive phase that is unresponsive to treatment with a mood stabilizer alone. Most clinicians will thus be familiar with the use of an antidepressant medication in combination with a mood stabilizer in the treatment of bipolar depression. Despite its frequent use, this is not a combination treatment without risk, with evidence suggesting the induction of both mania and increased frequency of cycling with antidepressants (27–32).

In an attempt to guide clinicians in the use of the ever more complex array of potential treatments for bipolar disorder, there have been published both expert consensus guidelines (5) and, more recently, evidence-based guidelines that recognize both the type and strength of evidence for specific treatments and the international differences in the approach to drug use in this illness (24). There is relatively little work that attempts to systematically assess actual clinical practice in the treatment of bipolar disorder, and such evidence as does exist may be locality specific and/or reflect evolving practice over time. That which does exist, however, gives some indication of increasing complexity of medication regimes in bipolar disorder but variability in the closeness of this to recommended practice and guidelines (33–38).

This chapter will consider, in turn, reasons that combination therapy might be required, the relationship of such combination treatment to illness phase, potential risks of combination treatment, and finally a summary of advantages and difficulties relating to various potential combinations of medications.

WHY COMBINE TREATMENT FOR BIPOLAR DISORDER?

There are a number of situations in which combination treatment of bipolar disorder might be indicated. Such circumstances may be more or less common dependent upon the phase of illness considered and this is examined with specific regard to illness phase in the next section. In addition to treatment of the mood swings that characterize the illness, it may be necessary to add specific treatments for particular groups of symptoms such as agitation or psychotic phenomena. A particularly significant feature of manic illness that often warrants treatment in its own right is sleep reduction. The need for specific use of antidepressants in bipolar depression has been alluded to previously. Anxiety symptoms may accompany both the depressive and manic phases of illness and may warrant symptomatic treatment when prominent. A further need for progressively more complex medical treatment may be difficulty in establishing euthymia following an acute illness episode or difficulty in maintaining euthymia without frequent relapses.

COMBINATION TREATMENTS IN RELATION TO ILLNESS SUBTYPE AND ILLNESS PHASE

The evolution of polypharmacological treatment initiated in an acute phase of illness will depend upon the context of the presentation. Use of more than one medication in a first manic presentation may arise from the need to control a combination of agitation, possible psychotic symptoms and elevated mood. Acute control of disturbed behavior is an initial high priority with fine tuning of mood-stabilizing medication following thereafter. There is an acknowledged contrast between European and North American practice in this regard with antipsychotic medications being used in the former case initially, mood-stabilizing treatment being added in thereafter. North American practice is focused more on the rapid introduction and upward titration of mood-stabilizing medication in this situation (5,24). The situation where a patient already on maintenance treatment has suffered a manic relapse is clearly somewhat different as, provided medication compliance has continued, the initial mood-stabilizing regime is already established at the point of relapse, additional medications being added to this to control the acute illness dependent upon the nature of its presentation. Similarly, the order of instituting different treatment modalities for a depressive episode will be dependent upon the stage in illness course in which the patient presents. The most common and readily recognized circumstance would be that of a depressive phase of illness in an individual who has already experienced a manic episode and is thus defined as bipolar. Less easy to prepare for and define is the initial presentation of a bipolar patient with a depressive phase that will, by definition, be initially treated as a unipolar depression. The likely use of combination treatment in this scenario is when depressed mood alters to the opposite (i.e., elevated) pole. While discontinuation of the antidepressant will be the normal first step in such situations, recurrence of low mood may indicate the need for further treatment. Should a mood stabilizer alone be unsuccessful in achieving this, there is a clear logic to re-introducing an antidepressant in combination with it.

Illness Subtype

Bipolar I disorder, with comparable duration and intensity of manic and depressive swings, may warrant the addition of specific treatments for either pole of the illness on top of an established mood-stabilizing regime dependent upon the responsiveness and severity of those individual episodes of abnormal mood. Should the illness prove resistant to effective prophylactic monotherapy, there is clearly a need for prophylactic treatments to be combined.

Bipolar II disorder, by contrast, is often characterized by more lengthy and persistent depressive episodes and relatively time limited and/or mild elevations in mood. It can thus be conceived that combination treatment in bipolar 2 disorder is more likely to require longer-term use of an antidepressant should mood stabilizer use (single or multiple) be insufficient to effectively control both poles of the illness.

Rapid cycling bipolar disorder is defined by the occurrence of four or more affective episodes in a 12-month period (39) and there is evidence to support better response of this subtype of illness to anticonvulsants, specifically valproate, than to lithium (6,40). Rapid cycling illness is often difficult to treat (40) and thus might be considered a form of bipolar illness more likely to result in the institution of combination treatment aimed at gaining greater control of fluctuations in mood. The relationship here between combination treatments that include antidepressants is complex, as antidepressants may be required for effective recovery from depressive swings but, in their own right, may precipitate or worsen rapid cycling (40–42).

Phases of Illness

Acute manic or mixed affective presentations include, in varying combinations, elevated mood, agitation and overactivity, reduced need for sleep, and psychotic symptoms. Initial treatment would normally be with (following the European and North American tradition, respectively) an antipsychotic medication with a mood stabilizer then introduced or rapidly titrated sodium valproate or lithium with supplementation with an antipsychotic if necessary. Concurrent with this initial antimanic treatment, there may be necessity for use of an hypnotic, benzodiazepines being generally preferred for this purpose. Benzodiazepines might also be necessary to further reduce the waking agitated state. Administration of all medications should normally be oral, but all the earlier-mentioned categories have specific drugs available for parenteral administration also in patients unwilling to accept oral treatment (5,24,43). The usual aim on gaining control of symptoms would be to gradually reduce combined treatment to arrive at maintenance medication with a single mood stabilizer. Both typical and atypical antipsychotics have antimanic properties in the acute phase (19,44–46). Continued symptoms in the face of adequate treatment with a first-line mood stabilizer or antipsychotic is an indication for the addition of further medication such as a second mood stabilizer or an antipsychotic in addition to the initial mood stabilizer. The combination of treatments for which most evidence exists is perhaps that of lithium and an anticonvulsant such as valproate or carbamazepine (21,23,47). Other investigated combinations with efficacy beyond that of monotherapy include those of a typical or an atypical antipsychotic with valproate or lithium (20,46,48,49).

Presentation of an individual already on established long-term treatment for bipolar disorder in a manic or hypomanic state will usually have treatment with any pre-existing mood stabilizer optimized and compliance ensured. Should such treatment prove inadequate, addition of an atypical antipsychotic or second mood stabilizer, as noted earlier, is appropriate (5,24).

Ongoing treatment resistance may warrant the addition of a third or subsequent antimanic agent with caution due to potential interactions.

Treatment of depression may be required in the following contexts. A patient may present with a depressive episode while not on mood-stabilizing medication but with a previous history of mania; alternatively, depression may occur within the context of pre-existing prophylactic treatment for bipolar disorder.

In the case of depression in an individual without prophylactic mood-stabilizing treatment, there is a significant risk of precipitating switch to mania if antidepressants are used unopposed by a mood stabilizer (24,27,28,41,42). Treatment should thus initially be with the establishment of mood-stabilizing/antimanic medication (lithium, an appropriate anticonvulsant or antipsychotic) (24,50) along with institution of an antidepressant, most appropriately an SSRI, there being evidence to suggest that this group of antidepressants have lesser propensity to result in a switch to mania (27,28,41,51). Use of an antipsychotic in the depressive phase of illness is appropriate, particularly where psychotic symptoms themselves are present (24). Monotherapy with a mood stabilizer may be sufficient to treat bipolar depression, although the evidence for this is limited (5,24). There is some evidence for lamotrigine having a particular role in bipolar depression, with the aim of improving depressed mood without tendency to induce mania (10,11).

The occurrence of a depressive episode in a patient taking prophylactic mood-stabilizing treatment warrants an initial assessment to ensure adequate serum levels of mood stabilizer where appropriate. It may be possible to address precipitating stressors in a practical or psychological sense without the need for antidepressants (24), but should depressive symptoms be severe, or the earlier-mentioned maneuvers not be effective, addition of an antidepressant is appropriate. Revision of any pre-existing antidepressant treatment should be considered as would be the case with unipolar depression, provided the protective presence of an antimanic agent is established. Detail of the relative merits of individual antidepressants in bipolar disorder has been reviewed in Chapter 22. There is little evidence specific to the management of treatment-resistant depression in bipolar disorder (24), the recommendation for management of this thus being that it should be treated in the same way as unipolar treatment-resistant depression in the context of mood-stabilizing/antimanic medication.

The final broad area of treatment in which combination medication may be indicated is that of prophylaxis. Monotherapies have been dealt with in other chapters and it is the addition of subsequent treatments to these strategies that will be considered here.

An individual on a simple monotherapy regime for prophylactic treatment will inevitably encounter stressful situations or changes in day-to-day life that may increase the risk of an acute episode due to stress or, for example, disruption of sleep–wake cycles. In these circumstances, short-term addition of a benzodiazepine to aid coping with anxiety or, alternatively, as an hypnotic may be an effective strategy to increase prophylactic defenses against an acute episode of illness. Such strategies might also be useful to tackle very early signs of recurrence. For individuals where such medication is insufficient, particularly with regard to manic relapse, short-term adjunctive treatment with an additional antimanic agent (e.g., an antipsychotic) may be appropriate.

Where strategies of short-term adjunctive treatment are insufficient to prevent relapse, longer-term combination treatment is appropriate, the choice of medications being logically dictated by the predominant illness pattern experienced by the patient. Where mania dominates the character of illness episodes, the most appropriate combinations with initial mood stabilizers would be the addition of one or, if necessary, progressively more medications with defined antimanic properties. Lithium, valproate, and antipsychotics, particularly atypical antipsychotics, would be appropriate in this case. When recurrent illness is more frequently characterized by depression, a second mood stabilizer such as lamotrigine (more effect in the depressive than the manic phase of illness) is appropriate. Further propensity to depression might be treated by the addition of an antidepressant in the longer term, provided there was no evidence of an increased risk of the individual switching to mania when compared with the usual course of their illness.

Where ongoing treatment resistance continues in the face of relatively straightforward combination therapy, there is evidence for the utility of clozapine as a further adjunctive measure (20).

As mentioned previously, rapid cycling bipolar illness is noted to be difficult to treat. Combination therapy in this situation may have both positive and negative aspects and requires close examination. Should antidepressants be thought to contribute to rapid cycling presentations they should be reduced and discontinued, further treatment focusing on combination mood stabilizer use. Choice of these medications should be guided by the character of relapses experienced by a patient. It is necessary to assess the benefit or otherwise of treatment regimes over a period (e.g., 6 months) that allows assessment of frequency of cycling (24).

Thyroid hormones: There is limited evidence only for the efficacy of supraphysiological thyroid hormone use in bipolar depression specifically. The use of this as strategy for augmentation in unipolar depression, however, is well recognized and thus its role in treatment-resistant bipolar depression may be justifiable where other measures have been ineffective (18,52–54).

Use of depot typical neuroleptics has a limited place in maintenance treatment (55), particularly where concordance issues arise, and thus the combination of these agents with other drugs used in a more short-term role for either pole of the illness warrants note. There are yet no specific data relating to the recently launched depot atypical antipsychotic risperidone.

HAZARDS OF COMBINATION TREATMENT

As with all complex pharmacological management, there is an increasing risk of the combined impact of side effects and of potential interactions between drugs as the number of medications taken by any individual progressively increases. Cross-checking of such possibilities and close follow-up of patients are thus essential, particularly when instituting new combination treatments. A number of possible problems warrant particular attention and should be considered alongside the potential advantages of the suggested combination therapies in the section on Drug Combinations.

Lithium combined with an SSRI may give increased risk of serotonergic side effects. Lamotrigine combined with valproate has a particular risk of increased likelihood of skin rashes including Stevens–Johnson syndrome and toxic epidermal necrolysis. A number of anticonvulsants and antipsychotic medications have the propensity to cause bone-marrow suppression, and thus hematological monitoring is warranted in such cases. Carbamazepine, in combination with other drugs, presents the clinician with the problem of liver enzyme induction, and thus the potential for plasma levels of these concurrently prescribed agents to be lowered. Although use of antidepressants in the context of antimanic treatment reduces the risk of switch to mania, it does not remove this and thus careful monitoring is required when antidepressants are introduced. It would seem reasonable to select an antidepressant with a shorter half-life such that, should there be a need for discontinuation, clearance from the patient's system will be reasonably rapid. Weight gain is a problem with many of the individual medications used in bipolar disorder, and combination treatment may thus compound this to an extent that patients may not tolerate. Prospective discussion of this issue is recommended, as is ongoing monitoring of weight and related concerns and ways in which they may be addressed. In embarking upon combination therapy there is a risk of progressive addition of medications—i.e., increasing polypharmacy—owing to some of those treatments employed being ineffective rather than incompletely effective. There can be no clear guidance on removal of apparently ineffective treatments when they have not yet been tried in combination with other drugs in a particular patient. Regular review of efficacy and tolerability with appropriate adjustments to medication regime is perhaps the only rational advice that can be given under such circumstances in a situation where specific evidence is lacking.

DRUG COMBINATIONS

With an increasing number of drugs with available evidence to suggest efficacy in bipolar disorder, there is an ever-increasing number of potential treatment combinations that could be considered. Table 1 summarizes potential benefits and recognized problems of a number of two-drug antimanic and/or mood-stabilizing combinations with specific reference to their use in bipolar illness (20,48,56–70). With any attempted combination therapy, it is essential that up-to-date information on known potential interactions be consulted. The risk of adverse effects and interactions clearly increases with the number of drugs combined, thus additional caution is needed when moving beyond the combination of two drugs, but it is hoped that the information given here will aid the choice of the components of combination therapies. This section does not attempt to give treatment algorithms—as this is a field that is developing rapidly a textbook is perhaps not the best place for such time-sensitive material. For additional guidance, the reader is referred to treatment guidelines currently in existence and to their subsequent revisions (5,24,27,43,51,71). The detailed nature of the individual mood stabilizers has already been considered in Chapter 14.

Combinations of these drugs with others for antidepressant, anxiolytic, or sedative actions have been considered in principle in preceding sections of this chapter. For details of the drugs themselves and their indications, see Chapters 14, 20 and 22.

Table 1 Recognized Benefits and Problems of 2-Drug Combinations in Bipolar Illness[a]

Problems	Actions / advantages								
	Lithium	Valproate	Carbamazepine	Typical antipsychotics	Atypical antipsychotics	Clozapine	Benzodiazepines	Lamotrigine	Topiramate
Lithium		Safe Possible synergism Possibly particularly useful in rapid cycling	Safe Possible synergism Possibly particularly useful in rapid cycling	Summative effects of drugs. Only very weak evidence for synergism.	Evidence for effectiveness of risperidone, olanzapine & quetiapine	Reports of efficacy	Well tolerated. Effective - possible alternative to neuroleptics, especially in acute mania	Well tolerated – specifically may have indication for depressive pole	Well tolerated, additional efficacy in treatment resistance
Valproate	No problem with interaction		Effective – possible synergism	Effective. Summative effects	Evidence for effectiveness of risperidone, olanzapine & quetiapine	Contradictory data regarding efficacy	As for lithium	Effective – especially in consideration of depressive pole	As lithium
Carbamaze-pine	Possible neurotoxicity in absence of raised lithium level	Reduction in plasma concentration of valproate. Possible inhibition of carabamazepine metabolism by valproate. Possible neurotoxicity		Effective Summative effects		Not safe	As for lithium	Insufficient data to conclude re benefits	As lithium
Typical antipsych-otics	Possible increase in neurotoxic effect. Possible increased risk of extrapyramidal effects. Increased risk of ventricular arrhythmias with thioridazine		Enhanced metabolism of antipsychotics		Little advantage	Little advantage	Enhanced sedative effects in acute phase		
Atypical antipsych-otics	Increased risk of ventricular arrhythmias with amisulpiride	Valproate and olanzapine – increased risk of neutropenia	Enhanced metabolism of antipsychotics	increased risk of adverse effects		Other than during crossover of treatment – not indicated	Enhanced sedative effect in acute phase		Some evidence for effective combination. Possible advantage of weight loss
Clozapine	Possible increase in neurological side effects	Possible neurotoxicity. Possible hepatic encephalopathy	Not safe – combined risk of haematological adverse effects.	increased risk of adverse effects	increased risk of adverse effects		Enhanced sedative effect		
Benzodiaz-epines			No specific adverse effect of combination	Enhanced sedation	Enhanced sedation	Enhanced sedation		Sedative and anxiolytic effects of benzodiazepine: summative	
Lamotrigine		Raised plasma level of lamotrigine Risk of rashes – including Stevens-Johnson syndrome. Very gradual introduction of lamotrigine.reuqired	Some reports of neurotoxicity – equivocal evidence. May lower plasma lamotrigine level						
Topiramate			Plasma topiramate level lowered						

[a]Blank cells indicate little specific research data available.

Other combination therapies are generally considered as add-ons to other regimes: thyroid hormone administration to supraphysiological (150% normal) levels (regardless of previous thyroid status) has some limited evidence for specific efficacy in rapid cycling bipolar disorder (52) as an augmentation strategy. This is also recognized in expert opinion as having a role in non-rapid cycling illness also (5). Bone-density monitoring should be considered in post-menopausal women in whom such strategy is employed. Additional treatments that are occasionally employed as augmentation strategies in bipolar disorder but for which specific evidence is relatively weak or lacking include the use of calcium antagonists, omega-3 fatty acids, adrenergic antagonists, and tiagabine for mania and the use of dopamine agonists, omega-3 fatty acids, inositol, buspirone, and calcium antagonists in depression (5,56,71).

SUMMARY

As in many illnesses, there is evidence to suggest that progressively more complex combination therapies are effective in gaining additional control of symptoms in patients who have been previously unresponsive or only partially responsive to treatment. Some strategies for such treatments are suggested here and are expanded upon in other treatment guidelines (5,24). Difficulty arises in that the more complex the treatment regime considered the fewer data specific to that combination that are available. There is an ongoing need for research into this area in order to inform practice in the future and it is an area in which evidence is likely to develop. A controlled trail of lithium and valproate as monotherapies and in combination is currently underway and may address more robustly the role of this particular combination in maintenance treatment (25,26). There is an obvious need for detailed discussion of combination therapies, their advantages, and disadvantages with the patients for whom they are being recommended, and while this section has dealt only with combination of pharmacological treatments, the role of psychological and psychotherapeutic interventions in bipolar disorder should be emphasized in its importance running alongside the drug regimes. Of particular relevance to combination drug treatment is evidence that work in a cognitive framework can increase concordance with medication regimes, thus optimizing the benefit derived from them at any particular level of complexity of treatment (72,73). A further treatment strategy that might also run alongside or as an alternative to combination medication therapies is ECT—see Chapter 25.

In conclusion, it should be acknowledged that, provided adverse effects and possible difficulties for a patient with any specific drug or combination of drugs allows, incremental complexity of combination treatment in bipolar disorder is warranted when adequate response to more simple treatment regimes has not been achieved.

REFERENCES

1. Bowden CL. New concepts in mood stabilization: evidence for the effectiveness of valproate and lamotrigine. Neuropsychopharmacology 1998; 19:194–199.
2. Davis JM, Janicak PG, Hogan DM. Mood stabilizers in the prevention of recurrent affective disorders: a meta-analysis. Acta Psychiatr Scand 1999; 100:406–417.
3. Bowden CL, Lecrubier Y, Bauer M, Goodwin G, Greil W, Sachs G, von Knorring L. Maintenance therapies for classic and other forms of bipolar disorder. J Affect Disord 2000; 59:S57–S67.

4. Nemeroff CB. An ever-increasing pharmacopoeia for the management of patients with bipolar disorder. J Clin Psychiatry 2000; 61:19–25.
5. Sachs GS, Printz DJ, Kahn DA, Carpenter D, Docherty JP. The expert consensus guideline series: medication treatment of bipolar disorder 2000. Postgrad Med 2000; Special Report:1–104.
6. Young AH, MacRitchie KAN, Calabrese JR. Treatment of bipolar affective disorder. Br Med J 2000; 231:1302–1303.
7. Sporn J, Sachs G. The anticonvulsant lamotrigine in treatment-resistant manic-depressive illness. J Clin Psychopharmacol 1997; 17:185–189.
8. Bowden CL, Calabrese JR, McElroy SL, Rhodes LJ, Keck PE Jr, Cookson J, Anderson J, Bolden-Watson C, Ascher J, Monaghan E, Zhou J. The efficacy of lamotrigine in rapid cycling and non-rapid cycling patients with bipolar disorder. Biol Psychiatry 1999; 45:953–958.
9. Botts SR, Raskind J. Gabapentin and lamotrigine in bipolar disorder. Am J Health Syst Pharm 1999; 56:1939–1944.
10. Calabrese JR, Bowden CL, McElroy SL, Cookson J, Andersen J, Keck PE Jr, Rhodes L, Bolden-Watson C, Zhou J, Ascher JA. Spectrum of activity of lamotrigine in treatment-refractory bipolar disorder. Am J Psychiatry 1999; 156:1019–1023.
11. Calabrese JR, Bowden CL, Sachs GS, Ascher JA, Monaghan E, Rudd GD. A double-blind placebo-controlled study of lamotrigine monotherapy in outpatients with bipolar I depression. Lamictal 602 Study Group. J Clin Psychiatry 1999; 60:79–88.
12. McElroy SL, Suppes T, Keck PE, Frye MA, Denicoff KD, Altshuler LL, Brown ES, Nolen WA, Kupka RW, Rochussen J, Leverich GS, Post RM. Open-label adjunctive topiramate in the treatment of bipolar disorders. Biol Psychiatry 2000; 47:1025–1033.
13. Walden J, Schaerer L, Schloesser S, Grunze H. An open longitudinal study of patients with bipolar rapid cycling treated with lithium or lamotrigine for mood stabilization. Bipolar Disord 2000; 2:336–339.
14. Calabrese JR, Keck PE Jr, McElroy SL, Shelton MD. A pilot study of topiramate as monotherapy in the treatment of acute mania. J Clin Psychopharmacol 2001; 21: 340–342.
15. Pande AC, Crockatt JG, Janney CA, Werth JL, Tsaroucha G. Gabapentin in bipolar disorder: a placebo-controlled trial of adjunctive therapy. Gabapentin Bipolar Disorder Study Group. Bipolar Disord 2000; 2:249–255.
16. Frye MA, Ketter TA, Kimbrell TA, Dunn RT, Speer AM, Osuch EA, Luckenbaugh DA, Cora-Ocatelli G, Leverich GS, Post RM. A placebo-controlled study of lamotrigine and gabapentin monotherapy in refractory mood disorders. J Clin Psychopharmacol 2000; 20:607–614.
17. Ghaemi SN, Goodwin FK. Use of atypical antipsychotic agents in bipolar and schizoaffective disorders: review of the empirical literature. J Clin Psychopharmacol 1999; 19:354–361.
18. Sachs GS, Thase ME. Bipolar disorder therapeutics: maintenance treatment. Biol Psychiatry 2000; 48:573–581.
19. Tohen M, Jacobs TG, Grundy SL, McElroy SL, Banov MC, Janicak PC, Sanger T, Risser R, Zhang F, Toma V, Francis J, Tollefson GD, Breier A. Efficacy of olanzapine in acute bipolar disorder. Arch Gen Psychiatry 2000; 57:841–849.
20. Suppes T, Webb A, Paul B, Carmody T, Kraemer H, Rush AJ. Clinical outcome in a randomized 1-year trial of clozapine versus treatment as usual for patients with treatment-resistant illness and a history of mania. Am J Psychiatry 1999; 156: 1164–1169.
21. Post RM, Ketter TA, Pazzaglia PJ, Denicoff K, George MS, Callahan A, Leverich G, Frye M. Rational polypharmacy in the bipolar affective disorders. Epilepsy Res Suppl 1996; 11:153–180.
22. Peselow ED, Fieve RR, Difiglia C, Sanfilipo MP. Lithium prophylaxis of bipolar illness. The value of combination treatment. Br J Psychiatry 1994; 164:208–214.

23. Solomon DA, Keitner GI, Ryan CE, Miller IW. Lithium plus valproate as maintenance polypharmacy for patients with bipolar I disorder: a review. J Clin Psychopharmacol 1998; 18:38–49.
24. Goodwin GM, Consensus Group of the British Association for Psychopharmacology. Evidence-based guidelines for treating bipolar disorder: recommendations from the British Association for Psychopharmacology. J Psychopharmacol 2003; 17:149–173.
25. Rendell JM, Juszczak E, Hainsworth J, Gucht EV, Healey C, Morriss R, Ferrier N, Young AH, Young H, Goodwin GM, Geddes JR. Developing the BALANCE trial—the role of the pilot study and start-up phase. Bipolar Disord 2004; 6:26–31.
26. Geddes J, Goodwin G, Cookson J. Bipolar disorder: clinical uncertainty, evidence-based medicine and large-scale randomised trials. Use of antipsychotic drugs and lithium in mania. Br J Psychiatry 2001:178 (Suppl 41): s191–s194.
27. Nolen WA, Bloemkolk D. Treatment of bipolar depression, a review of the literature and a suggestion for an algorithm. Neuropsychobiology 2000; 42:11–17.
28. Thase ME, Sachs GS. Bipolar depression: pharmacotherapy and related therapeutic strategies. Biol Psychiatry 2000; 48:558–572.
29. Goldstein TR, Frye MA, Denicoff KD, Smith-Jackson E, Leverich GS, Bryan AL, Ali SO, Post RM. Antidepressant discontinuation-related mania: critical prospective observation and theoretical implications in bipolar disorder. J Clin Psychiatry 1999; 60:563–567; quiz 568–569.
30. Compton MT, Nemeroff CB. The treatment of bipolar depression. J Clin Psychiatry 2000; 61 (Suppl 9): 57–67.
31. Moller HJ, Grunze H. Have some guidelines for the treatment of acute bipolar depression gone too far in the restriction of antidepressants? Eur Arch Psychiatry Clin Neurosci 2000; 250:57–68.
32. Ghaemi SN, Lenox MS, Baldessarini RJ. Effectiveness and safety of long-term antidepressant treatment in bipolar disorder. J Clin Psychiatry 2001; 62:565–569.
33. Verdoux H, Gonzales B, Takei N, Bourgeois M. A survey of prescribing practice of antipsychotic maintenance treatment for manic-depressive outpatients. J Affect Disord 1996; 38:81–87.
34. Fenn HH, Robinson D, Luby V, Dangel C, Buxton E, Beattie M, Kraemer H, Yesavage JA. Trends in pharmacotherapy of schizoaffective and bipolar affective disorders: a 5-year naturalistic study. Am J Psychiatry 1996; 153:711–713.
35. Ahmed Z, Anderson IM. Treatment of bipolar affective disorder in clinical practice. J Psychopharmacol 2001; 15:55–57.
36. Frye MA, Ketter TA, Leverich GS, Huggins T, Lantz C, Denicoff KD, Post RM. The increasing use of polypharmacotherapy for refractory mood disorders: 22 years of study. J Clin Psychiatry 2000; 61:9–15.
37. Frangou S, Raymont V, Bettany D. The Maudsley bipolar disorder project. A survey of psychotropic prescribing patterns in bipolar I disorder. Bipolar Disord 2002; 4: 378–385.
38. Lloyd AJ, Harrison CL, Ferrier IN, Young AH. The pharmacological treatment of bipolar affective disorder: practice is improving but could still be better. J Psychopharmacol 2003; 17:230–233.
39. American Psychiatric Association. Diagnostic and Statistical Manual of Mental Disorders. Washington: American Psychiatric Association Press, 1994.
40. Calabrese JR, Shelton MD, Rapport DJ, Kujawa M, Kimmel SE, Caban S. Current research on rapid cycling bipolar disorder and its treatment. J Affect Disord 2001; 67:241–255.
41. Peet M. Induction of mania with selective serotonin re-uptake inhibitors and tricyclic antidepressants. Br J Psychiatry 1994; 164:549–550.
42. Montgomery SA, Schatzberg AF, Guelfi JD, Kasper S, Nemeroff C, Swann A, Zajecka J. Pharmacotherapy of depression and mixed states in bipolar disorder. J Affective Disord 2000; 59:S39–S56.

43. Grunze H, Kasper S, Goodwin G, Bowden C, Baldwin D, Licht RW, Vieta E, Moller HJ. Disorders WTFoTGfB. World Federation of Societies of Biological Psychiatry Task Force on Treatment Guidelines for Bipolar Disorder. The World Federation of Societies of Biological Psychiatry (WFSBP) guidelines for the biological treatment of bipolar, disorders, part II: treatment of mania. World J Biol Psychiatry 2003; 4:5–13.
44. Cookson J. Use of antipsychotic drugs and lithium in mania. Br J Psychiatry 2001; 178 (Suppl 41): s148–s156.
45. Keck PE Jr, McElroy SL, Strakowski SM. Anticonvulsants and antipsychotics in the treatment of bipolar disorder. J Clin Psychiatry 1998; 59:74–81; discussion 82.
46. Sachs GS, Grossman F, Ghaemi SN, Okamoto A, Bowden CL. Combination of a mood stabilizer with risperidone or haloperidol for treatment of acute mania: a double-blind, placebo-controlled comparison of efficacy and safety. Am J Psychiatry 2002; 159: 1146–1154.
47. Denicoff KD, Smith-Jackson EE, Disney ER, Ali SO, Leverich GS, Post RM. Comparative prophylactic efficacy of lithium, carbamazepine, and the combination in bipolar disorder. J Clin Psychiatry 1997; 58:470–478.
48. Tohen M, Chengappa KN, Suppes T, Zarate CA Jr, Calabrese JR, Bowden CL, Sachs GS, Kupfer DJ, Baker RW, Risser RC, Keeter EL, Feldman PD, Tollefson GD, Breier A. Efficacy of olanzapine in combination with valproate or lithium in the treatment of mania in patients partially nonresponsive to valproate or lithium monotherapy. Arch Gen Psychiatry 2002; 59:62–69.
49. Muller-Oerlinghausen B, Retzow A, Henn FA, Giedke H, Walden J. Valproate as an adjunct to neuroleptic medication for the treatment of acute episodes of mania: a prospective, randomized, double-blind, placebo-controlled, multicenter study. European Valproate Mania Study Group. J Clin Psychopharmacol 2000; 20:195–203.
50. Bottlender R, Rudolf D, Strauss A, Moller HJ. Mood-stabilisers reduce the risk of developing antidepressant-induced maniform states in acute treatment of bipolar I depressed patients. J Affect Disord 2001; 63:79–83.
51. Grunze H, Kasper S, Goodwin G, Bowden C, Baldwin D, Licht R, Vieta E, Moller HJ. World Federation of Societies of Biological Psychiatry Task Force on Treatment Guidelines for Bipolar Disorder. World Federation of Societies of Biological Psychiatry (WFSBP) guidelines for biological treatment of bipolar disorders. Part I: treatment of bipolar depression. World J Biol Psychiatry 2002; 3:115–124.
52. Bauer MS, Whybrow PC. Rapid cycling bipolar affective disorder. II. Treatment of refractory rapid cycling with high-dose levothyroxine: a preliminary study. Arch Gen Psychiatry 1990; 47:435–440.
53. Nemeroff CB. Augmentation strategies in patients with refractory depression. Depress Anxiety 1996; 4:169–181.
54. Joffe RT, Sokolov ST, Singer W. Thyroid hormone treatment of depression. Thyroid 1995; 5:235–239.
55. Littlejohn R, Leslie F, Cookson J. Depot antipsychotics in the prophylaxis of bipolar affective disorder. Br J Psychiatry 1994; 165:827–829.
56. Freeman MP, Stoll AL. Mood stabilizer combinations: a review of safety and efficacy. Am J Psychiatry 1998; 155:12–21.
57. Ghaemi SN, Sachs GS. Long-term risperidone treatment in bipolar disorder: 6-month follow up. Int Clin Psychopharmacol 1997; 12:333–338.
58. Ghaemi SN, Sachs GS, Baldassano CF, Truman CJ. Acute treatment of bipolar disorder with adjunctive risperidone in outpatients. Can J Psychiatry Rev Canad Psychiatrie 1997; 42:196–199.
59. Guille C, Sachs GS, Ghaemi SN. A naturalistic comparison of clozapine, risperidone, and olanzapine in the treatment of bipolar disorder. J Clin Psychiatry 2000; 61:638–642.
60. Sokolski KN, Denson TF. Adjunctive quetiapine in bipolar patients partially responsive to lithium or valproate. Prog Neuropsychopharmacol Biol Psychiatry 2003; 27: 863–866.

61. Vieta E, Parramon G, Padrell E, Nieto E, Martinez-Aran A, Corbella B, Colom F, Reinares M, Goikolea JM, Torrent C. Quetiapine in the treatment of rapid cycling bipolar disorder. Bipolar Disord 2002; 4:335–340.
62. Delbello MP, Schwiers ML, Rosenberg HL, Strakowski SM. A double-blind, randomized, placebo-controlled study of quetiapine as adjunctive treatment for adolescent mania. J Am Acad Child Adolesc Psychiatry 2002; 41:1216–1223.
63. Frye MA, Ketter TA, Altshuler LL, Denicoff K, Dunn RT, Kimbrell TA, Cora-Locatelli G, Post RM. Clozapine in bipolar disorder: treatment implications for other atypical antipsychotics. J Affect Disord 1998; 48:91–104.
64. Vieta E, Torrent C, Garcia-Ribas G, Gilabert A, Garcia-Pares G, Rodriguez A, Cadevall J, Garcia-Castrillon J, Lusilla P, Arrufat F. Use of topiramate in treatment-resistant bipolar spectrum disorders. J Clin Psychopharmacol 2002; 22:431–435.
65. Chengappa KN, Rathore D, Levine J, Atzert R, Solai L, Parepally H, Levin H, Moffa N, Delaney J, Brar JS. Topiramate as add-on treatment for patients with bipolar mania. Bipolar Disord 1999; 1:42–53.
66. Guille C, Sachs G. Clinical outcome of adjunctive topiramate treatment in a sample of refractory bipolar patients with comorbid conditions. Prog Neuropsychopharmacol Biol Psychiatry 2002; 26:1035–1039.
67. Suppes T. Review of the use of topiramate for treatment of bipolar disorders. J Clin Psychopharmacol 2002; 22:599–609.
68. Vieta E, Goikolea JM, Olivares JM, Gonzalez-Pinto A, Rodriguez A, Colom F, Comes M, Torrent C, Sanchez-Moreno J. 1-year follow-up of patients treated with risperidone and topiramate for a manic episode. J Clin Psychiatry 2003; 64:834–839.
69. Vieta E, Sanchez-Moreno J, Goikolea JM, Torrent C, Benabarre A, Colom F, Martinez-Aran A, Reinares M, Comes M, Corbella B. Adjunctive topiramate in bipolar II disorder. World J Biol Psychiatry 2003; 4:172–176.
70. BMA/RPS. British National Formulary. London and Wallingford: British Medical Association/Royal Pharmaceutical Society, 2003.
71. American Psychiatric Association. Practice guideline for the treatment of patients with bipolar disorder (revision). Am J Psychiatry 2002; 159:1–50.
72. Scott J, Pope M. Nonadherence with mood stabilizers: prevalence and predictors. J Clin Psychiatry 2002; 63:384–390.
73. Scott J, Tacchi MJ. A pilot study of concordance therapy for individuals with bipolar disorders who are non-adherent with lithium prophylaxis. Bipolar Disord 2002; 4:386–392.

24

Expected Side-Effect Profile of Medications and Their Management

John W. Newcomer*, **Nuri B. Farber, Dan Haupt, and Peter Fahnestock**
Department of Psychiatry, Washington University School of Medicine, St. Louis, Missouri, U.S.A.

INTRODUCTION

This chapter aims to discuss common adverse events associated with the treatment of bipolar disorder, including some uncommon but important adverse events that deserve critical clinical consideration. It is not meant to be a compendium of all possible treatment-related adverse events, which are often referred to as side effects. While this chapter provides some discussion of treatment management issues, it should not be taken as a substitute for clinical judgment. Pharmacological treatments for bipolar disorder are associated with a large number of potential side effects, but these can be categorized into events with and without major clinical significance. The last section of this chapter will focus on adverse events, such as weight gain, related changes in insulin resistance, hyperglycemia, dyslipidemia, and the metabolic syndrome, that can potentially contribute to the most common causes of medical comorbidity and mortality in treated patients with psychiatric disorders.

Patients with severe mental illnesses, including bipolar disorder, experience increased mortality from medical causes, including particularly cardiovascular disease, in comparison to the general population (1). Because of this increased medical risk, clinicians should work to simultaneously maximize the clinical efficacy of bipolar treatment while minimizing side effects, such as weight gain and related changes in metabolic parameters, such as lipid levels and blood pressure, that could further increase risk for medical comorbidity in this high-risk population.

* Dr. Newcomer received grant support in 2004 and 2005 from NIMH, the National Alliance for Research on Schizophrenia and Depression (NARSAD), and the Sidney R. Baer Foundation, as well as investigator-initiated grant support from Pfizer Inc., Janssen Pharmaceutica, and Bristol-Myers Squibb (BMS). In addition, Dr. Newcomer has served as a consultant for BMS, Pfizer Inc., Janssen Pharmaceutica, AstraZeneca, GlaxoSmithKline, and Wyeth Research. Dr. Newcomer has no significant conflict of interest as defined by the Washington University School of Medicine Conflict of Interest Policy.

SIDE EFFECTS OF LITHIUM

Lithium continues to serve as the gold-standard mood stabilizer and a model for other agents being explored for their possible mood-stabilizing properties (2). Despite its narrow therapeutic index, lithium remains an important treatment for bipolar disorder. Adverse reactions to lithium that occur in >10% of patients include polydipsia, nausea, diarrhea, abnormal taste, and tremor (2). Less common side effects include polyuria, polydipsia, cognitive dulling, tremor, gastrointestinal distress, weight gain, acne, and hypothyroidism, with risk of most adverse events related to dose or plasma concentrations (2). For some patients, mild impairment in cognitive function is the most troubling side effect and is believed to be a major source of medication noncompliance. Sometimes, the clinician can find a dose that produces adequate control of bipolar disorder without producing this symptomatic complaint but this, unfortunately, is not always the case.

Monitoring of serum lithium levels allows for more precise adjustment of lithium dosing in order to potentially decrease the risk of serious adverse events. A 12-hour post-dose level between 0.8 and 1.2 mM is considered optimal for most individuals. Such standard lithium levels are more effective than lower levels during maintenance treatment, but tend to be associated with increased adverse effects (3), that can discourage patient compliance. Some individuals may benefit from slightly higher levels, but this benefit must be balanced with the increased likelihood of toxicity.

One common early mild neurologic side effect of lithium is a fine, rapid tremor. More severe neurological symptoms and signs, such as coarse motor tremor, dysarthria, ataxia, aphasia, vertigo, muscle twitching, and hyperreflexia can also be observed, and indicate toxicity. Mild toxicity occurs in most people in the 1.5–2.0 mM range. Additional signs of mild toxicity include nausea, vomiting, and mental sluggishness. A level of 4.0 mM is in the severe toxic range, is usually associated with acute renal failure, and requires the use of renal dialysis. Other consequences associated with severe toxicity include gross mental impairment (e.g., impaired consciousness, delirium, and coma), seizures, muscle fasciculations, hyperreflexia, and cardiac conduction delays (4). Although this symptomatology is usually reversible within 5 to 10 days, uncorrected lithium toxicity can result in death either from cardiac arrhythmias or viscous secretions in the respiratory tract. Evidence of even mild toxicity should prompt a decrease in lithium dosing, regardless of serum lithium levels (5). Of note, because lithium-related gastric irritation can produce nausea and vomiting in the absence of toxicity, these two symptoms alone may not herald the onset of toxicity (5).

Risk factors for side effects and toxicity during lithium therapy include pregnancy, organic brain disorder, reduced renal clearance with increasing age or renal disease, physical illness with diarrhea and/or vomiting, diuretic and/or other concomitant pharmacotherapy, and high sodium excretion and/or low sodium intake (6). In cases where toxicity occurs in an individual who has been on a stable dose of lithium, the clinician should determine the likely cause of the elevated lithium level. Major causes include: (1) deliberate or accidental overdose, (2) inadequate intake of free water in the setting of diabetes insipidus (see below), (3) decreased intake of sodium, (4) worsening renal function, and (5) drug–drug interactions. Several drugs are known to decrease lithium's renal clearance (7). Thiazide diuretics, by producing sodium loss in the kidneys, cause increased renal re-absorption of lithium. The prescribing of a thiazide diuretic should be accompanied by a decrease in the prescribed lithium dose. One approach is to initially decrease the lithium dose by 50% and then to adjust the dose upwards using lithium levels as a guide. Potassium-sparing diuretics (e.g., spironolactone and amiloride) and diuretics acting on the loop of Henle (e.g., furosemide and ethacrynic acid) appear to cause minimal increases in lithium retention. However, lithium toxicity can occur even with these "safer" diuretics if excessive volume depletion occurs. Angiotensin converting enzyme (ACE) inhibitors have also been noted to increase lithium levels possibly by inducing renal sodium depletion or by altering the rennin–angiotension–aldosterone system. Use of non-steroidal anti-inflammatory drugs (NSAIDs) also has been associated with increases in lithium levels. Because they can be obtained without a prescription, clinicians must be especially careful in asking about their potential use. Aspirin and acetaminophen appear to not have this effect and may be better choices if they can be substituted for an NSAID in a particular patient. A recent retrospective population-based study of drug-induced lithium toxicity in the elderly (8) concluded that the use of loop diuretics or ACE inhibitors increased the risk of hospitalization for lithium toxicity. While neither thiazide diuretics nor NSAIDs were strongly linked with an increase in risk of hospitalization due to lithium toxicity in this study, the use of surrogate indicators of toxicity and other methodological limitations suggest that clinicians should remain cautious when prescribing these agents (8).

Possible metabolic-endocrine abnormalities, renal impairment, and cardiac abnormalities on electrocardiogram (ECG) have been linked to lithium use, and are briefly discussed below (9). Lithium can produce several metabolic-endocrine disturbances. Discussed further in Section "Side Effects Associated with Metabolic Adverse Events," weight gain over 12 months of $\geq$5% of total baseline body weight frequently occurs. Hyperparathyroidism has also been noted to occur, possibly due to lithium disrupting the ability of serum calcium levels to control parathyroid secretion. The lithium-induced endocrine disturbance that requires the greatest clinical attention is hypothyroidism. Although reports of lithium-induced hypothyroidism range from 5% to 35% due to variability in the criteria for diagnosis and the sensitivity of laboratory tests, the prevalence of clinical hypothyroidism is estimated to be more likely in the range of 5% and more common in women (10). Lithium's hypothyroid effect appears to occur by several mechanisms, the primary one being a decrease in the release of thyroid hormones. This effect does not persist after the cessation of lithium therapy. Monitoring should occur prior to initiating lithium treatment and at routine intervals, usually yearly, throughout treatment. Probing for clinical evidence of hypothyroidism (e.g., cold intolerance, hair loss, constipation, and dry skin) and obtaining yearly thyroid stimulating hormone (TSH) measurements usually suffice to detect its presence. Given that several symptoms of hypothyroidism (e.g., weight loss, fatigue, cognitive impairment, apathy, and poor mood) mimic symptoms of affective disorder, clinicians should consider obtaining a TSH in individuals who appear to have poorly controlled affective illness. TSH measures can vary over time in normal individuals. Thus, it is usually best to verify an abnormal result with a second TSH level, and possibly a free thyroxine (T_4) level. Given the long half-life of thyroid hormones, verification of changes in levels should occur after a 3-month interval. Because the effect of lithium is reversible, thyroid supplementation (and not lithium discontinuation) is considered appropriate for those individuals found to be hypothyroid.

Nephrogenic diabetes insipidus is a common side effect of lithium treatment, estimated to occur in 50% of patients in one study (11). Nephrogenic diabetes insipidus is mainly a result of lithium inhibition of the distal tubule response to antidiuretic hormone. A subset of these patients will develop overt polyuria and polydipsia. In a minority of cases, significant volume depletion with concomitant rises in serum lithium levels can occur if a patient does not replace the fluid loss with adequate amounts of water. Amiloride can be used for symptomatic relief of nephrogenic diabetes insipidus in significantly affected individuals. Epithelial cellular swelling and glycogen deposition in the distal nephron has been associated with this impairment in renal tubular concentrating ability. The changes are reversible upon the cessation of lithium treatment. In the vast majority of patients, the inability to concentrate urine and its associated histological findings do not appear to predict subsequent permanent impairment in renal function (i.e., chronic renal insufficiency) (11–13).

These acute histological changes need to be differentiated from a second type of histological change that has been noted to occur in some lithium-treated patients. Initial reports of interstitial nephritis during lithium therapy raised concerns that chronic lithium treatment could produce irreversible nephrotoxicity (14) and have encouraged several investigators to examine this potential link. This chronic focal interstitial nephropathy is distinct from the acute histological changes discussed above. The prevalence of these interstitial changes in humans and their importance for renal functioning is still undetermined. In general, the better-designed studies tend to not find an association between long-term lithium treatment and renal insufficiency (15). However, concern still exists that these results are missing a subgroup of individuals who develop chronic renal insufficiency secondary to lithium exposure. One recent retrospective analysis (16) found that 20% of patients on long-term lithium developed evidence of renal insufficiency, defined as serum creatinine ≥1.5 mg/dL, after 11 to 15 years of lithium exposure.

Episodes of acute lithium toxicity, and the presence of medications or diseases known to adversely affect renal function (e.g., diabetes mellitus, hypertension) have been associated with individuals who subsequently develop renal insufficiency. Reduction in the dose or discontinuation of lithium leads to improved renal function in at least half of individuals. This improvement might be greatest in patients with creatinine clearance greater than 40 mL/min (17). Until research better delineates if specific subgroups of patients are at risk of developing chronic renal insufficiency, the clinician should obtain baseline measures of serum creatinine prior to the initiation of lithium treatment in all patients and continue to monitor serum creatinine periodically (every 6–12 months) throughout treatment. Evidence of increasing creatinine levels should prompt a careful evaluation of the patient's renal function and whether the dose of lithium should be decreased or another medication used in its place.

As noted above, lithium toxicity is associated with conduction delays and cardiac arrhythmias. However, lithium treatment within the clinical dose range has minimal effects in persons with normal cardiac function. A large number of individuals (estimated to be 20–30% of treated patients) will develop T-wave flattening and inversion. The effect on T-waves is believed to be secondary to lithium's accumulation inside of cardiac myocytes with subsequent intracellular hypokalemia. The decrease in intracellular potassium prolongs re-polarization resulting in a flatter T-wave. The effect does not produce symptoms and usually disappears with cessation of treatment. However, with toxic doses of lithium the lengthening of re-polarization, indicated by increases in the QT interval, can increase the theoretical risk for ventricular arrhythmias. Similar effects may also be significant at therapeutic doses but only in the setting of ventricular irritability; for this reason, lithium should be avoided in patients with frequent premature ventricular contractions and other high-risk conditions such as recent myocardial infarction or congestive heart failure. In part because the QT prolonging effect of lithium does not occur at therapeutic levels, routine ECG monitoring is not generally indicated.

Lithium can also directly affect the sinus node producing a sinus bradycardia. The exact mechanism by which lithium produces this effect is unknown. While the bradycardia is usually asymptomatic, it can have serious consequences in susceptible individuals. High-risk individuals include persons over the age of 50, those with history of syncope, transient ischemic attacks, palpitations, dyspnea on exertion, angina, or known cardiac disease that could affect sinus node function. Such individuals should receive a screening ECG to rule out sinus node dysfunction. If lithium treatment is indicated for such individuals, Holter monitoring is frequently needed to further assess safety. In severely affected individuals for whom lithium is the only treatment option, implantation of a pacemaker might allow for the safe use of this salt (18–20).

Lithium is also a teratogen and is classified as a Category D drug (21) that is typically not used in pregnant women. Lithium treatment in the first trimester is associated with a 4–12% chance of major congenital malformations, in comparison to a 2–4% risk in an untreated comparison group (22). Its ability to produce Ebstein's fetal cardiac malformation (0.1–0.2% absolute risk) during the first trimester of pregnancy is well known. Because of these risks, its use in the first trimester must be carefully weighed (9,23). Clinicians should rule out the possibility of pregnancy by history or laboratory exam prior to initiating lithium treatment in women of childbearing age. Use of lithium in the later months of pregnancy and during parturition is complicated by fluctuations in fluid balance and the renal clearance of lithium. Lithium levels need to be followed closely (e.g., every 2 weeks) and the dose adjusted appropriately. Finally, because lithium is secreted into breast milk, women are urged to not breast-feed their infants.

The potential adverse events associated with lithium therapy and the narrow therapeutic index underscore the need for careful selection of appropriate patients. Both the patient and their prescribing physician need to be able to work together to closely monitor adverse events during treatment.

SIDE EFFECTS OF ANTIEPILEPTIC DRUGS USED FOR BIPOLAR DISORDER

Introduction

Antiepileptic medications are being used increasingly in bipolar patients because of their potential mood-stabilizing properties. A large number of anticonvulsants are currently being evaluated for potential use in bipolar disorder, but evidence to date suggests that not all will be efficacious. Discussion will be restricted to the three agents with the greatest amount of positive clinical data and experience—valproate, lamotrigine, and carbamazepine. Data for side effects come primarily from large trials of patients taking these agents for seizure disorders (24).

Valproate

Approved by the U.S. Food and Drug Administration in 1995, valproate was the first anticonvulsant recognized as a mood stabilizer. In the United Kingdom, valproate semi-sodium was licensed for the acute treatment of mania in 2001 (25). Valproate is generally well tolerated and has been associated with a lower incidence of side effects in comparison to lithium in the treatment of bipolar patients (26). Valproate's common dose-related side effects are sedation, gastrointestinal effects (e.g., anorexia, nausea, dyspepsia, indigestion, vomiting, and diarrhea), benign elevations in hepatic transaminase, and neurological symptoms (most commonly tremor). Modest weight gain, dizziness, and asthenia are also common, as are benign changes in menstrual cycle. Gastrointestinal complaints, benign hepatic transaminase elevations, and sedation are more likely to occur at the initiation of treatment and usually subside with dose reduction and/or time. Gastrointestinal complaints may be more frequent during treatment with valproic acid and sodium valproate than during use of an enteric-coated divalproex sodium formulation (27). While rare, hepatotoxicity, pancreatitis, and thrombocytopenia are potentially serious side effects associated with valproate, requiring vigilance on the part of the treating clinician (9). Based in part on the risk of neural tube defects, use of valproate should be avoided in pregnant women (28).

Lamotrigine

Lamotrigine has been increasingly used in the treatment of bipolar disorder, perhaps due to the fact that it might have less adverse cognitive and metabolic effects and it might be more efficacious against the depressive phase of the illness. Dizziness, diplopia, ataxia, blurred vision, nausea, vomiting, ataxia, somnolence, and headache are some of the more commonly occurring side effects. Since most of these effects are dose related, dose reduction may minimize these effects (24,29). Clinicians should be aware that the combination of valproate and lamotrigine could increase plasma concentrations of lamotrigine, whereas the combination of carbamazepine and lamotrigine results in lower lamotrigine concentrations.

The most serious potential side effects of lamotrigine are dermatologic events, including Stevens–Johnson syndrome and toxic epidermal necrolysis. A benign allergic rash can be seen in approximately 10% of patients (30). Available data suggest that Stevens–Johnson syndrome and toxic epidermal necrolysis are rare events (31) that occur early in the course of treatment (usually within the first 2 months) and may be more frequent with rapid dose escalation and in patients taking valproate (30,32). Thus, it is recommended that the drug be slowly increased to its therapeutic dose over the initial 2 months. This slow titration might limit usefulness in acutely ill patients. Although Stevens–Johnson syndrome and toxic epidermal necrolysis are rare (31), their initial presentation might be difficult to distinguish from more benign drug rashes, resulting in treatment discontinuation by some clinicians when a rash appears. It can be helpful to screen prospective patients for rash prior to initiation of treatment in order to avoid unnecessary discontinuation related to a preexisting rash.

Carbamazepine

Carbamazepine is a tricyclic compound that is structurally similar to imipramine, with many of the same adverse effects, especially at high doses (e.g., conduction delays, serotonin syndrome when used with a monoamine oxidase inhibitor, and hypotension). It has been in use for approximately four decades for the treatment of trigeminal neuralgia, and was approved as an anticonvulsant in 1974 in the United States (33). While it was the first anticonvulsant that was used clinically to treat people with bipolar disorder, it has never been evaluated in a double-blind, placebo-controlled, randomized trial in the treatment of any phase of bipolar disorder. Accordingly, it is not approved for uses related to bipolar disorder by the U.S. FDA. As with other anticonvulsants, carbamazepine produces dose-related CNS adverse events. These effects include diplopia, blurred vision, fatigue, nausea, vertigo, nystagmus, ataxia, and sedation. These effects may be self-limited, or may be improved by, dose reduction. In a recently reported study (34), the most commonly reported side effects of carbamazepine included headache (22%), dizziness (16%), and rash (13.0%). While the rash is usually benign, in rare cases a clinically significant exfoliative dermatitis can develop. Hyponatremia has also been reported (35). Because carbamazepine has also been reported to rarely produce leucopenia, thrombocytopenia, and liver enzyme elevations, most clinicians will usually obtain platelet counts, white blood cell counts, and liver function measures before initiating treatment and at several points (e.g., every 3 months) throughout the first year of treatment. Disturbances are usually mild and transient, though rarely they can be severe. Severe blood dyscrasias (e.g., anaplastic anemia and agranulocytosis) are rare (i.e., four occurrences in children were reported to the manufacturer from 1980 to 1989) and can result in fatality in approximately one in 575,000 treated patients per year (36). Probably the most complex medical aspect of carbamazepine treatment is the induction of multiple hepatic cytochrome P450 enzymes after brief treatment (e.g., approximately 2 weeks), resulting in the need to adjust (i.e., increase) the dose of this agent and other medications. Like valproate, carbamazepine has also been linked to neural tube defects and thus should be avoided during pregnancy.

SIDE EFFECTS OF ANTIPSYCHOTIC MEDICATIONS USED FOR BIPOLAR DISORDER

The use of antipsychotic medications for the treatment of mania was established many years ago using typical or first-generation antipsychotics. Recent evidence indicating effectiveness of second-generation agents for this indication, as well as for mixed states and possibly for relapse prevention using some agents, has increased the use of newer antipsychotics in the treatment of bipolar disorder. Key adverse events with older agents that limited their use included extrapyramidal symptoms, including tardive dyskinesia. This is particularly important in light of evidence that suggests that patients with bipolar disorder may be particularly vulnerable to tardive dyskinesia (37). In addition, antipsychotic treatment-emergent depression has been reported in approximately 10–20% of bipolar and schizoaffective patients treated with first generation antipsychotics (38–40). This may also be a risk in up to 10% of patients treated with some second-generation agents, although more research is needed in this area (41).

Risperidone

Risperidone was the first front-line second-generation antipsychotic introduced in the U.S. market. Like the other second-generation antipsychotics which followed, risperidone is less likely to cause extrapyramidal side effects within the therapeutic dose range, in comparison to first-generation antipsychotics, and therefore may be more appropriate as a maintenance antipsychotic than first-generation agents, especially in those patients who are sensitive to these effects (42–44). However, higher-than-currently recommended doses of risperidone are associated with an increased risk of extrapyramidal side effects, consistent with the actions of any dopamine type 2 (D_2) receptor antagonist (45).

As discussed in Section "Side Effects Associated with Metabolic Adverse Events," patients taking risperidone can gain a mean of 2.1 kg over 10 weeks of treatment (46). Common side effects of risperidone include insomnia (approximately 8% of patients), anxiety, agitation, and headache. Probably due to antagonism of α_1 adrenergic receptors, orthostatic hypotension can occur, particularly at the onset of treatment and with rapid dose titration (45). Less common but potentially troubling side effects include dizziness, nausea/vomiting, and somnolence (47). Case reports have linked risperidone with an apparently rare risk of neuroleptic malignant syndrome (NMS), a potentially life-threatening syndrome also associated with first-generation and other second-generation agents (48–51). It should be noted that there are no good data indicating the incidence rate at which any second-generation antipsychotic agent may cause NMS, with the current literature limited to case reports. However, it is important to note that NMS is a theoretical possibility whenever a D_2 dopamine receptor antagonist is given.

Olanzapine

Introduced after risperidone in the United States, olanzapine treatment offers somewhat more sedation than risperidone at comparable antipsychotic doses, providing a potential advantage in inpatient treatment settings or in unstable outpatients where sedation can be a desirable element of the treatment response. Like risperidone, olanzapine treatment is associated with dose-dependent extrapyramidal symptoms, although once again this risk is lower than with conventional agents (52). An important adverse event associated with antipsychotic therapy, discussed for all of the individual agents together in a separate section (Section "Side Effects Associated with Metabolic Adverse Events") below, is the weight gain that can occur to varying degrees with different antipsychotic treatments. Olanzapine treatment is associated with the largest risk for significant weight gain compared to all other second-generation agents except clozapine, with patients reported to gain a mean of more than 6 kg/year (53). The important clinical significance of this adverse event is also discussed in Section "Side Effects Associated with Metabolic Adverse Events."

Olanzapine, like most currently available antipsychotic agents, binds to a number of different biogenic amine receptors in addition to therapeutic actions at D_2 dopamine receptors, contributing to a complex profile of potential adverse events. Side effects occurring in roughly 5–10% of olanzapine-treated patients include postural hypotension, constipation, dizziness, and akathisia (52). Some of the more potentially serious side effects uncommonly associated with olanzapine include diarrhea, vomiting, unsteadiness, difficulty walking, or unusual muscle weakness. Case reports have associated the use of olanzapine with apparently rare incidents of NMS (54).

Amisulpride

Amisulpride has been available in France since 1988, although its launch into other European countries did not start until 1997, and it is not licensed in the United States. Amisulpride treatment is associated with a number of potential adverse events that can occur more commonly with active treatment than with placebo. Discussed below, amisulpride treatment is associated with modest impact on body weight during short- and long-term therapy (approximately 1.5 kg mean 1-year weight gain) (55), and this limited weight gain potential would predict that amisulpride might be associated with a relatively low risk of adverse metabolic events, although the limited availability of metabolic data makes it difficult to draw firm conclusions (56). Coulouvrat and Dondey-Nouvel (57) analyzed the results of 11 studies comprising a total of 1933 patients, concluding that amisulpride displayed a number of advantages over conventional antipsychotics from a safety standpoint. One key concern with amisulpride is that it can cause significant plasma prolactin elevations, but it is not apparent whether this is associated with higher rates of related adverse endocrine events than observed during treatment with other antipsychotics.

Insomnia, anxiety, and agitation are common side effects of amisulpride (occurring in 5–10% of patients), while less common adverse effects include somnolence, constipation, nausea, vomiting, and xerostomia, which may occur in up to 2% of patients (58). NMS has been reported with amisulpride (59). In a study in which amisulpride 400 mg daily was administered to healthy volunteers, no notable extrapyramidal complications were observed in the group overall, with some mild adverse effects on psychomotor and cognitive performance (60). In comparison to conventional antipsychotics, amisulpride has been associated with lower use of anti-Parkinsonian medication and with fewer dropouts due to side effects (61).

Quetiapine

Quetiapine has increasingly been used for the treatment of psychosis and other psychiatric conditions based on its efficacy in psychosis and mania, and in part on the potential therapeutic value of its sedating effect, which is at least comparable to that of olanzapine and greater than some other agents. As with many other antipsychotics, somnolence is the most common side effect of quetiapine. In clinical trials with quetiapine, this led to withdrawal from treatment in 1.4% of patients (62). In addition, excessive sedation has been reported as a result of quetiapine overdose (63). In the elderly, somnolence, dizziness, and orthostatic hypotension are the most common side effects of quetiapine (64). Quetiapine is reportedly associated with a mean of approximately 2 to 3 kg of weight gain over 1 year of treatment (65).

The general side-effect profile of quetiapine is similar to that of other second-generation antipsychotic medications, with the notable exception of a low incidence of extrapyramidal events across the dose range tested in large clinical trials. Side effects occurring in roughly 5–10% of patients include headache, dizziness, tachycardia, constipation, dry mouth, dyspepsia, and orthostatic hypotension (65). Early concerns, based on pre-clinical evidence, about a potential risk of cataracts during quetiapine treatment have not received further support in the extensive post-marketing experience with this agent. Case reports have associated the use of quetiapine with rare incidents of NMS (66).

Ziprasidone

Ziprasidone is one of the newest antipsychotic agents, and has found a particularly useful role in the treatment of patients sensitive to or already suffering from weight gain and resultant metabolic side effects (see Section "Side Effects Associated with Metabolic Adverse Events"). Ziprasidone has a side-effect profile that is generally like that of other second-generation agents including a low incidence of extrapyramidal side effects. However, there are several key exceptions to the adverse event profile that are worth noting. Discussed in Section "Side Effects Associated with Metabolic Adverse Events," ziprasidone is one of the newer second-generation antipsychotic drugs that is associated with less short- and long-term weight gain (e.g., a mean of approximately 1 kg over 1 year) (67–71), and this may be related to a similarly low level of metabolic risk. Compared to some other second-generation agents, ziprasidone produces less sedation, although this remains the most common side effect of treatment, as with all antipsychotic agents. In addition, ziprasidone is currently the only second-generation antipsychotic associated with significant inhibition of serotonin and norepinephrine reuptake (72), theoretically minimizing the likelihood of treatment-emergent depression, although clinical proof of this concept remains to be demonstrated. Somnolence, nausea, and mild or moderate headache are the most common adverse events during ziprasidone treatment (73). First-dose postural hypotension presumed to relate to α_1 adrenergic blockade has occurred in a minority of patients taking ziprasidone. Other side effects occurring in roughly 5–10% of patients include muscle weakness, constipation, dyspepsia, diarrhea, akathisia, and dizziness (74,75). Early concerns about the potential clinical significance of a modest prolongation of the corrected QT interval (QTc) on ECG measurements performed in clinical trials with ziprasidone have been tempered by the lack of evidence for potential drug–drug interactions that might worsen such an effect (76), by the absence of any reported adverse clinical outcomes attributable to QTc prolongation (e.g., torsades de pointes) (77,78), and by an appreciation that modest QTc prolongation in general is not clearly associated with ventricular arrhythmia and death (79). Ziprasidone use does not routinely require baseline ECG assessments or ECG monitoring. Compared to conventional antipsychotics, and similar to other second-generation agents, ziprasidone may offer fewer adverse effects on cognitive function (73). Case reports have associated the use of ziprasidone with rare incidents of NMS (80). Finally, unlike the primary metabolism of other atypical antipsychotics, aldehyde oxidase-mediated reduction to a dihydrometabolite is the primary metabolic pathway of ziprasidone. Recent efforts to systematically identify drugs that could inhibit this enzyme have reported no routinely encountered clinically significant inhibitors of aldehyde oxidase. This is in contrast to most other therapeutic agents discussed in this chapter, which are primarily metabolized through cytochrome P450 enzyme systems that can be induced or inhibited by other commonly encountered medications.

Aripiprazole

Aripiprazole is the newest antipsychotic agent in the United States. Some data suggest that it functions clinically as a partial agonist at the D_2 dopamine receptor, rather than as a full antagonist. Discussed in Section "Side Effects Associated with Metabolic Adverse Events," aripiprazole, like ziprasidone, offers a favorable weight gain profile in comparison to other second-generation agents (approximately 1 kg of weight gain after 1 year) (81). In general, Phase II and III trials with aripiprazole demonstrated a favorable safety profile, with a low risk of significant adverse effects, including extrapyramidal side effects, weight gain, cardiovascular abnormalities, hyperprolactinemia, hypercholesterolemia, or glucose dysregulation (82–86). Relatively common side effects (occurring in 5–10 % of cases or more) include somnolence, headache, muscle weakness, insomnia, lightheadedness, nausea, akathisia, and subjective anxiety (87). The most troublesome common side effect caused by aripiprazole tends to be nausea, which may precipitate vomiting. Vomiting has been found to occur in 12% of patients receiving aripiprazole (vs. 7% of patients receiving placebo). Fortunately, this is usually time-limited (i.e., first week of treatment) (88,89). There have been no case reports to date linking aripiprazole with NMS. However, this may simply be due to the medication's recent introduction. As noted above, NMS is a theoretically possible effect of any D_2 dopamine receptor antagonist.

Clozapine

Clozapine was the first "atypical" or second-generation antipsychotic developed, and remains in several ways the archetype of the class, with no notable extrapyramidal side effects at clinical dosages. Due to risk, albeit low, for life-threatening adverse reactions, described below, it is approved only for use after other antipsychotic agents have been tried and found to be ineffective. Clozapine is also unique among antipsychotic agents in demonstrating efficacy for "treatment-resistant" schizophrenic patients (most rigorously defined as those patients who have failed to respond to two or more other antipsychotic agents) (90). Clozapine is also the first antipsychotic to demonstrate efficacy for the prevention of suicide in schizophrenia patients (91).

The most common side effects of clozapine are prominent sedation (39% of patients) and dizziness/vertigo (19% of patients) (92). Excessive salivation (sialorrhea) occurs to some degree in 31% of patients (92); in some cases, this can be quite disturbing to patients and difficult to treat, with antimuscarinic agents reported to be helpful in some patients (93). Other common side effects, occurring in roughly 5–10% of patients, include headache, tremor, constipation, diaphoresis, dry mouth, and syncope. Orthostatic hypotension occurs in 9% of patients, and this effect may be particularly concerning in elderly patients. Less common but notable side effects include nausea/vomiting, diarrhea, and urinary abnormalities (92).

One potentially life-threatening adverse event of clozapine is agranulocytosis, a syndrome of bone marrow suppression characterized by a marked decrease in the number of granulocytes, with resultant immunosuppression. The risk of agranulocytosis has led to strict regulations regarding the monitoring of neutrophil levels in patients receiving clozapine; agranulocytosis is defined as an absolute neutrophil count of less than $500\,mm^{-3}$ (92).

An uncommon but noteworthy adverse event associated with clozapine is an increasing risk of seizures as dose is increased (e.g., 4–5% incidence at >500 mg/day). Clozapine is associated with a substantial risk of clinically significant weight gain, and related metabolic dysfunction, including diabetes mellitus and dyslipidemia (94,95). Clozapine has rarely been associated with NMS in case reports (96).

SIDE EFFECTS OF ANTIDEPRESSANTS FOR BIPOLAR DISORDER

Introduction

Newer antidepressants have provided clinicians with treatment options that offer similar efficacy in comparison to tricyclic and heterocyclic antidepressants, with a more tolerable side effect profile. For example, these agents lack the cardiac toxicity potential of tricyclic antidepressants and are subsequently much less lethal in the event of overdose. While additional research remains to be done, recent as well as older literature suggests that antidepressant medications might increase suicidal ideation during the initial phase of treatment response in patients with unipolar depression. Concerns in this area underscore the need for particularly close monitoring of all patients for adverse events and clinical response during the early course of treatment.

Uncontrolled case-report data have long suggested a potential risk of "inducing" mania when treating bipolar patients with antidepressant medications, with clinical suspicion heightened for noradrenergic reuptake inhibitors. However, this has not been consistently shown in controlled prospective studies, and the issue remains controversial (97). There is also a clinical suspicion that antidepressants may induce rapid cycling in patients with bipolar disorder (98), and that noradrenergic agents may be preferentially responsible. Again, close monitoring and clinical judgment will remain critical to successful treatment in the absence of clear evidence concerning the risk for these and other potential adverse events.

Selective Serotonin Reuptake Inhibitors

Due to their relatively selective binding profile, selective serotonin reuptake inhibitors (SSRIs) are well tolerated by most people. Of the most common side effects, ejaculatory failure or delay, nausea, and diarrhea are probably the most troubling. Other common side effects include dry mouth, somnolence, dizziness, headache, diarrhea, fatigue, and insomnia (99–102). Withdrawal phenomenon (e.g., paresthesia, irritability) have been reported for SSRIs, particularly from agents with relatively shorter half-lives, and careful attention should be paid during discontinuation from these agents. Fluoxetine, with its longer half-life, has been associated with fewer reports of withdrawal symptoms upon discontinuation. In addition to withdrawal, clinicians should be aware of the infrequent but potentially serious risk of serotonin syndrome, especially when combing SSRIs with other agents that can increase serotonin levels in the brain. Finally, clinicians should be aware that protein binding, hepatic metabolism, and metabolite activity differ across antidepressants, and this may have clinical significance in some patients (103). SSRIs are eliminated via a combination of hepatic and renal metabolism and special attention should be paid to the choice of agent and dosing in patients with renal or hepatic impairment. With regard to hepatic metabolism, different agents across this class are inhibitors to varying degrees of different hepatic cytochrome P450 microsomal isoenzymes, leading to potential pharmacokinetic interactions with drugs that are metabolized by these isoenzymes. These interactions are under intense and ongoing study and clinicians should consult published databases whenever they are unsure about whether a potential interaction exists or not.

Bupropion

Common side effects produced by bupropion in placebo-controlled trials and during post-marketing surveillance include anorexia, dry mouth, rash, sweating, tinnitus, tremor, abdominal pain, agitation, anxiety, dizziness, insomnia, myalgia, nausea, palpitations, pharyngitis, and urinary frequency (104). The activating effects of bupropion should be considered and monitored in treating bipolar patients. However, bupropion has been reported to have a lower risk for transition from depression to mania in comparison to other antidepressants. The most clinically significant side effect of bupropion is seizures. Bupropion has a reported seizure incidence of 0.4% at doses less than 450 mg/day and 4% at doses of 450–600 mg/day.

The sustained-release preparation has an incidence of 0.1% at doses up to 300 mg/day. In light of these data, caution is indicated when considering bupropion use in patients with a history of seizure, brain injury or EEG abnormality, or recent history of alcohol withdrawal. Bupropion can also affect serum lithium and valproate levels enough to require dosage adjustment with these two other agents.

Venlafaxine

Side effects reported in $>10\%$ of patients taking venlafaxine include migraine, postural hypotension, tachycardia, increased appetite, weight gain, arthralgia, substernal chest pain, chills, fever, neck pain, ecchymosis, edema, amnesia, confusion, depersonalization, vertigo, pruritus, abnormal accommodation, and mydriasis (105). One of the most medically troubling and common potential side effects of venlafaxine is sustained elevation of diastolic blood pressure. Patients taking venlafaxine should have their blood pressure monitored regularly.

Mirtazapine

Somnolence is a particularly common side effect during mirtazapine treatment, occurring in more than half of treated patients. Clinicians are often tempted to start antidepressants at very low doses and titrate slowly. Some evidence suggests that this should be avoided with mirtazapine. At doses lower than 15 mg, the antihistamine effect is potentially maximal but the serum concentration may be too low to block (this should be an "alpha" symbol) α_2 adrenergic receptors. This leads to "unopposed" sedation effects that might be partially compensated for above 15 mg when α_2 adrenergic blockade begins. Thus, raising the dose of mirtazapine may partially alleviate somnolence. Other common side effects include dry mouth, increased appetite, constipation, and potentially significant levels of weight gain.

SIDE EFFECTS ASSOCIATED WITH METABOLIC ADVERSE EVENTS

Increased rates of obesity (106), T2DM (107), and cardiovascular disease in patients with bipolar disorder (1) make it important for clinicians to distinguish between side effects that present tolerability issues (less severe, generally self-limited and manageable) and those that present more important safety issues that could contribute to medical morbidity and mortality. For example, increases in weight and adiposity are well-established risk factors for T2DM (108). Patients with bipolar disorder tend to have higher prevalence of overweight and obesity (106), possibly related to lifestyle factors such as reduced access to healthy foods and medical care as well as the effect of many psychotropic medications on weight and adiposity. This increased prevalence of obesity may be related to the increased rates of T2DM and cardiovascular disease in this population.

While medications used for treatment of severe mental illness may contribute to these comorbid medical conditions, severe mental illness in itself may be a risk factor for medical comorbidity. Several major neuropsychiatric illnesses, including depression, schizophrenia, Alzheimer's dementia, and bipolar affective disorder have been associated with impaired glucose regulation and elevated rates of diabetes mellitus (109).

Mental Disorders and Diabetes Mellitus

Available data suggest that depression increases the risk of developing insulin resistance and T2DM, and that T2DM may increase the risk of developing depression (94,110–114). Investigators have reported similarly elevated rates of diabetes in patients with bipolar disorder compared to general population samples (107). Similar relationships between diabetes and schizophrenia have been observed (109). A recent cross-sectional study in 26 hospitalized first-episode antipsychotic-naïve schizophrenic patients found that 15% of these patients had impaired fasting glucose (115). Compared to control subjects matched for lifestyle and anthropometric measures, schizophrenia patients exhibited higher mean fasting glucose concentrations (95.8 vs. 88.2 mg/dL), insulin levels (9.8 vs. 7.7 μU/mL), and cortisol levels [499.4 vs. 303.2 nmol/L] (115). The elevated plasma cortisol levels observed in this sample probably contributed to some of the increase in insulin resistance and plasma glucose, with hypercortisolemia not typically observed in treated patients with schizophrenia (116), so that this study may overestimate the degree of insulin resistance and hyperglycemia that might persist past the acute state. In any case, this study complements earlier reports in support of the view that patients with schizophrenia and perhaps other major mental disorders may have increased risk for insulin resistance and T2DM, independent of exposure to antipsychotic medications.

The risk factors and underlying causes for developing diabetes mellitus in the setting of a preexisting psychiatric condition, or for developing a psychiatric condition in the setting of preexisting diabetes mellitus, are incompletely understood. In the past several years, investigators have begun to focus on some of the disease, lifestyle and treatment factors that may contribute to this important comorbidity.

Complicating our understanding of the association between diabetes and psychiatric conditions are reports indicating that many of the medications used to treat conditions such as bipolar disorder and schizophrenia can contribute to changes in whole-body glucose metabolism. This section will focus on the evidence associating commonly used treatments for bipolar disorder with adverse metabolic outcomes that could contribute to increased risk for T2DM and cardiovascular disease.

Antidepressant Treatment and Diabetes Mellitus

Pharmacological treatments for depression have been associated with changes in whole-body glucose metabolism (117–119). These same treatments may also cause changes in weight and adiposity, which could in turn decrease insulin sensitivity. Treatment-related changes in glucose metabolism can interact in a complex manner with the effect of depression itself on the risk for diabetes mellitus. An improvement in glucose control that can occur with the resolution of depression, independent of specific treatments, complicates the study of the specific glycemic effects of individual medications. For example, treatment with cognitive behavioral therapy can improve glycemic control (120). Improvement in glycemic control has also been reported during successful treatment of depression, even with medications associated with adverse effects on glucoregulation (118). Clinical response to treatment and medication effects have been confounded in most studies of drug effects on glucose metabolism that have been reported to date.

Selective serotonin reuptake inhibitors have generally been reported to reduce blood glucose levels. Most of the available data in this regard describe the use of fluoxetine in diabetic patients with depression, where fluoxetine treatment has been associated with significant reductions in weight, fasting glucose, and lipids (94, 121–123). Goodnick et al. (124) published the results of an open label study of the use of sertraline in patients with T2DM and depression. Patients treated with sertraline had improved dietary compliance and lowered glycated hemoglobin values. Despite the generally positive effects in these reports, potential worsening of glucose control may be possible with any treatment in the setting of increases in adiposity, and SSRI therapy can modestly increase weight in many individuals with some uncontrolled case reports of hyperglycemia (125).

Mood Stabilizers and Diabetes Mellitus

Some potential effects of mood stabilizers on glucose metabolism may be related to the weight gain they can induce. There may also be direct effects of these agents on glucose metabolism. Valproate, for example, has been associated with insulin resistance and elevated plasma insulin levels (126). Administration of lithium to patients diagnosed with manic depression has been associated with improved glucose tolerance, and withdrawal of lithium has been associated with worsening of glucose tolerance (127). In contrast, lithium therapy has been associated with decreased insulin sensitivity in a study of 13 patients with mania (128). Lithium has also been associated with case reports of hyperglycemia. One case described hyperglycemia that was likely associated with lithium toxicity in a severely ill hospitalized patient who died within a week of development of hyperglycemia (129). Another case report described a patient with Type 1 diabetes mellitus whose hyperglycemia waxed and waned with the patient's lithium level (130). In a letter, Johnston (131) described hyperglycemia associated with lithium toxicity, and diabetic ketoacidosis (DKA) without lithium toxicity in another patient. Both patients had previously normal urine and plasma glucose levels, and both died during their hospitalizations. In healthy volunteers, 3 weeks of lithium treatment did not result in any significant changes during an insulin challenge test (132). Another study observed a hypoglycemic effect of lithium in patients with Types 1 and 2 diabetes, but did not screen or evaluate subjects for the presence of comorbid psychopathology (133). In general, this literature has been limited by the lack of controlled studies.

Antipsychotics and Diabetes Mellitus

Certain antipsychotic medications can cause significant weight gain, which is a growing concern given the known health consequences of obesity. Obesity and weight gain are also major risk factors for insulin resistance and diabetes (134), leading to concerns about the weight gain induced by some psychotropic treatment regimens, particularly certain antipsychotic medications. In addition, hyperglycemia-related events have been reported during treatment with second-generation antipsychotics in the absence of obesity or substantial weight gain (135,136), suggesting that weight gain may be an important but not exclusive factor contributing to risk in this area.

There has been skepticism expressed about whether the weight gain associated with antipsychotic treatment is related to risk for hyperglycemia. The hypothesis that weight gain is only a risk factor in the general population, but not related to the risk of diabetes during antipsychotic treatment (137), would seem to depend on unknown protective factors to block the adverse effects of adiposity that have been well-established in a variety of species and human populations. Given the evidence for higher, rather than lower, prevalence of diabetes in psychiatric populations, it seems unlikely that such protective factors are operating in individuals with psychiatric illness. More generally, weight gain is a key risk factor for insulin resistance and the metabolic syndrome, potentially affecting many more individuals than frank T2DM (138).

Comparing drug effects relative to placebo, weight gain observed in various trials, and head-to-head comparisons all indicate that the relative incidence and magnitude of weight gain vary among the different specific antipsychotic medications. Studies of the long-term effects of antipsychotic drugs on weight, in contrast to short-term effects, are more relevant to clinical practice, where long-term treatment is the routine. Pooled doses of aripiprazole and ziprasidone have been associated with mean weight gain of approximately 1 kg/year; amisulpride with approximately 1.5 kg/year; quetiapine and risperidone with 2–3 kg/year; and olanzapine with more than 6 kg/year (47,53,55,65,75,88,139). Mean weight gain of more than 10 kg was observed in patients treated with olanzapine at doses between 12.5 and 17.5 mg, the highest doses tested in large-scale pivotal trials (53).

Insulin Resistance, Diabetes Mellitus, and Antipsychotic Treatment

A range of evidence suggests that treatment with certain antipsychotic medications, in comparison to no treatment or treatment with alternative antipsychotics, is associated with increased risk of insulin resistance, hyperglycemia, and T2DM (95,140). Of note, similar observations were made concerning phenothiazine treatment (141). Interpretation of the older and newer literature in this area has been complicated by reports that patients with major mental disorders like schizophrenia have an increased prevalence of abnormalities in glucose regulation (e.g., insulin resistance) prior to the introduction of antipsychotics (142). However, early studies did not control for age, weight, adiposity, ethnicity, or diet, with most experts hypothesizing that differences between patients and controls on key factors such as diet and activity level can contribute to at least some of the abnormalities observed.

Evidence spanning case reports and prospective observational studies (typically useful for hypothesis generation), retrospective database analyses (often useful for hypothesis testing, but methodological issues can limit interpretability, discussed below), and controlled experimental studies including randomized clinical trials (generally recognized as hypothesis testing) have identified an association between certain antipsychotic medications and adverse metabolic events that include hyperglycemia, dyslipidemia, insulin resistance, exacerbation of preexisting Type 1 diabetes mellitus (T1DM) and T2DM, new onset T2DM, and DKA (56,95,140). Adverse effects on glucose and lipid metabolism (e.g., diabetes and dyslipidemia) have more frequently and consistently been associated with treatment using clozapine and olanzapine. Relatively fewer and discrepant reports have described similar events in association with quetiapine or risperidone treatment. Current evidence detailing limited short- and long-term weight gain is consistent with no current evidence for adverse effects on metabolic outcomes for ziprasidone, amisulpride, and aripiprazole (109,140,143).

Although the relative risk of diabetes during treatment appears to match the rank order of weight gain liability with the different agents, weight gain may not explain all observed metabolic adverse events. Newcomer et al. (116) measured effects of conventional and atypical antipsychotics on glucose regulation in chronically treated non-diabetic patients with schizophrenia compared to untreated healthy controls, with all patient and control groups matched for adiposity and age. Using a modified oral glucose tolerance test, patients receiving olanzapine and clozapine demonstrated significantly higher fasting and post-load plasma glucose values compared to patients receiving conventional antipsychotics or untreated healthy controls. The risperidone-treated group did not differ from the conventional antipsychotic group, but had higher post-load glucose levels than the controls. Both olanzapine- and clozapine-treated patients had higher calculated insulin resistance in comparison to those treated with conventional agents, while risperidone-treated patients and typical antipsychotic-treated patients did not differ from the controls. Retrospective analyses of clozapine-, olanzapine-, and risperidone-associated cases of new onset diabetes in the FDA MedWatch database have suggested that while the majority of new-onset T2DM cases were associated with substantial weight gain or obesity, approximately 25% were not (135,136,144).

Analyses of case reports to the FDA MedWatch database concerning clozapine, olanzapine, and risperidone have also suggested that most new-onset T2DM cases occur within the first 6 months of treatment initiation, are typically associated with substantial weight gain or obesity (i.e., 75%), and affect individuals without a family history of diabetes in as many as half of cases, with some cases having a close temporal relationship between treatment initiation and discontinuation and the development and/or resolution of the adverse event (135,136,144).

The most important level of evidence for an association between antipsychotics and metabolic outcomes concerns controlled experimental studies and randomized clinical trials. Growing evidence supports the key observation that treatments producing the largest increases in weight and adiposity are also associated with the most consistent and clinically significant adverse effects on insulin sensitivity, blood glucose, and blood lipids. Five studies have reported significant increases in plasma insulin, suggesting decreased insulin sensitivity (i.e., insulin resistance) during olanzapine treatment in comparison to various control conditions (116,145–148), and some of these report a significant increase in insulin resistance during olanzapine therapy compared with baseline levels (146,147). Two studies report elevated insulin levels in 31–71% of patients receiving olanzapine treatment (149,150), while significant improvements in insulin resistance and beta-cell function were also observed in a study of 40 patients with schizophrenia following the switch from olanzapine to risperidone therapy (151). These studies are consistent with the evidence from general population samples that conditions which increase adiposity will tend to be associated with increases in insulin resistance, potentially leading to compensatory insulin secretion in those persons with pancreatic beta-cell reserve and hyperglycemia in those individuals with relative beta-cell failure.

Several other reports are representative of the generally consistent results of controlled studies on this topic. A pooled analysis of safety data from short-term (4–6 weeks) controlled trials of aripiprazole in schizophrenia found that changes in fasting serum glucose concentrations were similar between patients treated with aripiprazole and placebo (89). A 26-week controlled study of aripiprazole for relapse prevention in 310 patients with schizophrenia found no clinically significant change from baseline in fasting glucose concentration (152). A 6-week randomized study of atypical antipsychotics in 56 patients with schizophrenia (153) showed significant changes in triglyceride levels from baseline with olanzapine, clozapine, and quetiapine therapy. However, quetiapine-treated patients ($n = 14$) showed only a modest increase in triglyceride levels from baseline at week 6 (11.64 mg/dL, $p < 0.05$), with a mean increase approximately three times larger during clozapine (36.28 mg/dL) and olanzapine (31.23 mg/dL) therapy.

Fasting glucose, insulin, and lipid parameters have been assessed in a randomized, double-blind, 6-week study comparing olanzapine and ziprasidone therapy in 269 inpatients with an acute exacerbation of schizophrenia or schizoaffective disorder (154). Significant increases from baseline in median fasting plasma insulin levels ($p < 0.0001$) and HOMA calculated insulin resistance ($p < 0.0001$) were observed during olanzapine but not ziprasidone treatment. Median body weight increased by 7.2 lb (3.3 kg) from baseline with olanzapine treatment compared with 1.2 lb [0.5 kg] with ziprasidone, and median body weight was significantly higher in the olanzapine group than the ziprasidone group at endpoint ($p < 0.0001$). In this relatively young sample, with a significant compensatory hyperinsulinemic response, fasting plasma glucose did not change significantly in either olanzapine- or ziprasidone-treated subjects. Significant increases from baseline in median fasting total cholesterol (20 mg/dL, $p < 0.0001$), LDL cholesterol (13 mg/dL, $p < 0.0001$), and triglyceride (26 mg/dL, $p = 0.0003$) levels were observed with olanzapine therapy. In contrast, minimal changes were observed with ziprasidone therapy.

In the first published example of a prospective randomized evaluation of drug effects on the incidence of the metabolic syndrome, pooled data were used from two 26-week double-blinded, randomized, controlled trials (152,155), evaluating the effects of aripiprazole compared to placebo and olanzapine in a total of 624 subjects. In a pooled analysis of the two trials (156), the cumulative incidence of metabolic syndrome (±SE) varied across the different treatment conditions, with an incidence of 19.2% ± 4.0% during olanzapine treatment, 12.8% ± 4.5% on placebo treatment, and 7.6% ± 2.3% on treatment with aripiprazole. A log-rank test indicated significant differences among the three incidence rates ($p = 0.003$)(aripiprazole vs. olanzapine, 69% relative risk reduction) (156,157).

RECOMMENDATIONS AND CONCLUSION

The principles of primary prevention (preventing the occurrence of risk factors) and secondary prevention (preventing the worsening of existing risk factors) suggest the importance of efforts to lower the risk of adverse events that could occur in the treatment of bipolar disorder. This prevention approach may be particularly important when considering the risk factors for morbidity and mortality associated with metabolic syndrome, diabetes mellitus, and cardiovascular disease. Weight gain, hyperlipidemia, and abnormalities in glucose metabolism are modifiable factors that might be prevented or reversed with appropriate interventions. For example, combination therapies that could increase weight gain risk should be avoided when possible, and if an atypical antipsychotic is used, selection of one with low liability for weight gain and metabolic abnormalities should be considered, especially in patients with preexisting risk factors for diabetes and cardiovascular disease (e.g., family history, obesity). Close monitoring of patients from the outset of treatment is critical for early identification of treatment-induced weight gain and metabolic adverse events. In many patients, education coupled with modifications in diet and exercise regimen can prevent or mitigate these effects. Switching medications is an option for patients who experience persistent weight gain or related adverse metabolic effects during treatment.

In order to optimize the individual patient's treatment, clinicians need to consider not just efficacy, but also the number and severity of adverse effects. Pharmacotherapy of bipolar disorder can be associated with many side effects, some which are important and can affect medical outcomes, and some which are less important and may be self-limited. Finally, individual patients' risk factors for medical comorbidity are an important consideration when weighing clinical benefit and risks.

REFERENCES

1. Osby U, Brandt L, Correia N, Ekbom A, Sparen P. Excess mortality in bipolar and unipolar disorder in Sweden. Arch Gen Psychiatry 2001; 58:844–850.
2. Frye MA, Gitlin MJ, Altshuler LL. Treating acute mania. J Fam Pract 2003 March (suppl):S10–S13.
3. Gelenberg AJ, Kane JM, Keller MB, Lavori P, Rosenbaum JF, Cole K, Lavelle J. Comparison of standard and low serum levels of lithium for maintenance treatment of bipolar disorder. N Engl J Med 1989; 321:1489–1493.
4. Jefferson JW, Greist JH, Ackerman DL, et al. Lithium Encyclopedia for Clinical Practice. 2nd ed. Washington, DC: American Psychiatric Press, 1987.
5. Hollister LE, Czernansky JG. Clinical Pharmacology of Psychotherapeutic Drugs. 3rd ed. New York: Churchill Livingstone Inc., 1990.
6. Lenox RH, Manji HK. Lithium. In: Schatzberg AF, Nemeroff CB, eds. Essentials of Clinical Psychopharmacology. 1st ed. Washington, DC: American Psychiatric Publishing, Inc., 2001:207.
7. Harvey NS, Merriman S. Review of clinically important drug interactions with lithium. Drug Saf 1994; 10:455–463.
8. Juurlink DN, Mamdani MM, Kopp A, Rochon PA, Shulman KI, Redelmeier DA. Drug-induced lithium toxicity in the elderly: a population-based study. J Am Geriatr Soc 2004; 52:794–798.
9. American Psychiatric Association. Practice guidelines for the treatment of patients with bipolar disorder. Am J Psychiatry 2002; 159(suppl):4–50.
10. Jefferson JW. Lithium: the present and the future. J Clin Psychiatry 1990; 51(suppl):4–8; discussion 17–19.
11. Boton R, Gaviria M, Batlle DC. Prevalence, pathogenesis, and treatment of renal dysfunction associated with chronic lithium therapy. Am J Kidney Dis 1987; 10: 329–345.
12. Goodwin FK, Jamison KR. Manic-Depressive Illness. New York: Oxford University Press, 1990.
13. Walker RG. Lithium nephrotoxicity. Kidney Int Suppl 1993; 42:S93–S98.
14. Hestbech J, Hansen HE, Amdisen A, Olsen S. Chronic renal lesions following long-term treatment with lithium. Kidney Int 1977; 12:250.
15. Schou M. Forty years of lithium treatment. Arch Gen Psychiatry 1997; 54:9–13; discussion 14–15.
16. Lepkifker E, Sverdlik A, Iancu I, Ziv R, Segev S, Kotler M. Renal insufficiency in long-term lithium treatment. J Clin Psychiatry 2004; 65:850–856.
17. Presne C, Fakhouri F, Noel LH, Stengel B, Even C, Kreis H, Mignon F, Grunfeld JP. Lithium-induced nephropathy: rate of progression and prognostic factors. Kidney Int 2003; 64:585–592.
18. Jefferson JW. Update on lithium in clinical practice: an interview with James W. Jefferson, M.D. Curr Affect Illness 1991; 10:5–14.
19. Mitchell JE, Mackenzie TB. Cardiac effects of lithium therapy in man: a review. J Clin Psychiatry 1982; 43:47–51.

20. Roose SP, Bone S, Haidorfer C, Dunner DL, Fieve RR. Lithium treatment in older patients. Am J Psychiatry 1979; 136:843–844.
21. Briggs GG, Freeman RK, Yaffe SJ. Drugs in Pregnancy and Lactation. 3rd ed. Baltimore, MD: Williams & Wilkins, 1990.
22. Cohen LS, Friedman JM, Jefferson JW, Johnson EM, Weiner ML. A reevaluation of risk of in utero exposure to lithium. JAMA 1994; 271:146–150.
23. Licht RW, Vestergaard P, Kessing LV, Larsen JK, Thomsen PH. Psychopharmacological treatment with lithium and antiepileptic drugs: suggested guidelines from the Danish Psychiatric Association and the Child and Adolescent Psychiatric Association in Denmark. Acta Psychiatr Scand Suppl 2003; 419:1–22.
24. French JA, Kanner AM, Bautista J, Abou-Khalil B, Browne T, Harden CL, Theodore WH, Bazil C, Stern J, Schachter SC, Bergen D, Hirtz D, Montouris GD, Nespeca M, Gidal B, Marks WJ, Jr., Turk WR, Fischer JH, Bourgeois B, Wilner A, Faught RE Jr, Sachdeo RC, Beydoun A, Glauser TA. Efficacy and tolerability of the new antiepileptic drugs I: treatment of new onset epilepsy: report of the Therapeutics and Technology Assessment Subcommittee and Quality Standards Subcommittee of the American Academy of Neurology and the American Epilepsy Society. Neurology 2004; 62:1252–1260.
25. Macritchie K, Geddes JR, Scott J, Haslam D, Lima M, Goodwin G. Valproate for acute mood episodes in bipolar disorder (review). Cochrane Database Syst Rev 2003; 1: 1–13.
26. Vencovsky E, Soucek K, Zatecka I. Comparison of the side-effects of lithium and dipropylacetamide (Depamide). Cesk Psychiatr 1983; 79:223–227.
27. Wilder BJ, Karas BJ, Penry JK, Asconape J. Gastrointestinal tolerance of divalproex sodium. Neurology 1983; 33:808–811.
28. Gupta S. Safety in treating bipolar disorder. J Fam Pract 2003; March (suppl):S26–S29.
29. Bowden CL, Asnis GM, Ginsberg LD, Bentley B, Leadbetter R, White R. Safety and tolerability of lamotrigine for bipolar disorder. Drug Saf 2004; 27:173–184.
30. Guberman AH, Besag FM, Brodie MJ, Dooley JM, Duchowny MS, Pellock JM, Richens A, Stern RS, Trevathan E. Lamotrigine-associated rash: risk/benefit considerations in adults and children. Epilepsia 1999; 40:985–991.
31. Calabrese JR, Sullivan JR, Bowden CL, Suppes T, Goldberg JF, Sachs GS, Shelton MD, Goodwin FK, Frye MA, Kusumakar V. Rash in multicenter trials of lamotrigine in mood disorders: clinical relevance and management. J Clin Psychiatry 2002; 63:1012–1019.
32. Rzany B, Correia O, Kelly JP, Naldi L, Auquier A, Stern R. Risk of Stevens–Johnson syndrome and toxic epidermal necrolysis during first weeks of antiepileptic therapy: a casecontrol study. Study Group of the International Case Control Study on Severe Cutaneous Adverse Reactions. Lancet 1999; 353:2190–2194.
33. Israel M, Beaudry P. Carbamazepine in psychiatry: a review. Can J Psychiatry 1988; 33:577–584.
34. Ketter TA, Kalali AH, Weisler RH. A 6-month, multicenter, open-label evaluation of beaded, extended-release carbamazepine capsule monotherapy in bipolar disorder patients with manic or mixed episodes. J Clin Psychiatry 2004; 65:668–673.
35. Gandelman MS. Review of carbamazepine-induced hyponatremia. Prog Neuropsychopharmacol Biol Psychiatry 1994; 18:211–233.
36. Seetharam MN, Pellock JM. Risk-benefit assessment of carbamazepine in children. Drug Saf 1991; 6:148–158.
37. Hunt N, Silverstone T. Tardive dyskinesia in bipolar affective disorder: a catchment area study. Int Clin Psychopharmacol 1991; 6:45–50.
38. Kohler CG, Lallart EA. Postpsychotic depression in schizophrenia patients. Curr Psychiatry Rep 2002; 4:273–278.
39. Tohen M, Vieta E, Calabrese J, Ketter TA, Sachs G, Bowden C, Mitchell PB, Centorrino F, Risser R, Baker RW, Evans AR, Beymer K, Dube S, Tollefson GD,

Breier A. Efficacy of olanzapine and olanzapine–fluoxetine combination in the treatment of bipolar I depression. Arch Gen Psychiatry 2003; 60:1079–1088.

40. Tohen M, Zhang F, Keck PE, Feldman PD, Risser RC, Tran PV, Breier A. Olanzapine versus haloperidol in schizoaffective disorder, bipolar type. J Affect Disord 2001; 67: 133–140.
41. Kessler RC, McGonagle KA, Zhao S, Nelson CB, Hughes M, Eshleman S, Wittchen HU, Kendler KS. Lifetime and 12-month prevalence of DSM-III-R psychiatric disorders in the United States. Results from the National Comorbidity Survey. Arch Gen Psychiatry 1994; 51:8–19.
42. Chouinard G, Jones B, Remington G, Bloom D, Addington D, MacEwan GW, Labelle A, Beauclair L, Arnott W. A Canadian multicenter placebo-controlled study of fixed doses of risperidone and haloperidol in the treatment of chronic schizophrenic patients. J Clin Psychopharmacol 1993; 13:25–40.
43. Umbricht D, Kane JM. Medical complications of new antipsychotic drugs. Schizophr Bull 1996; 22:475–483.
44. Kopala LC, Good KP, Honer WG. Extrapyramidal signs and clinical symptoms in first-episode schizophrenia: response to low-dose risperidone. J Clin Psychopharmacol 1997; 17:308–313.
45. Green B. Focus on risperidone. Curr Med Res Opin 2000; 16:57–65.
46. Allison DB, Mentore JL, Heo M, Chandler LP, Cappelleri JC, Infante MC, Weiden PJ. Antipsychotic-induced weight gain: a comprehensive research synthesis. Am J Psychiatry 1999; 156:1686–1696.
47. Janssen Pharmaceutica Products LP. Risperdal (risperidone). Package insert. In: http://www.risperdal.com/files/risperdal.pdf ed; 2003.
48. Singer S, Richards C, Boland RJ. Two cases of risperidone-induced neuroleptic malignant syndrome [letter]. Am J Psychiatry 1995; 152:1234.
49. Bonwick RJ, Hopwood MJ, Morris PL. Neuroleptic malignant syndrome and risperidone: a case report. Aust N Z J Psychiatry 1996; 30:419–421.
50. Gleason PP, Conigliaro RL. Neuroleptic malignant syndrome with risperidone. Pharmacotherapy 1997; 17:617–621.
51. Bajjoka I, Patel T, O'Sullivan T. Risperidone-induced neuroleptic malignant syndrome. Ann Emerg Med 1997; 30:698–700.
52. Eli Lilly and Company. Zyprexa [package insert]. Indianapolis, IN, 2004.
53. Nemeroff CB. Dosing the antipsychotic medication olanzapine. J Clin Psychiatry 1997; 58(suppl 10):45–49.
54. Filice GA, McDougall BC, Ercan-Fang N, Billington CJ. Neuroleptic malignant syndrome associated with olanzapine. Ann Pharmacother 1998; 32:1158–1159.
55. Leucht S, Wagenpfeil S, Hamann J, Kissling W. Amisulpride is an "atypical" antipsychotic associated with low weight gain. Psychopharmacology (Berl) 2004; 173:112–115.
56. Newcomer JW. Second-generation (atypical) antipsychotics and metabolic effects: a comprehensive literature review. CNS Drugs 2005; 19(suppl.):1–93.
57. Coulouvrat C, Dondey-Nouvel L. Safety of amisulpride (Solian): a review of 11 clinical studies. Int Clin Psychopharmacol 1999; 14:209–218.
58. Green B. Focus on amisulpride. Curr Med Res Opin 2002; 18:113–117.
59. Bottlender R, Jager M, Hofschuster E, Dobmeier P, Moller HJ. Neuroleptic malignant syndrome due to atypical neuroleptics: three episodes in one patient. Pharmacopsychiatry 2002; 35:119–121.
60. Ramaekers JG, Louwerens JW, Muntjewerff ND, et al. Psychomotor, cognitive, extrapyramidal, and affective functions of healthy volunteers during treatment with an atypical (amisulpride) and a classic (haloperidol) antipsychotic. J Clin Psychopharmacol 1999; 19:209–221.
61. Leucht S, Pitschel-Walz G, Engel RR, Kissling W. Amisulpride, an unusual "atypical" antipsychotic: a meta-analysis of randomized controlled trials. Am J Psychiatry 2002; 159:180–190.

62. Green B. Focus on quetiapine. Curr Med Res Opin 1999; 15:145–151.
63. Harmon TJ, Benitez JG, Krenzelok EP, Cortes-Belen E. Loss of consciousness from acute quetiapine overdosage. J Toxicol Clin Toxicol 1998; 36:599–602.
64. Yeung P, Hellewell JSE, Raniwalla J, Atkinson. Seroquel: extrapyramidal symptoms and tolerability profile in the elderly. In: Poster Presentation. CINP, 1998.
65. AstraZeneca. Seroquel (quetiapine). Package insert. In: http:/www.fda.gov/medwatch/SAFETY/2004/Seroquel-lbl.pdf ed; 2004.
66. Bourgeois JA, Babine S, Meyerovich M, Doyle J. A case of neuroleptic malignant syndrome with quetiapine. J Neuropsychiatry Clin Neurosci 2002; 14:87.
67. Kroeze WK, Hufeisen SJ, Popadak BA, Renock SM, Steinberg S, Ernsberger P, Jayathilake K, Meltzer HY, Roth BL. H1-histamine receptor affinity predicts short-term weight gain for typical and atypical antipsychotic drugs. Neuropsychopharmacology 2003; 28:519–526.
68. Daniel DG, Zimbroff DL, Potkin SG, Reeves KR, Harrigan EP, Lakshminarayanan M. Ziprasidone 80 mg/day and 160 mg/day in the acute exacerbation of schizophrenia and schizoaffective disorder: a 6-week placebo-controlled trial. Ziprasidone Study Group. Neuropsychopharmacology 1999; 20:491–505.
69. Keck PJ, Buffenstein A, Ferguson J, Feighner J, Jaffe W, Harrigan EP, Morrissey MR. Ziprasidone 40 and 120 mg/day in the acute exacerbation of schizophrenia and schizoaffective disorder: a 4-week placebo-controlled trial. Psychopharmacology (Berl) 1998; 140:173–184.
70. Arato M, O'Connor R, Meltzer HY. A 1-year, double-blind, placebo-controlled trial of ziprasidone 40, 80 and 160 mg/day in chronic schizophrenia: the Ziprasidone Extended Use in Schizophrenia (ZEUS) study. Int Clin Psychopharmacol 2002; 17:207–215.
71. Hirsch SR, Kissling W, Bauml J, Power A, O'Connor R. A 28-week comparison of ziprasidone and haloperidol in outpatients with stable schizophrenia. J Clin Psychiatry 2002; 63:516–523.
72. Schmidt AW, Lebel LA, Howard HR Jr, Zorn SH. Ziprasidone: a novel antipsychotic agent with a unique human receptor binding profile. Eur J Pharmacol 2001; 425: 197–201.
73. Green B. Focus on ziprasidone. Curr Med Res Opin 2001; 17:146–150.
74. Physicians' Desk Reference. PDR 2005. 59 ed. 2005.
75. Pfizer. Geodon (ziprasidone HCl). Package insert. In: http://www.pfizer.com/download/uspi_geodon.pdf ed; 2004.
76. Harrigan EP, Miceli JJ, Anziano R, Watsky E, Reeves KR, Cutler NR, Sramek J, Shiovitz T, Middle M. A randomized evaluation of the effects of six antipsychotic agents on QTc, in the absence and presence of metabolic inhibition. J Clin Psychopharmacol 2004; 24:62–69.
77. Glassman AH, Bigger JT Jr. Antipsychotic drugs: prolonged QTc interval, torsade de pointes, and sudden death. Am J Psychiatry 2001; 158:1774–1782.
78. Nemeroff CB, Masand PS, Lieberman JA, Newcomer JW, Harvey P, Daniel D, Schatzberg AF, Weiden P. Oral ziprasidone in the treatment of schizophrenia, schizoaffective disorder, and bipolar mania: a clinical update. CNS Spectr. In press.
79. Montanez A, Ruskin JN, Hebert PR, Lamas GA, Hennekens CH. Prolonged QTc interval and risks of total and cardiovascular mortality and sudden death in the general population: a review and qualitative overview of the prospective cohort studies. Arch Intern Med 2004; 164:943–948.
80. Murty RG, Mistry SG, Chacko RC. Neuroleptic malignant syndrome with ziprasidone. J Clin Psychopharmacol 2002; 22:624–626.
81. DeLeon A, Patel NC, Crismon ML. Aripiprazole: a comprehensive review of its pharmacology, clinical efficacy, and tolerability. Clin Ther 2004; 26:649–666.
82. Kane JM, Carson WH, Saha AR, McQuade RD, Ingenito GG, Zimbroff DL, Ali MW. Efficacy and safety of aripiprazole and haloperidol versus placebo in patients with schizophrenia and schizoaffective disorder. J Clin Psychiatry 2002; 63:763–771.

83. Potkin SG, Saha AR, Kujawa MJ, Carson WH, Ali M, Stock E, Stringfellow J, Ingenito G, Marder SR. Aripiprazole, an antipsychotic with a novel mechanism of action, and risperidone vs placebo in patients with schizophrenia and schizoaffective disorder. Arch Gen Psychiatry 2003; 60:681–690.
84. Petrie JL, Saha AR, McEvoy JP. Aripiprazole, a new atypical antipsychotic: phase 2 clinical trial results [abstr]. Eur Neuropsychopharmacol 1997; 7(suppl 2):S227.
85. Daniel DG, Saha AR, Ingenito G, et al. Aripiprazole, a novel antipsychotic: overview of a phase II study result [abstr]. Int J Neuropsychopharmacol 2000; 3(suppl 1):S157.
86. Lieberman JA, Carson WH, Saha AR, et al. Meta-analysis of the efficacy of aripiprazole in schizophrenia. Poster presented at XXIIIrd Collegium Internationale Neuropsychopharmacologicum Congress, Montreal, Canada, June 23–27, 2002.
87. Bristol-Myers Squibb. Abilify [package insert], 2004.
88. Otsuka America Pharmaceutical & Bristol-Myers Squibb. Abilify (aripiprazole). Package insert. In: http://www.bms.com/cgi-bin/anybin.pl?sql=select%20PPI%20from%20TB_PRODUCT_PPI%20where%20_SEQ=101&key=PPI ed; 2004.
89. Marder SR, McQuade RD, Stock E, Kaplita S, Marcus R, Safferman AZ, Saha A, Ali M, Iwamoto T. Aripiprazole in the treatment of schizophrenia: safety and tolerability in short-term, placebo-controlled trials. Schizophr Res 2003; 61:123–136.
90. Kane J, Honigfeld G, Singer J, Meltzer H. Clozapine for the treatment-resistant schizophrenic. A double-blind comparison with chlorpromazine. Arch Gen Psychiatry 1988; 45:789–796.
91. Meltzer HY, Alphs L, Green AI, Altamura AC, Anand R, Bertoldi A, Bourgeois M, Chouinard G, Islam MZ, Kane J, Krishnan R, Lindenmayer JP, Potkin S. Clozapine treatment for suicidality in schizophrenia: International Suicide Prevention Trial (InterSePT). Arch Gen Psychiatry 2003; 60:82–91.
92. Novartis Pharmaceuticals Corporation. Clozaril. Package insert, 2002.
93. Rogers DP, Shramko JK. Therapeutic options in the treatment of clozapine-induced sialorrhea [review]. Pharmacotherapy 2000; 20:1092–1095.
94. Haupt DW, Newcomer JW. Abnormalities in glucose regulation associated with mental illness and treatment. J Psychosom Res 2002; 53:925–933.
95. American Diabetes Association. Consensus development conference on antipsychotic drugs and obesity and diabetes. Diabetes Care 2004; 27:596–601.
96. DasGupta K, Young A. Clozapine-induced neuroleptic malignant syndrome. J Clin Psychiatry 1991; 52:105–107.
97. Lewis JL, Winokur G. The induction of mania. A natural history study with controls. Arch Gen Psychiatry 1982; 39:303–306.
98. Simpson HB, Hurowitz GI, Liebowitz MR. General principles in the pharmacotherapy of antidepressant-induced rapid cycling: a case series. J Clin Psychopharmacol 1997; 17:460–466.
99. Bourin M, Chue P, Guillon Y. Paroxetine: a review. CNS Drug Rev 2001; 7:25–47.
100. Pollock BG. Citalopram: a comprehensive review. Expert Opin Pharmacother 2001; 2:681–698.
101. Baldwin DS. Escitalopram: efficacy and tolerability in the treatment of depression. Hosp Med 2002; 63:668–671.
102. Calil HM. Fluoxetine: a suitable long-term treatment. J Clin Psychiatry 2001; 62(suppl 22): 24–29.
103. Cassano P, Fava M. Tolerability issues during long-term treatment with antidepressants. Ann Clin Psychiatry 2004; 16:15–25.
104. Settle EC Jr. Bupropion sustained release: side effect profile. J Clin Psychiatry 1998; 59(suppl 4):32–36.
105. Danjou P, Hackett D. Safety and tolerance profile of venlafaxine. Int Clin Psychopharmacol 1995; 10(suppl 2):15–20.
106. Elmslie JL, Silverstone JT, Mann JI, Williams SM, Romans SE. Prevalence of overweight and obesity in bipolar patients. J Clin Psychiatry 2000; 61:179–184.

107. Regenold WT, Thapar RK, Marano C, Gavirneni S, Kondapavuluru PV. Increased prevalence of type 2 diabetes mellitus among psychiatric inpatients with bipolar I affective and schizoaffective disorders independent of psychotropic drug use. J Affect Disord 2002; 70:19–26.
108. Koh-Banerjee P, Wang Y, Hu FB, Spiegelman D, Willett WC, Rimm EB. Changes in body weight and body fat distribution as risk factors for clinical diabetes in US men. Am J Epidemiol 2004; 159:1150–1159.
109. Haupt DW, Newcomer JW. Hyperglycemia and antipsychotic medications. J Clin Psychiatry 2001; 62:15–26.
110. Gavard JA, Lustman PJ, Clouse RE. Prevalence of depression in adults with diabetes. An epidemiological evaluation. Diabetes Care 1993; 16:1167–1178.
111. Anderson RJ, Freedland KE, Clouse RE, Lustman PJ. The prevalence of comorbid depression in adults with diabetes: a meta-analysis. Diabetes Care 2001; 24:1069–1078.
112. Eaton WW, Armenian H, Gallo J, Pratt L, Ford DE. Depression and risk for onset of type II diabetes. A prospective population-based study. Diabetes Care 1996; 19: 1097–1102.
113. Kawakami N, Takatsuka N, Shimizu H, Ishibashi H. Depressive symptoms and occurrence of type 2 diabetes among Japanese men. Diabetes Care 1999; 22:1071–1076.
114. Moldin SO, Scheftner WA, Rice JP, Nelson E, Knesevich MA, Akiskal H. Association between major depressive disorder and physical illness. Psychol Med 1993; 23:755–761.
115. Ryan MC, Collins P, Thakore JH. Impaired fasting glucose tolerance in first-episode, drug-naive patients with schizophrenia. Am J Psychiatry 2003; 160:284–289.
116. Newcomer JW, Haupt DW, Fucetola R, Melson AK, Schweiger JA, Cooper BP, Selke G. Abnormalities in glucose regulation during antipsychotic treatment of schizophrenia. Arch Gen Psychiatry 2002; 59:337–345.
117. Lustman PJ, Freedland KE, Griffith LS, Clouse RE. Fluoxetine for depression in diabetes: a randomized double-blind placebo-controlled trial. Diabetes Care 2000; 23: 618–623.
118. Lustman PJ, Griffith LS, Clouse RE, Freedland KE, Eisen SA, Rubin EH, Carney RM, McGill JB. Effects of nortriptyline on depression and glycemic control in diabetes: results of a double-blind, placebo-controlled trial. Psychosom Med. 1997; 59:241–250.
119. Goodnick PJ, Henry JH, Buki VM. Treatment of depression in patients with diabetes mellitus. J Clin Psychiatry 1995; 56:128–136.
120. Lustman PJ, Griffith LS, Freedland KE, Kissel SS, Clouse RE. Cognitive behavior therapy for depression in type 2 diabetes mellitus. A randomized, controlled trial. Ann Intern Med 1998; 129:613–621.
121. Potter van Loon BJ, Radder JK, Frolich M, Krans HM, Zwinderman AH, Meinders AE. Fluoxetine increases insulin action in obese nondiabetic and in obese non-insulin-dependent diabetic individuals. Int J Obes Relat Metab Disord 1992; 16:79–85.
122. Gray DS, Fujioka K, Devine W, Bray GA. Fluoxetine treatment of the obese diabetic [published erratum appears in Int J Obes 1992; 16(9):717]. Int J Obes Relat Metab Disord 1992; 16:193–198.
123. O'Kane M, Wiles PG, Wales JK. Fluoxetine in the treatment of obese type 2 diabetic patients. Diabet Med 1994; 11:105–110.
124. Goodnick PJ, Kumar A, Henry JH, Buki VM, Goldberg RB. Sertraline in coexisting major depression and diabetes mellitus. Psychopharmacol Bull 1997; 33:261–264.
125. Petty KJ. Hyperglycemia associated with paroxetine [letter]. Ann Intern Med 1996; 125:782.
126. Isojarvi JI, Rattya J, Myllyla VV, Knip M, Koivunen R, Pakarinen AJ, Tekay A, Tapanainen JS. Valproate, lamotrigine, and insulin-mediated risks in women with epilepsy. Ann Neurol 1998; 43:446–451.
127. van der Velde CD, Gordon MW. Manic-depressive illness, diabetes mellitus, and lithium carbonate. Arch Gen Psychiatry 1969; 21:478–485.

128. Heninger GR, Mueller PS. Carbohydrate metabolism in mania before and after lithium carbonate treatment. Arch Gen Psychiatry 1970; 23:310–319.
129. Martinez-Maldonado M, Terrell J. Lithium carbonate-induced nephrogenic diabetes insipidus and glucose intolerance. Arch Intern Med 1973; 132:881–884.
130. Waziri R, Nelson J. Lithium in diabetes mellitus: a paradoxical response. J Clin Psychiatry 1978; 39:623–625.
131. Johnston BB. Diabetes mellitus in patients on lithium [letter]. Lancet 1977; 2:935–936.
132. Grof E, Arato M, Grof P, Brown GM, Lane J, Saxena B. Effects of lithium, nortriptyline and dexamethasone on insulin sensitivity. Prog Neuropsychopharmacol Biol Psychiatry 1984; 8:687–690.
133. Hu M, Wu H, Chao C. Assisting effects of lithium on hypoglycemic treatment in patients with diabetes. Biol Trace Elem Res 1997; 60:131–137.
134. Pi-Sunyer FX. Medical hazards of obesity. Ann Intern Med 1993; 119:655–660.
135. Koller E, Schneider B, Bennett K, Dubitsky G. Clozapine-associated diabetes. Am J Med 2001; 111:716–723.
136. Koller EA, Doraiswamy PM. Olanzapine-associated diabetes mellitus. Pharmacotherapy 2002; 22:841–852.
137. Boehm G, Racoosin JA, Laughren TP, Katz R. Consensus development conference on antipsychotic drugs and obesity and diabetes: response to consensus statement. Diabetes Care 2004; 27:2088–2089; author reply 2089–2090.
138. Park YW, Zhu S, Palaniappan L, Heshka S, Carnethon MR, Heymsfield SB. The metabolic syndrome: prevalence and associated risk factor findings in the US population from the Third National Health and Nutrition Examination Survey, 1988–1994. Arch Intern Med 2003; 163:427–436.
139. Kinon BJ. The routine use of atypical antipsychotic agents: maintenance treatment. J Clin Psychiatry 1998; 59(suppl 19):18–22.
140. Casey DE, Haupt DW, Newcomer JW, Henderson DC, Sernyak MJ, Davidson M, Lindenmayer JP, Manoukian SV, Banerji MA, Lebovitz HE, Hennekens CH. Antipsychotic-induced weight gain and metabolic abnormalities: implications for increased mortality in patients with schizophrenia. J Clin Psychiatry 2004; 65:4–18.
141. Thonnard-Neumann E. Phenothiazines and diabetes in hospitalized women. Am J Psychiatry 1968; 124:978–982.
142. Kasanin J. The blood sugar curve in mental disease. Arch Neuro Psychiatry 1926; 16: 414–419.
143. Yang SH, McNeely MJ. Rhabdomyolysis, pancreatitis, and hyperglycemia with ziprasidone. Am J Psychiatry 2002; 159:1435.
144. Koller EA, Cross JT, Doraiswamy PM, Schneider BS. Risperidone-associated diabetes mellitus: a pharmacovigilance study. Pharmacotherapy 2003; 23:735–744.
145. Melkersson KI, Hulting AL. Insulin and leptin levels in patients with schizophrenia or related psychoses—a comparison between different antipsychotic agents. Psychopharmacology (Berl) 2001; 154:205–212.
146. Ebenbichler CF, Laimer M, Eder U, Mangweth B, Weiss E, Hofer A, Hummer M, Kemmler G, Lechleitner M, Patsch JR, Fleischhacker WW. Olanzapine induces insulin resistance: results from a prospective study. J Clin Psychiatry 2003; 64:1436–1439.
147. Glick ID, Fryburg D, O'Sullivan RL, Siu C, Simpson G. Ziprasidone's benefits versus olanzapine on weight gain and insulin resistance. American Psychiatric Association 154th Annual Meeting, 2001 May.
148. Simpson G, Weiden P, Pigott TA, Romano S. Ziprasidone vs olanzapine in schizophrenia: 6-month continuation study. Eur Neuropsychopharmacol 2002; 12:S310.
149. Melkersson KI, Dahl ML. Relationship between levels of insulin or triglycerides and serum concentrations of the atypical antipsychotics clozapine and olanzapine in patients on treatment with therapeutic doses. Psychopharmacology (Berl) 2003; Nov; 170(2): 157–166. Epub 2003 Jul 8.

150. Melkersson KI, Hulting AL, Brismar KE. Elevated levels of insulin, leptin, and blood lipids in olanzapine-treated patients with schizophrenia or related psychoses. J Clin Psychiatry 2000; 61:742–749.
151. Berry S, Mahmoud R. Improvement of insulin indices after switch from olanzapine to risperidone. Eur Neuropsychopharmacol 2002; 12:S316.
152. Pigott TA, Carson WH, Saha AR, Torbeyns AF, Stock EG, Ingenito GG. Aripiprazole for the prevention of relapse in stabilized patients with chronic schizophrenia: a placebo-controlled 26-week study. J Clin Psychiatry 2003; 64:1048–1056.
153. Atmaca M, Kuloglu M, Tezcan E, Ustundag B. Serum leptin and triglyceride levels in patients on treatment with atypical antipsychotics. J Clin Psychiatry 2003; 64:598–604.
154. Simpson GM, Glick ID, Weiden PJ, Romano SJ, Siu CO. Randomized, controlled, double-blind multicenter comparison of the efficacy and tolerability of ziprasidone and olanzapine in acutely ill inpatients with schizophrenia or schizoaffective disorder. Am J Psychiatry 2004; 161:1837–1847.
155. McQuade RD, Jody D, Kujawa M, Carson WH, Iwamoto T. Long-term weight effects of aripiprazole versus olanzapine. Poster presented at the American Psychiatric Association, San Francisco, 2003.
156. L'Italien GJ. Pharmacoeconomic impact of antipsychotic-induced metabolic events. Am J Manage Care 2003; 3:S38–S42.
157. Casey DE, L'Italien GJ, Waldeck R, Cislo P, Carson WH. Metabolic syndrome comparison between olanzapine, aripiprazole, and placebo. Poster presented at the American Psychiatric Association, San Francisco, 2003.

25

Electroconvulsive Therapy in Bipolar Disorders and Other Brain Stimulation Methods: Vagus Nerve Stimulation, Transcranial Magnetic Stimulation, Magnetic Seizure Therapy and Deep Brain Stimulation

M. Kosel
Department of Psychiatry, University of Bonn, Bonn, Germany

Thomas E. Schlaepfer
Department of Psychiatry, University Hospital, Bern, Switzerland, University of Bonn, Bonn, Germany, and Johns Hopkins University, Baltimore, Maryland, U.S.A.

INTRODUCTION

Five brain stimulation techniques are being actively researched at the present moment as treatments for neuropsychiatric disorders. Only one of them, electroconvulsive therapy (ECT), is a clinically established treatment for different psychiatric disorders, including depression, mania, and catatonia. The four other methods, deep brain stimulation (DBS), transcranial magnetic stimulation (TMS), magnetic seizure therapy (MST), and vagus nerve stimulation (VNS) are currently at different stages of research as potential clinical treatments of several psychiatric disorders, most importantly for treatment of refractory depression (TMS, MST, DBS, and VNS) and obsessive–compulsive disorder (DBS) and not in widespread clinical use. Even if their clinical utility is not yet established, they are valuable as research tools in the search of the underlying neurobiology of the investigated disorders and they may well mature into treatment options for patients that are resistant to conventional interventions. The important research activity in basic mechanisms of disease accompanying the clinical studies of these new brain stimulation techniques, in animal models as well as in humans will be of relevance to bipolar disorders, which are a heterogeneous category of clinical entities as defined according to the Diagnostic and Statistical Manual of the American Psychiatric Association, Fourth Edition (DSM IV) (1). The main categories are: (a) bipolar I disorders, (b) bipolar II disorders, (c) rapid cycling, and (d) bipolar disorders not otherwise specified. To date, there is no unifying model available explaining the underlying psychopathological mechanisms.

As discussed in previous chapters, the main and first line treatment options in bipolar disorders are pharmacological strategies, and, most important to an efficient long-term therapy of these chronic disorders, combined psychotherapeutic strategies such as psychoeducation, interpersonal- and cognitive-behavioral therapy. ECT has a clearly defined, however generally underestimated, place in the treatment plan of bipolar disorders. In this chapter, we will review data on ECT, TMS, MST, VNS, and DBS in bipolar disorders. The main focus will be the discussion of the indications and their justification in the treatment of bipolar disorders by ECT, since the other brain stimulation methods are in relatively early stages of research considering their clinical applicability in those disorders.

ELECTROCONVULSIVE THERAPY

History

Modern ECT refers to the induction of seizures in patients under anesthesia and myorelaxation by electrical stimuli applied to the skin of the head by surface electrodes with the aim to diminish the expression of defined psychiatric symptoms in specific disorders. Due to space limitations, we are unable to discuss general technological or procedural aspects of ECT. These topics are thoroughly and exhaustively discussed elsewhere (2).

Interestingly enough, ECT remains today one of the most controversial treatments in psychiatry despite its excellent efficacy and manageable side effect profile. Among mental health professionals and the general public, different opinions are expressed, ranging from its appraisal as a live-saving and possibly first-line treatment in a number of indications, which is not offered often enough to patients to complete objection to its use, to declaring it an outright ineffective, brain damaging, barbarian, and inhumane treatment. Patients who underwent ECT therapy, however, rarely take the latter stance. ECT having commenced its career in U.S. movies as helpful remedy for personal distress in the middle of the last century has become a progressively more negative and cruel treatment, leaving the impression of a brutal, harmful, and abusive maneuver with doubtful benefit (3–7). Such discrepancies in the view of the usefulness are mirrored by the differences in rates of use in different countries, but also of regional differences. In the Vienna-area, Austria, 0.07 ECT sessions were administered in 1994/1995 to 1000 people of the general population. In the province of Quebec, Canada, the same number augmented from 0.47 in 1988 to 1.0 in 2001. In the United States of America, in 1975, 58,667 patients have been treated with ECT, in 1980, 31,540 and in 1986, 36,558. This corresponds to rates of 2.72, 1.38, and 1.52 patients treated per 10,000 in the general population. In England, this rate was 2.32 in 1999 and in Italy 0.11 in 1992 (8).

ECT was introduced as a clinical treatment exactly 70 years ago. In the 1934s, Ladislas Joseph von Meduna, a Hungarian neuropsychiatrist, hypothesized, that convulsions in patients with schizophrenia would reduce their symptoms. Pharmacological induction of seizures using intramuscular injections of camphor and pentylenetetrazol proved unreliable, difficult to administer, and had multiple side effects, whereas antipsychotic effects could be clearly documented. After 1937, Cerletti and Bini introduced ECT as a method to reliably induce seizures. Within a few years,

ECT became the dominant somatic treatment for schizophrenia and depression. From the 1950s on, the use of ECT began to decline. Two reasons might have accounted for this: (A) many pharmacological agents to treat psychosis, mania, and depression became available and (B) ECT was portrayed in society at large as a cruel and inhumane treatment (9).

Significant improvements in the technique of ECT have since been made, including the use of muscle relaxants in combination with short anesthesia and pre-oxygenation of the patient, the use of electroencephalogram (EEG) recordings and significantly improved stimulators, measures which contributed to greatly reducing the morbidity and side effects of this treatment. ECT has gained popularity again in the last 15 years due to its consistently and clearly demonstrated efficacy in mood disorders (2). The move from sine wave ECT to brief pulse stimulation during the 1980s significantly reduced the severity of cognitive side effects of the treatment, and provided the first clear demonstration that the type of electrical current applied to the scalp was a major determinant of side effects (10). Recent research has extended this finding by showing that electrode placement interacts with electrical dosage in determining efficacy as well as side effects (11). In the scientific literature, ECT is generally considered as a very efficient treatment with a broad indication especially in cases refractory to pharmacotherapy. According to the recommendations for treatment, training and privileging of ECT of the American Psychiatric Association (2), ECT may be indicated as a primary or secondary treatment in major depression, mania, and schizophrenia based on substantial scientific evidence.

General Recommendations for the Use of ECT

In the ECT-task force report of the American Psychiatric Association published in 2001, general recommendations concerning the use of ECT have been made (2). In general, the indication to treat a patient with ECT has to be made on an individual basis evaluating the patient's diagnosis, type and severity of symptoms, treatment history, consideration of the anticipated risk and benefits of ECT, and alternative treatment options and patient preference. No diagnosis should automatically lead to treatment with ECT. Primary use of ECT prior to a psychotropic medication include the following considerations:

a. a need for rapid, definitive response because of the severity of a psychiatric or medical condition;
b. a higher risk of other treatments compared to the risks of ECT;
c. a history of poor medication response or good ECT response in one or more previous episodes of the illness; and
d. the patient's preference.

However, in most cases, ECT is used after treatment failure with psychotropic medications.

Diagnostic indications are based on either compelling data supporting the efficacy of ECT or on a strong consensus in the field supporting the use of ECT. These include major depression, single episode (296.2×) and major depression, recurrent (296.4×), as well as bipolar major depression, including bipolar disorder, depressed (296.5×) and bipolar disorder, mixed (296.6). ECT is also an efficacious treatment for mania, including bipolar disorder, mania (296.4×) and bipolar disorder, mixed (296.6×). Finally, psychotic exacerbations in schizophrenia are considered as a principal diagnostic indication when psychotic symptoms in the present episode have an abrupt or recent onset, in the catatonic subtype (295.20) and when there is a history of a favorable response to ECT. It is also considered an efficacious treatment for related psychotic disorders [schizophreniform disorder (295.40) and schizoaffective disorder (295.70)] and finally, it may be useful in patients with psychotic disorders not otherwise specified (298.9) when the clinical features are similar to those of other major diagnostic indications.

For other diagnoses, the efficacy data for ECT are not conclusive or only a partial consensus exists in the field supporting its use. In such cases, standard treatments have to be implemented first. The use of ECT in psychiatric conditions other than those mentioned above is not adequately substantiated and should be carefully justified. ECT may be effective in treating deliria of various etiologies, including toxic and metabolic and also in the management of severe secondary affective and psychotic conditions with symptoms similar to those of primary psychiatric diagnoses. Other conditions include Parkinson's disease, neuroleptic malignant syndrome, and intractable seizure disorder.

If there is no response to an index ECT course, the response to the treatment can be potentiated to several means. Electrode placement can be switched from unilateral to bilateral, the stimulus intensity can be increased, and medication with anticonvulsant properties can be diminished or stopped. Continuation treatment (during the 6 months following the remission of an index episode) with ECT is indicated if the patient has a history of illness that has been responsive to ECT and

a. pharmacotherapy alone has not been effective in treating index episodes or in preventing relapse or recurrence;
b. pharmacotherapy cannot safely be administered; and
c. the patient prefers treatment with ECT and agrees to receive continuation ECT.

Maintenance therapy (longer than 6 months past the end of the index episode) with ECT is generally indicated in patients receiving continuation ECT. It should be assessed at least every 6 months (2).

ECT has an established and important role in the management of life-threatening conditions such as depressive stupor, catatonia, and neuroleptic malignant syndrome (12).

Adverse Effects and Side Effect Profile of ECT

As mentioned above, the technique of ECT has continuously been revised since its inception in the 1930s and its safety profile has been improved considerably. It is difficult to estimate the rate of ECT-related mortality. A reasonable current estimate is one case of treatment-related death per 10,000 patients or one per 80,000 treatments; rates which might be higher in patients with severe medical conditions. The rate of mortality is considered to be the same as that associated with minor surgery and occurs immediately after the seizure or during the postictal recovery period. Leading causes of death and significant morbidity are cardiovascular and pulmonary causes. Therefore, patients must be carefully assessed before the application of ECT and ECT procedures should accordingly be modified. Other sources of morbidity are prolonged seizures (lasting longer than 3 min) and status epilepticus. Inadequate oxygenation during prolonged seizures (motor or EEG activity) increases the risk of hypoxia and cerebral dysfunction as well as cardiovascular complications. Prolonged seizures need to be terminated pharmacologically with an anesthetic agent or a benzodiazepine. Prolonged apnea is a rare event occurring primarily in patients who have a slow metabolism of succinylcholine. It is critical to maintain adequate oxygenation during prolonged apnea, which will usually resolve within 30 to 60 minutes. Headache is a common side effect of ECT. During and shortly after the postictal recovery period, it is observed in up to 45% of the patients. It is mild in most patients and treatment is symptomatic with aspirin, acetaminophen, non-steroidal anti-inflammatory drugs (NSAIDs), sumatriptan, or more potent analgesics (2). Muscle sores following ECT have also been reported and can be treated symptomatically with aspirin, acetaminophen, or NSAIDs if severe. The prevalence of nausea is estimated to be between 1% and 23% and can be treated symptomatically.

A small number of patients with depression or mixed affective states may switch into hypomania or mania during the ECT course. On some patients, also the severity of manic symptoms may worsen under ECT treatment. There is no established strategy for managing manic symptoms that emerge during an ECT course. Some of the patients may develop postictal delirium. Spontaneous recovery may take from 5 to 45 minutes, but pharmacological intervention with 5–10 mg of diazepam is indicated because of the subjective severity of this disorder.

Cognitive side effects are an important limitation of the use of ECT. Type and severity of cognitive alterations change rapidly with time following each treatment. They are most severe during the postictal period and are correlated with the technique of administration ECT. Bilateral electrode placement, sine wave stimulation, high electrical dosage relative to seizure threshold, closely spaced treatment sessions, higher numbers of treatments, and high dosage of barbiturate anesthetic agents are each independently associated with more intense cognitive side effects compared with right unilateral electrode placement, brief pulse waveform, lower electrical intensity, more widely spaced treatments, fewer treatments, and lower dosage of barbiturate anesthesia.

ECT selectively results in anterograde and retrograde amnesia. Usually, the extent of retrograde amnesia reduces substantially with increasing time since ECT. In some patients, the recovery from retrograde amnesia will be incomplete and there are reports that ECT can even result in persistent or permanent memory loss (2).

The question whether ECT might cause permanent brain changes such as neuronal loss is certainly crucial. To date, there is no conclusive evidence whatsoever that modern, brief pulse ECT performed under general anesthesia and hyperoxygenation has such effects. One recent report on a non-human primate model of ECT designed to mimic clinical ECT demonstrated absence of neuropathological lesions (13).

ECT AS IN THE TREATMENT OF BIPOLAR DISORDERS

Indications/Guidelines

Recently, the American Psychiatric Association published a revised practice guideline for the treatment of patients with bipolar disorder (14). In manic or mixed episodes, recommended first-line treatments are pharmacological. When first-line medication treatment at optimal doses fails to control symptoms, ECT may be considered for patients with severe or treatment-resistant mania or if preferred by the patient. This recommendation is made with substantial clinical confidence [scale of three levels: (a) substantial clinical confidence, (b) moderate clinical confidence, (c) on the basis of individual circumstances]. ECT is considered a potential treatment for patients experiencing mixed episodes or for patients experiencing severe mania during pregnancy (based on moderate clinical confidence). In depressive episodes, ECT is recommended with substantial clinical confidence as a reasonable alternative first-line treatment (besides pharmacological treatment with lithium or lamotrigine) in patients with life-threatening inanition, suicidality, or psychosis. For patients with severe or treatment-resistant depression or depression with psychotic or catatonic features, ECT should be considered. It is a potential treatment for patients experiencing mixed episodes or for patients experiencing severe mania during pregnancy based on moderate clinical confidence. No recommendation is made to treat rapid cycling with ECT. Concerning maintenance therapy, the first-line treatments are pharmacological. Maintenance sessions of ECT may also be considered for patients whose acute episode responded to ECT. This recommendation is made with moderate clinical confidence.

In the guidelines of the World Federations of the Societies of Biological Psychiatry (WFSBP), the use of ECT in the treatment of bipolar disorder is less extensively discussed. ECT is considered the most successful non-pharmacological treatment modality in depression. This view is supported by Level B evidence [on a scale ranging from A to D where A represents good research-based evidence and B fair research-based evidence, including evidence from at least two randomized, double-blind controlled trials which, however, fail on a criterion (e.g., they have a small sample size or no placebo control) or from one randomized, double-blinded study and at least one prospective, large-scale naturalistic study]. The major role of ECT is seen in very severe and psychotic depression or in depression with severe psychomotor retardation. The risk of switch to mania is estimated to be about 7%. It is underlined that the readiness to use ECT is quite different in different countries, reflecting mainly public opinion and not its usefulness (15). Concerning mania, ECT is regarded as the most efficacious treatment modality when other approaches have failed. ECT is frequently chosen and anecdotally found effective. This appreciation is based on level C evidence [one randomized double-blinded study with comparator, one prospective open-label (POL) study, or two POLs with >10 participants]. ECT as a treatment of mania should accordingly be considered in patients accepting this treatment and who have not responded to previous drug treatments. In this guideline, ECT is not discussed as a treatment of rapid cycling (16).

Evidence of Efficacy

The best available evidence of the efficacy of ECT is as a treatment of depressive disorder. ECT is considered as the most effective antidepressant treatment with a remission rate in major depression cited as greater than 80% (17). To ascertain the benefits and harms of ECT, the U.K. ECT Review Group made a meta-analysis of data of short-term efficacy (at the end of an ECT treatment course) from randomized controlled trials including patients suffering from depressive illness. Real ECT was significantly more effective than simulated ECT [six trials, 256 patients, standardized effect size (SES) −0·91, 95% CI −1·27 to −0·54, trials published between 1963 and 1980]. Treatment with ECT was significantly more effective than pharmacotherapy (18 trials, 1144 participants, SES −0·80, 95% CI −1·29 to −0·29, trials published between 1962 and 2000). Bilateral ECT was more effective than unipolar ECT (22 trials, 1408 participants, SES −0·32, 95% CI −0·46 to −0·19). It was concluded that ECT is an effective short-term treatment for depression, being probably more effective than drug therapy. Bilateral ECT is moderately more effective than unilateral ECT, and high-dose ECT is more effective than low dose. The reviewers noted that data on cognitive functioning were far from comprehensive. They tentatively concluded that cognitive impairments associated with ECT treatment mostly reflect changes in memory—i.e., temporary anterograde amnesia and retrograde amnesia and that memory deficits were not limited to personal autobiographical memory. ECT seems to cause more memory impairment than simulated ECT or drug therapy and some variations in the method of ECT also have an effect on the degree of cognitive impairment produced: bilateral ECT produces greater impairment than unilateral ECT, treatment three times a week more than twice a week, and high-dose ECT produces more impairment than does low-dose ECT. There is, however, little evidence from randomized studies that sine wave causes more memory impairment than brief pulse (18). Several trials included in this metaanalysis were conducted in patients suffering from bipolar depression. There was, however, no analysis comparing the outcome in bipolar and unipolar depression. In another recently published metaanalysis, controlled studies published from 1978 onward were analyzed comparing ECT with other treatments for depression. Fifteen studies were identified which fulfilled the inclusion criteria: (1) the study dates from 1978 onward; (2) the study population is depressed patients; (3) an observer depression rating scale was used; (4) means and standard deviations of the rating scale scores were available; and (5) ECT was compared with another treatment. The effect of ECT was shown to be superior after a full course compared to fewer treatment sessions. No evidence was found for a superior speed of action of ECT or for a difference in efficacy between sine wave and brief pulse stimulation. ECT was shown to be superior to medication and simulated ECT. Some evidence was found that psychosis predicted better response to ECT. In this metaanalysis, as in the one by the U.K.-ECT study group, no mention is made concerning bipolar depression (19).

In a large, double-blind study including 228 patients, results support the hypothesis, that ECT might act faster and that fewer ECT applications are needed in bipolar than in unipolar depression to achieve similar control of symptoms (20).

ECT is considered as highly effective in the treatment of mania, even if controlled evidence is lacking (21). In a review study assessing studies published between 1942 and 1992, 80% of 589 patients with mania showed remission or marked clinical improvement (22). ECT has an equivalent or superior efficacy in acute manic state compared to lithium and chlorpromazine. This view is supported by a series of retrospective studies including either naturalistic case series or comparisons of outcome using ECT with outcome using lithium carbonate or chlorpromazine. In three prospective comparative studies published between 1988 and 1994, the hypothesis of acute effectiveness of ECT in mania is supported as well as likely superiority of ECT against lithium therapy or combined lithium–haloperidol treatment (2). In a retrospective study, the lengths of hospital stay of manic or patients with mixed episode were assessed and a comparison made between patients treated with ECT and patients treated exclusively with pharmacotherapy. The use of ECT during hospitalization for mania was associated with longer stays. However, this effect disappeared when the time before the instauration of ECT was not taken into account (23).

In rapid cycling, reports on ECT remain scant and results are conflicting. In some studies, ECT is reported inefficient or even as inducing rapid cycling. There are however case reports available that indicate also therapeutic efficacy (24). Recent studies in patients with mixed affective states indicate that ECT is effective in this condition, even in medication-resistant episodes (25–27).

Continuation and Maintenance Treatment with ECT

Relapse after a successful ECT-treatment course is still a major limitation of this treatment. Actually, in depressed patients refractory to adequate medication trials, the relapse rate is still estimated to be about 50%, the majority occurring after 6 months (28). Therefore, maintenance therapy after a successful course of ECT is mandatory, by drug treatment, by maintenance ECT, or by a combined therapy. In a review by Vaidya et al. (29), the topic of continuation and maintenance ECT is addressed. Most research on continuation and maintenance ECT from 1945 to 1999 has consisted of nine naturalistic studies, 25 case reports, five retrospective studies, and six prospective studies, with however as main flaws the lack of matched control groups and the absence of well-defined outcome measures. Four controlled prospective studies are available and one with a single-blind, randomized design. There are 15 reports available, published between 1949 and 2000, where bipolar patients were included. In an analysis, responders and non-responders could not be distinguished based on whether they were in a manic or in a depressed phase. The only generalization, which the reviewers could make from the included reports, is that maintenance ECT can be safely used in bipolar patients. It reduces hospitalizations in treatment-resistant patients. However, patient's characteristics that predict positive outcomes or the influence of parameters such as concomitant medication, seizure duration, or quality of seizure, are not known. There is controversy about how long maintenance treatment should last, more or less than 6 months. Bipolar patients appear to need more frequent maintenance sessions than unipolar patients. It is advised that inter-treatment intervals should not be greater than 1 to 3 weeks (29).

The maintenance ECT practice at the Mayo Clinic, Rochester, USA, was reviewed for the year 2000 in a retrospective study. Forty-three patients had received maintenance ECT for at least 1 year. The reviewed patients had unipolar non-psychotic depression ($n = 19$), unipolar psychotic depression ($n = 15$), bipolar disorder ($n = 4$), and schizoaffective disorder ($n = 5$). They had multiple medication or psychotherapy trials or both and multiple hospitalizations before receiving maintenance therapy. The data showed that patients sustained initial post-index ECT depression ratings and had even a slight drop over time, had improved functional status, and showed no cognitive deterioration as measured with the Mini Mental State Examination (MMSE). In the year before maintenance ECT (excluding the time of the index treatments), there was a collective total of 817 psychiatric hospital days compared to a total of 139 psychiatric hospital days during the time of maintenance ECT, which averaged 29 months/patient. However, data did not include patients who were not given maintenance ECT at least for 1 year. As conclusion, there seems to be a subset of patients that benefits from maintenance ECT, which is considered efficacious and safe (30).

Special Patient Populations

In a Cochrane review, the efficacy and safety of ECT (compared to simulated ECT or antidepressants) in depressed elderly was assessed. Articles published between 1966 and 2000 were analyzed. Randomized, controlled trials on depressed elderly

(> 60 years) with or without concomitant conditions like cerebrovascular disease, dementia of the Alzheimer's type, vascular dementia, or Parkinson's disease were included. Only three randomized trials could be included, one on the efficacy of real ECT vs. simulated ECT, one on the efficacy of unilateral vs. bilateral ECT, and the other comparing the efficacy of ECT once a week with ECT three times weekly. All studies had major methodological shortcomings, and data essential to perform a quantitative analysis were mostly lacking. Although in one study, it was concluded that real ECT was superior over simulated ECT, these conclusions need to be interpreted cautiously. Only results from the second trial (unilateral vs. bilateral ECT) could be analyzed, not convincingly showing efficacy of unilateral ECT over bilateral ECT. Randomized evidence on the efficacy and safety of ECT in depressed elderly with concomitant dementia, cerebrovascular disorders, or Parkinson's disease is completely lacking. Possible side effects could not be adequately examined because of the lack of randomized evidence and the methodological shortcomings. The reviewers concluded that none of the objectives of the review could be adequately tested because of the lack of firm, randomized evidence. They call for a well-designed randomized controlled trial in which the efficacy of ECT is compared to one or more antidepressant (31). However, the application of ECT in the elderly is widely assessed in prospective follow-up studies albeit without randomization or control conditions, in retrospective studies and in case reports. It is also on the grounds of this broadly based clinical experience that ECT is considered as an efficient treatment with an acceptable side effect profile in the elderly (2).

A review article by Rey and Walter (32) assessed efficacy and safety of ECT in young people (under 18). Sixty reports were identified with a total of 396 patients. Most of them were single case reports, without controlled studies. Rates of improvement were 63% for depression, 80% for mania, 42% for schizophrenia, and 80% for catatonia. The authors concluded that ECT in the young seems similar in effectiveness and in side effects to ECT in adults.

In New South Wales, Australia, 1.53 patients aged 14 to 18 in 100,000 adolescents were treated annually from 1990 to 1999, a total of 84 courses (826 ECTs) in 72 patients, according to a retrospective study. An increase in the use of ECT in involuntarily hospitalized females was observed between the period from 1990 to 1995 compared to 1996 to 1999. Marked improvement or resolution of symptoms after a completed course of ECT occurred in patients suffering from psychotic depression (after 83% of completed courses), mania (100%), bipolar disorder (89%), mood disorders generally (72%), and catatonic schizophrenia (80%), but only after 24% of courses in patients with schizophrenia spectrum disorders. Adverse events included headache (after 61% of courses), confusion (20%), subjective memory problems (19%), and manic switch (4%). Prolonged seizures (longer than 3 minutes) were observed in three of the 826 treatments. ECT is viewed by the authors as an efficient treatment especially in mood disorders, with generally minor adverse events (33).

NEW BRAIN STIMULATION METHODS FOR BIPOLAR DISORDERS UNDER RESEARCH

Of the four other brain stimulation methods (VNS, TMS, MST, and DBS), studies to evaluate a clinical efficacy in bipolar disorder have only been conducted with TMS at the time. However, the other methods appear to have mood modulating properties, which might prove interesting by further evaluating their extent and mechanisms.

Transcranial Magnetic Stimulation

Transcranial magnetic stimulation refers to a technique of delivering magnetic pulses to the cerebral cortex with a stimulating coil, which is directly applied to the head. The equipment consists of two parts: a stimulator, which generates brief pulses of strong electrical currents whose frequency and intensity can be varied, and the stimulation coil. Single, paired, or repetitive magnetic pulses (rTMS) can be delivered. The magnetic field generated at the coil has a peak strength comparable to the magnetic field generated by a magnetic resonance imaging device. It passes unimpeded through scalp and scull, inducing an electrical current in the underlying tissues that depolarizes neurons up to a distance of 2 to 3 cm. Therefore, only superficial structures of the brain can be directly interfered with. However, distant effects of the application of TMS for example on regional cerebral blood flow can be measured (34,35). TMS can transiently disrupt or induce activity in focal brain regions, depending on the region stimulated. Applied to the visual cortex for example, strong TMS can produce phosphenes, and a stimulus of lower intensity induces transient scotomas (36). Also other functions, such as linguistic processing, can be investigated with rTMS (37).

Recently, three meta-analyses assessing the relevance of the antidepressant effect of TMS have been published. In the meta-analysis published by Burt et al. (38) three categories of studies were analyzed: open and uncontrolled trials, sham or otherwise controlled trials, and comparisons of rTMS and ECT. In the uncontrolled studies, the degree of therapeutic change was estimated to be relatively modest. The average reduction in Hamilton Depression Rating Scale (HDRS) scores or Montgomery–Asberg Depression Rating Scale (MADRS) scores was only 37% (SD = 29, unweighted mean). The meta-analysis concerning the controlled studies yielded similar conclusions: among the 23 comparisons between rTMS stimulation and a supposed less or non-therapeutic condition, the combined effect size (Cohen's *d*) was 0.67, whereas the point estimate for the Cohen's *d* (432 individual cases, unadjusted) was 0.79 ($p < 0.0001$). The magnitude of therapeutic effects was estimated to be doubtful, since the average (unweighted) percentage change in HDRS scores in the active condition was 23.9% (SD = 24.9), while the sham or control condition resulted in a percentage improvement of 7.3% (SD = 25.1). Three studies (39–41) comparing rTMS with ECT in a total of 112 cases were analyzed and yielded a combined Cohen's *d* of 0.21 favoring ECT. The average percent improvement in HDRS scores in the rTMS conditions was 47.1%, double the magnitude of the therapeutic effect of the meta-analysis comparing TMS with sham or control condition. The authors suggested that rTMS conditions in these studies were longer than the ones usually administered and that sample characteristics may have predisposed to a favorable rTMS response. The average percentage improvement of ECT was only 54.5%, unusually low for this form of treatment since high dosage right unilateral and bilateral ECT averaged at about 70% improvement in recently published studies (11).

Martin et al. (42) conducted a systematic review of randomized controlled trials that compared rTMS with sham in patients with depression. A total of 14 trials (324 patients) were included. The pooled analysis using the HDRS scores showed an effect in favor of rTMS compared with sham after 2 weeks of treatment (standardized mean difference =−0.35; 95% CI −0.66 to −0.04), but this was not significant at the 2-week follow-up (standardized mean difference −0.33; 95% CI −0.84 to 0.17). They concluded that current trials provide insufficient evidence to support the *clinical* use of rTMS in the treatment of depression.

These meta-analyses confirmed earlier results of a meta-analysis where also a statistical significant difference was found between rTMS and sham condition with limited therapeutic effect (43). In the meta-analysis by McNamara et al. (44), rTMS was found to have more pronounced antidepressant effect than placebo conditions with a number needed to treat of 2–3 with a 95% confidence interval 1.6–4.0, total, in fife suitable trials for meta-analysis including 81 patients.

Two studies comparing ECT with rTMS not included in the above meta-analysis have also been published recently. In one 25 and in the other 41 patients were included. They both did not find differences in efficacy between ECT and rTMS (45,46). In the study by Dannon et al. (46), data gathered at 3- and 6-month follow-up points suggest that the clinical gains obtained with rTMS last at least as long as those obtained with ECT. The results of these studies should, however, be considered as not yet definitive and they should be viewed bearing in mind the conclusions in the meta-analysis by Burt et al. (38), cited above.

Other recently published studies assessing therapeutic outcome do not warrant different conclusions concerning the antidepressant efficacy of TMS than the ones drawn from the meta-analyses mentioned above. These studies have generally low numbers of assessed patients. In some reports, there is no difference of efficacy between sham conditions and the real stimulation condition (47–49), whereas in others real stimulation conditions yields better antidepressant efficacy (50). Patient parameters probably predictive for a better response to rTMS are still not clearly established. Psychotic features, higher age, bad previous response to rTMS, and certain brain physiological markers assessed by functional neuroimaging (51,52) might be associated with a diminished antidepressant effect of rTMS (53).

The specific antidepressant efficacy of rTMS in bipolar disorder has also been assessed. Results are however contradictory and preliminary. In a double-blind, controlled study, 10 patients received 20 sessions of rTMS and 10 patients received 10 sessions of sham rTMS followed by 20 sessions of rTMS. Sham rTMS was found to have no effect. The real group showed statistically significant improvement compared to the control group after 2 weeks of stimulation. Both patient groups responded similarly to TMS after 2 weeks of real stimulation. Additional stimulation of another 2 weeks did not change the antidepressant response (54). Twenty-three depressed patients suffering from bipolar I (12 patients), bipolar II (nine patients), and bipolar disorder mixed state (two patients) were randomly assigned to receive either daily left prefrontal rTMS (5 Hz, 110% motor threshold, 8 seconds on, 22 seconds off, during 20 minutes) or placebo stimulation each weekday morning during 2 weeks. No difference could be found in the rate of responders as defined by an HDRS <10 or the mean HDRS change from baseline over the 2 weeks. The stimulation was well tolerated with no significant adverse events or induction of mania (55).

Only few studies assessing antimanic properties of rTMS have been conducted. Sixteen patients with mania according to DSM-IV were stimulated at 80% of their motor threshold and given 10 daily consecutive sessions of 20 trains per session. Frequency was 20 Hz for 2 seconds per train; inter-train interval was 1 minute. The stimuli were given over the right prefrontal cortex or the left prefrontal cortex, randomly assigned. Evaluation of the clinical efficacy was based on assessment with the brief psychiatric rating scale, mania subscale, and the Young Mania Rating Scale. Significantly more improvement was observed in patients treated with right than with left prefrontal TMS. It was concluded that right prefrontal TMS had antimanic properties (56). In a subsequent controlled study, 19 patients completed a course of right TMS (11 patients) vs. sham right rTMS (eight patients) according to the same parameters as outlined above. Right TMS was no more effective than sham rTMS. The authors concluded, that possibly the previous results were due to an effect of left rTMS to worsen mania (57).

Compared to ECT, MST, DBS, and VNS, rTMS can be considered as relatively safe, since it is noninvasive and the induction of convulsions are not required for a treatment. Therefore, side effects linked to anesthesia and convulsion do not occur. There are, however, side effects directly linked to the application of rTMS or occurring till a few hours later. Of major concern is involuntarily induced epileptic seizure. Potential side effects of minor importance include local pain during application, changes in the auditory performance due to the noise generated in the coil, and headache as well as the concern of alterations of cognitive functions.

The risk of causing a seizure is the primary safety concern with TMS. Even if this risk is primarily associated with rTMS, also single pulse stimulation has been reported to produce seizures in patients with large cerebral infarcts, contusions, or other structural brain lesions. According to Wassermann (58), in patients with completely subcortical lesions, no seizures are reported. According to the same author, there are a few articles reporting the induction of seizures in epilepsy patients without gross lesions.

Mainly short-term observations concerning cognitive function after TMS administration are available. rTMS can produce transient disruption of various cerebral functions, depending on the site of stimulation. Observations reported include a significant decrease in a memory subtest within an hour after stimulation with 150 trains of rTMS at 15 Hz and 120% motor threshold delivered at four different positions (37). Commenting this results, Lorberbaum and Wassermann (59) conclude that these cognitive effects were due to sub-convulsive epileptic activity or that the threshold for adverse effects on memory might be near that of seizure. Recent studies confirm that the application of TMS is not associated with significant cognitive side effects (48,49,60).

No significant changes in auditory threshold were observed in a study involving 12 depressed subjects undergoing rTMS during 4 weeks when assessed for 4 weeks after the end of the study (61).

The application of TMS may cause local pain resulting from direct stimulation of muscles underlying the coil and from stimulation of facial and scalp nerves. It is generally more painful at higher intensities and frequencies. About 5–20% of subjects experience subsequently tension headache (62).

The International Society for Transcranial Stimulation (ISTS) has published guidelines concerning the application and the managing of risks of rTMS in order to assure the safety of subjects and patients and to guarantee minimal standards (63,64). It is clear that the use of rTMS should comply with regulations put forward by local regulatory bodies, medical professional organizations, and medical licensing boards (64).

Magnetic Seizure Therapy

Magnetic seizure therapy is a method using rTMS at convulsive parameters in order to induce therapeutic seizures under general anesthesia in the same setting as the one used for ECT (for a review, see Ref. 65). The following reasons led to the development of MST. (a) ECT is considered as one of the most efficient treatments of depression, especially of drug resistant depression (18). The induced convulsion is necessary to the antidepressant effect of ECT. Indeed, the benefit of induced convulsions in psychiatric disorders led initially to the development of ECT. Therefore, a method capable to reliably induce convulsions has a great potential to have also antidepressant and other clinically useful properties. (b) During the last 65 years, the application of ECT has been steadily improved and the side effect profile of ECT changed dramatically. However, at least one-third of patients treated with ECT experience significant memory loss (3). The cognitive impairments are directly related to the applied dose of current passing through the brain. They also depend on the location of the electrodes, bilateral stimulation causing more important cognitive impairment than unilateral (11,66). This could be due to the electrical currents passing through both hippocampi when bilateral stimulation is applied. Indeed, the hippocampi are important regions implied in episodic memory (67). A method inducing seizures not impairing memory would therefore be a potentially important step in improving the available physical treatment of depression and other psychiatric disorders.

The first therapeutic magnetic seizure in a psychiatric patient was induced at the University Hospital in Bern, Switzerland, in 2000 (68). Results of a randomized, within-subject, double-masked trial comparing ECT and MST in 10 patients indicate that MST appears to have less subjective and objective side effects, is associated with faster recovery of orientation, and is superior to ECT on measures of attention, retrograde amnesia, and category fluency (69). This could be due to the fact that MST allows a more focused stimulation of the brain to induce seizures. Recently, the successful treatment by MST of a patient suffering from-difficult-to-treat major depression has been reported (70). This methodology is still in a very early phase. The antidepressant efficacy of MST remains to be proved in appropriate trials. Technical problems have to be solved in order to further develop powerful and reliable stimulators. However, if the antidepressant effect could be confirmed and if MST could be shown to have a better side effect profile than ECT, this new form of magnetic brain stimulation could get an important place in the treatment of depression, and probably also bipolar depression.

Vagus Nerve Stimulation

Vagus nerve stimulation refers generally to the electrical stimulation of the left vagus nerve at the cervical level. Stimuli are generated and delivered by the VNS Therapy® System (VNS-TS) manufactured by Cyberonics Inc., Houston, Texas, U.S.A. Two helical electrodes are wrapped around the left vagus nerve and are linked to a pulse generator, which is similar to a cardiac pacemaker in size and shape. The generator is implanted subcutaneously in the chest wall below the left clavicle. It can be programmed by telemetry. VNS is the only brain stimulation technique where the stimulation is not applied directly to the central nervous system. The left vagus nerve, which carries about 80% of afferent fibers, is used to modulate indirectly brain structures belonging to the vagal projection system. By this technique, the state of excitability of the brain is influenced but also structures of the limbic system implicated in mood regulation.

The first clinical investigations of VNS in humans with the VNS-TS were carried out in 1988 (71). The development of the VNS-TS was initiated on the basis of animal model experiments showing that stimulation of the vagus nerve aborted or reduced seizures (72). Since 1988, more than 20,000 VNS-TS have been implanted in patients suffering from of epilepsy. The U.S.-Food and Drug Administration (FDA) approved VNS in 1997 as an adjunctive therapy in reducing the frequency of seizures in adults and adolescents over 12 years of age with partial onset seizures that are refractory to antiepileptic medications (73). In a recent Cochrane review, two randomized double-blind trials (both sponsored by Cyberonics Inc.) were analyzed with regard to reduction in seizure frequency and side effects in patients suffering from drug-resistant partial epilepsy. The reviewers drew the conclusion that VNS appeared to be an effective treatment for the adjunctive treatment of medication-resistant partial seizures and that it was well tolerated with a substantially different adverse effects profile than antiepileptic drugs. Statistically significant adverse effects associated with implantation were hoarseness, cough, pain, and paresthesia, and statistically significant adverse effects associated with therapeutic stimulation were hoarseness, cough, dyspnea, pain, and paresthesia (74).

The first implant of a VNS-TS system for treatment-resistant depression was performed in 1998 at the Brain Stimulation Laboratory of the Medical University of South Carolina. Clinical observations of improved mood in VNS-treated patients suffering from epilepsy lead to focused investigations of the effect of VNS on comorbid symptoms of depression and anxiety in epilepsy patients. Twenty adult patients were assessed before and 3 months after VNS implantation and compared to a control group on stable antiepileptic drug treatment not treated with VNS. The VNS group showed a significant decrease in mood scales [Cornell Dysthymia Rating Scale, HDRS, Beck depression inventory] but not in the Hamilton Rating Scale for anxiety. No significant differences between the two groups were found across time (75). Mood improvement could also be documented in a study where 28 patients treated for 6 months with VNS were assessed with several self-rating scales. Although Beck depression inventory scores did not improve at a statistically significant level, other indicators of general mood improved (a rating scale measuring dysphoria and anxiety) (76). Since the publication of results of an open-label, multicenter pilot study (D01-study) involving 60 patients suffering from depression, VNS has gained considerable interest as a potential treatment of relative drug-resistant major depressive episodes (MDEs). Results of these investigations as well as from a 1-year follow-up of 30 patients are promising (77,78) and in 2001, VNS was approved for a CE mark (indicating compliance with safety and environmental regulations) in the member countries of the European Union for treatment of adults with treatment-resistant or treatment-intolerant chronic or recurrent depression, including unipolar and bipolar depression.

In the D01 study, 30 patients were included and 30 patients were later added (77,79). Patients with a DSM-IV diagnosis of major depressive disorder or bipolar I or II disorder were included who suffered currently from an MDE. The MDE had to be longer than 2 years in duration or the patient had to have at least four MDEs in his or her lifetime. Patients had to score at least 3 on the antidepressant treatment history form indicating that they had failed to at least two medication trials during the current MDE using different medication classes. It was required that no substantial clinical improvement was detected in a psychotherapy trial of at least 6 weeks. The score on the Hamilton depression rating 28-item scale had to be at least 20 and scores on the global assessment of function scale had to be 50 at maximum. Those with bipolar disorder had to have resistance, intolerance, or a medical contraindication to lithium. Exclusion criteria included atypical or psychotic features in the current MDE; a history of schizophrenia, schizoaffective disorder, or other non-mood disorder psychosis; current rapid-cycling bipolar disorder; a current secondary diagnosis or signs of delirium, dementia, amnesia, or other cognitive disorder; and clinically significant current suicidal intent. Six patients were diagnosed with bipolar I disorder, 10 with bipolar II disorder, 28 with unipolar recurrent disorder, and 16 with unipolar disorder, single episode. During the acute study (baseline period before VNS and 12-week period after the implantation) medication regimens were kept stable, except that that medication dosage could be decreased, but not increased (79). Among the 59 patients who completed the acute phase of the study, the diagnosis (unipolar vs. bipolar) was not identified as a prognostic factor by logistic regression based on the assessment of symptoms of depression by the HDRS (79).

In a follow-up study, the first 30 included patients were assessed until 9 months after the 3-month acute study. During this period, changes in psychotropic medication and VNS parameters were allowed. The response rate (defined as at least 50% reduction in baseline HDRS score) was 40% (12/30) and the remission rate (HDRS score less than 10) increased from 17% (5/30) after the acute phase study to 29% (8/28) (78). There continued to be evidence of sustained or even enhanced response to VNS in patients reaching the 2-year mark (54% of responders in 24 patients) (73).

The acute phase of a double-blind, controlled study involving 235 patients (in 20 sites in the United States) with chronic or recurrent pharmacoresistant depression was completed in October 2001. Antidepressant efficacy did not differ at a statistically significant level between the active ($n = 114$ patients) and the sham treatment group. At the 1-year follow-up (patients of the sham treatment group were switched to the real treatment group after the end of the acute study), 30% of the VNS-treated patients ($n = 205$) responded to the treatment as defined by a 50% reduction of the HRDS score. A matched group of 124 depressed patients were treated during 1 year with the best available treatment. In this group, only 13% fulfilled the response criteria (data on file, Cyberonics Inc.). First data on results in an open-label European multicenter study following the same protocol as the D01 study has become available recently (80). Antidepressant effects seem to be considerably higher in this study, a partial explanation for this difference seems to be the higher degree of treatment resistance of patients in the American D01 study.

Mortality in patients treated with VNS was assessed in a 2-year extension of a study of mortality and sudden, unexpected, unexplained death in epilepsy in the cohort of patients receiving VNS for the treatment of epilepsy. One thousand eight hundred and nineteen individuals were followed for a total of 3176 person-years from implantation. The rates for sudden, unexpected, unexplained death in epilepsy under VNS treatment were found to be similar to those reported from clinical trials with new drugs and cohorts of patients with severe epilepsy. The rate of sudden, unexpected, unexplained death of 5.5 per 1000 person-years over the first 2 years of treatment dropped to 1.7 thereafter (81). Postoperative infection is estimated to occur in approximately 3–6% of patients (82). Intraoperative ventricular asystole during the initial testing of the VNS-TS device is reported in nine patients. These episodes resolved without further negative consequences for the patients (83). The occurrence of such phenomena in patients with epilepsy was estimated to be 0.1% (84).

The following side effects (percentage of a population of 95 patients) were reported (only side effects occurring in at least 10% of patients): Voice alteration (66%), cough (45%), pharyngitis (35%), pain (28%), dyspnea (25%), headache (24%), dyspepsia (18%), vomiting (18%), paresthesia (18%), nausea (15%), accidental injury (13%), fever (12%), infection (12%). Only voice alteration and dyspnea were significantly higher in this stimulation group compared with the 103 patients in the low (placebo) stimulation group. One implanted patient of the high stimulation group had postictal Cheyne–Stokes respiration which recurred also after device deactivation (85).

Isolated complications of VNS such as chronic diarrhea (86), Horner syndrome (87), posture-dependent stimulation of the phrenic nerve (88), spasm of the sternocleidomastoid muscle (89), worsening of preexisting obstructive sleep apnea (90), increased risk of aspiration among children with severe mental and motor retardation coupled with a need for assistance with feeding (91), and swallowing difficulties in children (92) have been reported. Side effects are primarily a function of output current and, to a lesser extent, pulse duration and duty cycle. Duty cycles less than or equal to 50% appear to be safe and effective. Side effects seem to respond to a reduction in pulse duration, e.g., from 500 μs to 250 μs (93). Microwave transmission, cellular phones, and airport systems do not affect the NCP system. However, the manufacturer advises reasonable caution in avoiding devices that generate strong electric or magnetic fields. He indicates that therapeutic radiation, external defibrillation, extracorporal shockwave lithotripsy, and electrocautery surgery may damage the pulse generator's circuitry. Magnetic resonance imaging should not be performed with a magnetic resonance body coil in the transmit mode. According to the manufacturer's guidelines, an MRI should be done only using a transmit and receive type head of coil and specific precautions have to be respected (94).

In the studies on depression, the most common adverse side events at 1-year post-implantation were voice alteration (21%), and dyspnea and neck pain (each 7%). No patient discontinued due to adverse events. One patient, however, had the generator explanted due to lack of efficacy at 11 months post-implantation. An episode of deep venous thrombophlebitis and one episode of hypomania resulted in hospitalizations and were judged by the investigators as possibly related to stimulation. One patient received ECT treatment with the VNS-TS implanted but switched off. No complications were reported (78). The effect of VNS on cognitive functions was assessed in 27 treatment-resistant depressed patients taking part in the studies cited. They were assessed with a neurocognitive test battery before and 10 weeks after the start of VNS. No deterioration in any neurocognitive measure was detected. Motor speed (finger tapping), performance of the digit symbol test, verbal fluency, logical reasoning, working memory, and response inhibition improved (95). Effects of VNS on memory appear however to be complex. VNS could enhance recognition memory in humans (96). There are indications that VNS might deteriorate reversibly figural but not verbal memory (97).

Compared to other antidepressant treatment modalities, the cost profile of VNS could be beneficial, if effective maintenance therapy could be achieved with either a reduction in the use of concomitant drugs or a reduction in other costs, such as hospitalization for depression relapses. However, in the treatment of drug-refractory epilepsy, a seizure-free state is rarely achieved and VNS is mostly combined with antiepileptic drug maintenance therapy (98).

Deep Brain Stimulation

Deep brain stimulation is a technique, which allows to directly stimulate brain areas using microelectrodes with a diameter on the order of a millimeter. These electrodes are stereotactically targeted to the structures planned to be stimulated. The electrodes are linked to a multipolar pulse generator similar in size to a cardiac pacemaker and implanted subcutaneously below the clavicles. The stimulators are programmed using telemetry. The most important field of application of DBS are movement disorders, especially Parkinson's disease. Indeed, DBS of the thalamus received CE-mark approval in 1993 for the treatment of tremor and in 1997, approval by the U.S.-Food and Drug Administration (FDA). To treat movement disorders other than (or in addition to) tremor by stimulating the sub-thalamic nucleurs (STN) or the globus pallidus internus was approved in Europe in 1998 (CE-mark) and in 1998 in the United States (FDA approval) (99). Investigational uses in neurology include epilepsy, pain, dystonia, brain injury, and vegetative states (100).

In psychiatry, DBS is being investigated as a potential treatment of refractory obsessive–compulsive disorder (OCD). Available results indicate that DBS might have substantial benefits in otherwise very difficult to treat patients (101–103). There are also several reports that DBS produces marked affective changes in movement disorder patients. It may induce depressive symptoms and even suicidality (104,105) but also mood improvement (106) and even manic states (107,108). Important methodological problems (site of stimulation, stimulation parameters, patient population, which might benefit from this technique) as well as ethical problems remain to be resolved. An application of DBS in bipolar disorders remains at the present moment highly hypothetical. In intractable OCD, the success of disrupting dysfunctional corticobasal brain circuits by stereotactic psychosurgery laid the ground to test whether function lesions induced by high-frequency DBS would have similar clinical effects. Such experience is lacking in bipolar disorder, where pathophysiological mechanisms appear to be less clear.

DISCUSSION AND CONCLUSIONS

Scientifically based psychiatrists consider ECT as a highly effective treatment that is most certainly underused in bipolar disorders. In psychiatry, it is among the treatments that have been most intensely and for the longest time investigated. For the large majority of patients, ECT is a save therapy and the sometimes prominent side effects are in most cases transitory. It is also important to note, that these side effects are of minor importance when treating potentially life-threatening disorders (109) with a mortality rate of up to 20% in the case of depression (110). In a study assessing the patients' views on the benefits of and possible memory loss from ECT, over 80% of patients from the Royal College of Psychiatrists in the U.K. were satisfied with ECT. However, memory loss that was persistent at least 6 months after a treatment course was considered as clinically relevant in at least one-third of the patient population (3).

There are relatively few controlled clinical trials published where actual diagnostic criteria are applied and modern ECT techniques used, for example brief or ultrabrief electrical pulses. This applies especially for bipolar disorders. It is not possible to date to differentiate the efficacy of ECT in unipolar and bipolar depression, since the available data are not conclusive. Also recent controlled trials in mania, which besides depression and some forms of schizophrenia is considered a primary indication for ECT [according to the ECT-Task Force Report of the American Psychiatric Association (2)], are rare. One explanation of the relative lack of such studies might be the lack of funding from companies for obvious reasons (5).

Challenges facing the field of convulsive therapy today include maintaining response following an effective course of ECT and minimizing cognitive side effects. Still, it is of obvious importance to investigate the underlying mechanisms of the treatment in order to understand effect and side effects better and thus to improve acceptance of the therapy for patients and the public at large. Concerning the application of ECT, there is an ongoing discussion about the best compromise between side effect profile and clinical efficacy, e.g., whether it is best to administer high dosage unilateral or lower dosage bilateral ECT, whether fixed dose or individually adapted dose ECT should be administered, etc. Another problem of the field is that indications and use of ECT are in many countries not based on the scientific evidence but on political considerations (5,8). The confidence of patients, health care professionals, and society at large in ECT has to be increased by the application of high-quality standards (111) and maximal transparence in the communication with concerned patients and their surrounding persons.

Besides its clinical usefulness, ECT remains an important research tool. Its precise mechanism of action, which is obviously different from that of pharmacological treatments, remains a secret to be discovered. This will continue to provide insights into the research on pathophysiological mechanisms of the disorders, in which ECT is effective. Such exciting new developments include the modulation of gene expression, intracellular signaling, or neurogenesis (112–114).

During the last few years, several novel methods using electrical stimulation of the brain have been developed and investigated as treatments of depression. They are at different stages of development. Until now, none of them has been approved by the U.S.-FDA as a treatment for major depression or bipolar disorders. MST has to be considered as a promising but still very experimental technique where antidepressant efficacy and major technical problems still need to be addressed. Until now, no data have been published concerning the use of DBS as an antidepressant or antimanic treatment. VNS is a standard technique to treat drug treatment refractory partial onset epilepsy. Preliminary data indicate that it has an antidepressant effect at medium term (after 1 year). As for rTMS, definite results of large multicenter studies establishing clearly an antidepressant effect are still lacking and concerning mania, only a few trials with conflicting results are available. Besides, main open questions about the use of rTMS concern technical questions (where to stimulate, at which parameters, frequency, and for how long), diagnostic ones (age of patients, psychotic vs. non-psychotic depression) as well as the place of rTMS in the antidepressant treatment armamentarium (rTMS as only treatment or as add-on treatment, rTMS as maintenance therapy after a course of ECT). Besides the clinical aspects, all these techniques offer exciting research tools that, hopefully, allow the investigation of the neurobiology of depression and other psychiatric disorders.

REFERENCES

1. Diagnostic and Statistical Manual of Mental Disorders (DSM IV). Washington DC: American Psychiatric Association, 1994.
2. ECT Task Force of the American Psychiatric Association: the Practice of Electroconvulsive Therapy. Washington DC: American Psychiatric Press, 2001.
3. Rose D, Fleischmann P, Wykes T, Leese M, Bindman J. Patients' perspectives on electroconvulsive therapy: systematic review. BMJ 2003; 326(7403):1363.
4. McDonald A, Garry Walter G. The portrayal of ECT in American movies. J ECT 2001; 17(4):264–274.
5. Fink M. ECT has much to offer our patients: it should not be ignored. World J Biol Psychiatry 2001; 2(1):1–8.

6. Reisner AD. The electroconvulsive therapy controversy: evidence and ethics. Neuropsychol Rev 2003; 13(4):199–219.
7. Youssef H, Youssef F. The death of electroconvulsive therapy. Adv Ther 2001; 18(2): 83–89.
8. Banken R. L'utilisation des électrochocs au Québec. Montréal: Agence d'évaluation des technologies et des modes d'intervention en santé (AETMIS), © Gouvernement du Québec, 2003, 2002:xvii–103.
9. Beyer JL, Weiner RD, Glenn MD. Electroconvulsive Therapy. Washington: American Psychiatric Press, 1998.
10. Weiner RD, Rogers HJ, Davidson JR, Squire LR. Effects of stimulus parameters on cognitive side effects. Ann NY Acad Sci 1986; 462:315–325.
11. Sackeim HA, Prudic J, Devanand DP, Nobler MS, Lisanby SH, Peyser S, Fitzsimons L, Moody BJ, Clark J. A prospective, randomized, double-blind comparison of bilateral and right unilateral electroconvulsive therapy at different stimulus intensities. Arch Gen Psychiatry 2000; 57(5):425–434.
12. McCall WV. Electroconvulsive therapy in the era of modern psychopharmacology. Int J Neuropsychopharmacol 2001; 4:315–324.
13. Dwork AJ, Arango V, Underwood M, Ilievski B, Rosoklija G, Sackeim HA, Lisanby SH. Absence of histological lesions in primate models of ECT and magnetic seizure therapy. Am J Psychiatry 2004; 161(3):576–578.
14. American Psychiatric Association. Practice guideline for the treatment of patients with bipolar disorder (revision). Am J Psychiatry 2002; 159(4 suppl):1–50.
15. Grunze H, Kasper S, Goodwin G, Bowden C, Baldwin D, Licht R, Vieta E, Moller HJ. World Federation of Societies of Biological Psychiatry (WFSBP) guidelines for biological treatment of bipolar disorders. Part I: treatment of bipolar depression. World J Biol Psychiatry 2002; 3(3):115–124.
16. Grunze H, Kasper S, Goodwin G, Bowden C, Baldwin D, Licht RW, Vieta E, Möller HJ. The World Federation of Societies of Biological Psychiatry (WFSBP) guidelines for the biological treatment of bipolar disorders, part II: treatment of mania. World J Biol Psychiatry 2003; 4:5–13.
17. Kellner CH, Fink M. The efficacy of ECT and "treatment resistance." J ECT 2002; 18:1–2.
18. The UK ECT Review Group. Efficacy and safety of electroconvulsive therapy in depressive disorders: a systematic review and meta-analysis. Lancet 2003; 361:799–808.
19. Han Kho KH, van Vreeswijk MF, Simpson S, Zwinderman AH. A meta-analysis of electroconvulsive therapy efficacy in depression. J ECT 2003; 19(3):139–147.
20. Daly JJ, Prudic J, Devanand DP, Nobler MS, Lisanby SH, Peyser S, Roose SP, Sackeim HA. ECT in bipolar and unipolar depression: differences in speed of response. Bipolar Disord 2001; 3(2):95–104.
21. Keck PE Jr, Mendlwicz J, Calabrese JR, Fawcett J, Suppes T, Vestergaard PA, Carbonell C. A review of randomized, controlled clinical trials in acute mania. J Affect Disord 2000; 59(suppl 1):S31–S37.
22. Mukherjee S, Sackeim HA, Schnur DB. Electroconvulsive therapy of acute manic episodes: a review of 50 years' experience. Am J Psychiatry 1994; 151(2):169–176.
23. Volpe FM, Tavares A. Impact of ECT on duration of hospitalizations for mania. J ECT 2003; 19(1):17–21.
24. Kho KH. Treatment of rapid cycling bipolar disorder in the acute and maintenance phase with ECT. J ECT 2002; 18(3):159–161.
25. Devanand DP, Polanco P, Cruz R, Shah S, Paykina N, Singh K, Majors L. The efficacy of ECT in mixed affective states. J ECT 2000; 16(1):32–37.
26. Ciapparelli A, Dell'Osso L, Tundo A, Pini S, Chiavacci MC, Di Sacco I, Cassano GB. Electroconvulsive therapy in medication-nonresponsive patients with mixed mania and bipolar depression. J Clin Psychiatry 2001; 62(7):552–555.

27. Gruber NP, Dilsaver SC, Shoaib AM, Swann MC. ECT in mixed affective states: a case series. J ECT 2000; 16(2):183–188.
28. Bourgon LN, Kellner CH. Relapse of depression after ECT: a review. J ECT 2000; 16(1):19–31.
29. Vaidya NA, Mahableshwarkar AR, Shahid R. Continuation and maintenance ECT in treatment-resistant bipolar disorder. J ECT 2003; 19(1):10–16.
30. Russell JC, Rasmussen KG, O'Connor MK, Copeman CA, Ryan DA, Rummans TA. Long-term maintenance ECT: a retrospective review of efficacy and cognitive outcomes. J ECT 2003; 19:4–9.
31. Van der Wurff FB, Stek ML, Hoogendijk WL, Beekman AT. Electroconvulsive therapy for the depressed elderly. Cochrane Database Syst Rev 2003; 2(CD003593).
32. Rey JM, Walter G. Half a century of ECT use in young people. Am J Psychiatry 1997; 154(5):595–602.
33. Walter G, Rey JM. Has the practice and outcome of ECT in adolescents changed? Findings from a whole-population study. J ECT 2003; 19(2):84–87.
34. Bohning DE, Shastri A, Wassermann EM, Ziemann U, Lorberbaum JP, Nahas Z, Lomarev MP, George MS. BOLD-fMRI response to single-pulse transcranial magnetic stimulation (TMS). J Magn Res Imag 2000; 11:569–574.
35. Catafau AM, Perez V, Gironell A, Martin JC, Kulisevsky J, Estorch M, Carrio I, Alvarez E. SPECT mapping of cerebral activity changes induced by repetitive transcranial magnetic stimulation in depressed patients. A pilot study. Psychiatry Res Neuroimag Sec 2001; 106:151–160.
36. Hallett M. Transcranial magnetic stimulation and the brain. Nature 2000; 406:147–150.
37. Flitman SS, Grafman J, Wassermann EM, Cooper BA, O'Grady J, Pascual-Leone A, Hallett M. Linguistic processing during repetitive transcranial magnetic stimulation. Neurology 1998; 50:175–181.
38. Burt T, Lisanby SH, Sackeim HA. Neuropsychiatric applications of transcranial magnetic stimulation: a meta analysis. Int J Neuropsychopharmacol 2002; 5(1):73–103.
39. Grunhaus L, Dannon PN, Schreiber S, Dolberg OH, Amiaz R, Ziv R, Lefkifker E. Repetitive transcranial magnetic stimulation is as effective as electroconvulsive therapy in the treatment of nondelusional depressive disorder: an open study. Biol Psychiatry 2000; 47:314–324.
40. Grunhaus L, Schreiber S, Dolberg OT, Polak D, Dannon PN. A randomized controlled comparison of electroconvulsive therapy and repetitive transcranial magnetic stimulation in severe and resistant nonpsychotic major depression. Biol Psychiatry 2003; 53(4):324–331.
41. Pridmore S, Bruno R, Turinier-Shea Y, Reid P, Rybak M. Comparison of unlimited numbers of rapid transcranial magnetic stimulation (rTMS) and ECT treatment sessions in major depressive episode. Int J Neuropsychopharmacol 2000; 3:129–134.
42. Martin JL, Barbanoj MJ, Schlaepfer TE, Thompson E, Perez V, Kulisevsky J. Repetitive transcranial magnetic stimulation for the treatment of depression. Systematic review and meta-analysis.. Br J Psychiatry 2003; 182:480–491.
43. Holtzheimer PE, Russo J, Avery DH. A meta-analysis of repetitive transcranial magnetic stimulation in the treatment of depression. Psychopharmacol Bull 2001; 35(4): 149–169.
44. McNamara B, Ray JL, Arthurs OJ, Boniface S. Transcranial magnetic stimulation for depression and other psychiatric disorders. Psychol Med 2001; 31(7):1141–1146.
45. Janicak PG, Dowd SM, Martis B, Alam D, Beedle D, Krasuski J, Strong MJ, Sharma R, Rosen C, Viana M. Repetitive transcranial magnetic stimulation versus electroconvulsive therapy for major depression: preliminary results of a randomized trial. Biol Psychiatry 2002; 51(8):659–667.
46. Dannon PN, Dolberg OT, Schreiber S, Grunhaus L. Three- and six-month outcome following courses of either ECT or rTMS in a population of severely depressed individuals—preliminary report. Biol Psychiatry 2002; 51(8):687–690.

47. Boutros NN, Gueorguieva R, Hoffman RE, Oren DA, Feingold A, Berman RM. Lack of a therapeutic effect of a 2-week sub-threshold transcranial magnetic stimulation course for treatment-resistant depression. Psychiatry Res 2002; 113(3):245–254.
48. Loo CK, Mitchell PB, Croker VM, Malhi GS, Wen W, Gandevia SC, Sachdev PS. Double-blind controlled investigation of bilateral prefrontal transcranial magnetic stimulation for the treatment of resistant major depression. Psychol Med 2003; 33(1):33–40.
49. Moser DJ, Jorge RE, Manes F, Paradiso S, Benjamin ML, Robinson RG. Improved executive functioning following repetitive transcranial magnetic stimulation. Neurology 2002; 58(8):1288–1290.
50. Herwig U, Lampe Y, Juengling FD, Wunderlich A, Walter H, Spitzer M, Schonfeldt-Lecuona C. Add-on rTMS for treatment of depression: a pilot study using stereotaxic coil-navigation according to PET data. J Psychiatr Res 2003; 37(4):267–275.
51. Nadeau SE, McCoy KJ, Crucian GP, Greer RA, Rossi F, Bowers D, Goodman WK, Heilman KM, Triggs WJ. Cerebral blood flow changes in depressed patients after treatment with repetitive transcranial magnetic stimulation: evidence of individual variability. Neuropsychiatry Neuropsychol Behav Neurol 2002; 15(3):159–175.
52. Mottaghy FM, Keller CE, Gangitano M, Ly J, Thall M, Parker JA, Pascual_Leone A. Correlation of cerebral blood flow and treatment effects of repetitive transcranial magnetic stimulation in depressed patients. Psychiatry Res 2002; 115(1–2):1–14.
53. Gershon AA, Dannon PN, Grunhaus L. Transcranial magnetic stimulation in the treatment of depression. Am J Psychiatry 2003; 160:835–845.
54. Dolberg OT, Dannon PN, Schreiber S, Grunhaus L. Transcranial magnetic stimulation in patients with bipolar depression: a double blind, controlled study. Bipolar Disord 2002; 4(suppl 1):94–95.
55. Nahas Z, Kozel FA, Anderson B, George MS. Left prefrontal transcranial magnetic stimulation (TMS) treatment of depression in bipolar affective disorder: a pilot study of acute safety and efficacy. Bipolar Disord 2003; 5(1):40–47.
56. Grisaru N, Chudakov B, Yaroslavsky Y, Belmaker R. Transcranial magnetic stimulation in mania: a controlled study. Am J Psychiatry 1998; 155:1608–1610.
57. Kaptsan A, Yaroslavsky Y, Applebaum J, Belmaker RH, Grisaru N. Right prefrontal TMS versus sham treatment of mania: a controlled study. Bipolar Disord 2003; 5(1): 36–39.
58. Wassermann E. Side effects of repetitive transcranial magnetic stimulation. Depression Anxiety 2000; 12:124–129.
59. Lorberbaum JP, Wassermann EM. George MS, Belmaker R, eds. Safety Concerns of TMS, in Transcranial Magnetic Stimulation in Neuropsychiatry. Washington, DC: American Psychiatric Press, 2000:141–161.
60. Martis B, Alam D, Dowd SM, Hill SK, Sharma RP, Rosen C, Pliskin N, Martin E, Carson V, Janicak PG. Neurocognitive effects of repetitive transcranial magnetic stimulation in severe major depression. Clin Neurophysiol Official J Int Fed Clin Neurophysiol 2003; 114(6):1125–1132.
61. Loo C, Sachdev P, Elsayed H, McDarmont B, Mitchell P, Wilkinson M, Parker G, Gandevia S. Effects of a 2- to 4-week course of repetitive transcranial magnetic stimulation (rTMS) on neuropsychologic functioning, electroencephalogram, and auditory threshold in depressed patients. Biol Psychiatry 2001; 49:615–623.
62. George MS, Lisanby SH, Sackeim HA. Transcranial magnetic stimulation. Arch Gen Psychiatry 1999; 56:300–311.
63. Wassermann EM. Risk and safety of repetitive transcranial magnetic stimulation: report and suggested guidelines from the International Workshop on the Safety of repetitive transcranial magnetic stimulation, June 5–7, 1996. Electroencephalogr Clin Neurophysiol 1998; 108:1–16.
64. Belmaker B, Fitzgerald P, George MS, Lisanby SH, Pascual-Leone A, Schlaepfer TE, Wassermann E. Managing the risks of Repetitive Transcranial Stimulation Interna-

tional Society for transcranial stimulation consensus statement. CNS Spectr 2003; 8(7):489.

65. Lisanby SH, Morales O, Payne N, Kwon E, Fitzsimons L, Luber B, Nobler MS, Sackeim HA. New developments in electroconvulsive therapy and magnetic seizure therapy. CNS Spectr 2003; 8(7):529–536.
66. Sackeim HA, Prudic J, Devenand DP, Kiersky JE, Fitzsimons L, Moody BJ, McElhiney MC, Coleman EA, Settembrino JM. Effects of stimulus intesity and electrode placement on the efficacy and cognitive effects of electroconvulsive therapy. N Engl J Med 1993; 328:839–846.
67. Hasselmo ME, McClelland JL. Neural models of memory. Curr Opin Neurobiol 1999; 9(2):184–188.
68. Lisanby SH, Schlaepfer TE, Fisch HU, Sackeim HA. Magnetic seizure therapy of major depression. Arch Gen Psychiatry 2001; 58:303–304.
69. Lisanby SH, Luber B, Schlaepfer TE, Sackeim HA. Safety and feasibility of magnetic seizure therapy (MST) in major depression: randomized within-subject comparison with electroconvulsive therapy. Neuropsychopharmacology 2003; 28(10):1852–1865.
70. Kosel M, Frick C, Lisanby SH, Fisch HU, Schlaepfer TE. Magnetic seizure therapy (MST) improves mood in refractory major depression. Neuropsychopharmacology 2003; 28(11):2045–2048.
71. Penry JK, Dean JC. Prevention of intractable partial seizures by intermittent vagal stimulation in humans: preliminary results. Epilepsia 1990; 31(suppl 2):S40–S43.
72. Terry R, Tarver WB, Zabara J. An implantable neurocybernetic prosthesis system. Epilepsia 1990; 31(suppl 2):S33–S37.
73. Carpenter LL, Friehs GM, Price LH. Cervical vagus nerve stimulation for treatment-resistant depression. Neurosurg Clin N Am 2003; 14(Apr):275–282.
74. Privitera MD, Welty TE, Ficker DM, Welge J. Vagus Nerve Stimulation for Partial Seizures. Vol. Issue 3. Oxford: The Cochrane Library, 2002.
75. Harden CL, Pulver MC, Ravdin LD, Nikolov B, Halper JP, Labar DR. A pilot study of mood in epilepsy patients treated with vagus nerve stimulation. Epilepsy Behav 2000; 1:93–99.
76. Hoppe C, Helmstaedter C, Scherrmann J, Elger CE. Self-reported mood changes following 6 months of vagus nerve stimulation in epilepsy patients. Epilepsy Behav 2001; 2:225–342.
77. Rush AJ, George MS, Sackeim HA, Marangell LB, Husain MM, Giller C, Nahas Z, Haines S, Simpson RK, Goodmann R. Vagus nerve stimulation (VNS) for treatment-resistant depression: a multicenter study. Biol Psychiatry 2000; 47:276–286.
78. Marangell LB, Rush AJ, George MS, Sackeim HA, Johnson CR, Husain MM, Nahas Z, Lisanby SH. Vagus nerve stimulation (VNS) for major depressive episodes: one year outcomes. Biol Psychiatry 2002; 51:280–287.
79. Sackeim HA, Rush AJ, George MS, Marangell LB, Husain MM, Nahas Z, Johnson CR, Seidman S, Giller C, Haines S, Simpson RK, Goodman RR. Vagus nerve stimulation (VNS) for treatment-resistant depression: efficacy, side effects, and predictors of outcome. Neuropsychopharmacology 2001; 25:713–728.
80. Schlaepfer TE, Wagner M, Kosel M, Frick C. Vagus nerve stimulation for major depression—results from the European Multicenter Trial D03. 42nd Annual Meeting of the American College of Neuropsychopharmacology, San Juan, Puerto Rico, 2003.
81. Annegers JF, Coan SP, Hauser WA, Leestma J. Epilepsy, vagal nerve stimulation by the NCP system, all-cause mortality, and sudden, unexpected, unexplained death. Epilepsia 2000; 41:453–549.
82. Ben-Menachem E. Vagus nerve stimulation, side effects, and long-term safety. J Clin Neurophysiol 2001; 18:415–418.
83. Schachter SC. Vagus nerve stimulation therapy summary—five years after FDA approval. Neurology 2002; 59(suppl 4):S15–S20.

84. Tatum WO, Moore DB, Stecker MM, Baltuch GH, French JA, Ferreira JA, Carney PM, Labar DR, Vale FL. Ventricular asystole during vagus nerve stimulation for humans. Neurology 1999; 52:1267–1269.
85. Handforth A, DeGiorgio CM, Schachter SC, Uthman BM, Naritoku DK, Tecoma ES, Henry TR, Collins SD, Voughn BV, Gilmartin RC, Labar DR, Morris GL, Salinsky MC, Osorio I, Ristanovic RK, Labiner DM, Jones JC, Murphy JV, Ney GC, Wheless JW. Vagus nerve stimulation for partial-onset seizures: a randomized active-control trial. Neurology 1998; 51:48–55.
86. Sanossian N, Haut S. Chronic diarrhea associated with vagal nerve stimulation. Neurology 2002; 58:330.
87. Kim W, Clancy RR, Liu GT. Horner syndrome associated with implantation of a vagus nerve stimulator. Am J Ophthalmol 2001; 131:383–384.
88. Leijten FS, Van Rijen PC. Stimulation of the phrenic nerve as a complication of vagus nerve pacing in a patient with epilepsy. Neurology 1998; 51:1224–1225.
89. Iriarte J, Artieda J, Alegre M, Schlumberger E, Urrestarazu E, Pastor MA, Viteri C. Spam of the sternocleidomastoid muscle induced by vagal nerve stimulation. Neurology 2001; 57:2319–2320.
90. Malow BA, Edwards J, Merzec M, Sagher O, Fromes G. Effects of vagus nerve stimulation on respiration during sleep. Neurology 2000; 55:1450–1454.
91. Lundgren J, Ekberg O, Olsson R. Aspiration: a potential complication to vagus nerve stimulation. Epilepsia 1998; 39:998–1000.
92. Schallert G, Foster J, Lindquist N, Murphy JV. Chronic stimulation of the left vagal nerve in children: effect on swallowing. Epilepsia 1998; 39:1113–1114.
93. Heck C, Helmers SL, DeGiorgio CM. Vagus nerve stimulation therapy, epilepsy and device parameters: scientific basis and recommendations for use. Neurology 2002; 59(S4):S31–S37.
94. Physician's Manual. NeuroCybernetic Prothesis System NCP Pulse Generator Models 100 and 101. Houston, USA: Cyberonics, 2001.
95. Sackeim HA, Keilp JG, Rush AJ, George MS, Marangell LB, Dormer JS, Burt T, Lisanby SH, Husain MM, Cullum CM, Oliver N, Zboyan H. The effects of vagus nerve stimulation on cognitive performance in patients with treatment-resistant depression. Neuropsychiatry Nerupsychiol Behav Neurol 2001; 14:53–62.
96. Clark KB, Naritoku DK, Smith DC, Browning RA, Jensen RA. Enhanced recognition memory following vagus nerve stimulation in human subjects. Nat Neurosci 1999; 2: 94–98.
97. Helmstaedter C, Hoppe C, Elger CE. Memory alterations during acute high-intensity vagus nerve stimulation. Epilepsy Res 2001; 47:37–42.
98. George MS, Sackeim HA, Rush AJ, Marangell LB, Nahas Z, Husain MM, Lisanby SH, Burt T, Goldman J, Ballenger JC. Vagus nerve stimulation: a new tool for brain research and therapy? Biol Psychiatry 2000; 47:287–295.
99. Andrews RJ. Neuromodulation I. Techniques—deep brain stimulation, vagus nerve stimulation, and transcranial magnetic stimulation. Ann NY Acad Sci 2003; 993: 1–13; discussion 48–53.
100. Greenberg BD, Rezai AR. Mechanisms and the current state of deep brain stimulation in neuropsychiatry. CNS Spectr 2003; 8(7):522–526.
101. Cosyns P, Gabriels L, Nuttin B. Deep brain stimulation in treatment refractory obsessive compulsive disorder. Verh K Acad Geneeskd Belg 2003; 65(6):385–399; discussion 399–400.
102. Gabriels L, Cosyns P, Nuttin B, Demeulemeester H, Gybels J. Deep brain stimulation for treatment-refractory obsessive–compulsive disorder: psychopathological and neuropsychological outcome in three cases. Acta Psychiatr Scand 2003; 107(4):275–282.
103. Nuttin B, Cosyns P, Demeulemeester H, Gybels J, Meyerson B. Electrical stimulation in the anterior limbs of internal capsules in patients with obsessive–compulsive disorder. Lancet 1999; 354:1526.

104. Thobois S, Mertens P, Guenot M, Hermier M, Mollion H, Bouvard M, Chazot G, Broussolle E, Sindou M. Subthalamic nucleus stimulation in Parkinson's disease: clinical evaluation of 18 patients. J Neurol Neurosurg Psychiatry 2002; 249(5):529–534.
105. Berney A, Vingerhoets F, Perrin A, Guex P, Villemure JG, Burkhard PR, Benkelfat C, Ghika J. Effect on mood of subthalamic DBS for Parkinson's disease: a consecutive series of 24 patients. Neurology 2002; 59(9):1427–1429.
106. Straits-Troster K, Fields JA, Wilkinson SB, Pahwa R, Lyons KE, Koller WC, Troster A. Health-related quality of life in Parkinson's disease after pallidotomy and deep brain stimulation. Brain Cogn 2000; 42(3):399–416.
107. Herzog J, Reiff J, Krack P, Witt K, Schrader B, Muller D, Deuschl G. Manic episode with psychotic symptoms induced by subthalamic nucleus stimulation in a patient with Parkinson's disease. Mov Disord 2003; 18(11):1382–1384.
108. Kulisevsky J, Berthier ML, Gironell A, Pascual-Sedano B, Molet J, Pares P. Mania following deep brain stimulation for Parkinson's disease. Neurology 2002; 59(9): 1421–1424.
109. Cuijpers P, Smit F. Excess mortality in depression: a meta-analysis of community studies. J Affect Disord 2002; 72(3):227–236.
110. Wulsin LR, Vaillant GE, Wells VE. A systematic review of the mortality of depression. Psychosom Med 1999; 61(1):6–17.
111. Eranti SV, McLoughlin DM. Electroconvulsive therapy—state of the art. Br J Psychiatry 2003; 182:8–9.
112. Madsen TM, Treschow A, Bengzon J, Bolwig TG, Lindvall O, Tingstrom A. Increased neurogenesis in a model of electroconvulsive therapy. Biol Psychiatry 2000; 47(12): 1043–1049.
113. Coyle JT, Duman RS. Finding the intracellular signaling pathways affected by mood disorder treatments. Neuron 2003; 38(2):157–160.
114. Altar CA, Laeng P, Jurata LW, Brockman JA, Lemire A, Bullard J, Bukhman YV, Young TA, Charles V, Palfreyman MG. Electroconvulsive seizures regulate gene expression of distinct neurotrophic signaling pathways. J Neurosci 2004; 24(11): 2667–2677.

26

Role of Psychotherapy in the Management of Bipolar Disorder

Michael E. Thase
Department of Psychiatry, University of Pittsburgh School of Medicine, Western Psychiatric Institute and Clinic, Pittsburgh, Pennsylvania, U.S.A.

INTRODUCTION

Bipolar affective disorder has long been considered to be the most "biological" of the mood disorders and, perhaps because of this perception, research investigating the role of psychotherapy historically has been relatively short lived. Indeed, whereas there has been evidence that several forms of psychotherapy are effective treatments of major (unipolar) depressive disorder for more than two decades (see, e.g., Refs. 1, 2), comparable evidence of the utility in bipolar disorder has only begun to emerge within the past 5 years. Increased interest in studying this application of psychotherapy has been driven in part by evidence that psychosocial risk factors (such as level of social support or exposure to adverse life events) affect the longitudinal course of bipolar affective disorder (3–5). The importance of medication non-adherence to longer-term treatment outcomes and the obvious link between patients' thoughts and feelings about their condition and medication non-compliance provided another rationale (6–9). Ultimately, the limited efficacy of standard pharmacological strategies provided the most compelling rationale for taking seriously the potential role of adjunctive psychotherapies. In this respect, it should be kept in mind that the utility of various focused forms of adjunctive psychotherapy had been well established in schizophrenia by the mid-1980s (10–12). The results of these controlled trials, no doubt, helped to put to rest overly reductionistic approaches to the therapeutics of severe mental disorders.

BACKGROUND

It is fair to say that before the introduction of antipsychotic medications or lithium salts, there was ample clinical evidence that insight-oriented psychotherapies were not effective treatments of mania. In fact, Fromm-Reichmann (13) concluded that psychoanalytic psychotherapy was even less useful in manic depression than in schizophrenia. The predominant view was that mania was not responsive to psychoanalysis because it was the product of relatively primitive defenses, basically an unconsciously motivated escape from the intolerable introjections underlying depression. One can only imagine the futility of trying to conduct a psychoanalytic session with a grandiose, sleep-deprived, restless, and potentially assaultive manic individual! Hard-earned psychotherapeutic gains made during depressive episodes or periods of euthymia likewise seemed to "go out the window" when patients subsequently cycled into mania. It is not surprising that, within the context of the futility of psychoanalysis, Cade's (14) discovery of the efficacy of lithium salts and emerging evidence of a high degree of heritability (15) ushered in the predominant view that this "biological" illness was best—if not exclusively—treated with somatic therapies.

Despite such biological hegemony, many clinicians continued to use psychotherapy as an adjunct to pharmacotherapy, specifically to address the personal and social consequences of bipolar affective disorder (see, e.g., the review by Goodwin and Jamison (16)). Although definitive data from controlled studies were lacking, clinical experience suggested that group and individual psychotherapies could be used productively to help patients address issues such as denial of the illness, ambivalence about accepting the need for treatment, and disappointments/frustrations arising from the impact of the illness on achieving one's life goals. Drawing from first-hand experience, Jamison (17) poignantly illustrated that psychotherapy can have an important, even life-saving, role in prevention of suicide.

During the 1990s, four psychotherapies for bipolar disorder were introduced by modifying approaches that were initially developed for patients with schizophrenia (18,19) or depressive disorders (20,21). Each of these interventions embraced biopsychosocial models of psychopathology; the approaches primarily differ in their emphasis on psychoeducational (PE) (22), family-dyadic (23), cognitive-behavioral (24), and interpersonal (25) aspects of bipolar affective disorder. A number of clinical trials testing these so-called specific psychotherapies now have been completed and, as will be reviewed in more detail subsequently, for the first time, an evidence-based case for the role of psychosocial treatment can be made.

Issues in Studying the Efficacy of Psychotherapy for Bipolar Disorder

As reviewed in detail by Swartz et al. (26), several issues complicate studying the effects of psychotherapy in bipolar disorder. These issues are discussed in what follows, along with some suggested solutions or ideas to at least lessen the impact of these complications on the validity of treatment studies.

Duration of Therapy

As many of the potential benefits of an adjunctive psychotherapy would be expected to develop over time, studies must necessarily be conducted across many months or even years in order to evaluate the predicted effects. As such, even pilot research studies, which are generally necessary to determine the promise and feasibility of an intervention *before* larger-scale investigations can be undertaken, may take several years to complete. The only suggested solution to this problem is acceptance: this type of research cannot be done quickly!

Phase of Illness

Research strategies that follow psychopharmacologic paradigms typically focus on one discrete phase of illness, i.e., a depressive or manic index episode. Of course, distinctions between bipolar I and bipolar II forms of the illness, taking into account the mixed and rapid cycling presentations of both of these subtypes, are relevant to such treatment research. Not only does this "phase-specific" approach reduce the number of potentially eligible patients, but also polarity of the index episode also tends to affect the likelihood of particular outcomes and influences the choices of concomitant pharmacotherapies. If the goals of the experimental therapy are truly phase specific (i.e., "does Beck's model of cognitive therapy hasten remission of bipolar depression?"), only a subset of bipolar patients would be eligible to participate; the only solution available to address this problem may be to conduct a multicenter trial. Alternatively, the investigator may choose to focus on outcomes that are relevant across phases of illness. For example, if the goals of psychotherapy are longitudinal, time to any type of relapse is an appropriate outcome. Across phases of illness, assessments of global adjustment, functional status, quality of life, composite measures of symptom burden, and days lost to illness also are relevant outcomes.

Exclusion Criteria

There has been a tendency in psychopharmacological research to exclude patients with complicating or comorbid conditions as a means to maximize the homogeneity of the study group. In conventional terms, the internal validity of an experiment is enhanced by reducing the known sources of variance that can adversely affect (i.e., moderate) outcome. It is hard to argue with this conventional wisdom! However, three problems result from use of extensive sets of exclusion criteria. First, as only a minority of people with bipolar affective disorder are "free" of complications such as anxiety or a substance abuse disorders, it is hard to find a sufficient number of people with relatively uncomplicated disorders who are both eligible and willing to participate. Second, highly exclusive studies run the risk of losing generalizability to the broader group of people who are treated in day-to-day clinical practice. Third, and most importantly, as case complexity typically conveys negative prognostic information (i.e., people with highly comorbid bipolar disorders tend to have a lower probability of recovering or staying well with standard treatment), the sensitivity of a study to detect an additive effect may be limited by a "ceiling effect." In other words, the lower a study group's inherent risk of relapse, the less the likelihood of showing the effect of an adjunctive therapy. Thus, beyond enhancing feasibility and generalizability, it is suggested that more inclusive studies will be more feasible, have greater generalizability, and have greater design sensitivity to detect additive effects for adjunctive psychotherapies.

The solution to the problems imposed by restrictive entry criteria begins with questioning the need for each particular exclusion criterion. Feasibility and external generalizability should only be sacrificed when it is clear that the decision *not to exclude* a participant would jeopardize the chances for a successful experiment.

Decisions About Pharmacotherapy

Adopting overly restrictive pharmacotherapy protocols is a parallel example of relying too heavily on the conventional research methods. Of course, it is again useful to have experimental control over potentially confounding variables, and significant between-group differences in medications utilized could adversely affect design sensitivity. However, this concern must be balanced against the issues of feasibility and generalizability. Specifically, as only a minority of bipolar patients can be managed affectively with relatively simple treatment plans, studies that impose highly restrictive medication protocols (e.g., monotherapy with lithium or divalproex or withdrawal of adjunctive antipsychotic or benzodiazepines within 4 weeks of stabilization, etc.) will prove to be infeasible. Even if a sufficiently large patient population could be screened to identify a sufficient number of patients who are responsive to relatively simple treatment regimens, the generalizability of this rarefied study group to "real-world" patients would be questionable.

It is, therefore, recommended that when the primary question of the research is the efficacy of psychotherapy, the pharmacotherapy protocol should be standardized but flexible. For example, pharmacotherapy could follow a "menu of reasonable choices" outlined in practice guidelines or published treatment algorithms, which are tailored to the needs of the individuals [see, e.g., the treatment approaches outlined by the American Psychiatric Association (27) or Sachs and Thase (28)]. In a clinical research setting that provides expert care, it is extremely unlikely that a systematic bias in treatment selection would emerge. There is, of course, the perennial concern that clinicians would prescribe more vigorous pharmacotherapy to the patients in a control group, which might inadvertently neutralize detecting an advantage for the psychotherapy (2). Thus, it is important to document that treatment as "usual" in the experimental and control groups is comparable. In the unlikely event that the groups actually differ with respect to treatment received, these differences can be counted as secondary outcomes and any potential impact on outcome can be examined post hoc via stratification, much the same as a failure of randomization is addressed.

What is the Best Control Group?

The standard control group for psychopharmacologic research, i.e., double-blind administration of an identically appearing inert placebo, permits the effects of the passage of time, repeated measurement, the expectations of the patient and the treating clinician, and the supportive aspects of patient care to be estimated in relation to the active effect of the medication. Unfortunately, there is no comparably satisfactory control group for psychotherapy research. A waiting list control group is the easiest to implement and does permit the effects of the passage of time and repeated assessment to be taken into account.

A waiting list control condition does not, however, account for the non-specific elements of the helping relationship, nor are the patients' and clinicians' expectations for benefit taken into account. In fact, it could be argued that stasis is the expectation conveyed by assignment to a waiting list control condition (i.e., "I should wait patiently until it's my turn to receive therapy."). As such, a design using random assignment to a waiting list control group has excellent sensitivity to detect an additive effect, but little capacity to differentiate the impact of the specific vs. the non-specific aspects of the clinical intervention. A design that contrasts an adjunctive psychotherapy versus a waiting list control group of "treatment as usual only" group is thus most appropriate for an initial trial, i.e., before adjunctive treatment efficacy has been established.

Once the efficacy is established, the principal alternative to a waiting list control group involves developing a so-called pseudotherapy, i.e., an intervention that provides comparable amounts of therapeutic support and similar expectations for improvement, without the specific or technical interventions that define the model of psychotherapy that is being tested. The principal limitations of a pseudotherapy control group center around the capacity of the research team to maintain equipoise and to ensure that the allegiance of the therapists is comparable. Namely, if the same therapists are conducting the experimental and psychotherapy interventions, it is very likely that they will expect the "name brand" to be a better treatment than "brand X." Studies of the social psychology of experiments provide ample documentation that such differences in expectations do affect results (29). In order for a pseudotherapy to truly accomplish the aims of an adequate control group, both therapists and patients alike must find the rationale for the control intervention to be convincing and therapists must have the same espirit de corps and expectations for benefit as those conducting the "name brand" intervention. This requires a level of attention to detail and protocol development that are usually far greater than the time and resources available to the researchers.

Once efficacy is established in relation to an appropriate "attention-control" condition, the most appropriate second design alternative involves designation of one form of psychotherapy as a standard of comparison. This approach not only controls for non-specific factors, but also permits allegiance artifact to be minimized by ensuring that both therapies are competently administered and supervised. The principal strength of a study design that compares two forms of "name-brand" psychotherapy is that it permits evaluation of both relative efficacy and potential mode-specific benefits (i.e., dysfunctional thoughts, marital or family functioning, or adherence). The major drawback of a study comparing two active psychotherapies is the probability of what methodologist call Type 2 error. Generally, one would like at least an 80% chance of detecting the expected difference between treatments, which results in a "false negative" rate of $<20\%$. However, modern studies of antidepressant therapies amply document that it takes literally hundreds of subjects in each arm of a study in order to have adequate statistical power to differentiate between active therapies (30). Few studies of the efficacy of psychotherapy have 50 subjects per arm, let alone the 200+ that might be necessary to conduct an adequately powered comparison of, say, cognitive behavioral and family-focused therapies (FFTs). The standard therapy control group thus should be utilized only when there is evidence from earlier studies that the intervention has efficacy *and* if resources are sufficient to ensure enrollment of enough subjects to have adequate statistical power.

REVIEW OF CONTEMPORARY TREATMENT STRATEGIES AND RELEVANT RESEARCH

Psychotherapies that have been tested in randomized controlled trials (RCTs) of bipolar disorder include (i) psycho education, (ii) cognitive behavior therapy (CBT), (iii) family focused therapy, and (iv) interpersonal and social rhythm therapy (IPSRT). Although these approaches utilize a number of common strategies, they differ with respect to intensity (i.e., the "dose" of therapy utilized) and areas of emphasis and, hence, might be expected to have differential impact on the illness.

Psychoeducation

Perry et al. (31) developed a relatively brief PE therapy and tested it within the context of conventional ambulatory mental health care in the United Kingdom. The intervention consisted of 7 to 12 individual sessions that addressed the importance of medication adherence, recognition of prodromal symptoms, and use of early intervention to forestall impending episodes. In this add-on design, all patients

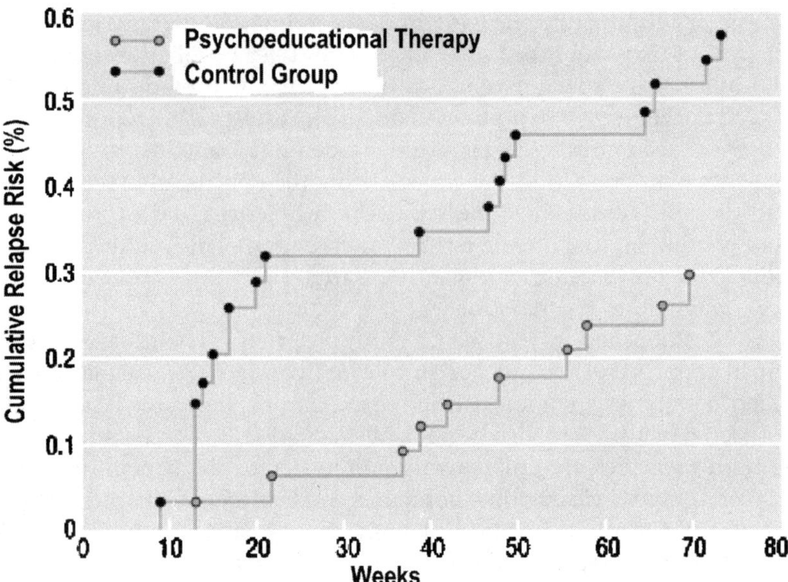

Figure 1 Survival analysis of relapse risks across 1.5 years of follow-up. *Source:* Adapted from Ref. 31.

continued to receive maintenance pharmacotherapy under the direction of their treating psychiatrist. A total of 69 remitted patients with bipolar I disorder were randomly assigned to receive either PE therapy or a treatment as usual alone. The primary endpoint of this study was time to relapse across 18 months of follow-up.

When compared with the control group, PE therapy significantly reduced the risk of manic relapse (i.e., 18% vs. 46%) and significantly delayed the time to first manic relapse (Fig. 1). The investigators found that additional benefits of PE included improvements in patients' social and vocational functioning. Interestingly, the effect of the PE intervention on the risk of depressive relapses was not as marked (i.e., 31% vs. 48%) and did not reach statistical significance. However, as a 17% difference in depression relapse rates would, if reliable, have public health significance, this may well represent a Type 2 error.

A second major controlled trial of PE was conducted by Colom et al. (32). This Barcelona-based research group compared a more extensive course of group PE (up to 21 sessions provided across 5 months) versus a pseudotherapy control intervention, which consisted of a like number of unstructured group sessions. The study group consisted of 120 euthymic bipolar outpatients. All patients had been remitted for at least 6 months prior to randomization and continued to receive maintenance pharmacotherapy during the 24-month duration of the study. The investigators found that group PE significantly reduced the number of recurrences of both depression and mania and increased the duration of sustained remission. At the end of the follow-up, 92% of the control group had suffered a recurrence when compared with 67% of the PE group (Fig. 2).

Two ongoing studies are evaluating PE provided as a component of broader disease management programs. Results of the first trial, a multi-site Veterans Administration collaborative study conducted by Bauer et al. (33), are not yet available. The centerpiece of this study is the Life Goals Program, a two-phase structured group

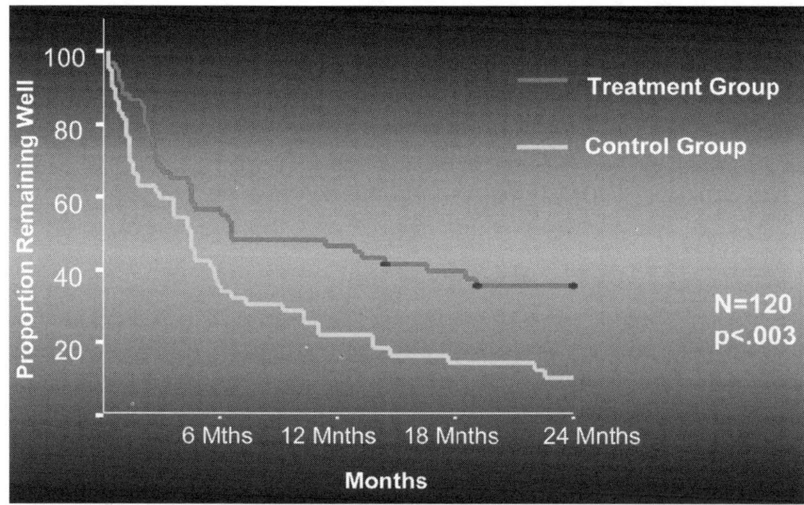

Figure 2 Efficacy of group PE therapy: survival analysis of relapse risks across 2 years of follow-up. *Source:* Adapted from Ref. 32.

therapy (22). The first phase of the program consists of five sessions of PE. The second phase focuses on identification of longer-term goals and use of stepwise behavioral approaches to facilitate goal attainment.

In the second trial, Simon et al. (34,35) evaluated a disease management program added to conventional ambulatory therapy provided by a managed care organization. The intervention was implemented by an experienced psychiatric nurse and included care planning, monthly telephone monitoring of symptoms and medication, feedback and co-ordination of care with the mental health treatment team; a structured, PE-focused group therapy also was available to patients in the experimental condition (34). The investigators randomized more than 400 patients with bipolar disorder (type I or II) during the 3-year research project, using a treatment as usual control group. In a report of the first 12 months of outcome, patients receiving the added PE intervention experienced significantly lower mean mania ratings, as well as a significant reduction days spent manic (GE Simon, personal communication). However, consistent with the findings of Perry et al. (31), depression ratings and days spent depressed were not significantly reduced by the experimental program.

Cognitive Behavior Therapy

This approach builds upon PE through the systematic use of self-monitoring diaries, daily homework assignments, stepwise behavioral assignments, and cognitive restructuring exercises to promote identification and remediation of negative thoughts (24). Although usually conducted as an individual therapy, CBT can be modified to be provided in groups. Several controlled studies of CBT have been completed during the past few years.

To date, two controlled studies of CBT have been completed; both studies were conducted in the United Kingdom. In the first trial, Scott et al. (35) randomly assigned 42 outpatients with bipolar disorder (type I or II) to receive either 20 sessions of CBT (across 6 months) or a waiting list control group. Patients receiving

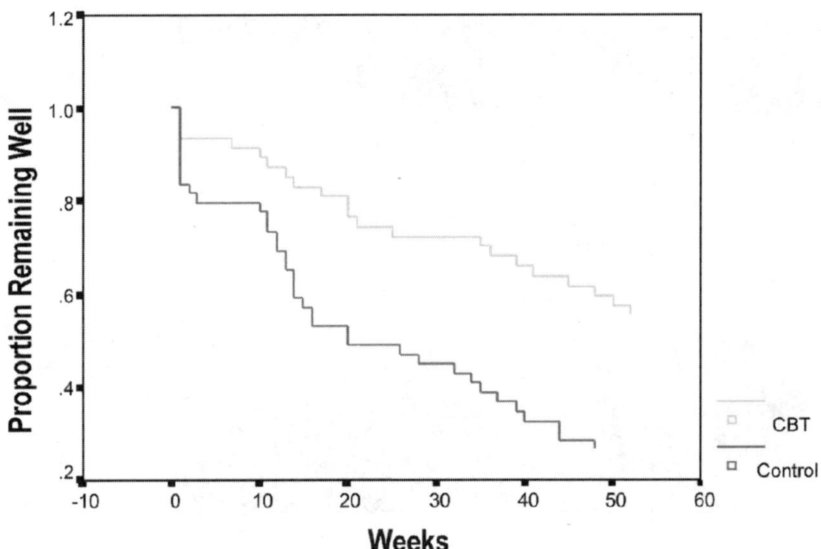

Figure 3 Efficacy of CBT: survival analysis of relapse risks across 1 year. *Source:* Adapted from Ref. 36.

CBT experienced significantly greater reduction of depressive symptoms by the end of the 6-month protocol, although the reduction in manic symptoms did not differ when compared with the waiting list control group. The patients receiving CBT also experienced significant improvements in social and vocational functioning. As the study group was predominately afflicted by depressive symptoms, this trial probably did not have the power to detect a significant effect on the less prevalent manic symptoms. At the end of the randomized study, the patients who completed 6 months of treatment in the control group also received CBT. A total of 18 months follow-up was available for 29 CBT-treated participants. Using a mirror-image (within-subjects) approach to analysis, there was a 60% reduction in episodes of mania and depression following CBT when compared with the preceding 18 months.

In the second study, Lam et al. (36) randomly assigned 103 outpatients with bipolar I disorder to receive either added CBT or treatment as usual alone. Although patients were considered to be "stabilized" at the time of study entry, most patients had residual depressive symptoms. The CBT group received an average of 14 sessions during the first 6 months, with two subsequent "booster" sessions. Across the 12-month study, the CBT-treated group experienced significantly fewer episodes of illness; 75% of the control group suffered at least one relapse as compared to only 44% in the CBT group (Fig. 3). There were also significant reductions in hospital admissions and days hospitalized in the CBT group.

Family-Focused Therapy

This strongly PE approach was developed by investigators at the University of California at Los Angeles and the University of Colorado and can be flexibly adapted for use with either nuclear families or couples. The methods of FFT include helping families to develop acceptance that the interpersonal difficulties are attributable to the illness (not laziness, indifference, or "badness"), improving communication skills, and adopting a stepwise approach to problem solving (23). For research

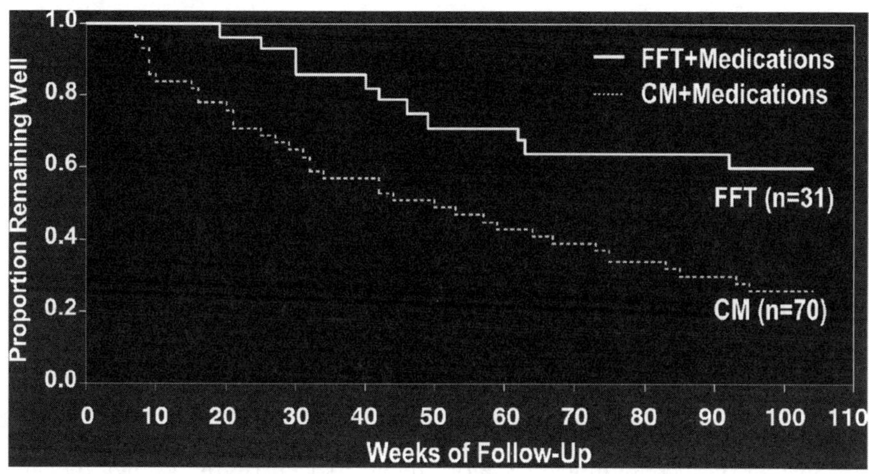

Figure 4 Efficacy of FFT: survival analysis of relapse risks across 2 years of follow-up. *Source:* Adapted from Ref. 39.

applications, the FTT protocol consists of up to 21 sessions conducted across 9 months.

In the first controlled study, 101 recently remitted outpatients with bipolar I disorder were randomly assigned to either FFT ($n = 31$) or a less intensive crisis management condition ($n = 70$) (37,38). Family therapy resulted in a significant reduction in relapse risk and a significant increase in well days when compared with the control group (Fig. 4). Family therapy also resulted in significantly lower levels of both depressive and manic symptoms across 24 months of follow-up. Overall, 73% of the control group relapsed as compared to only 45% of those treated with FFT (38).

In the second trial, 53 patients with bipolar I disorder were randomized to receive either FFT or a similarly intensive course of individual supportive therapy (39). The treatments appeared to be similarly effective during the first year of the study. However, during the second and third years of the study, a significant difference in re-hospitalization rates emerged. Specifically, 60% of the group that received individual therapy ultimately required re-hospitalization as compared to only 12% of the FFT-treated group.

Interpersonal and Social Rhythm Therapy

IPSRT (25) combines the methods of one of the best-studied psychotherapies for depression with behavioral strategies intended to help patients better regulate their daily routines and adopt less chaotic lifestyles. In addition to PE and disease management strategies, IPSRT focuses on (i) the link between life events and mood swings; (ii) developing more regular daily rhythms; (iii) identification and management of potential precipitants of rhythm dysregulation, with special attention to interpersonal triggers; and (iv) grief work to assist mourning of the loss of the "healthy" self (40).

A relatively large trial of IPSRT was conducted by Frank and colleagues at the Western Psychiatric Institute and Clinic of the University of Pittsburgh. A total of 175 acutely ill (i.e., manic, depressed, or mixed episodes) bipolar I patients were treated by specialist teams consisting of an expert psychiatrist and a psychotherapist trained in both IPSRT and disease-management approaches. Medications were selected according to a "best practices" treatment algorithm. The investigators randomly assigned half of the study group to receive at least 12 weeks of IPSRT; the remainder of the study group received a like number of sessions of intensive clinical management (ICM). This initial phase of the study continued until patients achieved 4 weeks of stable remission (both mania and depression). A total of 125 patients (71% of the intent-to-treat study group) achieved stable remission; the average time to stable remission was almost 19 weeks. Thereafter, a second randomization was undertaken to determine the treatment assignment for the 2-year-long maintenance phase. Patients thus could have received one of four treatment sequences: (i) IPSRT (acute) followed by IPSRT (maintenance), (ii) IPSRT followed by ICM, (iii) ICM followed by IPSRT, and (iv) ICM followed by ICM. The final results have not yet been published but are currently under editorial review. Several interesting preliminary findings have emerged from interim analyses. For example, although the patients receiving IPSRT developed significantly more regular social rhythms, they did not experience any greater reduction of depressive or manic symptoms during acute-phase therapy, nor was the probability or speed of recovery from the index episode enhanced in any way (40). During the first year of the maintenance phase, a trend was observed for higher relapse risk among the patients who switched from IPSRT to ICM when compared with the group that received IPSRT across the whole program (41). Curiously, the opposite trend was observed in the sub-group of stabilized patients who had IPSRT added to their treatment plan during the maintenance treatment phase. Thus, there was a significant treatment type by treatment sequence interaction, such that the groups that had the same psychosocial treatment across the entire study had significantly longer survival than the groups that underwent a change in treatment assignment at the start of the maintenance phase (41). The authors concluded that changes in the treatment milieu could adversely affect the outcome of bipolar disorder and that, when treatment has been effective, ensuring the stability of the treatment plan can improve outcomes.

CONCLUSIONS

The number of RCTs of psychotherapy for bipolar disorder has increased substantially during the past 5 years. Cumulatively, the data demonstrate that psychotherapy added to ongoing pharmacological management can play an important role in the longer-term management of bipolar disorder. In fact, the magnitude of the effects of adjunctive psychotherapy is generally moderately large (Table 1) (26) and approach or exceed the effect sizes of treatments such as divalproex (42), olanzapine (43), or lamotrigine (44).

Almost all of the evidence that has emerged to date has pertained to the value of psychotherapy during maintenance treatment of bipolar disorder. This is noteworthy because (i) there is ample evidence that focused psychotherapies are effective treatments of unipolar depression (1,45) and (ii) there is still great need to develop effective, well-tolerated therapies for bipolar depression (46). However, only two of the studies, reviewed herein, address acute-phase outcomes. On the one hand, the study of Frank et al. (40) failed to find any added effect on depressive symptoms during the acute phase of their trial of IPSRT. On the other hand, although preliminary, the findings of Scott et al. (35) did suggest that CBT reduced depressive symptoms.

Table 1 Effect Sizes of Psychosocial Treatments in Published Studies

Form of psychotherapy	Outcome/endpoint	Effect size[a] (Cohen's *w* or *d*)	Number needed to treat[b]
PE (31)	Manic relapse	0.30	4
PE (31)	Depressive relapse	0.16	7
PE (32)	Relapse during treatment phase	0.22	5
PE (32)	Relapse (2-year follow-up phase)	0.32	4
Care management (GE Smith, personal communication)	Number of weeks with manic symptoms	0.14	7
Family therapy (38)	Relapse (2 years)	0.17	6
Cognitive therapy (36)	Relapse (1 year)	0.32	4
Cognitive therapy (35)	Relapse (1.5 years/ mirror image)	0.45	3
Family therapy (39)	Relapse (2 years)	>0.5	2

Source: Adapted from Ref. 26.
[a]Effect size (*w* or *d*) of <0.20 is considered small; 0.2–0.5 is considered moderate; >0.5 is considered large 43.
[b]Number needed to treat refers to the number of patients who would need to be treated in order to prevent one adverse outcome 44.

A more extensive study of the effect of several forms of psychotherapy for bipolar depression is ongoing as part of the Systematic Treatment Enhancement Program for Bipolar Disorders (STEP-BD) (47). In this trial, 40% of the planned 300 participants will receive pharmacotherapy and three sessions of PE and 60% will be randomly assigned to received CBT, FFT, or IPSRT. Once completed in late 2005, this will be the first adequately powered trial to evaluate the effects of psychotherapy specifically for bipolar depression. The study also will provide interesting preliminary data contrasting the three psychotherapies.

The modern, disease-specific psychotherapies developed or adapted for treatment of bipolar disorder share a number of common themes, including PE, assertive management of medication side effects, self-monitoring of mood states and sleep patterns, "shoring up" of the patient's social support system, and identification and treatment of symptoms (48). It is possible that a considerable portion of the outcome variance associated with a specific therapy of bipolar disorder actually is explained by non-specific factors. The specific elements of the particular models of psychotherapy thus would be manifest either (i) over and above the impact of these non-specific factors or (ii) via more efficient or efficacious delivery of the benefits of these common elements. To date, only the studies of Colom et al. (32) and Rea et al. (40) permit differentiation of specific from non-specific effects. Although both of these studies documented relatively large specific effects, it is not clear that either trial ensured that the "standard therapy" was administered with high credibility and similar expectations for success.

The impact of the specific elements of treatment models thus cannot yet be distinguished from the effects of the common or non-specific elements of psychotherapy. However, now that the therapeutic effects of adding focused psychotherapy to pharmacotherapy have been convincingly documented, a new generation of

Table 2 Ten Key Elements of Enhanced Clinical Intervention

Education about the mood disorder
Education about medications used to treat the disorder
Education about basic sleep and social rhythm hygiene
Education regarding the use of rescue medications
Careful review of symptoms
Careful review of side effects
Medical and behavioral management of side effects
24-hr on-call service
Discussion of early warning signs of impending episodes
Nonspecific support

Source: Adapted from Ref. 26.

research can be designed in order to address issues of treatment specificity. This issue has public health implications over and above questions of theoretic importance. Specifically, whereas it is likely that only highly trained psychotherapists can administer CBT or FFT, it is equally likely that group PE interventions can be provided by less experienced or less highly trained clinicians. Questions of cost effectiveness consequently will need to be addressed in the next generation of research. A modest therapeutic effect that can be administrated inexpensively to a large number of people ultimately may have as much value to the overall state of public health as a treatment with a large effect that is contingent upon the availability of a skilled psychotherapist.

With this issue in mind, our group at the University of Pittsburgh Medical Center has undertaken a study of a relatively low-intensity PE therapy called Enhanced Clinical Intervention (ECI). This approach builds upon the approaches of Bauer and McBride (22) and Simon et al. (34) and consists of 10 elements that are adapted to the specific needs of the patients (Table 2). The study is being conducted in six clinical settings, selected to ensure adequate representation of African-Americans, elders, youth, and rural patient groups. There are few exclusion criteria, and a semistandardized but highly flexible pharmacotherapy protocol is utilized. Results of this study, which will be available in 2007, will help to evaluate the value of less intensive (and less expensive) psychosocial interventions in real-world setting.

ACKNOWLEDGMENTS

This research has been supported in part by the National Institute of Mental Health Grants MH-30915 and MH-29618, as well as Contract MH-80001.

REFERENCES

1. Depression Guideline Panel. Clinical Practice Guideline Number 5. Depression in Primary Care. Treatment of Major Depression. Vol 2. AHCPR Publication No. 93–0551. Rockville, MD: U.S. Department of Health and Human Services Agency for Health Care Policy and Research, 1993.
2. Thase ME. Psychopharmacology in conjunction with psychotherapy. In: Snyder CR, Ingram RE, eds. Handbook of Psychological Change: Psychotherapy Processes and Practices for the 21st Century. New York: John Wiley & Sons, 2000:474–497.

3. Butzlaff RL, Hooley JM. Expressed emotion and psychiatric relapse: a meta analysis. Arch Gen Psychiatry 1998; 55:547–552.
4. Johnson SL, Roberts JE. Life events and bipolar disorder: implications from biological theories. Psychol Bull 1995; 117(3):434–449.
5. Johnson SL, Winett CA, Meyer B, et al. Social support and the course of bipolar disorder. J Abnorm Psychol 1999; 108:558–566.
6. Cochran S. Preventing medication non-compliance in the outpatient treatment of bipolar affective disorders. J Consult Clin Psychol 1984; 52:873–878.
7. Colom F, Vieta E, Martinez-Aran A, et al. Clinical factors associated with treatment noncompliance in euthymic: bipolar patients. J Clin Psychiatry 2000; 61:549–555.
8. Greenhouse WJ, Meyer B, Johnson SL. Coping and medication adherence in bipolar disorder. J Affect Disord 2000; 59:237–241.
9. Scott J, Pope M. Non-adherence with mood stabilizers: prevalence and predictors. J Clin Psychiatry 2002; 65:384–390.
10. Falloon J, Boyd J, McGill C, et al. Family management in prevention of morbidity in schizophrenia: clinical outcomes of a two-year longitudinal study. Arch Gen Psychiatry 1985; 42:887–896.
11. Hogarty GE, Anderson CM, Reiss DJ, et al. Family psychoeducation, social skills training, and maintenance chemotherapy in the aftercare treatment of schizophrenia. I. One-year effect of a controlled study on relapse and expressed emotion. Arch Gen Psychiatry 1986; 43:633–642.
12. Lieberman RP, Mueser KT, Wallace CJ, et al. Training skills in the psychiatrically disabled: learning coping and competence. Schizophr Bull 1986; 12:631–647.
13. Fromm-Reichmann F. Intensive psychotherapy of manic-depressives. Confinia Neurol 1949; 9:158–165.
14. Cade JFL. Lithium salt in the treatment of psychotic excitement. Med J Aust 1949; 2:349–352.
15. Rosanoff AJ, Handy L, Plesset IR. The etiology of manic-depressive syndromes with special reference to their occurrences in twins. Am J Psychiatry 1935; 91:725–762.
16. Goodwin F, Jamison K. Manic-Depressive Illness. New York, NY: Oxford University Press, 1990.
17. Jamison KR. An Unquiet Mind: a Memoir of Moods and Madness. New York: Random House, 1995.
18. Anderson CM, Hogarty GE, Reiss DJ. Family treatment of adult schizophrenic patients: a psycho-educational approach. Schizophr Bull 1980; 6:490–505.
19. Goldstein MJ, Miklowitz DJ. The effectiveness of psychoeducational family therapy in the treatment of schizophrenic disorders. J Marital Fam Ther 1995; 21:361–376.
20. Beck AT, Rush AJ, Shaw BF, et al. Cognitive Therapy of Depression. New York, NY: Guilford Press, 1979.
21. Klerman GL, Weissman MM, Rounsaville BJ, et al. Interpersonal Psychotherapy of Depression. New York, NY: Basic Books, 1984.
22. Bauer MS, McBride L. Structured Group Psychotherapies for Bipolar Disorder: the Life Goals Program. New York: Springer, 1996.
23. Miklowitz DJ, Goldstein MJ. Bipolar Disorder: a Family Focused Treatment Approach. New York: Guilford Press, 1997.
24. Basco MR, Rush AJ. Cognitive-Behavioral Therapy for Bipolar Disorder. New York: Guilford Press, 1996.
25. Frank E, Kupfer DJ, Ehlers CL, et al. Interpersonal and social rhythms therapy for bipolar disorders: integrating interpersonal and behavioral approaches. Behav Ther 1994; 17:143–149.
26. Swartz HA, Frank E, Kupfer DJ. Psychotherapy of bipolar disorder. In: Stein DJ, Kupfer DJ, Schatzberg AF, eds. Textbook of Mood Disorders. Arlington, VA: American Psychiatric Publishing, Inc. In press.

27. American Psychiatric Association. Practice guideline for the treatment of patients with bipolar disorder (revision). Am J Psychiatry 2002; 159(suppl 1).
28. Sachs GS, Thase ME. Bipolar Disorder. A Systematic Approach to Treatment. London, England: Martin Dunitz Ltd., 2000.
29. Rosenthal R. Experimenter Effects in Behavioral Research. New York: Appleton-Century-Crofts, 1966.
30. Thase ME. Comparing the methods used to compare antidepressants. Psychopharmacol Bull 2002; 36(suppl 1):4–17.
31. Perry A, Tarrier N, Morriss R, et al. Randomised controlled trial of efficacy of teaching patients with bipolar disorder to identify early symptoms of relapse and obtain treatment. Br Med J 1999; 318:149–153.
32. Colom F, Vieta E, Martinez-Aran A, et al. A randomized trial on the efficacy of group psychoeducation in the prophylaxis of recurrences in bipolar patients whose disease is in remission. Arch Gen Psychiatry 2003; 60:402–407.
33. Bauer MS, Williford WO, Dawson EE, et al. Principles of effectiveness trials and their implementation in VA Cooperative Study #430: "reducing the efficacy-effectiveness gap in bipolar disorder." J Affect Disord 2001; 67:61–78.
34. Simon GE, Ludman E, Unuetzer J, et al. Design and implementation of a randomized trial evaluating systematic care for bipolar disorder. Bipolar Disord 2002; 4: 226–236.
35. Scott J, Garland A, Moorhead S. A pilot study of cognitive therapy in bipolar disorders. Psychol Med 2001; 31:459–467.
36. Lam DH, Watkins ER, Hayward P, et al. A randomized controlled study of cognitive therapy for relapse prevention for bipolar affective disorder: outcome of the first year. Arch Gen Psychiatry 2003; 60:145–152.
37. Miklowitz DJ, Simoneau TL, George EA, et al. Family-focused treatment of bipolar disorder: one year effects of a psychoeducational program in conjunction with pharmacotherapy. Biol Psychiatry 2000; 48:582–592.
38. Miklowitz DJ, George EL, Richards JA, et al. A randomized study of family-focused psychoeducation and pharmacotherapy in the outpatient management of bipolar disorder. Arch Gen Psychiatry 2003; 60:904–912.
39. Rea MM, Tompson MC, Miklowitz DJ, et al. Family-focused treatments versus individual treatments for bipolar disorder: results of a randomized clinical trial. J Consult Clin Psychol 2003; 71:482–492.
40. Frank E, Swartz HA, Kupfer DJ. Interpersonal and social rhythm therapy: managing the chaos of bipolar disorder. Biol Psychiatry 2000; 48:593–604.
41. Frank E, Swartz HA, Mallinger AG, et al. Adjunctive psychotherapy for bipolar disorder: effects of changing treatment modality. J Abnorm Psychol 1999; 108:579–587.
42. Bowden C, Calabrese JR, McElroy S, et al. A randomized, placebo-controlled, 12-month trial of divalproex and lithium in treatment of outpatients with bipolar I disorder. Arch Gen Psychiatry 2000; 57:481–489.
43. Tohen M, Chengappa KNR, Suppes T, et al. Relapse prevention in bipolar I disorder: 18-month comparison of olanzapine plus mood stabiliser v. mood stabiliser alone. Br J Psychiatry 2004; 184:237–245.
44. Goodwin GM, Bowden CL, Calabrese JR, et al. A pooled analysis of 2 placebo-controlled 18-month trials of lamotrigine and lithium maintenance in bipolar I disorder. J Clin Psychiatry 2004; 65:432–441.
45. Thase ME. Depression-focused psychotherapies. In: Gabbard GO, ed. Treatment of Psychiatric Disorders. Vol.2. 3rd ed. Washington, DC: American Psychiatric Press Inc., 2001:1181–1227.
46. Thase ME, Sachs GS. Bipolar depression: pharmacotherapy and related therapeutic strategies. Biol Psychiatry 2000; 48(6):558–572.

47. Sachs GS, Thase ME, Otto MW, et al. Rationale, design, and methods of the systematic treatment enhancement program for bipolar disorder (STEP-BD). Biol Psychiatry 2003; 53:1028–1042.
48. Milkowitz DJ. Psychosocial issues in bipolar depression. In: Kupfer D, ed. Bipolar Depression: the Clinician's Reference Guide (BD-CRG). Montvale, NJ: Current Psychiatry, 2004:61–78.

27

Toward an Integrated View: Algorithms in Bipolar Disorder

Heinz Grunze

Department of Psychiatry, Ludwig-Maximilians University, Munich, Germany

INTRODUCTION

Until the 1990s, the development of treatment guidelines was not a topic for bipolar disorder. At that time, bipolar disorder was a clearly and restrictive-defined illness and the treatment options were limited. Since then the understanding of bipolar disorder broadened, and in parallel, the number of medications proving efficacy in at least one phase of the illness drastically increased. Thus, not only diagnosis, but also treatment became more complex and there was an obvious need to give treating clinicians some kind of guidance. Especially during the recent years, a plenty fold of national guidelines has been developed, for example, the Canadian (1,2), the Dutch (3), the Austrian (4), the Australian and New Zealand (5), the Danish (6), the German (7), the APA practice guidelines (8), the North American Expert consensus Guideline series (9), the Texas consensus conference algorithm (10), and the BAP guidelines (11), and this list is far from being complete. Besides those national treatment recommendations, the World Federation of Societies of Biological Psychiatry (WFSBP) developed multinational guideline series for the acute treatment of bipolar depression, mania, and maintenance treatment (12–14).

Whereas most guidelines appear rather uniform when it comes to treatment recommendations for acute mania, diverging opinions can be observed concerning the treatment of bipolar depression and maintenance treatment.

For bipolar depression, some national guidelines (e.g., Refs. 7,11) prefer the concomitant use of a mood stabilizer and a (modern) antidepressant, mainly a SSRI or bupropion, where licensed. Others, e.g., the Dutch (3), the 2005 Canadian Network for Mood and Anxiety Disorders (CANMAT) Guidelines for treatment of bipolar Disorder, which are currently in preparation, or the APA 2002 practice guideline (8) appear more reluctant concerning antidepressants, or do not cover the topic of antidepressant (6). In the APA guidelines, antidepressants are only mentioned as an adjunct treatment in severe depression when mood stabilizer monotherapy is not successful. This view has also been picked up by a recent expert consensus (15) where, in line with the APA guidelines, lamotrigine and lithium monotherapy were favored as first choice. This potential over-ranking of mood stabilizers and devaluation of antidepressants still remains a matter of ongoing discussion (16,17).

A recent review of Vestergaard (18) examined treatment discrepancies between European and North American guidelines for maintenance treatment. This review compared the British (11), a German (7), and the Danish (6) guidelines with the APA practice guidelines for the treatment of patients with bipolar disorder 2002 (8). It highlights some differences concerning the comprehension of the illness based on different diagnostic systems (ICD-10 vs. DSM-IV), the time of initiation of maintenance treatment and the first choice for the pharmacological management. There seems a tendency in the European guidelines to give priority to bipolar I disorder and to extrapolate the recommendations to other, mostly "atypical" called forms of bipolar disorder. The APA guidelines reflect more a categorical diagnostic thinking by including more extensive treatment recommendations for bipolar II disorder and rapid cycling as specified in DSM-IV. However, it is apparent that controlled evidence is scarce for these forms of bipolar disorder as recently reviewed by Hadjipavlou (19). Concerning initiation of maintenance treatment, the APA guidelines strongly recommend maintenance treatment after the first manic episode, whereas European guidelines are more conservative by either delaying initiation after the second episode (6) or only consider early maintenance following a very disruptive first manic episode. As far as the first choice pharmacological treatment is concerned, both the European and the North American guidelines recommend lithium. In addition, the APA guidelines also recommend valproate alongside with lithium as a first-line choice. This may reflect both the differences in clinical experience and use of valproate and different interpretations of the so far only well-controlled valproate maintenance study by Bowden et al. (20). Despite recent controlled studies, olanzapine and lamotrigine are not yet recommended in all guidelines corresponding to their level of scientific evidence. This may be as well due to a tendency to give priority to medications that are more familiar to treating clinicians as well as to a mismatch between the rapidly increasing evidence for these new medications and the frequency of updates of treatment recommendations.

STRENGTHS AND WEAKNESSES OF GUIDELINES FOR BIPOLAR DISORDER

Similar to the diversity of the cultural background, the methods of forming guidelines and their implementations differ. Several approaches might be used for forming guidelines: expert opinion, surveys, consensus panels, and systematic literature search. This may finally lead either to general guidelines, more specific recommendations or even detailed treatment algorithms. However, especially if they are formed on a national basis, they clearly focus on local treatment habits, resources and needs and are difficult to translate in another setting. Thus, it became increasingly popular to create "evidence based" guidelines as the probably smallest common denominator by which cultural differences can be bridged. Basing guidelines only on published evidence may additionally also minimize the influence and bias of opinion-leaders.

But why it is still difficult to develop guidelines for bipolar disorders based only on methodologically sound trials or meta-analyses? At least on the level of second-line treatments, evidence becomes sparse. A recent literature survey showed that between 1988 and 1995 only 1194 bipolar patients took part in clinical trials, regardless whether it was for mania, bipolar depression or maintenance, whereas more than

12,000 patients were exposed to atypical antipsychotics in different schizophrenia studies (21). In addition, previous trials of "older" drugs usually do not satisfy the methodological criteria proposed by EMEA, FDA, or other authorities. For example, despite the fact that lithium is considered as the gold standard and widely used as a comparator, there has been no placebo-controlled, conclusive study of lithium in mania prior to the valproate study of Bowden (22), where lithium served as an active comparator. Another disadvantage of purely evidence-based recommendations is that they will not reflect and apply to the real world patient due to the selected nature of patients in clinical trials. It has been estimated that not more than 20% of originally screened patients will get randomized in clinical studies in bipolar disorder (23). This weakness of guidelines was recognized in the recently published guidelines of the British Association for Psychopharmacology stating, "guidelines are systematically derived statements that are aimed at helping individual patient and clinician decisions. The principal recommendation should apply to the *average* patient." Another weakness of purely evidence-based guidelines is that most studies considered are large scale clinical trials with the purpose of approving newly launched medications. These studies either show what they are supposed to show or, in case they are negative, often do not get into the public domain. Few exceptions exist as a publication of the failed studies on gabapentin in mania (24) or the failed studies of lamotrigine (25); however, these examples are likely to be outnumbered several times by skeletons in the closet. Thus, it is almost impossible to give a fair judgment of a drug not being aware of negative trials.

Another problem of selectivity in these trials is that they are almost exclusively focusing on the homogenous population of bipolar I patients. Thus, any conclusions are difficult to derive for manifestations other than this typical form. This lack of evidence becomes especially obvious when trying to formulate guidelines for bipolar II patients or other so-called "atypical manifestations."

Furthermore, comorbidities are usually an exclusion criterion in controlled studies, but clinical reality in the real world patient. Clinicians may be disappointed if they discover that there is an obvious gap of efficacy described in controlled studies and effectiveness in real world patients. A frequently cited example for this is the lithium maintenance study of Mario Maj (26), where in the intent-to-treat analysis, only 23% of bipolar I patients remained relapse free during the 5-year observational period. This is contrasting the outcome of earlier controlled and thus selective lithium maintenance study showing response rates of more than 80%.

Finally, there is still a very obvious lack of methodologically well-controlled studies on combination treatment. A survey of Frye et al. (27) showed that only 3.3% of affectively ill patients received three or more medications on release from hospital in the early 1970s, but 43.8% in the early 1990s. This clinical tendency to polypharmacotherapy is so far insufficiently covered by controlled studies, with the exception of recent acute mania studies of valproate (28) and atypical antipsychotics (e.g., Refs. 29–31). In conclusion, guidelines based solely on published evidence from controlled studies may not translate into clinical useful treatment, mainly due to:

1. Lack of methodologically acceptable studies, especially for older agents or treatment modalities where a placebo control is unethical (e.g., ECT).
2. A bias in the available literature on controlled studies leaving out failed studies.

3. A discrepancy of the population studied in controlled studies compared to "real world patients."
4. Their focus on monotherapy ignoring to some degree the clinical practice of (skillful?) polypharmacy.

Guidelines incorporating clinical experience, however, may focus more on the real world patient and also consider the broadening of the bipolar diagnosis. They may give priority to drugs familiar to treating physicians and also utilize experience with long-term treatment exceeding the usual duration of a controlled study. However, this approach is not unproblematic when opinion, for example of a large community of psychiatrists, as with the North American consensus guidelines (9), is their sole basis. This approach may either risk to picture just general (sometimes outdated) treatment habits or, when choosing only a few experts, it may be biased towards a special treatment ideology. Even worse, financial interest of pharmaceutical companies may interfere when it comes to grading different medications.

Additionally, with the rapid progress in clinical research, many guidelines are already outdated when they are published. Based on evidence, many new substances, e.g., latest generation atypical antipsychotics, should be ranked much higher in current treatment guidelines as they are. However, a lack of clinical experience and some skepticism of experts may prevent a higher ranking.

In conclusion, it should be clear in a physician's mind that guidelines are never absolute truth but they all have several shortcomings. Therefore, guidelines should distinguish between the levels of evidence for a specific treatment and the strength of recommendation as, for example, the BAP guidelines do (11). Another weakness of the most current guidelines is that they concentrate on the pharmacological treatment of bipolar disorder, due to a relative poverty of controlled data for additional treatments like ECT, TMS, psychoeducation, and psychotherapy. However, this may change with future guidelines, as there is cumulative evidence from methodologically sound studies underlining the importance of psychotherapy and psychoeducation.

THE WFSBP GUIDELINES SERIES ON THE TREATMENT OF BIPOLAR DISORDER

With the diversity of national treatment habits, it is usually difficult to transfer treatment recommendations easily from one country to another. When a comprehensive opinion on the treatment of bipolar disorder is demanded, such a project can only be accomplished by an international scientific society with worldwide presence. The WFSBP recently published guidelines on the acute treatment of bipolar depression (12), mania (13), and maintenance treatment of bipolar disorder (14). As this constitutes the first multicultural attempt of guidelines, their content and the process to achieve consensuses may deserve a closer look.

In principle, the WFSBP guidelines are based on a consensus among the presidents of the national societies of biological psychiatry and renowned experts from all over the world, representing different treatment expertise and cultural backgrounds.

The WFSBP guidelines for the treatment of bipolar disorder consist of three separate parts, which were published between 2002 and 2004. The focus of all three parts of the guidelines is psychopharmacological treatment, as the evidence for other treatment options, e.g., psychotherapy, is still sparse and developed just recently.

Acknowledging its special burden, the first part of the guidelines series was dedicated to the acute treatment of bipolar depression (12). The second part was dedicated to the acute treatment of mania (13) and the final part reviewed maintenance and prophylactic treatment options (14).

The common ground of these guidelines is expert opinion. However, compared to other guidelines that are compiled by a handpicked small number of experts and where the initiative was started or at least supported by a pharmaceutical company, this guideline may be less biased through selection processes. A first draft was compiled by the secretary, the chair and the two co-chairs of the task force. Grading of treatment options was primarily done according to peer-reviewed published scientific evidence, but to ensure actuality, also recent proceedings of major scientific conferences were considered. To become a recommended treatment, however, not only the scientific evidence was of importance, but also the clinical practicability and access to medication. This first draft of the respective guideline was then sent out for comments and corrections to all acting presidents of the National Societies of Biological Psychiatry, and their feedback was integrated into a second version of the guidelines. In addition, well-renowned international experts for bipolar disorder were asked to comment on the guidelines. With this broad basis of opinions, consisting of the 54 presidents of National Societies of Biological Psychiatry and several experts from different cultural background, it is reasonable to assume that a potential bias has been minimized. By communicating and discussing topics through e-mail without the need to attend a meeting, and by publication in the official journal of the WFSBP, the whole guideline process could be conducted without any sponsorship from pharmaceutical companies.

The second draft of the guidelines incorporating the feedback was then extensively reviewed by the chair and the two co-chairs of the WFSBP task force before publication in the *World Journal of Biological Psychiatry*.

Scientific evidence was graded according to four levels (A–D), adapting and modifying the so-called PORT criteria (32). The same criteria were also applied for the WFSBP guidelines on the treatment of unipolar depression (33,34). The highest scientific evidence (level A) was reached if a medication could prove efficacy in at least three methodologically sound trials including at least one placebo controlled trial and at least two comparison trials with another standard treatment. In these trials, criteria such as sufficient sample size, duration of trial, randomized and concealed distribution to either treatment, and double-blind conditions should have been met. Level B was achieved if a substance showed efficacy in at least two controlled studies against an established comparator, or one double-blind controlled study and supporting data from a large prospective naturalistic study. Level C reflected efficacy shown in one RDB study and at least one prospective study (>10 patients), whereas level D was given if evidence is purely based on prospective case studies with a minimum of 10 patients, or large-scale retrospective chart analyses and support by expert opinion.

These criteria appear rather soft, especially when compared, e.g., to evidence-based guidelines of schizophrenia or several medical conditions. But it turned out that not a single medication could already meet even these soft level A criteria in the first guideline on bipolar depression. For the treatment of acute mania, at least lithium, valproate, several atypical antipsychotics, and, of the typical antipsychotics, chlorpromazine and haloperidol did satisfy level A criteria. For long-term treatment, only lithium, lamotrigine, and olanzapine were able to fulfill level A criteria. Thus, it becomes very obvious that compared to other disorders, the evidence base

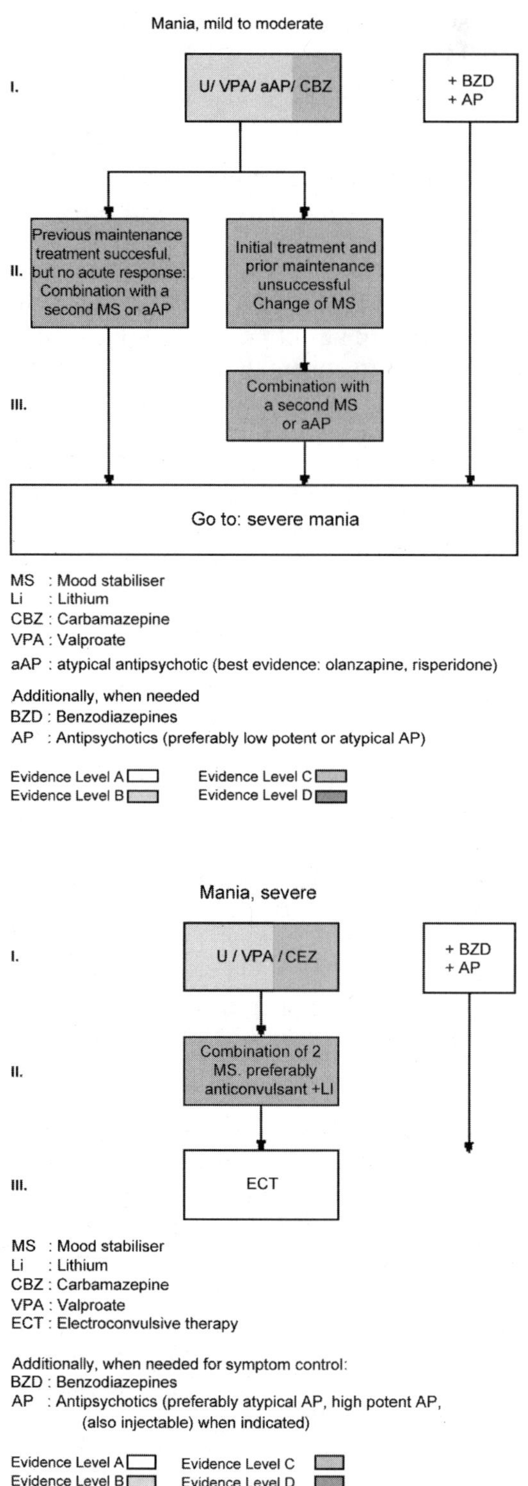

Figure 1 A suggested treatment algorithm for acute mania. *Source*: From Ref. 13.

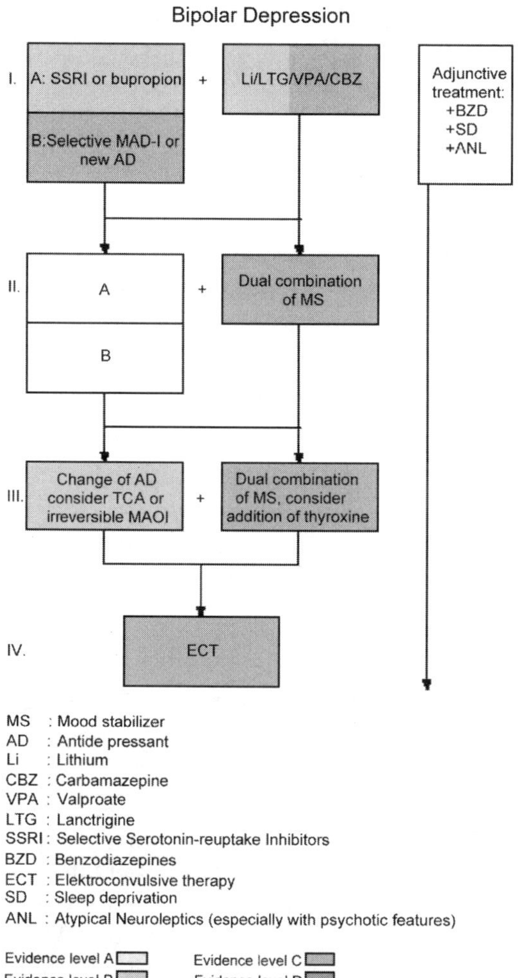

Figure 2 A suggested treatment algorithm for bipolar depression. *Source*: From Ref. 12.

for the psychopharmacological treatment of bipolar disorder is still very limited, especially for the acute treatment of bipolar depression.

To ensure practicability of the guidelines, the guidelines were not drafted by medication but by clinical symptomatology (e.g., euphoric mania, mixed states, hypomania, mania within a rapid cycling course). As a synthesis of evidence base and clinical practicability, the following treatment algorithms as depicted in Figures 1–3 were finally developed.

THE BRITISH ASSOCIATION FOR PSYCHOPHARMACOLOGY GUIDELINE

A slightly different approach was chosen for the guidelines of the British Association of Psychopharmacology (BAP) that was published in 2003. They are also based

Bipolar I disorder without rapid cycling	*Bipolar I with rapid cycling*	*Bipolar II disorder without rapid cycling*	*Bipolar II with rapid cycling*	*Schtzoaffective disorder (bipolar type)*
Lithium (A)	Combination of lithium and carbamazepine (C) or valproate (C)	Lithium (C)	Lamotrigine (C)	Lithium(C) in schtzo-dominant type: Atypical antipsychotics (A)
Mania-dominant type: Atypical anti psychotics (especially olanzapine (A)), Depression-dominant type: lamotrigine (A)	Mania-dominant type: lithium (C), olanzapine (D) Depression-dominant type: lamotrigine (D)	Carbamazepine (D)	Valproate (D)	Carbamazepine (C)
Valproate (B)	Carbamazepine (D) dozapine (D)	Lamotrigine (-), valproate (-) with prominent depressions: modem antidepressants (-)	Carbamazepine (-), lithium (-)	Valproate (D), Atypical antipsychotics (-)
Carbamazepine (B), with severe manias: classical, antipsychotics, clozapine, fisperidone (D) with prominent depressions: modern antidepressants in combination with a mood stabilizer (D), maintenance ECT (D)	Nimodipine (B)	Atypical antipsychotics (-), maintenance ECT (-)	Nimodipine (-), atypical antipsychotics (-)	Classical antipsychotics (-), maintenance ECT (-)

Figure 3 Treatment choices for maintenance treatment of different forms of bipolar disorder. *Source*: From Ref. 14.

on literature search and expert opinion. The different treatment options were discussed during a one-day conference where both British national experts and international experts were invited as presenters or discussants. In addition, interest groups, e.g., scientific advisors of pharmaceutical companies and consumer groups, were attending as observers. The proceedings of this meeting were then drafted as a first manuscript and commented by the participating experts. The final version was then consented by all participants. Although these British guidelines are again mainly focusing on the pharmacological treatment they also integrated recommendations beyond evidence based medicine, as access to and standards of health care. Besides purely scientific aspects, this may also strengthen the political impact of such guidelines. Keeping the stigmatization of bipolar patients, the lack of knowledge about bipolar disorder in the general public, and the continuous cut of public research support in mind, treatment guidelines should probably go also beyond specifying studies and their scientific evidence in order to change something to the better.

CONCLUSIONS

When drafting a guideline, someone learns more about uncertainty and limitations than about undisputable scientific evidence. This seems to be especially true for bipolar disorder. Even when a solid evidence base can be identified, that does not mean that this translates into clinical practicability and usefulness. In the author's opinion, some general recommendations when compiling future guidelines should be considered:

1. Expert consensus should be independent from sponsorship and be based on a broad number of experts, who are at least partially selected by a mechanism that is independent from the guideline (e.g., including all presidents of National Societies of Biological Psychiatry). This may limit a suspected bias to some degree.
2. Start from the evidence base and clearly state what the evidence says, then comment on the clinical usefulness as a separate issue (not mixing evidence and opinion).
3. Update the guidelines frequently, most guidelines are already outdated when published.
4. With the growing body of scientific evidence, future guidelines may not only concentrate on pharmacological treatment but should also integrate the evidence and finally comment about psychotherapy, psychoeducation, and new treatments like repetitive transcranial magnetic stimulation (rTMS) or vagus nerve stimulation (VNS).

When it comes to the recommendations of recent guidelines, there is—at least for the pharmacological treatment—an obvious merger of opinion. Concerning bipolar depression, there is still some discrepancy between many European guidelines and North American guidelines; this may be related to the lack of evidence that is especially true for the treatment of bipolar depression. Here, it is absolutely true that "one good experiment is worth a hundred expert opinions," and hopefully the number of good studies will grow within the next years. This may form a more solid platform of evidence on which clinical utility and practicability can be discussed and, finally, treatment recommendations can be given.

REFERENCES

1. Kusumakar V, Yatham LN, Haslam DR, Parikh SV, Matte R, Silverstone PH, Sharma V. Treatment of mania, mixed state, and rapid cycling. Can J Psychiatry 1997; 42(suppl 2):79–86.
2. Sharma V, Yatham LN, Haslam DR, Silverstone PH, Parikh SV, Matte R, Kutcher SP, Kusumakar V. Continuation and prophylactic treatment of bipolar disorder. Can J Psychiatry 1997; 42(suppl 2):92–100.
3. Nolen WA, Knoppert-van der Klein EAM, Bouvy PF, Honig A, Klompenhouwer JL, De Wit A, Ravelli DP. Richtlijn bipolaire stoornissen. Boom, Amsterdam 2001.
4. Kasper S, Haushofer M, Zapotoczky HG, Aschauer H, Wolf R, Bonelli M, Wuschitz A. Konsensus-statement: Diagnostik und Therapie der bipolaren Störung. Neuropsychiatrie 2002; 13:100–108.
5. Royal Australian and New Zealand College of Psychiatrists Clinical Practice Guidelines Team for Bipolar Disorder. Australian and New Zealand clinical practice guidelines for the treatment of bipolar disorder. Aust N Z J Psychiatry 2004; 38:280–305.
6. Licht RW, Vestergaard P, Kessing LV, Larsen JK, Thomsen PH. Psychopharmacological treatment with lithium and antiepileptic drugs: suggested guidelines from the Danish Psychiatric Association and the Child and Adolescent Psychiatric Association in Denmark. Acta Psychiatr Scand Suppl 2003; 419:1–22.
7. Grunze H, Walden J, Dittmann S, Berger M, Bergmann A, Bräunig P, Dose M, Emrich HM, Gastpar M, Greil W, Möller H-J, Uebelhack R. Psychopharmakotherapie bipolarer affektiver Erkrankungen. Nervenarzt 2002; 73:4–17.

8. Zarin D, Pincus HA, McIntyre JS. APA Practice Guideline For The Treatment Of Patients With Bipolar Disorder 2002. http://www.psych.org/clin_res/pg_bipolar.cfm
9. Sachs GS, Printz DJ, Kahn DA, Carpenter D, Docherty JP. The Expert Consensus Guideline Series: Medication Treatment of Bipolar Disorder 2000. A Postgraduate Medicine Special Report 2000:1–104.
10. Suppes T, Dennehy EB, Swann AC, Bowden CL, Calabrese JR, Hirschfeld RM, Keck PE Jr, Sachs GS, Crismon ML, Toprac MG, Shon SP. Report of the Texas Consensus Conference Panel on medication treatment of bipolar disorder 2000. J Clin Psychiatry 2002; 63:288–299.
11. Goodwin GM. Evidence-based guidelines for treating bipolar disorder: recommendations from the British Association for Psychopharmacology. J Psychopharmacol 2003; 17:149–173.
12. Grunze H, Kasper S, Goodwin G, Bowden CL, Baldwin D, Licht RW, Vieta E, Möller H-J. WFSBP Task Force on Treatment Guidelines for Bipolar Disorders. The World Federation of Societies of Biological Psychiatry (WFSBP) Guidelines for the Biological Treatment of Bipolar Disorders. Part I: Treatment of bipolar depression. World J Biol Psychiatry 2002; 3:115–124.
13. Grunze H, Kasper S, Goodwin G, Bowden CL, Baldwin D, Licht RW, Vieta E, Möller H-J. WFSBP Task Force on Treatment Guidelines for Bipolar Disorders. The World Federation of Societies of Biological Psychiatry (WFSBP) Guidelines for the Biological Treatment of Bipolar Disorders. Part II: Treatment of mania. World J Biol Psychiatry 2003; 4:5–13.
14. Grunze H, Kasper S, Goodwin G, Bowden CL, Möller H-J. WFSBP Task Force on Treatment Guidelines for Bipolar Disorders. The World Federation of Societies of Biological Psychiatry (WFSBP) Guidelines for the Biological Treatment of Bipolar Disorders. Part III: Maintenance treatment. World J Biol Psychiatry 2004; 5:120–135.
15. Calabrese JR, Kasper S, Johnson G, Tajima O, Vieta E, Yatham E, Young AH. International Consensus Group on Bipolar I Depression Treatment Guidelines. J Clin Psychiatry 2004; 65:571–579.
16. Möller H-J, Grunze H. Have some guidelines for the treatment of acute bipolar depression gone too far in the restriction of antidepressants? Eur Arch Psychiatry clin Neurosci 2000; 250:57–68.
17. Möller H-J, Grunze H. Do recent efficacy data on the drug treatment of acute bipolar depression support the position that drugs other than antidepressants are the treatment of choice? A conceptual review. Eur Arch Psychiatry Clin Neurosci. In press.
18. Vestergaard P. Guidelines for maintenance treatment of bipolar disorder: are there discrepancies between European and North American recommendations? Bipolar Disord 2004; 6:519–522.
19. Hadjipavlou G, Mok H, Yatham LN. Pharmacotherapy of bipolar II disorder: a critical review of current evidence. Bipolar Disord 2004; 6:14–25.
20. Bowden CL, Calabrese JR, McElroy SL, Gyulai L, Wassef A, Petty F, Pope HG, Chou JC, Keck PE, Rhodes LJ, Swann AC, Hirschfeld RM, Wozniak PJ. A randomized, placebo-controlled 12-month trial of divalproex and lithium in treatment of outpatients with bipolar I disorder. Divalproex Maintenance Study Group. Arch Gen Psychiatry 2000; 57:481–489.
21. Ghaemi N, Sachs G, Goodwin FK. What is to be done? Controversies in the diagnosis and treatment of manic-depressive illness. World J Biol Psychiatry 2000; 2:65–74.
22. Bowden CL, Brugger AM, Swann AC, Calabrese JR, Janicak PG, Petty F, Dilsaver SC, Davis JM, Rush AJ, Small JG, Garza-Trevino ES, Risch SC, Goodnick PJ, Morris DD. Efficacy of divalproex vs lithium and placebo in the treatment of mania. The Depakote Mania Study Group. JAMA 1994; 271:918–924.
23. Licht RW, Gouliaev G, Vestergaard P, Frydenberg M. Generalisability of results from randomised drug trials. A trial on antimanic treatment. Br J Psychiatry 1997; 170: 264–267.

24. Pande AC, Crockatt JG, Janney CA, Werth JL, Tsaroucha G. Gabapentin in bipolar disorder: a placebo-controlled trial of adjunctive therapy. Gabapentin Bipolar Disorder Study Group. Bipolar Disord 2000; 2:249–255.
25. Goldsmith DR, Wagstaff AJ, Ibbotson T, Perry CM. Lamotrigine: a review of its use in bipolar disorder. Drugs 2003; 63:2029–2050.
26. Maj M, Pirozzi R, Magliano L, Bartoli L. Long-term outcome of lithium prophylaxis in bipolar disorder: a 5-year prospective study of 402 patients at a lithium clinic. Am J Psychiatry 1998; 155:30–35.
27. Frye MA, Ketter TA, Leverich GS, Huggins T, Lantz C, Denicoff KD, Post RM. The increasing use of polypharmacotherapy for refractory mood disorders: 22 years of study. J Clin Psychiatry 2000; 61:9–15.
28. Müller-Oerlinghausen B, Retzow A, Henn F, Giedke H, Walden J. Valproate as an adjunct to neuroleptic medication for the treatment of acute episodes of mania. A prospective, randomized, double-blind, placebo-controlled multicenter study. J Clin Psychopharmacol 2000; 20:195–203.
29. Tohen M, Chengappa KN, Suppes T, Zarate CA Jr, Calabrese JR, Bowden CL, Sachs GS, Kupfer DJ, Baker RW, Risser RC, Keeter EL, Feldman PD, Tollefson GD, Breier A. Efficacy of olanzapine in combination with valproate or lithium in the treatment of mania in patients partially nonresponsive to valproate or lithium monotherapy. Arch Gen Psychiatry 2002; 59:62–69.
30. Sachs GS, Grossman F, Ghaemi SN, Okamoto A, Bowden CL. Combination of a mood stabilizer with risperidone or haloperidol for treatment of acute mania: a double-blind, placebo-controlled comparison of efficacy and safety. Am J Psychiatry 2002; 159: 1146–1154.
31. Yatham LN, Grossman F, Augustyns I, Vieta E, Ravindran A. Mood stabilisers plus risperidone or placebo in the treatment of acute mania. International, double-blind, randomised controlled trial. Br J Psychiatry 2003; 182:141–147.
32. Lehman AF, Steinwachs DM. Translating research into practice: the Schizophrenia Patient Outcomes Research Team (PORT) treatment recommendations. Schizophr Bull 1998; 24:1–10.
33. Bauer M, Whybrow PC, Angst J, Versiani M, Moller HJ. World Federation of Societies of Biological Psychiatry (WFSBP) Guidelines for Biological Treatment of Unipolar Depressive Disorders, Part 2: Maintenance treatment of major depressive disorder and treatment of chronic depressive disorders and subthreshold depressions. World J Biol Psychiatry 2002; 3:69–86.
34. Bauer M, Whybrow PC, Angst J, Versiani M, Möller H-J. WFSBP Task Force on Tretment Guidelines for Unipolar Depressive Disorders. World Federation of Societies of Bioplogical Psychiatry (WFSBP) Guidelines for Biological Treatment of unipolar depressive disorder, Part 1: Acute and continuation treatment of major depressive disorder. World J Biol Psychiatry 2002; 3:4–43.

Index